AYURVEDIC HERBS

The Comprehensive Resource for Ayurvedic Healing Solutions

VIRENDER SODHI, MD (AYURVED), ND

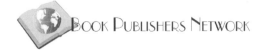

Book Publishers Network
P.O. Box 2256
Bothell • WA • 98041
Ph • 425-483-3040
www.bookpublishersnetwork.com

Copyright © 2014 by Dr. Virender Sodhi

All rights reserved. No part of this book may be reproduced, stored in, or introduced into a retrieval system, or transmitted in any form, or by any means (electronic, mechanical, photocopying, recording, or otherwise) without the prior written permission of the publisher and/or author except by a reviewer who may quote brief passages in a review.

The scanning, uploading, and distribution of this book via the internet or via any other means without the permission of the publisher and/or author is illegal and punishable by law. Please purchase only authorized electronic editions and do not participate in or encourage electronic piracy of copy written materials.

10 9 8 7 6 5 4 3 2 1

Printed in the United States of America

LCCN 2014907442
ISBN 978-1-940598-31-4

Cover design: Laura Zugzda
Interior design: Stephanie Martindale and Leigh Faulkner
Indexer: Carolyn Acheson

Table of Contents

Preface v
Introduction vii
Acknowledgments ix

1. Adhatoda Vasica 1
2. Aegle Marmelos 9
3. Andrographis Paniculata 25
4. Asparagus Racemosus 41
5. Azadirachta Indica 53
6. Bacopa Monnieri 73
7. Berberis Aristata 87
8. Boerhaavia Diffusa 97
9. Boswellia Serrata 103
10. Centella Asiatica 121
11. Cedrus Deodara 137
12. Cissus Quadrangularis 143
13. Commiphora Mukul 151
14. Convolvulus Pluricaulis 163
15. Crataeva Nurvala 169
16. Curcuma Longa 175
17. Cyperus Rotundus 195
18. Didymocarpus Pedicellata 201
19. Dioscorea Bulbifera 205
20. Eclipta Alba 211
21. Embelia Ribes 219
22. Glycyrrhiza Glabra 227
23. Gymnema Sylvestre 243
24. Inula Racemosa 251
25. Momordica Charantia 257
26. Mucuna Pruriens 267
27. Nigella Sativa 277
28. Ocimum Sanctum 289
29. Phyllanthus Amarus 303
30. Phyllanthus Emblica 311
31. Picrorhiza Kurroa 327
32. Piper Longum 337
33. Piper Nigrum 345
34. Pterocarpus Marsupium 353
35. Rubia Cordifolia 361
36. Shilajit 369
37. Sida Cordifolia 377
38. Solanum Nigrum 383
39. Swertia Chirayita 389
40. Terminalia Bellerica 395
41. Terminalia Chebula 405
42. Tribulus terrestris 417
43. Trigonella foenum-graecum 429
44. Withania Somnifera 437

Index 459

Preface

Never before, in the history of primary medicine, have the interest in and use of Ayurvedic and herbal medicine been so great on a global scale as they are today.

Ayurvedic medicine is defined as *the* traditional medicine of India by the World Health Organization (WHO). "Ayurveda" is the main form of primary care for hundreds of millions of Indians.

Complementary and Traditional medicine are used as primary care medicine by more than half the world's population; most households in the world utilize natural supplements on a day-to-day basis. The use of herbal medicine, although traditional in many Eastern cultures, had been only a minor fad in Western medicine until recent decades. This trend has been shifting, however, with the emergence of rigorous studies and research on the effects of traditional remedies on chronic diseases, including diabetes, cardiovascular disease, hypertension, auto-immune disease, cancer—just to name a few.

The purpose of this book is to enlighten people regarding the practical use and efficacy of Ayurvedic Herbal Medicine.

Introduction

This book has been in the process of planning, research and writing for over 25 years.

In 1980, when I graduated with a medical degree from Dayanand Ayurvedic Medical College in Jalandhar, India, I knew I wanted to write a book on herbs. At that time, I knew the various herbs well, but had not yet figured out their practical uses that would be most efficacious in clinical application.

Over the years, I have gained much experience and confidence in my use of herbal medicine through treating thousands of people with a variety of chronic diseases. These have included:

- **Reversal of diabetes in patients with Type I and Type II diabetes.** Working together with patients we have been able to diminish the use of exogenous insulin in Type I diabetes up to 80 percent and restore normal sugar metabolism in Type II diabetes without dependence on oral hypoglycemic drugs.

- **People with auto-immune diseases,** who were on immune-modifying drugs such as Enbrel, Remicade, Methotrexate, Prednisone, etc., were able to manage their illness without the need of these highly toxic medications and over time return to a normal life. I have followed some of these patients for 15-20 years without relapses, as long as they have followed the principles of Ayurvedic medicine. Lupus, psoriasis, psoriatic arthritis, hepatitis B, hepatitis C, ulcerative colitis, Crohn's disease, heart disease, are some of the chronic diseases I have been able to treat successfully with the use of herbs, Ayurvedic diet, and lifestyle modifications, yoga, exercise, and breathing exercises (pranayama).

- **Women with known breast cancer have gone into remission.**

- **Patients on 4-5 antihypertensive drugs** who come to my clinic will, within a period of three to nine months, be off all these drugs and enjoying life, following an Ayurvedic lifestyle.

How did my life's work begin? Growing up in the Himalayas was my first introduction to the world of herbal medicine. My father was a keen observer of medicinal plants. As young as the age of five, I remember being on walks with him when he would stop by a plant and say something like: "This plant is called *Gotu Kola*. Look at the shape of its leaves; it looks like a brain. This herb is used as a brain tonic…. Look at this. This is *berberis*; it is good for the liver." He would ask us to chew on the leaves or fruits of these plants to experience the taste and feel in the mouth of the medicine. This was fascinating to me as a young boy. By the age of nine or ten, I was collecting samples of herbs in bottles and labeling them by the disease they treated. These experiences completely chiseled the basic knowledge of herbs into my brain.

Today, as a physician, I am an avid reader of research studies. The scientific descriptions of Ayurvedic medicine have seemed beyond our modern comprehension for a long time, but with new biochemical, genetic, and clinical studies this knowledge is becoming more accessible. I have found the classical wisdom of Ayurvedic medicine to be very scientific in nature. With this growing base of knowledge and comprehension, I have been able to use the herbs with better understanding and broader application today than ever in the past.

Over the last few years, I have been engaged in an Integrative Oncology fellowship with Dr. Mark Rosenberg. We have been seeing lots of cancer patients. During this time, I have been able to apply the Ayurvedic principles to help these people with greater success.

In this book, readers will find that I have collected the general knowledge of the extensive research and theoretical applications of herbs as may be found in monographs. But, one may find that the true benefit of this text is in the description of uses of herbal medicine in clinical practice. Under the section "Dr. Sodhi's experience," the reader will find how I have been able to use these herbs with traditional and scientific knowledge on a case-by-case basis.

There are vast annals of research out there on herbs, but taken as a whole this information is rarely comprehensible. With this book, I have dared to dive into the depths of the scientific ocean and pull out a few pearls that can inform the prudent clinician regarding the practical use of Ayurvedic herbal medicine in our modern world. I hope readers will find this book a resource to help them bring humankind to a healthier place.

The Ayurvedic model describes the job of a physician as: Swasthasya swasthya rakshanam, meaning "health is inherent; our work is to help maintain it." If one studies the classical Ayurvedic texts, one rarely finds them talking about disease. Rather, the texts put forward the concept of "syndromes." These are complex interactions of physiological/functional imbalances that lead to incidence of disease. When the physician reverses those syndromes through Ayurvedic diet and lifestyle, yoga, exercise and pranayama, while also modifying thought processes (including the way people relate to themselves, their relationships, and their environment), and of course, through herbal medicine, one is able to restore balance, and thus cure disease. This is described as the restoration of the inherent health of the individual.

As an Ayurvedic and Naturopathic physician, my goal is to help humanity attain a disease-free society.

Acknowledgments

My parents would have been very happy to see their son's book published. I am sure they are sending their blessings from heaven. This book would not have been possible without the encouragement of my mother, Mrs. Veena Sodhi; and my father, Mr. Dharampal Singh Sodhi, who were very instrumental in encouraging me to become a doctor. They insisted that I must learn the traditional knowledge of medicine, explaining that Natural medicine—specifically herbal medicine—holds the true power of permanent healing, while all other manufactured forms are temporarily palliative and rarely promote permanent healing.

I would like to thank my wife, Rekha Sodhi. She has stood by my side for over 30 years and made great personal sacrifices for the greater good of all. When I decided to migrate to the United States, she stayed behind with my son, Gunny, for three years in India. This was very hard on all of us. She has dedicated her life to our family and to holistic medicine. She currently runs the Panchakarma center at our Bellevue, Washington, clinic.

I am wholeheartedly grateful to be a part of a holistic family. Together we are upholding our culture, tradition, and dream for empowering all with holistic medicine. I cherish my brothers who have been doing this work with me. I want to acknowledge them individually for their unique contributions:

The animal whisperer of the family, Dr. Tejinder Sodhi, is a pioneering holistic veterinarian. He has been the founding president of the holistic chapter of Veterinary Medicine in Washington State. Then, he went on to become president of Washington Association of Holistic Veterinary Medicine, as well as Washington State Veterinary Medical Association. He continues to see animal patients of all shapes and sizes at his Bellevue and Lynnwood clinics. His wife, Dr. Sushma Sodhi, who manages the Veterinary clinic, is a PhD who did her post-doctorate studies in microbiology at the University of Washington.

Jitender Sodhi, along with his lovely wife, Pankaj Sodhi, manages Ayush Herbs in India, where we grow our own herbs. We have been able to induct the art of Ayurvedic formulations into the modern methods of medicine-making. With the aid of innovative research and the application of classical knowledge, we have been able to extract herbal medicine by novel methods to ensure the highest quality and quantity of medicinal compounds in a formula without separating these compounds from the whole herb. This is essential for the effectiveness of these formulae because traditional wisdom teaches us that plants are conscious beings, therefore true intelligence for healing is in the whole herbs and not in an individualized compound. He manages the farms of Ayush and coordinates with farmers to produce organic herbs.

My youngest brother, Dr. Shailender Sodhi, is also an Ayurvedic and Naturopathic Doctor. He is currently practicing with me at our Bellevue clinic, as well as serving as the President of Ayush Herbs Inc. He is also a deeply passionate medical practitioner and educator. Heartfelt thanks to Dr. Anju Sodhi, my sister-in-law, as well as a wonderful Ayurvedic and Naturopathic Doctor working with us at our Bellevue clinic.

My son Gunny has also played a part in supporting the family's dream. Though he has not taken on medicine as his practice, Gunny has chosen to apply his knowledge and skills in business toward helping us cultivate and grow the impact of Ayurvedic medicine and Natural medicine, as a whole, in the West. He recently married his beautiful wife, Dr. Kirat Sodhi, a dentist.

Rishi Sodhi, my second son, may not be here with us any longer but he always inspired me with his mental acuity and intelligence. Losing my child taught me how fragile we all are! It taught me to live in the moment and to make the best of it. May his soul rest in peace.

I owe a debt of gratitude to my colleagues and teachers, in Ayurvedic, Allopathic and Naturopathic medicine, for supporting and challenging me in the best way possible. I can recall numerous conversations and inspirations that have guided me to this stage in my life. In writing this book, I have had much help and a lot of inspiration. I would like to acknowledge my past resident, Dr. Kalyan Kadam, who has put in hundreds of hours of research and collecting references. Another student whom I want to thank is Dr. Anup Mulakaluri.

Finally, my sincere gratitude to all of my patients, for so many of them have inspired me to deepen my study and my practice of medicine. They have induced my curiosity and desire to learn and discover novel ways of applying Ayurveda towards the treatment and cure of conditions that I would not have imagined possible otherwise.

Thank you, love you, be healthy. OM Shanti.

Virender Sodhi

Virender Sodhi, MD (Ayurved), ND

CEO

Ayush Herbs, INC

Clinical Director of Ayurvedic, Naturopathic and Medical Clinic

1

Adhatoda vasica

Introduction

Adhatoda vasica, a small evergreen shrub, has a multitude of uses in traditional Ayurveda and is best known for its effectiveness in treating respiratory conditions. The leaf buds of vasica are chewed, sometimes with ginger, by yogis or sadhus, and this has a stimulant effect on the respiratory system.

As an antispasmodic and an expectorant, vasica has been used for centuries with much success in treating asthma, chronic bronchitis, and other respiratory conditions. More recently, this herb has been studied for its potential in treating tuberculosis.[1] All parts of *Adhatoda vasica* have medicinal value. A powdered form of the herb, boiled in sesame oil, is used to heal ear infections and to arrest bleeding. Boiled leaves of vasica, in the form of a poultice, are used to treat rheumatic pain and to relieve the pain of urinary tract infections.

Adhatoda vasica also is believed to have abortifacient properties and is commonly used in some parts of India to stimulate uterine contractions, which speeds childbirth. This plant, too, is used to stem bleeding in conditions such as peptic ulcers, gingivitis, excessive menstrual bleeding, and hemorrhoids.[2]

Synonymous Names

English: Malabar Nut
Hindi: Adosa
Sanskrit: Vasaka

Adhatoda is known by a variety of ethnic and regional names, including the above, as well as Adulsa, Arusha, Justicia adhatoda, Adulsa Arusa, Adathodai, Bakash, Adalodakam, Adusoge, Addasaramu, Lion's Muzzle, and Stallion's Tooth.

Habitat

Native to India and the foothills of the Himalayas, Malaysia, and Sri Lanka, Adhatoda vasica is cultivated in tropical areas and grows to an elevation of 1300 meters above sea level. Adhatoda grows well in a wide variety of soils but thrives especially in dry areas.

Botanical Characteristics

Adhatoda vasica is a small, evergreen, perennial shrub, which reaches an average height of 3 meters. Its branches are opposite and ascending. The broad, leathery leaves, which sometimes are used as an insecticide, measure from 10 to 15 centimeters in length and are about 4 centimeters in width. They are pubescent—light green on top and darker green beneath. The leaves grow in an opposite formation and are entirely lanceolate and shortly petiolate, tapering toward both apex and base. When dry, the leaves become brownish-green and have a bitter taste. Their smell is similar to strong tea.

The stem of Adhatoda is soft and makes good charcoal. The flowers are large, dense, and terminal spikes with attractive white petals, streaked with purple on the lower lip. The fruit is a small, clavate, longitudinally channeled capsule containing four globular seeds. The leaves, roots, flowers, and bark are all used for medicinal purposes.

Chemical Composition

The wide variety of pharmacological uses of Adhatoda is believed to be the result of its rich concentration of alkaloids.[2,3] The prominent alkaloid in Adhatoda's leaves is the quinazoline alkaloid known as vasicine.[4,5,6,7]

In addition to vasicine, the leaves and roots of Adhatoda contain the alkaloids L-vasicinone, deoxyvasicine, maiontone, vasicinolone and vasicinol.[8,9] Research indicates that these chemicals are responsible for Adhatoda's bronchodilatory effect.[10,11]

The chemical constitution of Adhatoda also includes phytosterols and triterpenes including daucosterol, a-amyrin, and epitaraxerol. The following flavonoids have been isolated from Adhatoda's leaves and flowers: apigenin, astragalin, kaempferol, quercetin, vitexin, isovitexin, violanthin, 2"-O-xylosylvitexin, rhamnosylvitexin, and 2'-hydroxy-4-glucosyloxychalcone.[12,13]

The oil isolated from Adhatoda's leaves has been found to contain more than 50 fatty acids and hydrocarbons. The richest concentration of these is in the form of decane. Also present are the hydroxyalkanes 37-hydroxyhexatetracont-l-en-15-one and 29-methyltriacontan-l-ol, and linolenic, arachidonic, linoleic, palmitic and oleic acids.[14,15] A ketone, 4-heptanone, forms the major compound in the volatile oil isolated from Adhatoda's flowers.[16] Also present are at least 36 other compounds, including 3-methylheptanone.[17]

Pharmacological Activity

Anti-tubercular Activity

Adhatoda has been studied for its potential in fighting tuberculosis.[18] Chemical synthesis of one of Adhatoda's alkaloids, vasicine, produces bromhexine and ambroxol—two widely used mucolytics. Both of these chemicals have a pH-dependent growth inhibitory effect on mycobactrium tuberculosis. Indirect effects of Adhatoda on tuberculosis include increased lysozyme and rifampicin levels in bronchial secretions, lung tissue, and sputum, suggesting that Adhatoda may play an important adjunctive role in the treatment of tuberculosis.[19,20]

Aqueous extracts of leaves of *Acalypha indica, Adhatoda vasica, Allium cepa, Allium sativum,* and *Aloe vera* were tested in-vitro for their activity against two multi-drug-resistant (MDR) isolates of Mycobacterium tuberculosis and Mycobacterium fortuitum. Extracts from isolates of all of the five plants—Acalypha indica, Adhatoda vasica, Allium cepa, Allium sativum, and Aloe vera—exhibited anti-tuberculosis activity.

In L-J medium, the proportion of inhibition of the plant extracts mentioned above is 95%, 32%, 37%, 72%, and 32%, respectively, for MDR isolate DKU-156; and 68%, 86%, 79%, 72%, and 85%, respectively, for another MDR isolate, JAL-1236. For another Mycobacterium tuberculosis, H37Rv, inhibition was found to be 68%, 70%, 35%, 63%, and 41%, at 4% v/v concentration in L-J medium In BacT/ALERT medium also, extracts of these plants showed significant inhibition against M. tuberculosis.[21]

Anti-asthmatic and Bronchodilatory Activity

Adhatoda has been used in traditional Indian medicine for thousands of years to treat respiratory disorders. Both vasicine and vasicinone—the primary alkaloid constituents of Adhatoda—are well established as therapeutical respiratory agents.[22] Extracts of Adhatoda's leaves and roots are useful in treating bronchitis and other lung and bronchiole disorders, as well as common coughs and colds. A decoction of Adhatoda leaves has a soothing effect on irritation in the throat and acts as an expectorant to loosen phlegm in the respiratory passages.

A 1999 study evaluating the antitussive activity of Adhatoda extract in anesthetized guinea pigs and rabbits and in unanesthetized guinea pigs showed that the plant has good antitussive activity.[23] Administered intravenously, it was 20%–40% as active as codeine when coughing was induced mechanically and electrically in the study animals. The antitussive activity of Adhatoda was similar to codeine against coughing induced by irritating aerosols.[24]

Investigations using vasicine showed bronchodilatory activity both in-vitro and in-vivo. Vasicinone showed bronchodilatory activity in vitro but bronchoconstrictory activity in vivo, suggesting that it probably is biotransformed in-vivo, causing bronchoconstriction. In combination, the two alkaloids showed bronchodilatory activity both in-vivo and in-vitro.[25]

Vasicine also exhibited strong respiratory stimulant activity, moderate hypotensive activity, and a cardiac-depressant effect, whereas vasicinone was devoid of these activities. The cardiac-depressant effect was reduced significantly when using a mixture of vasicine and vasicinone.[26,27]

Anti-parasitic Activity

Adhatoda vasica has been used commonly in the indigenous system of medicine of Naga tribes in India for curing intestinal worm infections. The anticestodal efficacy of Adhatoda vasica leaf extract has been established in the Hymenolepis diminuta rat experimental model. The efficacy of Adhatoda was better than praziquantel.[28]

Anti-allergy Activity

Adhatoda has been found to reduce ovalbumin and PAF-induced allergic reactions. An extract containing the alkaloid vascinol and 20% vasicine inhibited ovalbumin-induced allergic reactions by about 37% at a concentration of 5 mg.[29] Vasicinone has been shown to be a potent anti-allergen in tests on mice, rats, and guinea pigs.[30]

Studies have shed more light on Ambroxol, a widely used secretolytic agent originally developed from vasicine, a natural alkaloid in Adhatoda vasica, extracts of which have been used to treat bronchitis, asthma, and rheumatism. Ambroxol has been reported to inhibit IgE-dependent mediator secretion from human mast cells and basophils, which are key effector cells of allergic inflammation. Ambroxol attenuated basophil IL-4 and IL-13 secretions, and in addition, ambroxol reduced IgE-dependent p38 MAPK (mitogen-activated protein kinase) phosphorylation in basophils. These results clearly show that ambroxol is more potent and effective at inhibiting IgE-dependent basophil mediator release and p38 MAPK activity.[31] Thus, it may have a role in cancer prevention.

Abortifacient and Uterotonic Activity

Because Adhatoda has abortifacient and uterotonic properties, it is useful for inducing abortion and for stimulating uterine contractions to speed childbirth. Studies on human subjects have shown that the alkaloid vasicine has significant uterotonic activity.[32] This action seems to be influenced by the presence or absence of certain estrogens.

In research on the activity of vasicine in stimulating uterine contractions, human myometrial strips taken from the uterus of pregnant and non-pregnant women alike were treated with Adhatoda. The herb was found to induce uterine contractions, with an effectiveness similar to that of the drug oxytocin.[33,34]

Similar results in humans were observed in a survey study conducted in two towns of Uttar Pradesh, India, in 1987. During the research period, local women anecdotally confirmed the anti-reproductive properties of Adhatoda.[35]

Animal studies, too, have demonstrated vasica's abortifacient properties. Aqueous or 90% ethanol plant extracts were given orally to test rats and guinea pigs for 10 days after insemination. Leaf extracts of Adhatoda vasica were 100% abortive at doses equivalent to 175 mg/kg.[36]

Adhatoda also was shown to have an abortifacient effect on guinea pigs, with varied effectiveness depending on the stage of pregnancy. The effects were more marked when estrogens were used as a priming influence—indicating that the actions of vasicine probably were mediated via the release of prostogladins.[37]

Wound-healing Activity

The effectiveness of Adhatoda in promoting wound healing was evaluated in an animal study.[38] For the purposes of the study, wounds were created along the vertebral columns of buffalo calves, followed by application of alcoholic and chloroform extracts of Adhatoda in a powdered form.

Compared to control animals, the calves treated with Adhatoda vasica showed significantly improved healing. Vasica improved breaking strength, tensile strength, absorption, and extensibility in the wound repair tissue. In addition, the levels of elastin, collagen, hydroxyproline, hexosamine, and zinc were greatly increased in the animals treated with Adhatoda. The alcoholic extract of the herb was found to be the most effective.[39]

Cholagogue Activity

In laboratory experiments on cats and dogs, Adhatoda was found to increase bile activity when the animals were given an intravenous dose of 5 mg/kg. In dogs, the amount of excreted bile increased by 40%–100%. The animals also showed an increase in excretion of bilirubin.[40]

Anti-ulcer Activity

Adhatoda was studied for its anti-ulcerogenic activity against ulcers induced by ethanol, pylorus ligation, and aspirin. Adhatoda leaf powder showed a considerable degree of anti-ulcer activity in experimental rats as compared to controls. The highest degree of activity was observed in the ethanol-induced ulceration model.[41]

These results suggest that in addition to its classically established pharmacological activities, Adhatoda has immense potential as an anti-ulcer agent. Further research showed that a syrup of Adhatoda improved symptoms of dyspepsia.[42]

Anti-bacterial Activity

Adhatoda's anti-bacterial properties have been evaluated clinically.[43] A leaf extract was investigated for anti-bacterial activity using paper disc and dilution methods. In-vitro screening showed a strong activity of Adhatoda's alkaloids against the bacteria Pseudomonas aeruginosa. Significant anti-bacterial activity against the Gram-positive bacteria strains Streptococcus faecalis, Staphylococcus aureus, Staph epidermidis, and the gram-negative E. coli also were noted.[44]

In another study, Adhatoda was tested for its capacity to inhibit the growth of bacteria in untreated water. At pH 7, growth of the bacterial population was inhibited by 82%. At pH 6.5, several coliform bacterial strains also were inhibited. These findings suggest a possible application of Adhatoda in improving the quality of drinking water.⁴⁵

Insecticidal Activity

Adhatoda has been used for centuries in India as an insecticide. Its leaves have been shown to control insect pests in oil seeds, in both laboratory and warehouse conditions.⁴⁶ Research has shown Adhatoda's alkaloid, vasicinol, to have an anti-fertility effect against several insect species by causing blockage of the oviduct.⁴⁷ The same study showed that essential oils taken from Adhatoda reduced feeding activity in specific granary pests. Research also has proven Adhatoda's effectiveness as an insect repellent.⁴⁸

Ethnoveterinary Usage

Adhatoda has been used successfully in veterinary medicine for thousands of years in India.⁴⁹ It is effective for a variety of animal conditions including coughs, colds, and diseases such as abscesses, anthrax, throat diseases, asthma, tuberculosis, jaundice, scabies, urticaria, rheumatism, pneumonia, hematuria, and contagious abortion.

Dr. Sodhi's Experience

While growing up in the foot hills of Himalayas, we sucked on the flowers of Adhatoda for the nectar. Honeybees swarmed around the plants of Adhatoda. Honey from these flowers has a distinctive whitish color and was considered therapeutic for common cold, asthma, allergies, and tuberculosis. Locals smoked the dried leaves for asthma and chronic cough. They had a saying, "If there is Adhatoda plant, nobody can dare to cough." It is interesting that this herb has powerful antitussive properties, as powerful as codeine for aerosol irritants but without the side-effects of narcotics. Leaves were smoked close to houses for the insect-repellent properties.

I used this herb extensively for allergies, with great success in combination with *Emblica officinalis, Tinospora cordifolia,* Holy basil and three bitters, which I designed for my allergies. This combination has tremendous success in treating allergies.

Also, herb balls made from leaves of Adhatoda are used as poultices in inflammatory conditions of the joints, making it helpful in treating rheumatoid arthritis, systemic lupus erythematosus, fibromyalgia, polymyalgia, and even osteoarthritis. Natives use the combination of Adhatoda vasica and Vites negundo leaves for the same purpose.

Safety Profile

Excessive doses of vasica may cause diarrhea and vomiting. The herb should not be used by pregnant women, because of its capacity to induce abortion. No adverse effects of using Adhatoda in concert with other drugs or medicines have been observed.

Dosage

Liquid extract: 2–5 ml
Leaf juice: 10–20 ml
Flower juice: 10–20 ml
Root decoction: 40–80 ml
Extract 10: 1 100 mg twice per day

Ayurvedic Properties

Adhatoda vasica pacifies vitiated pitta and kapha and has therapeutic action against cough, bronchitis, asthma, inflammation, hemorrhage, hemorrhoids, eye diseases, and bloody diarrhea.

Guna: Laghu (light), ruksha (dry)
Rasa: Tikta (bitter), kashaya (astringent)
Veerya: Shita (cold)
Vipaka: Katu (pungent)
Dosha: Pacifies kapha and pitta

Notes

1. R. N. Chopra, *Indigenous Drugs of India* (Calcutta: Academic Publishers, 1982).

2. A. Sharafkhaneb, S. Velamuri, V. Badmeev, C. Lan, and N. Hanania, "The potential role of natural agents in treatment of airway inflammation," *Ther Adv Respiratory Disease*, 2007, 1(2): 105–120.

3. S. P. Jain, S. C. Singh, and H. S. Puri, "Medicinal plants of Neterhat, Bihar, India,"*International Journal of Pharmacognosy*, 1994, 32:44.

4. Ubonwan Pongprayoon Claeson, Torbjorn Malmfors, Gearg Wikman, and Jan G. Bruhn, "Adhatoda vasica: A critical review of ethnopharmocoligical and toxicological data," *Journal of Ethnopharmacology*, 2000, 72:1–20.

5. M. P. Jain and V. K. Sharma, "Phytochemical investigation of roots of Adhatoda vasica," *Planta Medica*, 1982, 46: 250.

6. P. K. Lahiri and S. N. Pradhan, "Pharmacological investigation of vasicinol, an alkaloid from Adhatoda vasica Nees," *Indian Journal of Experimental Biology*, 1964, 2:219.

7. O. P. Gupta, K. K. Anand, B. J. Ghatak, and C. K. Atal, "Pharmacological investigations of vasicine and vasicinone—the alkaloids of Adhatoda vasica," *Indian Journal of Medical Research*, 1977, 66(4):680.

8. Jain and Sharma, Note 5.

9. K. L Dhar, M. P. Jain, S. K. Koulm, and C. K. Atal, "Vasicol, a new alkaloid from Adhatoda vasica," *Phytochemistry*, 1981, 20(2):319.

10. H. L. Bhalla and A. Y. Nimbkar, "Preformulation studies III. Vasicinone, a bronchodilatory alkaloid from Adhatoda vasica Nees (absorption, potency and toxicity studies)," *Drug Dev. Indian. Pharm*, 1982, 8(6):833.

11. A. H. Amin and D. R. Mehta, "A bronchodilator alkaloid (vasicinone) from Adhatoda vasica Nees," *Nature*, 1959 (Oct. 24), 184(Suppl. 17):1317.

12. A. Mullar, S. Antus, M. Bittinger, et al., "Chemistry and pharmacology of the antiasthmatic plants, Galpinia glauca, Adhatoda vasica, Picrorrizha kurroa," *Planta Medica*, 1993, 59S.A586.

13. A. O. Prakash, V. Saxena, S. Shukla, R. K. Tewari, S. Mathur, A. Gupta, S. Sharma, and R. Mathur, "Anti implantation activity of some indigenous plants in rats," *Acta Eur Fertility*, 1985 (Nov.–Dec.), 16(6):411–448.

14. H. P. Bhartiya and P. C. Gupta, "A chalcone glycoside from the flowers of Adhatoda vasica," *Phytochemistry*," 1982, 21(1):247.

15. R. S. Singh, T. N. Misra, H. S. Pandey, and B. P. Singh, Aliphatic hydroxyketones from Adhatoda vasica," *Phytochemistry*, 1991, 30(11):3799.

16. S. Ahmed El-Sawi, F. Abd El-Megeed Hashem, and A. M. Ali, "Flavonoids and antimicrobial volatiles from Adhatoda vasica Nees. *Pharmacy and Pharmacology Letters*, 1999, 9(2):52.

17. El-Sawi et al., Note 16.

18. V. C. Barry, M. L. Conalty, H. J. Rylance, and F. R. Smith, "Antitubercular effect of an extract of Adhatoda vasica," *Nature*, 1955 (July 16), 176(4472):119–120.

19. M. Narimaian, M. Badalyan, V. Panosyan, E. Gabrielyan, A. Panossian, G. Wikman, and H. Wagner, "Randomized trial of a fixed combination (KanJang) of herbal extracts containing Adhatoda vasica, Echinacea purpurea and Eleutherococcus senticosus in patients with upper respiratory tract infections," *Phytomedicine*, 2005 (Aug.), 12(8):539–547.

20. J. M. Grange and N. J. C. Snell, "Activity of bromhexine and ambroxol, semi-synthetic derivatives of vasicine from the Indian shrub Adhatoda vasica, against Mycobacterium tuberculosis in vitro," *Journal of Ethnopharmacology*, 1996, 50(1):49.

21. R. Gupta, B. Thakur, P. Singh, H. B. Singh, V. D. Sharma, V.M. Katoch, and S. V. Chauhan, "Anti-tuberculosis activity of selected medicinal plants against multi-drug resistant Mycobacterium tuberculosis isolates," *Indian J Med Res.*, 2010 (June), 131:809–813.

22. W. Dorsch and H. Wagner, "New antiasthmatic drugs from traditional medicine?" *Int Arch Allergy Appl Immunol*, 1991, 94(1–4):262–265.

23. J. N. Dhuley, "Antitussive effect of Adhatoda vasica extract on mechanical or chemical stimulation-induced coughing in animals," *J Ethnopharmacol.*, 1999 (Nov. 30), 67(3):361–365.

24. Dhuley, Note 23.

25. Gupta et al., Note 7.

26. Gupta et al., Note 7.

27. H. L. Bhalla and A. Y. Nimbkar, "Preformulation studies III. Vasicinone, a bronchodilatory alkaloid from Adhatoda vasica Nees (absorption, potency and toxicity studies), *Drug Dev. Indian. Pharm.*, 1982, 8(6):833.

28. Jain, Singh, and Puri, Note 3.

29. J. K. Paliwa, A. D. Dwivedi, S. Sihgh, and R. C. Gupta, "Pharmacokinetics and in-situ absorption studies of a new anti-allergic compound 73/602 in rats," *Int J Pharm.*, 2000 (March 20), 197(1–2):213–220.

30. H. Wagner, "Search for new plant constituents with potential antiphlogistic and antiallergic activity," *Planta Med.*, 1989 (June), 55(3):235-241. (review)

31. B. F. Gibbs, "Differential modulation of IgE-dependent activation of human basophils by ambroxol and related secretolytic analogues," *Int J Immunopathol Pharmacol.*, 2009 (Oct.–Dec.), 22(4):919–927.

32. C. K. Atal, "The chemistry and pharmacology of vasicine, a new oxytocic and abortifacient," Regional Research Laboratory, CSIR, Jammu-Tawi, India, 1980.

33. O. P. Gupta, et al, "Vasicine, alkaloid of Adhatoda vasica, a promising uterotonic abortifacient, *Indian Journal of Experimental Biology*, 1978, 16(10):1075.

34. Atal, Note 32.

35. Gupta et al., Note 33.

36. D. Nath, N. Sethi, R. K. Singh, and A. K. Jain. "Commonly used Indian abortifacient plants with special reference to their teratologic effects in rats," *J Ethnopharmacol*, 1992 (April), 36(2):147–154.

37. Atal, Note 32.

38. M. K. Bhargava, H. Singh, and A. Kumar, "Evaluation of Adhatoda vasica as a wound healing agent in buffaloes, Clinical, mechanical and biochemical studies," 1988, *Indian Veterinary Journal*, 65(1):33.

39. Bhargava et al., Note 38.

40. M. I. Rabinovich, A. I. Leskov, and A. S. Gladkikh, "Cholegogic properties of peganine," *Vrachei*, 1966: 181.

41. N. Shrivastava, A. Srivastava, A. Banerjee, and M. Nivasarkar, "Anti-ulcer activity of Adhatoda vasica Nees," *J Herb Pharmacother*, 2006, 6(2):43–49.

42. G. N. Chaturvedi, N. P. Rai, R. Dhani, and S. K. Tiwari, "Clinical trial of Adhatoda vasica syrup (vasa) in the patients of non-ulcer dyspepsia (Amlapitta)," 1983, *Ancient Science of Life*, 3(1):19.

43. A. H Brantner and A. Chakraborty, "In vitro anti-bacterial activity of alkaloids isolated from Adhatoda vasica Nees," *Pharmacy and Pharmacology Letters*, 1998, 8(3):137.

44. V. K. Patel and H. Venkatakrishna-Bhatt, "In vitro study of antimicrobial activity of adhatoda vasika Linn (leaf extract) on gingival inflammation—a preliminary report," *Indian J Med Sci.*, 1984 (April), 38(4):70–72.

45. S. Kumar and K. Gopal, "Screening of plant species for inhibition of bacterial population of raw water," *Journal of Environmental Science and Health*, 1999, A34(4):975.

46. A. S. Srivastava, H. P. Saxena, and D. R. Singh, "Adhatoda vasica, a promising insecticide against pests of storage," *Lab. Dev*, 1965, 3(2):138.

47. B. P. Saxena, K. Tikku, and C. K. Atal, "Insect antifertility and antifeedant alleochemics in Adhatoda vasica," *Insect Sci. Appl.*, 1986, 7(4):489.

48. C. K. Kokate, J. L. D'Cruz, R. A. Kumar, and S. S. Apte, "Anti-insect and juvenoidal activity of phytochemicals derived from Adhatoda vasica Nees," *Indian Journal of Natural Products*, 1985, l(1–2):7.

49. M. K Jha, "The folk veterinary system of Bihar—a research survey," NDDB, 1992, Anand, Gujrat.

Additional Resources

R. K. Maikhuri and A..K. Gangwar, "Ethnobiological notes on the Khasi and Garo tribes of Meghalaya, Northeast India." *Economic Botany*, 1965, 47:345.

M. Rajani and K. Pundarikakshudu, "A note on the seasonal variation of alkaloids in Adhatoda vasica Nees," *International Journal of Pharmacognosy*, 1996, 34(4):308–309.

G. S. Pahwa, U. Zutshi U, and C. K. Atal, "Chronic toxicity studies with vasicine from Adhatoda vasica Nees in rats and monkeys," *Indian J Exp Biol.*, July 25, 1987, 7:467–470.

Arun K. Yadav and Vareishang Tangpu, "Anticestodal activity of *Adhatoda vasica* extract against *Hymenolepis diminuta* infections in rats," *Journal of Ethnopharmacology*, Sept. 2008, 119 (2): 322–332.

2

Aegle marmelos

Introduction

Aegle marmelos, commonly known as Bael, is a fruit-bearing tree indigenous to the hills and plains of central and southern India. This tree is an object of honor in the Hindu religion. The god Shiva is said to live under the Bael tree, so the tree often is planted in temple gardens, and its leaves are used in religious celebrations.

The aromatic fruit of Bael is widely enjoyed in India; eaten whole, dried, or made into a refreshing drink. The fruit promotes healthy digestion and is used medicinally to treat diarrhea, dysentery, and cholera.[1] Bael fruit also heals intestinal ulcers and possesses anti-viral, anti-microbial, and anti-inflammatory properties. Further, Bael is used to treat reproductive abnormalities such as miscarriage, placental retention, and vaginal hemorrhage. Ayurvedic practitioners use Bael to relieve tachycardia, bradycardia, swelling of the throat, hemorrhagic septicemia, pneumonia, polyuria, and lumbar fracture.[2]

The leaves, bark, and roots of Bael have medicinal value, too. The roots, in the form of a decoction, are used to treat melancholia, intermittent fevers, and heart palpitations. The bitter-tasting leaves are used in the form of a poultice to relieve ophthalmic disorders, generalized inflammation, febrile delirium and acute bronchitis. The fresh leaves of Bael are used to stimulate a weak heart, and to relieve dropsy and beriberi.[3]

A juice extracted from the leaves of Bael is used in treating diabetes. This bitter, pungent juice, when mixed with honey, relieves catarrh and fever. Another Bael-leaf preparation, with black pepper, is used to treat jaundice associated with edema and constipation. The leaf decoction is said to alleviate asthma. The young leaves and shoots of the Bael tree are consumed as a vegetable in Thailand and as a seasoning for food in Indonesia, where they are believed to reduce appetite.

Synonymous Names

English: Bengal quince
Hindi: Bael, bel, beli
Sanskrit: Bilva, Shivaphala
Aegle marmelos also is known by the names Bilwa, Bel, Kuvalam, Koovalam, Madtoum, Beli fruit, Stone apple, and Wood apple.

Habitat

A subtropical species, *Aegle marmelos* grows to an altitude of 1200 meters (4,200 feet). It is cultivated throughout India, as well as in Sri Lanka, the northern Malay Peninsula, Java, and the Philippines. Bael also is found in many areas of Southeast Asia. It will not bear fruit in areas that do not have a long, dry season.

Botanical Characteristics

Bael is a medium-sized, deciduous tree that grows to a height of 18 meters (54 feet). Its branches bear sharp spines about 2.5 mm in length. The leaves are trifoliate, and full of aromatic oil. The large, sweet-scented flowers are greenish-white in color and bloom from May to June. The corky bark is light gray.

The woody-skinned, smooth fruit of the Bael tree ranges in size from 5 to 15 cm in diameter. Some varieties of Bael fruit have extremely hard skin and must be cracked open with a hammer. Bael fruit has numerous seeds, which are densely covered with fibrous hairs and embedded in a thick, gluey, aromatic pulp. The fruit pulp bears 8 to 15 segments and generally is yellow, soft, sweet, and fragrant. It is eaten fresh, or it may be dried.

The Bael tree grows to maturity in about 60 years. Its typical girth is 1–1.5 m (3-4.5 feet). Bael is regenerated easily in its natural habitat and also can be grown in nurseries from seed and root cuttings.

Chemical Composition

Aegle marmelos is a member of the rutaceae family. The rind of the fruit and its pulp, its root-bark, leaves, and flowers are constituted with a bitter principle, volatile oils, pectin, and tannin. The wood-ash of the Bael tree is rich in minerals and phosphates.

Bael leaves have a high alkaloid content, the most prominent alkaloids of which are aegelenine and aegeline. The roots and aerial parts contain skimmianine. Anthraquinones present in Bael are 7,8-Dimethoxy-1-hydroxy-2-methyl anthraquinone and 6-hydroxy-l-methoxy-3-methyl anthraquinone.[4,5]

The fruit of Bael contains the coumarins marmelosin, allo-imperatorin, marmelide, and psoralen, and the roots contain umbelliferone, psoralen, xanthotoxin, dimethoxycoumarin, and scopoletin. The xylem yields a-xanthotoxol-8-O-beta-D-glucoside, and the seeds contain luvangetin.[6,7]

Bael fruit also contains tannic acid. The tannin content of the fruit and rind is 7%–9% and 18%–22%, respectively. The leaves also contain condensed tannins. Minor constituents include reducing sugar, essential oils, ascorbic acid, and various minerals.

Pharmacological Activity

Anti-diarrheal Activity

Clinical studies have demonstrated the effectiveness of Bael for treating irritable bowel syndrome (IBS), a condition that is becoming increasingly prevalent. In a randomized human clinical trial, an Ayurvedic preparation consisting of Aegle marmelos and the Ayurvedic herb Bacopa monnieri was compared to a standard therapy for IBS (clidinium bromide with chlordiazepoxide and psyllium husk) and a matching placebo. These results are significant in that treatment with herbal preparations generally does not produce side-effects. The symptoms of 57 patients (33.7%) improved after treatment with the Ayurvedic preparation, in contrast to 60 patients (35.5%) who improved with the standard therapy. At the end of the 6-week study, the Ayurvedic preparation containing Bael was shown to be as effective as traditional therapy in relieving IBS symptoms.[8]

The Ayurvedic preparation was the most useful in treating diarrhea-predominant IBS, compared to the placebo; however, long-term therapy (longer than 6 months) showed that neither treatment was better than the placebo in limiting relapse. In the author's view, however, the results can be improved significantly with nutritional and lifestyle changes, along with the use of Ayurvedic preparations.

The results of an animal study further demonstrated the anti-diarrheal properties of Bael fruit.

This study tested the anti-diarrheal potential of a chloroform extract of the roots of Bael. The extract was evaluated both in-vitro using agar dilution and disc diffusion techniques, and in-vivo using rats. Of the 35 diarrhea-causing bacterial strains evaluated, the extract was found to be active against Vibrio cholerae, Escherichia coli, and Shigella. This action was determined to be comparable to the drug ciprofloxacin. Animals treated with the root extract showed significant resistance against castor oil-induced diarrhea.[9]

Anti-bacterial, Anti-viral, Anti-parasitic and Anti-fungal Activity

The leaves of Aegle marmelos have been shown to have anti-microbial properties. In a spore germination assay, essential oils isolated from the leaves of Bael were observed to inhibit the growth of a variety of fungal isolates. Complete inhibition of the germination of all fungal spores was observed at 500 ppm, except for the most resistant fungal strain, Fusarium udum, which was inhibited 80% at 400 ppm. The essential oils of Bael also inhibited the growth of 21 different bacterial strains, including Gram-positive (cocci and rods), Gram-negative (rods), and 12 fungi including three yeast-like and nine filamentous strains.[10]

Further research into Bael's anti-microbial effects showed that the seed oil was effective against Vibrio cholerae, Klebsiella pneumonia, and Salmonella typhimurium. Anti-fungal activity was noted against Candida albicans, Aspergillus fumigates, and Trichophyton mentagrophytes. Ethanolic extract from the roots of the tree was effective against *Curvularia lanata, Aspergillus niger,* and *Rhizopus nodulens.*[11]

Lectins are a class of ubiquitous proteins/glycoproteins that are found abundantly in nature. Lectins have unique carbohydrate-binding property and hence have been exploited as drugs against various infectious diseases. Research has isolated one such novel lectin from the fruit pulp of Aegle marmelos. This isolated lectin was partially characterized, and its effect against Shigella dysenteriae infection was evaluated. The isolated lectin was found to be a dimeric protein with N-acetylgalactosamine, mannose, and sialic acid binding specificity. The effect of Aegle marmelos fruit lectin on the adherence of Shigella dysenteriae to human colonic epithelial cells (HT29 cells) was evaluated by Enzyme Linked Immune Sorbent Assay, and invasion was analyzed. The protective nature of the Aegle marmelos fruit lectin was assessed by analyzing apoptosis through the dual staining method. Aegle marmelos fruit lectin was found to significantly inhibit hemagglutination activity of Shigella, and its minimum inhibitory concentration was 0.625 µg/well. Further, at this concentration, lectin was found to inhibit Shigella dysenteriae adherence and invasion of HT29 cells and protect the HT29 cells from Shigella dysenteriae induced apoptosis. To conclude, Aegle marmelos lecitin inhibits adherence and invasion of Shigella to the HT29 cells thus, protects the host.[12]

Shigella dysenteriae continues to be a major health problem, which leads to death from diarrhea and dysentery, predominantly in children below the age of 5. Bacterial invasion of the colonic epithelium causes severe inflammation and dissemination of the bacteria generates abscesses and ulcerations. Periplasmic copper, zinc super oxide dismutase of Shigella protects it from exogenous superoxide produced by the host during its invasion. Hence, in this study, an attempt was made to study the effect of aqueous extract of Aegle marmelos on the host and pathogen defense.[13] A histology analysis of rats ileal loop showed the loss of virulence in aqueous extract of A. marmelos pre-treated Shigella, and their intracellular survival also was decreased when the active component was present in aqueous extract of A. marmelos, identified as imperatorin, confirmed by UV absorption spectrum and HPLC.

An increase in peripheral blood mononuclear cell viability and a decrease in intracellular bacterial count, along with a transmission electron microscope analysis of imperatorin-treated S. dysenteriae, succumbed to host oxidative stress. Loss of virulence is associated with attenuation of copper, zinc super oxide dismutase activity in Shigella, which was confirmed by using activity staining of bacterial cell lysate. Further, docking analysis has proved that imperatorin present in aqueous extract of A. marmelos inhibited copper, zinc super oxide dismutase. From the above study, it is concluded that Shigella succumb to oxidative stress (host defense) as a result of inhibition of copper, zinc super oxide dismutase (pathogen's defense) by imperatorin, an active compound aqueous extract of A. marmelos.

Patients with acquired immunodeficiency syndrome (AIDS) face great socioeconomic difficulties in obtaining treatment, so there is an urgent need for new, safe, and inexpensive anti-HIV agents. Traditional medicinal plants are a valuable source of novel anti-HIV agents and may offer alternatives to expensive medicines in the future. Various medicinal plants or plant-derived natural products have shown strong anti-HIV activity and are under various stages of clinical development in different parts of the world. This study was directed toward assessment of anti-HIV activity of various extracts prepared from Indian medicinal plants. The plants were chosen on the basis of similarity of chemical constituents with reported anti-HIV compounds or on the basis of their traditional usage as immunomodulators. The different extracts were prepared by Soxhlet extraction and liquid–liquid partitioning; 92 extracts were prepared from 23 plants. Anti-HIV activity was measured in a human CD4+ T-cell line, CEM-GFP cells infected with HIV-1NL4.3. Nine extracts of eight different plants significantly reduced viral production in CEM-GFP cells infected with HIV-1NL4.3. Aegle marmelos, Argemone mexicana, Asparagus racemosus, Coleus forskohlii, and Rubia cordifolia demonstrated promising anti-HIV potential and were investigated for their active principles.[14]

Tropical disease research by the World Health Organization has duly recognized traditional medicine as an alternative for antifilarial drug development. Polyphenolic compounds that are present in traditionally used herbal medicines are natural anti-oxidants; paradoxically, however, they may exert a pro-oxidant effect. The popular drug diethyl carbamazine citrate harnesses the innate inflammatory response and the consequent oxidative assault to combat invading microbes.

With this perspective, extracts of Vitex negundo L. (roots), Butea monosperma L. (leaves), Aegle marmelos Corr. (leaves), and Ricinus communis L. (leaves) were selected to explore the possible role of oxidative rationale in the antifilarial effect in-vitro.[15] Apart from the last of these, the other three plant extracts were reported to have polyphenolic compounds. A dose-dependent increase was found in the levels of lipid peroxidation and protein carbonylation for all three plant extracts except Ricinus communis L. (leaves). Such an increase in oxidative parameters also showed some degree of plant-specific predilection in terms of a relatively higher level of particular oxidative parameter. A high degree of correlation was observed between the antifilarial effect and the levels of corresponding oxidative stress parameters for these three plants. In contrast, an extract of Ricinus communis L. (leaves), which is relatively deficient in polyphenolic ingredients, recorded a maximum 30% loss of motility and also did not show any significant difference from the corresponding control levels in the various stress parameters.

Anti-diabetic Activity and Related Activity

Various studies have evaluated the effectiveness of Bael in treating diabetic disorders. An aqueous extract of Bael leaves was assessed for its ability to stimulate insulin release both in normoglycemic and in streptozotocin-diabetic rats. Treatment with the extract resulted in significant hypoglycemic activity in both models. Where the ability of the surviving cells to release more insulin and elevated levels of plasma insulin were measured, the extract was comparable to insulin in restoring blood glucose levels and normalizing body weight.[16]

In streptozotocin-induced diabetic rats, histopathological changes were seen in acinar cells and hepatocytes, along with a decrease in glycogen content of the liver. The extract of Bael appeared to have a regenerative effect on acinar cells of the pancreas and kidney glomeruli.[17] A similar action was observed in an alloxan-induced animal model of diabetes, in which the action was comparable to that of insulin.[18]

Another study evaluated the hypoglycemic and anti-oxidant effect of the aqueous extract of Bael leaves on diabetic rats.[19] Male albino rats were randomly divided into three groups— control, diabetic rats, and diabetic rats treated with Bael leaf extract. At the end of 4 weeks, glucose, urea, and glutathione-S-transferase (GST) in plasma, glutathione (GSH), and malondialdehyde (MDA) levels in erythrocytes were measured in all of the study groups. A decrease in blood glucose level was observed in the treated animals, compared to the untreated animals; however, the decrease did not reach the levels of the control group. The Bael-treated group animals showed an increase in erythrocyte glutathione (GSH) and a decrease in MDA compared to the Group Two animals. The plasma GST levels were elevated in diabetic rats compared to the control group. A decrease in GST was observed in the treated animals compared to the untreated diabetic animals. The above studies confirm that Bael leaf extracts may be useful in the long-term management of diabetes.

In a study[21] carried out to find the effects of Aegle marmelos leaf extract and insulin alone and in combination with pyridoxine on the cerebellar 5 hydroxytryptamine (5-HT) through the 5-HT(2A) receptor subtype, gene expression studies on the status of anti-oxidants-superoxide dismutase (SOD), glutathione peroxidase (GPx), 5-HT(2A) and 5-HT transporter (5-HTT), and immunohistochemical studies in streptozotocin-induced diabetic rats.[20] The 5-HT and 5-HT(2A) receptor-binding parameters, B(max) and K(d), showed a significant decrease (p<0.001) in the cerebellum of diabetic rats compared to the control group. Gene expression studies of SOD, GPx, 5-HT(2A), and 5-HTT in the cerebellum showed a significant down regulation (p<0.001) in the diabetic rats compared to the control group. Pyridoxine treated alone and in combination with insulin, Aegle marmelos to diabetic rats, reversed the B(max), K(d) of 5-HT, 5-HT(2A) and the gene expression of SOD, GPx, 5-HT(2A), and 5-HTT in the cerebellum to near control. The gene expression of 5-HT(2A) and 5-HTT was confirmed by immunohistochemical studies. Also, the Rotarod test confirmed the motor dysfunction and recovery by treatment. These data suggest the anti-oxidant and neuroprotective role of pyridoxine and A. marmelose through the upregulation of 5-HT through 5-HT(2A) receptor in diabetic rats. This suggests that pyridoxine treated alone and in combination with insulin and A. marmelose has a role in the regulation of insulin synthesis and release, normalizing diabetic-related oxidative stress and neurodegeneration, affecting the motor ability of an individual by serotonergic receptors through 5-HT(2A) function.

Phytotherapy has played an important role in the management of diabetes and related complications. In the following study, different fractions of Catharanthus roseus, Ocimum sanctum, Tinospora cordifolia, Aegle marmelos L., Ficus golmerata, Psoralea corlifolia, Tribulus terrestris, and Morinda cetrifolia were evaluated as possible inhibitors of aldose reductase (AR: a key enzyme implicated in cataractogenesis) and anti-oxidant agents. Anti-cataract activity of the selected plants was demonstrated using the "sugar induced lens opacity model," and the cytotoxicity studies were carried out using the MTT assay.

Among the tested plants, water extract of M. cetrifolia (IC50 0.132 mg/ml) exhibited maximum AR inhibitory activity as compared to other phytofractions, which showed the activity in an IC50 range of 0.176-0.0.82 mg/ml. All of the plant fractions showed considerable anti-oxidant potential. The sugar induced lens opacity studies revealed that M. cetrifolia possess significant anti-cataract potential to maintain lens opacity as compared to the glucose induced lens opacity in the bovine lens model. The extract of the selected plants showed moderate cytotoxicity against the HeLa cell line. Results of these studies may be useful in converting botanicals into therapeutic modalities.

The global epidemic of type 2 diabetes demands the rapid evaluation of new and accessible interventions. This study investigated whether Aegle marmelos fruit aqueous extract (AMF; 250, 500 and 1000 mg/kg) reduces insulin resistance, dyslipidemia and β-cell dysfunction in high-fat diet-fed streptozotocin (HFD-STZ)-induced diabetic rats by modulating peroxisome proliferator-activated receptor-γ (PPARγ) expression.[22] The serum levels of glucose, insulin, homeostasis model assessment of insulin resistance (HOMA-IR), homeostasis model assessment of β-cell function (HOMA-B), lipid profile, TNF-α and IL-6 were evaluated. Further, the TBARS level and SOD activity in pancreatic tissue and PPARγ protein expression in liver were assessed. In addition, histopathological and ultrastructural studies were performed to validate the effect of AMF on β-cells. The HFD-STZ treated rats showed a significant increase in the serum levels of glucose, insulin, HOMA-IR, TNF-α, IL-6, dyslipidemia with a concomitant decrease in HOMA-B and PPARγ expression. Treatment with AMF for 21 days in diabetic rats positively modulated the altered parameters in a dose-dependent manner. Further, AMF prevented inflammatory changes and β-cell damage along with a reduction in mitochondrial and endoplasmic reticulum swelling. These findings suggest that the protective effect of Aegle marmelos in type 2 diabetic rats is a result of the preservation of β-cell function and insulin-sensitivity through increased PPARγ expression.

Radioprotective Activity

The radioprotective effects of Bael extracts have been confirmed in laboratory research.[23] A hydroalcoholic extract of Aegle marmelos was evaluated in cultured human peripheral blood lymphocytes using the micronucleus assay method. Before experimental exposure to radiation, the lymphocytes were treated with various concentrations of Bael extract to determine the optimum protective dose. After treatment, the lymphocytes were exposed to 3 Gy gamma radiation. The micronucleus frequency in cytokinesis-blocked lymphocytes was evaluated after exposure to radiation. Treatment of the lymphocytes with different concentrations of the Aegle extract significantly reduced the frequency of radiation induced micronuclei. The greatest reduction was observed at a concentration of 5 microg/ml of extract. In further research, the lymphocytes were treated with 5 microg/ml Bael extract before exposure to various doses of gamma radiation. Varying levels of gamma radiation exposure in the control groups resulted in dose-dependent increases in lymphocytes bearing one, two, and multiple micronuclei. Lymphocytes treated with 5 microg/ml of extract showed a significantly reduced frequency of multiple nuclei compared to the irradiated controls.

To better understand the radioprotective activity of the Bael extract, research was conducted to evaluate free radical scavenging in-vitro. Bael extract inhibited free radicals in a dose-dependent manner up to a dose of 200 microg/ml on average, after which the effectiveness leveled off. These results demonstrate that Bael extract at 5 microg/ml protects human peripheral blood lymphocytes against radiation-induced DNA damage and genomic instability. The radioprotective activity of Bael may be a result of scavenging of radiation-induced free radicals and the resulting decrease in oxidative stress.

Another study investigated the radioprotective activity of a leaf extract from Bael in mice exposed to different doses of gamma radiation. Swiss albino male mice were administered various single doses of the extract before being exposed to radiation. The animals were monitored for symptoms of radiation sickness and mortality up to 30 days post-irradiation. Glutathione and lipid peroxidation were estimated in the surviving animals of both groups on day 31 after irradiation. The results of this study showed Bael extract to be non-toxic up to a single dose of 1750 mg kg(-1). The optimum radioprotective dose was five consecutive doses of 15 mg/kg, with the highest survival observed at 10 Gy radiation. Irradiation caused a dose-dependent decline in survival, whereas treatment of mice with Bael extract enhanced survival. This study confirms that treatment with Bael extract reduced the symptoms of radiation-induced sickness and increased survival rates.[24]

Anti-cancer Activity and Chemoprotective Activity

Chemoprevention is a novel approach to studying the anti-initiating and anti-tumor-promoting efficacy of medicinal plants and their active principles. One study investigated the chemopreventive potential of Aegle marmelos fruit extract in 7, 12-dimethylbenz[a]anthracene-induced skin carcinogenesis and its influence on oxidative stress and the anti-oxidant defense system.[25] The oral administration of A marmelos at 100 mg/kg body weight/day during peri-initiational, post-initiational, and peri- and post-initiational phases of papillomagenesis showed a significant reduction in tumor incidence, tumor yield, tumor burden, and the cumulative number of papillomas when compared with the carcinogen treated control. The average latent period increased significantly (7.88 weeks; control group) to 9.45, 11.11, and 11.54 weeks in different Aegle marmelos extract (AME) experimental groups. An enzyme analysis of the skin and liver showed a significant elevation in anti-oxidant parameters such as super-oxide dismutase, catalase, glutathione, and vitamin C in the AME-treated groups when compared with the carcinogen-treated control. The elevated level of lipid peroxidation in the positive control was inhibited significantly by AME administration. These results indicate that AME has the potential to reduce chemically induced skin papillomas by enhancing the anti-oxidant defense system.

Another study examined the inhibitory effects of Aegle marmelos methanolic extract on diethyl-nitrosamine (DEN) initiated and 2-acetyl amino-fluorene (2-AAF) promoted liver carcinogenesis in male Wistar rats.[26] Interestingly, it was found that A. marmelos (25 and 50 mg/kg body weight) resulted in a marked reduction of the incidence of liver tumors, which was further confirmed with histopathology. Further, to understand the underlying mechanisms of the chemoprevention potential of A. marmelos, the levels of hepatic anti-oxidant defense enzymes, ornithine decarboxylase (ODC) activity and hepatic DNA synthesis as a marker for tumor promotion, because a direct correlation between these marker parameters and carcinogenicity has been well documented. Treatment of male Wistar rats for five consecutive days with 2-AAF induced significant hepatic toxicity, oxidative stress and hyper-proliferation. Pre-treatment of A. marmelos extract (25 and 50 mg/kg body weight) prevented oxidative stress and toxicity by restoring the levels of anti-oxidant enzymes at both doses. The promotion parameters (ODC activity and DNA synthesis) induced by administering 2-AAF in the diet with partial hepatectomy (PH) also were significantly suppressed dose-dependently by A. marmelos. Therefore, it can be concluded that ultimately the protection against liver carcinogenesis by A. marmelos methanolic extract might be mediated by multiple actions, including restoration of cellular anti-oxidant enzymes, detoxifying enzymes, ODC activity, and DNA synthesis.

In one study, cancer chemopreventive properties were evaluated on 7, 12-dimethylbenz (a) anthracene (DMBA) induced skin papillomagenesis in Swiss albino mice.[27] A single topical application of DMBA, followed 2 weeks later by repeated application of croton oil until the end of the experiment (i.e., 16 weeks) caused a 100% tumor incidence. In contrast, mice treated with the Aegle marmelos extract (50 mg/kg b. wt./animal/day) in the peri-initiational phase (i.e., 7 days before and 7 days after DMBA application; Group IV) and the post-initiational phase (from the day of croton oil treatment until the end of the experiment; Group V), exhibited a significant reduction to 70% and 50% respectively. The cumulative number of papillomas after 16 weeks was 67 in the control group, but 26 and 23 in the animals treated with AME at peri-initiational and post-initiational stages, respectively. The tumor burden and tumor yield were decreased significantly (Group IV-3.7, 2.6; Group V- 4.6, 2.3) as compared to the carcinogen-treated control group (6.7, 6.7).

More than 20,000 lipid extracts of plants and marine organisms were evaluated in a human breast tumor T47D cell-based reporter assay for hypoxia inducible factor-1 (HIF-1) inhibitory activity.[28] In T47D cells, Aegle marmelos extract inhibited hypoxia induced HIF-1 activation with IC50 values of 0.063 and 0.068 µM, respectively. Aegle marmelos extract also suppressed hypoxic induction of the HIF-1 target genes GLUT-1 and VEGF. Mechanistic studies revealed that Aegle marmelos extract inhibited HIF-1 activation by blocking the hypoxia-induced accumulation of HIF-1α protein.

Cardioprotective Activity

The therapeutic effect of Aegle marmelos on the cardiovascular system has been demonstrated in laboratory research. An extract of Aegle marmelos root bark (100 p.g/ml) was shown to inhibit the spontaneous beating rate of cultured mouse myocardial cells by approximately 50%. Aurapten, a pure compound isolated from the extract, was found to be the most potent.[29]

An aqueous leaf extract of Aegle marmelos was studied for its ability to prevent isoprenaline-induced myocardial infarction in rats. The animals received pre-treatment with the extract for 35 days, after which myocardial infarction was induced by isoprenaline administered subcutaneously at an interval of 24 hours for 2 days. The post-treatment analysis showed that the activity of the creatinine kinase (CK) and lactate dehydrogenase (LDH) was increased significantly in serum and decreased significantly in the heart tissue of the isoprenaline-treated rats. Pre-treatment with Aegle marmelos extract decreased the activity of both CK and LDH in serum and showed protective action on the heart tissue.[30]

These research results also showed the activity of sodium-potassium dependent adenosine triphosphatase to be decreased significantly, whereas the activity of calcium-dependent adenosine triphosphatase was increased simultaneously in the hearts and aortas of the study animals. Pre-treatment with extract increased the activity of the sodium potassium-dependent adenosine triphosphatase and decreased the activity of calcium-dependent adenosine triphosphatase in the heart and aorta simultaneously. Cholesterol and triglyceride levels increased, while phospholipid levels decreased in the hearts and aortas of the isoprenaline-treated rats. In the pre-treated rats, the levels of cholesterol and triglycerides decreased, whereas phospholipids increased in the heart and aorta. These results suggest clinical relevance for Aegle marmelos extract in treating cardiovascular conditions.

The pathogenesis of diabetic cardiomyopathy (DCM) is complex, and the therapeutic options available to treat DCM are limited. This study was designed to investigate the effect of Aegle marmelos leaf extract on early-stage DCM in alloxan-induced diabetic rats.[31] Diabetes was induced in Wistar rats (150-200 g) by injecting alloxan (150 mg kg(-1); i.p.). Ethanol extract of Aegle marmelos leaves was administered at varying doses (100, 200, and 400 mg kg(-1)) and tolbutamide (100 mg kg(-1)) as standard. Fasting blood glucose (FBG), total cholesterol, thiobarbituric acid reactive substances (TBARS), reduced glutathione (GSH), catalase (CAT), superoxide dismutase (SOD), lactate dehydrogenase (LDH) and creatine kinase (CK) were determined by standard methods. Aegle marmelos extract (AME) was found to decrease the levels of FBG, total cholesterol, TBARS, LDH, and CK, and increase the levels of GSH, CAT, and SOD dose dependently as compared to diabetic control groups. The maximum dose-dependent decrease in TBARS (63.46%), LDH (34.04%), CK (53.14%) and increase in GSH (64.91%), CAT (59.34%), SOD (69.65%) was evident at an optimum dose of 200 mg kg(-1). Histopathological studies revealed salvage in the morphological derangements as indicated by the absence of necrosis and a marked decrease in inflammatory cells in AME-treated groups as compared to diabetic control. The conclusion is that treatment with AME attenuates the severity and improves the myocardium in early stages of alloxan-induced DCM at a dose of 200 mg kg(-1).[31]

In another study, The lipid-lowering effect of 50% ethanolic extract of the leaves of Aegle marmelos was evaluated in triton and diet-induced hyperlipidemia models of Wistar albino rats.[32] The extract at 125 and 250 mg/kg dose levels inhibited the elevation in serum cholesterol and triglycerides levels on Triton WR 1339 administration in rats. The extract at the same dose levels significantly attenuated the elevated serum total cholesterol and triglycerides with an increase in the high-density lipoprotein cholesterol in high-fat diet-induced hyperlipidemia rats. The standard drugs atorvastatin in the former study and gemfibrozil in the latter study showed slightly better effects. In the author's opinion, treatment of hyperlipidemia is multifactorial where nutrition is the hallmark for successful treatment.

Anti-ulcer Activity

Research has confirmed the anti-ulcer effectiveness of Aegle marmelos fruit. In one study, luvagetin, a pyranocouramin isolated from the seeds of the Aegle marmelos fruit, was tested for its ability to inhibit gastric ulcers. Rats and guinea pigs were given the substance orally before administering various ulcer-producing substances. Luvangetin showed a significant protective capacity against pylorus-ligated and aspirin-induced gastric ulcers in rats, as well as against cold-restraint stress induced gastric ulcers in rats and guinea pigs.[33]

Anti-inflammatory Activity

This study evaluated and compared the anti-inflammatory activity of the aqueous root bark extract of Aegle marmelos in experimental acute and chronic inflammatory animal models.[34] Aqueous extract of root bark of Aegle marmelos was prepared and tested for anti-inflammatory activity in albino rats weighing 150–280 grams. The animals were randomly divided into three groups of six each; one group served as the control and other two groups received indomethacin and Aegle marmelos orally 1 hour prior to experimentation. The in-vivo anti-inflammatory activity was studied using the acute (Carrageenan-induced paw edema) and chronic (cotton pellet-induced granuloma) animal models. Anti-inflammatory activity was expressed as percent inhibition (PI). Statistical analysis was performed using one-way analysis of variance (ANOVA) followed by Scheffe's post hoc test. P < 0.05 was considered statistically significant. The PI with indomethacin and Aegle marmelos in carrageenan-induced paw edema were 52.7% and 46%, and in cotton pellet-induced granuloma were 24.7% and 9.2%, respectively. Indomethacin showed highly significant anti-inflammatory activity in both models. Aegle marmelos, however, showed highly significant activity in the acute model but also showed anti-inflammatory activity in chronic model of inflammation. As Aegle marmelos showed significant antiinflammatory activity in the models studied, it can be a promising anti-inflammatory agent.

Aegeline or N-[2-hydroxy-2(4-methoxyphenyl) ethyl]-3-phenyl-2-propenamide is a main alkaloid isolated from Aegle marmelos collected in Yogyakarta Indonesia. This study investigated the effects of aegeline on the histamine release from mast cell. The study was performed by using (1) rat basophilic leukemia (RBL-2H3) cell line, and (2) rat peritoneal mast cells (RPMCs). DNP(24)-BSA, thapsigargin, ionomycin, compound 48/80 and PMA were used as inducers for histamine release from the mast cell.[35] Aegeline inhibited the histamine release from RBL-2H3 cells induced by DNP(24)-BSA. Indeed, aegeline showed strong inhibition when RBL-2H3 cells were induced by Ca(2+) stimulants such as thapsigargin and ionomycin. Aegeline is suggested to influence the intracellular Ca(2+) pool only, as it could not inhibit the (45)Ca(2+) influx into RBL-2H3 cells. Aegeline showed weak inhibitory effects on the histamine release from RPMCs, even though it still succeeds in inhibiting when the histamine release is induced by thapsigargin.

These findings indicate that aegeline altered the signaling pathway related to the intracellular Ca(2+) pool in which thapsigargin acts. Based on the results, the inhibitory effects of aegeline on the histamine release from mast cells depended on the type of mast cell and also involved some mechanisms related to intracellular Ca(2+) signaling events via the same target of the action of thapsigargin or the downstream process of intracellular Ca(2+) signaling in mast cells.

Aegle marmelos also has been investigated for its immunomodulatory effects. A propelargonidin extracted from an aqueous extract of unripe Bael fruit showed an inhibitory effect on classic immune response pathways. The extract had no effect on the alternative pathway of complement activation.[36]

Ophthalmic Activity

A study was designed to evaluate the intraocular pressure (IOP)-lowering activity of topical application of the aqueous extract of Aegle marmelos fruit in experimental animal models. The IOP-lowering effect of Aegle marmelos fruit extract in rabbits with experimentally elevated IOP also was compared to that of timolol 0.25%.[37] In rabbits with normal IOP, the Aegle marmelos fruit extract at a concentration of 1% showed the maximum IOP-lowering effect with a 22.81% reduction from the baseline IOP. The maximum IOP reduction achieved in water loading and steroid-induced models with the same concentration of Aegle marmelos was 27.57 and 28.41% from baseline, respectively. The efficacy was comparable to that of timolol after 45 minutes of water loading in the water-loading model, and during the first 2 hours of treatment in the steroid-induced model.

Anxiolytic and Anti-depressant Activity

The objective of this study was to evaluate the anxiolytic and anti-depressant activities of methanol extract of Aegle marmelos leaves, as well as its interaction with conventional anxiolytic and anti-depressant drugs using elevated plus maze and tail suspension test in mice. Albino mice were treated with Aegle marmelos (75, 150 and 300 mg/kg, po), imipramine (20 mg/kg, po), fluoxetine (20 mg/kg, po), and a combination of sub-effective dose of Aegle marmelos with imipramine or fluoxetine.[38.] Effects were observed on (a) time spent on, (b) number of entries into, (c) number of stretch attend postures, and (d) number of head dips in arms of elevated plus maze and on duration of immobility in the tail suspension test. Effects of pre-treatment with prazosin (0.062 mg/kg, po), haloperidol (0.1 mg/kg, po), and baclofen (10 mg/kg, po) also were studied on mice with Aegle marmelos induced decrease in duration of immobility. Effects of Aegle marmelos (75, 150 and 300 mg/kg po) were observed on loco-motor activity using a photoactometer. The results showed that Aegle marmelos significantly ($P<0.05$) and dose dependently increased the proportionate time spent on and the number of entries into open arms, and decreased the number of stretch attend postures and head dips in closed arms. A dose dependent and significant ($P<0.05$) anti-immobility effect was found in the mice treated with Aegle marmelos. A combination of Aegle marmelos (75 mg/kg, po) with imipramine (5 mg/ kg, po) or fluoxetine (5 mg/kg, po) also produced significant ($P<0.05$) anxiolytic and anti-depressant activity. Anti-depressant activity of Aegle marmelos (150 mg/kg, po) was significantly ($P<0.05$) decreased by prazosin, haloperidol, and baclofen. Methanol extract showed an insignificant ($P>0.05$) effect on the locomotor activity of mice. It is concluded that Aegle marmelos possesses potential anxiolytic and anti-depressant activities and enhances the anxio-lytic and anti-depressant activities of imipramine and fluoxetine.

Anti-fertility Activity

A 50% ethanolic extract of Aegle marmelos leaves was fed orally to male albino rats at dose levels of 200 and 300 mg/kg body wt./day for 60 days. Recovery was assessed for an additional 120 days.[39] Oral administration of Aegle marmelos did not cause a loss of body weight. The motility and sperm concentrations were reduced significantly, along with complete inhibition of fertility at a dose of 300 mg/kg. The level of serum testosterone also declined, and spermatogenesis was impaired. The number of normal tubules and height of epithelial cells of the caput and cauda were reduced significantly. The cross-sectional surface area of Sertoli cells and mature Leydig cells was reduced, along with a dose dependent reduction of preleptotene and pachytene spermatocytes. Thus, the anti-fertility effects of Aegle marmelos seemed to be mediated by disturbances in structure and function in testicular somatic cells including Leydig and Sertoli cells, resulting in an alteration in physio-morphological events of spermatogenesis. Complete recovery, however, was observed after a 120-day withdrawal.

Respiratory Tract Activity

Marmin or 7-(6',7'-dihydroxygeranyl-oxy)couma-rin is a compound isolated from Aegle marmelos. This study examined the effects of marmin on the contraction of guinea pig-isolated trachea stimulated by several inducer—namely, histamine, metacholine, compound 48/80. Also was evaluated its action against contraction induced by extracellular or intracellular calcium ion.[40] The possibility of marmin to potentiate the relaxation effect of isoprenaline also was studied. Marmin added in the organ bath at 10 minutes prior to the agonist-inhibited contractions elicited by histamine and metacholine in a concentration-dependent manner. Moreover, marmin antagonized the hista-mine induced contraction in a competitive manner.

Marmin mildly potentiated the relaxation effect of isoprenaline. In this study, marmin abrogated the contraction of tracheal smooth muscle induced by compound 48/80, an inducer of histamine release. Besides, marmin successfully inhibited CaCl(2)-induced contraction in Ca(2+)-free Krebs solution. Marmin also inhibited two phases of contraction that were consecutively induced by metacholine and CaCl(2) in Ca(2+)-free Krebs solution. Based on the results, the conclusion was that marmin could inhibit contraction of the guinea-pig tracheal smooth muscle, especially by interfering with the histamine receptor, inhibiting the histamine release from mast, inhibiting intracellular Ca(2+) release from the intracellular store and the Ca(2+) influx through voltage-dependent Ca(2+) channels.

Ethnoveterinary Usage

Bael is a highly esteemed herb in veterinary practice. All parts of the Bael tree—its fruit, leaves, roots, stems, and bark—help to cure dehydration and diarrhea in ruminants.[41] Bael also is useful in treating reproductive ailments such as miscarriage, vaginal hemorrhage, and placental retention. Preparations made from Bael have been found to be effective treatments for intestinal lesions, inflammation of the throat, pneumonia, and dysentery.

Dr. Sodhi's Experience

When considering treatment with Bael fruit, the practitioner should ask the following:

- Is there an intestinal infection?
- Are parasites present, or likely to be present?
- Is there diarrhea, dysentery, or colitis?
- Is there diabetes?
- Is there a problem with hearing related to aging and/or Meniere's disease?

Bael fruit is a sweet demulcent that has a specific action against protozoa. It also initiates antimicrobial activity against many bacteria and fungi strains. Bael is useful in treating parasitic infections when a more soothing therapy is needed for the colon than what might be provided by a bitter antiparasitic herb such as Neem (Azadirachta indica). Like Neem, Bael has a hypoglycemic effect. Bael is highly effective in treating colitis and dysentery, and is safe for treating diarrhea and dysentery in children.

I have observed extraordinary results in using Bael to treat cases of Giardia and amoebic dysentery. When frothy diarrhea and urine are present, Bael may be used with Shunthi (Zingiber officinale) and Pippli (Piper longum). In cases of dark yellow stool, inflamed anus, painful nausea, and burning in the stomach, Bael may be used with Neem. I have used Bael fruit, along with curcumin and boswellia serrata extract, to treat ulcerative colitis, Crohn's disease, and other inflammatory bowel diseases. This treatment has had a high success rate for these conditions, and those treated were able to eliminate their standard medical treatment of sulfasalazine, mesalazine, methortexate, mercaptopurine (6MP), and steroids.

Children enjoy Bael fruit because it is sweet. The fruit has a calming effect, so it can be used to treat anxiety. Research also suggests that Bael can be a treatment for age-related deafness and Meniere's disease. Its role in diabetes control merits investigation as well.

In my clinical experience, patients who have not responded to standard conventional treatment for Clostridium difficile responded well to Bael powder. The suggested dose of Bael fruit powder is 3–5 grams three times a day along with probiotics.

Safety Profile

Bael fruit generally is regarded as safe, although feeding large amounts to rats produced hepatic lesions, including vein abnormalities. The maximum tolerated dose of the 50% ethanolic extract of roots was 1000 mg/kg in adult albino mice.

The leaves of the Bael tree are said to cause abortion and sterility in women, so caution should be exercised by pregnant women and by those who may become pregnant. The bark is used in some areas as a fish poison. Like Neem, Bael fruit it is hypoglycemic, so it should not be taken by itself on an empty stomach. Long-term use of extract of Bael leaves at high doses can produce anti-spermatogenic activity.

Dosage

Fruit powder: 2–12 g
Infusion: 12–20 ml
Decoction: 28–56 ml
Fruit extract powder: 5:1 200mg-500 mg three times a day.

Ayurvedic Properties

Rasa: Tikta (bitter), kashaya (astringent)
Guna: Laghu (light), ruksha (dry)
Vipaka: Katu (pungent)
Veerya: Ushna (hot)
Dosha: Pacifies kapha and vata, and promotes pitta

Notes

1. J. Morton, *Bael Fruit*. In *Fruits of Warm Climates*, pp. 187–190. (Julia F. Morton, Miami, FL, 1987).
2. S. Pitre and S. K. Srivastava, "Pharmacological, microbiological and phytochemical studies on roots, Aegle marmelos" *Fitoterapia*, 1987, (3):194.
3. B. Bhavan, "Aegle marmelos," In *Bharatiya Vidya Bhavan Selected Medicinal Plants of India* (Mumbai, India: Chemexcil, 1992).
4. S. D. Srivastava, S. Srivastava, and S. K. Srivastava, "New anthraquinones from heartwood of Aegle marmelos," *Fitoterapia*, 1996, 67:83.
5. N. N. Barthakur and N. P. Arnold, "Central organic and inorganic constituents in bael (Aegle marmelos Correa) fruit," *Tropical Agriculture*, 1996, 66(1):65.
6. Muhammad Shaiq Ali and Muhamad Kashif Pervez, "Marmenol: A 7-geranyloxycoumarin from the leaves of Aegle marmelos corr," *Natural Product Research*, April 2004, 18(2): 141–146.
7. B. R. Sharma and Perveen Sharma, "Constituents of Aegle marmelos II. Alkaloids and Coumarin from fruits," *Plant Medica*, 1981, 43:102–103.
8. S. K. Yadav, A. K. Jain, S. N. Tripathi, and J. P. Gupta, "Irritable bowel syndrome: therapeutic evaluation of indigenous drugs," *Indian Journal of Medical Research*, 1989, 90:496.
9. R. Mazumder, S. Bhattacharya, A. Mazunder, A. K. Pattnaik, P. M. Tiwary, and S. Chaudhary, "Antidiarrhoeal evaluation of Aegle Marmelos (Correa) Linn. root extract," *Phytother Res.*, Jan. 2006, 20(1):82–84.
10. S. Patnaik, V. R. Subramanyam, and C. Kole, "Anti-bacterial and antifungal activity often essential oils in vitro," *Microbios*, 1996, 86(349):237.
11. K. Rusia and S. K. Srivastava, "Antimicrobial activity of some Indian medicinal plants, *Indian Journal of Pharmaceutical Sciences*, 1988, 50(I):57.
12. S. B. Raja, M. R. Murali, N. K. Kumar, and S. N. Devaraj, "Isolation and partial characterisation of a novel lectin from Aegle marmelos fruit and its effect on adherence and invasion of Shigellae to HT29 cells," *PLoS One,* Jan. 21, 2011, 6(1).

13. S. B. Raja, M. R. Murali, K. Roopa, and S. N. Devaraj, "Imperatorin a furocoumarin inhibits periplasmic Cu-Zn SOD of Shigella dysenteriae thereby modulates its resistance towards phagocytosis during host pathogen interaction,"*Biomed Pharmacother.*, Dec. 2, 2010. (Epub Dec 2, 2010)

14. S. Sabde, et al, "Anti-HIV activity of Indian medicinal plants," *J Nat Med.*, July 2011, 65(3–4):662-669. (Epub 2011 Mar. 3).

15. R. D. Sharma, et al, "Possible implication of oxidative stress in antifilarial effect of certain traditionally used medicinal plants in vitro against Brugia malayi microfilariae," *Pharmacognosy Res.*, Nov. 2010, 2(6):350–354.

16. P. V. Seema B. Sudha, P. S. Padayatti, A. Abraham, K. G. Raghu, and C. S. Paulose, "Kinetic studies of purified malate dehydrogenase in liver of streptozotocin-diabetic rats and the effect of leaf extract of Aegle marmelos (L.) Correa ex Roxb.," *Indian Journal of Experimental Biology*, 1996, 34(6):600.

17. A. V. Das, P. S. Padayatti, and C. S. Paulose, "Effect of leaf extract of Aegle marmelos (L.) Correa ex Roxb. on histological and ultrastructural changes in tissues of streptozotocin induced diabetic rats, "*Indian Journal of Experimental Biology*, 1996, 34(4):341.

18. P. T. Ponnachan, C. S. Paulose, and K. R. Panikkar, "Effect of leaf extract of Aegle marmelos in diabetic rats, *Indian Journal of Experimental Biology*, 1993, 31(4):34S.

19. S. Upadhya, K. K. Shanbbag, G. Suneetha, M. Balachandra Naidu, and S. Upadhya, "A study of hypoglycemic and anti-oxidant activity of Aegle marmelos in alloxan induced diabetic rats," *Indian J Physiol Pharmacol.*, Oct. 2004, 48(4):476–480.

20. P. M. Abraham, J. Paul, and C. S. Paulose, "Down regulation of cerebellar serotonergic receptors in streptozotocin induced diabetic rats: Effect of pyridoxine and Aegle marmelose," *Brain Res Bull.* Apr. 2010, 29, 82(1–2):87–94.

21. R. N. Gacche and N. A. Dhole, "Profile of aldose reductase inhibition, anti-cataract and free radical scavenging activity of selected medicinal plants: an attempt to standardize the botanicals for amelioration of diabetes complications," *Food Chem Toxicol.*, Aug. 2011, 49(8):1806–1813.

22. A. K. Sharma, S. Bharti, S. Goyal. S. Arora, S. Nepal, K. Kishore, S. Joshi, S. Kumari, and D. S. Arya, "Upregulation of PPARγ by Aegle marmelos ameliorates insulin resistance and β-cell dysfunction in high fat diet fed-streptozotoc in induced type 2 diabetic rats," *Phytother Res.*, Oct. 25, 2011, 10:1457–1465.

23. G. C. Jagetia, P. Venkatesh, and M. S. Baliga, "Evaluation of the radioprotective effect of Aegle marmelos (L.) Correa in cultured human peripheral blood lymphocytes exposed to different doses of gamma-radiation: a micronucleus study," *Mutagenesis*, July 2003, 18(4):387–393.

24. G. C. Jagetia, P. Venkatesh, and M. S. Baliga, "Evaluation of the radioprotective effect of bael leaf (Aegle marmelos) extract in mice," *Int J Radiat Biol.*, Apr. 2004, 80(4):281–290.

25. A. Agrawal, S. Jahan, D. Soyal, E. Goyal, and P. K. Goyal, "Amelioration of chemical-induced skin carcinogenesis by Aegle marmelos, an Indian medicinal plant, fruit extract," *Integr Cancer Ther.*, Aug. 23, 2011.

26. T. H. Khan and S. Sultana, "Effect of Aegle marmelos on DEN initiated and 2-AAF promoted hepatocarcinogenesis: a chemopreventive study," *Toxicol Mech Methods*," July 2011, 21(6):453–462. (Epub Mar 21, 2011).

27. A. Agrawal, P. Verma, and P. K. Goyal, "Chemomodulatory effects of Aegle marmelos against DMBA-induced skin tumorigenesis in Swiss albino mice," *Asian Pac J Cancer Prev.*, 2010, 11(5):1311–1314.

28. J. Li, F. Mahdi, L. Du, S. Datta, D. G. Naglea, and Y. D Zhou, "Mitochondrial respiration inhibitors suppress protein translation and hypoxic signaling via the hyperphosphorylation and inactivation of translation initiation factor eIF2α and elongation factor eEF2," *J Nat Prod.*, Sept. 23, 2011, 74(9):1894–1901.

29. N. Kakiuchi, L. R. Senaratne, and S.L. Huang, et al., "Effects of constituents of Beli (Aegle marmelos) on spontaneous beating and calcium paradox of myocardial cells," *Planta Medica*, 1991, S7(l):43.

30. P.S. Prince and M. Rajadurai, "Preventive effect of Aegle marmelos leaf extract on isoprenaline-induced myocardial infarction in rats: biochemical evidence," *J Pharm Pharmacol.*, Oct. 2005, 57(10):1353–1357.

31. R. Bhatti, S. Sharma, S. J. Singh, and M. P. Ishar, "Ameliorative effect of Aegle marmelos leaf extract on early stage alloxan-induced diabetic cardiomyopathy in rats," *Pharm Biol.*, Nov. 2011, 49(11):1137–1143.

32. C. Vijaya, M. Ramanathan, and B. Suresh, "Lipid lowering activity of ethanolic extract of leaves of Aegle marmelos (Linn.) in hyperlipidaemic models of Wistar albino rats," *Indian J Exp Biol.*, March 2009, 47(3):182–185.

33. R. K. Goel, R. N. Maiti, M. Manickam, and A. B. Ray, "Antiulcer activity of naturally occurring pyranocoumarin and isocoumarins and their effect on prostanoid synthesis using human colonic mucosa," *Indian Journal of Experimental Biology*, 1997, 35(10):1080.

34. J. M. Benni, M. K. Jayanthi, and R. N. Suresha, "Evaluation of the anti-inflammatory activity of Aegle marmelos (Bilwa) root," *Indian J Pharmacol.*, July 2011, 43(4):393–397.

35. A. E. Nugroho, S. Riyanto, M. A. Sukari, and K. Maeyama K., "Effects of aegeline, a main alkaloid of Aegle Marmelos Correa leaves, on the histamine release from mast cells," *Pak J Pharm Sci.*, July 2011, 24(3):359–367.

36. A. M. Abeysekera, K. T. D. De Silva, S. Samarsinghe, P. A. K. Seneviratne, A. J. J. Van Den Berg, and R. P. Labadie. "An immunomodulatory C-glucosylated propelargonidin from the unripe fruit of Aegle marmelos," *Fitoterapia* 67(4):367.

37. R. Agarwal, S. K. Gupta, S. Srivastava, R. Saxena, and S. S. Agrawal, "Intraocular pressure-lowering activity of topical application of Aegle marmelos fruit extract in experimental animal models," *Ophthalmic Res.*, 2009, 42(2):112–116.

38. S. Kothari, M. Minda, and S. D. Tonpay, "Anxiolytic and anti-depressant activities of methanol extract of Aegle marmelos leaves in mice," *Indian J Physiol Pharmacol*, Oct.–Dec., 2010, 54(4):318–328.

39. A. Chauhan and M. Agarwal, "Reversible changes in the antifertility induced by Aegle marmelos in male albino rats," *Syst Biol Reprod Med.*, Nov.–Dec. 2008, 54(6):240–246.

40. A. E. Nugroho, Y. Anas Y. P. N. Arsito, J. T. Wibowo, S. Riyanto, and M. A. Sukari, "Effects of marmin, a compound isolated from Aegle marmelos Correa, on contraction of the guinea pig-isolated trachea. *Pak J Pharm Sci.,* Oct. 2011, 24(4):427–433.

41. International Institute of Rural Reconstruction, "Ethnoveterinary medicine in Asia. An information kit on traditional animal health care practices, Part I, General Information" (Silang, Philippines: IIRR, 1994).

ANDROGRAPHIS PANICULATA

INTRODUCTION

Andrographis paniculata is a shrub found throughout India and other Asian countries. It has been called Indian Echinacea because of its high value in providing immune support. Historically, Andrographis has been used to address epidemics in the Indian subcontinent.

In China, India, and other countries of subtropical and Southeast Asia, Andrographis is used for medicinal purposes. The fresh and dried leaves, as well as the fresh juice of the whole plant, have been included in a variety of medical traditions. In Chinese herbalism, Andrographis supports healthy digestive, cardiovascular, and urinary systems. In Sweden, Andrographis is used as a primary herb during the winter season for its immune support.

Andrographis is a member of the plant family Acanthaceae. A prominent herb in Ayurvedic tradition, it is included in at least 26 Ayurvedic formulas. Andrographis is a significant "cold property" herb—to rid the body of heat (as in fevers) and to dispel toxins from the body. Research has confirmed that Andrographis, if properly administered, has a surprisingly broad range of pharmacological effects, some of which are extremely beneficial.

SYNONYMOUS NAMES

Andrographis is known in northeastern India as Maha-tita, which means "king of bitters." It also is called Bhui-neem because the plant, though much smaller in size than Neem, is similar in appearance and has a bitter taste like Neem. Because of its bitterness, it is known in Malaysia as Hempedu Bumi, which means "bile of earth." In Tamil it is called Sirunangai or Siriyanangai.

Other names include:
Sanskrit: Kalmegha, Bhunimba
Hindi: Kirayat
English: The Creat
Chinese: Chuan Xin Lian

HABITAT

Andrographis is found throughout tropical Asian countries, often in isolated patches, in a variety of habitats including plains, hill slopes, wastelands, farms, dry or wet lands, seashores, and even roadsides. Native populations of Andrographis are spread throughout south India and Sri Lanka, which likely represent the center of origin and diversity of the species. The herb also grows in northern India, Java, Malaysia, Indonesia, West Indies, and elsewhere in the Americas (where it probably was introduced as a non-native species). In addition, the species is found in Hong Kong, Penang, Malacca, Pangkor Island, Malaya, Thailand, West Java, Borneo, Celebes, Brunei, West Indies, Jamaica, Barbados, and the Bahamas.[1]

Andrographis is cultivated quite easily because it grows in all types of soil. Moreover, it grows in soil types where almost no other plant can be cultivated, most notably in "serpentine soil," which is relatively high in aluminum, copper and zinc. This hardiness helps to account for its wide distribution.

Unlike other species of its genus, Andrographis is common in most parts of India, including the plains and hilly areas up to 500 meters, which accounts for its wide use. Ever since ancient times, villages and ethnic communities in India have been using this herb to treat a variety of ailments.

Botanical Characteristics

Andrographis paniculata, an annual plant, is branched and erect, growing to an average height of 1/2 to 1 meter. The aerial parts of the plant—leaves and stems—are the source of the active phytochemicals used in treatment. Usually found in moist, shady areas, Andrographis has glabrous leaves and white flowers with rose-purple spots on the petals. The stem is dark green in color and quadrangular with longitudinal furrows and wings on the angles of the younger parts. The leaves are glabrous, lanceolate, and pinnate, measuring approximately 8 cm long and 2.5 cm wide. Andrographis flowers are small, with spreading axillary and terminal racemes or panicles. The capsules are linear-oblong and acute at both ends, measuring 1.9 cm x 0.3 cm. Its seeds are numerous, subquadrate, and yellowish brown.

Chemical Composition

Andrographis leaves contain the highest concentrations of andrographolide (2.39%), the most medicinally active phytochemical in the plant, and the seeds contain the lowest concentration.[2] Other medicinal chemicals present in the herb are also bitter principles— diterpenoids, deoxyandrographolide, -19ß-D-glucoside, and neo-andrographolide—all of which have been isolated from the leaves.[3]

The primary medicinal component of Andrographis is andrographolide. This substance has a bitter taste, is colorless crystalline in appearance, and is called a "diterpene lactone"—a chemical name that describes its ringlike structure. Besides the related bitters cited above, active components of Andrographis include 14-deoxy-11,12- didehydroandrographolide (andrographlide D), homoandrographolide, andrographan, andrographon, andrographosterin, and stigmasterol—the last of which was isolated from an Andrographis preparation.[4]

The active constituents of Andrographis usually are extracted using ethanol, and liquid extracts or tinctures are the most common method of dispensing the product. When consumed, andrographolides appear to accumulate in organs throughout the viscera. In one study, 48 hours after ingestion of the herb, the concentration of labeled andrographolide consisted of: 20.9%, brain; 14.9%, spleen; 11.1%, heart; 10.9%, lung; 8.6%, rectum; 7.9%, kidney; 5.6%, liver; 5.1%, uterus; 5.1%, ovary; and 3.2%, intestine.[5] Andrographolides are excreted fairly rapidly from the body via the urine and the gastrointestinal tract.

The wide tissue and organ distribution and the immune-stimulating and regulatory actions of Andrographis make it ideal in the prevention and treatment of many diseases and conditions.[6]

Pharmacological Activity

Anti-carcinogenic Activity

The anti-cancer potential of Andrographis paniculata has been studied in number of cell line and animal studies, including the following.[7,8,9,10] 20 patients with stage IV, end-stage cancer, one bladder, five breast, two prostate, one neuroblastoma, two non-small-cell lung, three colon, one mesothelioma, two lymphoma, one ovarian, one gastric, and one osteosarcoma.

Treated with: Transfer Factor Plus, 3 tablets 3 times per day, IMU Plus (non-denatured milk whey protein, 40 gm/day); intravenous (50–100 gm/day) and oral (1–2 gm/day) ascorbic acid; Agaricus Blazeii Murill teas (10 gm/day); immune modulator mix (a combination of vitamins, minerals, anti-oxidants, and immune-enhancing natural products); nitrogenated soy extract (high levels of genistein and dadzein) and Andrographis paniculata (500 mg twice daily).

Baseline NK function assay and TNF alpha and receptor levels were measured by ELISA from resting and phytohemagglutinin (PHA)-stimulated adherent and non-adherent peripheral blood mononuclear cell (PBMC). Total mercaptans and glutathione in plasma were taken and were compared to the levels measured 6 months later. Complete blood counts and chemistry panels were monitored routinely.

After 6 months, 16 of the 20 patients were still alive. The 16 survivors had significantly higher NK function than baseline ($p < .01$ for each) and TNF alpha levels in all four cell populations studied ($p < .01$ for each). Total mercaptans ($p < .01$) and TNF alpha receptor levels were reduced significantly ($p < .01$). Also, hemoglobin, hematocrit, and glutathione levels were elevated significantly. The only toxicity noted was occasional diarrhea and nausea. The quality of life improved for all survivors by SF-36 form evaluation. The combination of immunoactive nutraceuticals was effective in significantly increasing NK function, other immune parameters, and hemoglobin from peripheral blood mononuclear cells in patients with late-stage cancers.[11]

Andrographis paniculata extract along with whole-body hyperthermia was found to enhance the total white blood count in cyclophosphamide (CTX)- and radiation-treated animals compared to untreated control animals. Regression in solid tumor development was observed when cyclophosphamide- and radiation-exposed animals were treated with the extract in combination with whole-body hyperthermia. Myeloperoxidase activity in tumor tissue from cyclophosphamide and radiation-treated animals was also inhibited significantly when they were administered with Andrographis paniculata extract along with whole body hyperthermia. Production of cytokines such as IL-2, GM-CSF and tumor necrosis factor (TNF-alpha), which was reduced after combined CTX and radiation treatment, was increased significantly by the simultaneous treatment of extract and whole body hyperthermia.[12] This makes Andrographis an excellent choice as an adjuvant for patients who are going through chemotherapy and radiation treatments.

Studies using mice have shown that Andrographis stimulates the immune system in two crucial ways. First, it produces an antigen-specific response, stimulating the production of antibodies that counteract invading microbes. Second, Andrographis triggers a nonspecific immune response in which macrophage cells scavenge and destroy invaders. Because of these actions, Andrographis is effective against a variety of infectious and oncogenic (cancer-causing) agents.[13]

In the quest to combat the spread of cancerous cells, researchers are searching for substances that can cause cancer cells to mature more rapidly. In one study using mice, researchers searched for naturally occurring substances that would cause differentiation of leukemia cells. Andrographis was chosen because it contained terpenes that are known to cause such differentiation. This study demonstrated that Andrographis exerted potent cell differentiation-inducing activity on leukemia cells.[14] In addition to causing cancer cell maturity or differentiation, extracts from the leaves of the plant are cytotoxic (cell-killing) against some cancer cells. This cancer cell-killing ability was demonstrated against human epidermoid carcinoma (squamous cell carcinoma) of the skin lining of the nasopharynx and against lymphocytic leukemia cells. The study found that Andrapholide has a cancer cell killing ability superior to the levels of effectiveness recommended by the National Cancer Institute for a cytotoxic substance.[15]

Anti-viral Activity

Exciting research has indicated that Andrapholide extracts may have great promise for interfering with the viability of the HIV virus. Researchers have theorized that Andrographis extracts may disrupt the HIV virus' "signal transduction," in which the virus subverts the messaging capacities of normal cells, tricking them into producing more viral particles.[16] Using signal transduction technology (methods that investigate cell messaging systems), scientists found that Andrographis contains substances that destroy the communications mechanism of HIV. Andrographolide prevented transmission of the virus to other cells and stopped the progress of the disease by modifying cellular signal transduction. It was theorized that Andrographolide probably does this by inhibiting enzymes that facilitate the transfer of phosphates that act as the energy storehouses of the cell. During the cell cycle, phosphates are created or chemically changed and energy is produced. This energy is used in regulating the cell cycle and for the many cellular functions during reproduction of the cell. Andrographolide, thus, may interfere with key enzymes that result in viral reproduction.

Testing of Andrographolide demonstrated that extracts increased the ability of the HIV drug AZT to inhibit replication of HIV. The effect of the combination was greater than that of either compound alone. An added benefit is that lower doses of AZT could be used. Some researchers believe that Andrographolide extracts may be useful in combating other viruses, including the Ebola virus and the viruses associated with herpes, hepatitis, and influenza.

In a study examining 27 types of "heat clearing" and detoxifying medicinal herbs, researchers at the China Academy of Traditional Chinese Medicine in Beijing reported that Andrographis was one of the herbs that had an inhibitory effect on HIV replication.[17] Leukemia cells in particular have been shown to be highly sensitive to the effects of Andrographolide.[18]

Action Against Common Cold

A randomized, double-blind, placebo-controlled clinical study was conducted to evaluate the efficacy of an extract of Andrographis paniculata in patients with uncomplicated upper respiratory tract infection (URTI).[19] The assessment involved quantification of symptom scores by Visual Analogue Scale. Nine self-evaluated symptoms of cough, expectoration, nasal discharge, headache, fever, sore throat, earache, malaise/fatigue, and sleep disturbance were scored. A total of 223 patients of both sexes were randomized in two groups that received either extract of Andrographis paniculata (200 mg/day) or placebo in a double-blind manner.

In both the treatments, mean scores of all symptoms showed a decreasing trend from day 1 to day 3, but from day 3 to day 5, most of the symptoms in the placebo-treated group either remained unchanged (cough, headache, and earache) or were aggravated (sore throat and sleep disturbance), whereas in the extract of Andrographis paniculata-treated group all symptoms showed a decreasing trend. Within groups, mean scores of symptoms in both groups decreased significantly ($p <$ or $= 0.05$) from day 1 to day 3 and day 5, while from day 3 to day 5 all symptoms except expectoration in the placebo group did not improve significantly, whereas in the extract of Andrographis paniculata-treated group all symptoms except earache improved significantly (p < or = 0.05).

Comparing the mean between both groups, all symptoms at day 1 and day 3 were found to be the same, while at day 5 all symptoms except earache in the extract of Andrographis paniculata-treated group improved significantly (p < or = 0.05) over the placebo group. Similarly, within groups, overall scores of all symptoms in both groups decreased significantly (p < or = 0.05) from day 1 to day 3 and day 5, while from day 3 to day 5, the placebo group did not improve significantly, whereas the extract of Andrographis paniculata-treated group showed significant improvement (p < or = 0.05). In the between-groups analysis, the extract of Andrographis paniculata group showed significant reduction (p < or = 0.05) in overall symptom scores compared to the placebo group. Both the placebo and the extract of Andrographis paniculata-treated group had only a few minor adverse effects with no significant difference in occurrence (Z = 0.63; p > 0.05).[20]

The comparison of overall efficacy of the extract of Andrographis paniculata over the placebo was found to be significant (p < or = 0.05), and it was 2.1 times (52.7%) higher than the placebo. The findings of this study revealed that extract of Andrographis paniculata was effective in reducing symptoms of upper respiratory tract infection.[21]

The common cold was prevented with an extract of Andrographis in a pilot double-blind study. Students were given Kan Jang, a formulation including Andrographis, and were diagnosed for the presence or absence of colds during a 3-month period.[22] The study group received a dose of 200 mg/day. After one month there was no significant difference in the number of colds; however, after the third month of intake, the incidence of colds had decreased significantly compared to the placebo group. The students who took Andrographis had a rate of incidence of colds of 30% compared to 62% for the students who received the placebo. The relative risk of catching a cold indicated that the preventive effect could be a consequence of the presence of Andrographolide, which has proven immunostimulant effects.

The amount of Andrographis used in the above study was much less than that used in a prior study that produced even quicker results. In that study, patients were divided into two groups, one of which received 1200 mg/day of the herb. These patients already had colds with symptoms including nasal discharge, nasal stuffiness, sore throat, earache, cough, fever, headache, and malaise. At the beginning of the study, the patients receiving supplements and those receiving a placebo had similar symptoms. The symptoms, including tiredness, shivering, sore throat, and muscular aches, diminished significantly on the fourth day of treatment. The researchers concluded that treatment with 4% andrographolides accelerated recuperation of patients from the common cold.

Fever-reducing Activity

Andrographis also serves as a folk medicine remedy for fever, pain reduction, and intestinal disorders. Its ability to lower fever has been demonstrated independently in several laboratory studies. Studies of rats done in China showed that andrographolide, neoandrographolide, and dihydroandrographolide can lower the fever produced by different fever inducing agents, such as bacterial endotoxins (toxic chemicals released from bacteria), pneumococcus, hemolytic streptococcus, typhoid, paratyphoid, and the chemical 2,4-dinitrophenol.[23]

Researchers tested Andrographis to determine whether it did, in fact, work in these conditions.[24] Fever was induced in rats. Rectal body temperature was reduced for 30, 100, and 300 mg. of andrographolide/kg body weight. Although the analgesic (pain-killing) activity of andrographolide was weak compared to aspirin, the anti-pyretic (fever-reducing) activity was comparable to that of aspirin.

The study found that 300 mg/kg body weight of andrographolide was as effective as the same amount of aspirin. In fact, the extract was found to possess anti-ulcerogenic activity. It reduced the development of ulcers by 31%, while the standard ulcer drug, cimetidine, had an 85.43% reduction rate. Andrographolide caused a significant decrease in total stomach acidity and acid stomach juice secretion, without the cost and side effects associated with other ulcer therapies.[25]

In another study, Andrographis extracts produced results comparable to 200 mg of aspirin/kg. body weight.[26] The researchers also established a wide margin of safety in using the extracts, an indication of the lack of toxicity of the substance.

The anti-inflammatory effects of Andrographis compounds have been shown in many studies in which inflammation was produced by chemicals. Inflammation caused by histamine, dimethyl benzene, croton oil (hemolytic necrosis), and acute pneumocystis produced by adrenaline was significantly reduced or relieved.[27] This effect was observed for all major andrographolides: deoxyandrographolide, andrographolide, neoandrographolide, and dehydroandrographolide. Dehydroandrographolide had the most pronounced effect, followed by neoandrographolide and andrographolide. The mechanism seemed to involve the adrenal glands,. as the effect disappeared when the adrenal glands were removed from the experimental animals.[28]

A study was performed to evaluate the antinociceptive and anti-edematogenic properties of andrographolide isolated from the leaves of Andrographis paniculata using two animal models.[29] The antinociceptive activity was evaluated using the acetic acid-induced writhing and the hot-plate tests. Antiedematogenic activity was measured using the carrageenan-induced paw edema test. Subcutaneous (s.c.) administration of andrographolide (10, 25, and 50 mg/kg) did not affect the motor coordination of the experimental animals but produced significant ($p < .05$) antinociceptive activity when assessed using both tests. But 2 mg/kg naloxone failed to affect the 25 mg/kg andrographolide activity in both tests, indicating that the activity was modulated via nonopioid mechanisms. Further, andrographolide showed significant ($p < .05$) anti-edematogenic activity. In conclusion, the results suggest that andrographolide has antinociceptive and antiedematogenic activities; it may be useful for treating pain and inflammation after human studies are conducted.

Anti-malarial Potential

The anti-malarial potential of Andrographis and its components are of particular interest now because the associated bacteria are showing resistance to drugs. Although Andrographis and other herbs are not substitutes for antibiotics, these and other herbs could have a complementary effect when used along with antibiotics.

Malaria is still a prevalent disease in many tropical and subtropical countries, difficult to eradicate because the parasites that carry malaria become resistant to the drugs used. Extracts of Andrographis were evaluated against Plasmodium berghei, one of the parasites that transmit malaria. The extract was found to disrupt the multiplication of the parasites considerably.[30]

Two Andrographis components, neoandrographolide and deoxandrographolide, were found to be the most effective of the four. Pre-treating animals with neoandrographolide for 15 to 21 days prior to exposure, as well as after malarial infection, was found to be more effective than treatment that was started only after infection. The effects were better than treatment after infection with chloroquine, a commonly used anti-malarial drug. The researchers repeated the effects of Andrographis and reported that the protective action may be a result of reactivation of superoxide dismutase, a key anti-oxidant enzyme that protects the liver.

Anti-diarrheal Activity

Diarrhea-type diseases constitute one of the top 10 causes of death worldwide and a leading cause of death in children in developing countries, especially those under 5 years of age. The use of antibiotics is resulting in antibiotic-resistant strains of bacteria. Although many drugs are used to relieve the symptoms of diarrhea (kaolin-pectin, bismuth, Lomotil, loperamide hydrochloride, and others), a number of these have undesirable side-effects. Experiments on animals demonstrate that Andrographis can prevent or stop diarrhea. This inexpensive and easily obtained herbal remedy could benefit many, especially people in developing countries where diarrheal disease is almost catastrophic.

Andrographis extracts have had significant effects against the diarrhea associated with E. coli bacterial infections.[31] The herb's components, andrographolide and neoandrographolide, showed activity similar to that of loperamide (Imodium), the most common anti-diarrheal drug.

Acute bacterial diarrhea in patients was treated with a total dose of 500 mg andrographolide divided over three dosing periods per day for 6 days (2.5 to 3.0 mg/kg of body weight). This regimen was combined with rehydration. Of the 80 patients treated, 66 were cured—an 82.5% cure rate. Seven additional patients responded favorably to the treatment, and only seven patients (8.8%) did not respond. Effectiveness of the treatment was confirmed by laboratory tests of stool samples.[32] In another study, Andrographis was used to treat 1,611 cases of bacterial dysentery and 955 cases of diarrhea, with an overall effectiveness of 91.3%.[33]

In additional research, chronic inflammation of the colon was treated with a combination of Andrographis (60 g) and Rehmannia glutinosa (30 g), decocted. Rehmannia is a Chinese herb used to treat anemia and fatigue, and to promote the healing of injured bones. It also is a demulcent. The liquid part of the mixture was used as an enema at doses of 100 to 150 ml each night for 14 days. Of the total of 85 patients, 61 (72%) were considered clinically cured and 22 (26%) had symptomatic relief.[34]

Cardioprotective Activity

Andrographis has clot-dissolving properties compared to drugs used in the treatment of heart attacks. Andrographis may prevent some of the heart attacks or strokes that occur within one month of angioplasty. The process of blood clotting in the body is not yet fully understood. It is a delicate balance between the clotting necessary to achieve healing and the processes that could cause abnormal and unwanted clotting.

Andrographis extracts have been demonstrated to increase the time it takes for blood clots to form, thereby decreasing the risk of blood vessels closing (restenosis) after angioplasty procedures. In studies with rabbits receiving angioplasty, the herbal extract significantly prevented constriction of blood vessels. The rabbits received treatment for 3 days before angioplasty and for 4 weeks after surgery. Arterial narrowing occurred in 100% of animals not receiving Andrographis, but only 70% of those receiving Andrographis showed narrowing.[35] Narrowing caused by injury to the inner lining of the blood vessel and by high cholesterol in the diet also was found to be decreased by Andrographis. Thus, the herb may be effective in preventing repeated narrowing of vessels after coronary angioplasty.

80% to 90% of patients with destroyed heart muscle resulting from an acute myocardial infarction (heart attack), clots are found in the heart shortly after the beginning of symptoms. When heart muscle is deprived of its blood supply, and therefore of oxygen, the tissue dies. Physicians and researchers believe that the best treatment for this condition is to limit the size of the myocardial infarction to preserve the pump function of the heart. Agents that dissolve the clots and increase blood flow through the blocked artery are being sought constantly. Andrographis may prove to be an important part of the treatment plan in such cases.

Researchers at the Tongji Medical University in China demonstrated that Andrographis given to dogs one hour after development of myocardial infarction had less damage to the heart muscle.[36] In subsequent studies at the same university, researchers demonstrated by electrocardiograph that abnormal changes in heart readings were prevented by pre-treatment with angioplasty. Also, clumping of platelets (the blood particles that initiate clotting) was inhibited, and no clot (thrombus) that could cause infarction was induced.[37] An added effect of Andrographis was that it activated fibrinolysis, the natural process in the body that dissolves clots.[38]

Correcting high blood pressure is integral in preventing cardiovascular disease. Researchers have reported that an extract of Andrographis produced antihypertensive (blood pressure-lowering) effects.[39] The extract was given intravenously to hypertensive rats. Noradrenaline, a hormone secreted by the brain, acts to constrict blood vessels and increase heart rate, blood pressure, and blood sugar levels. Andrographis extract inhibited the increase in blood pressure that is caused by noradrenaline.

Researchers believe that the antihypertensive action of Andrographis relaxes the smooth muscle in the walls of blood vessels. This relaxation prevents the blood vessel from constricting and limiting blood flow to the heart, brain, and other body organs. The herbal therapy keeps blood, and therefore oxygen, flowing to the brain. Diminished blood flow to the brain can cause short-term memory loss, ringing in the ears, dizziness, headaches, depression, and impaired mental performance.

The effects of Andrographis are produced without toxicity and at a reasonable cost, making this herb a good option for cardiovascular therapy.

Anti-inflammatory Activity

The anti-inflammatory action of dehydroandrographolide increases synthesis and release of adrenocorticotrophic hormone (ACTH) of the pituitary gland of the brain. ACTH signals the adrenal gland to make cortisol, a natural anti-inflammatory.[40] In research done on the anti-inflammatory activity of naturally occurring products, Andrographis was found to inhibit edema (swelling resulting from fluid trapped in tissues). At a concentration of 200 mg/kg body weight, the extract significantly inhibited (by 60%) edema at 3 hours after administration. At 400 mg/kg body weight, 62.7% was inhibited.[41]

Persistent activation of nuclear factor NF kappa-B has been associated with the development of asthma. In one study, Andrographolide, the principal active component of the medicinal plant Andrographis paniculata, inhibited NF kappa-B activity.[42] Broncho-alveolar lavage fluid was assessed for total and differential cell counts as well as cytokine and chemokine levels. Serum IgE levels also were determined. Lung tissues were examined for cell infiltration and mucous hypersecretions and the expression of inflammatory biomarkers. Airway hyper-responsiveness was monitored by direct airway resistance analysis. Andrographolide dose dependently inhibited OVA-induced increases in total cell count, eosinophil count, and IL-4, IL-5, and IL-13 levels recovered in bronchoalveolar lavage fluid and reduced serum level of OVA-specific IgE. It attenuated OVA-induced lung tissue eosinophilia and airway mucous production, mRNA expression of E-selectin, chitinases, Muc5ac, and inducible nitric oxide synthase in lung tissues, and airway hyper-responsiveness to methacholine. In normal human bronchial epithelial cells, andrographolide blocked tumor necrosis factor-induced phosphorylation of inhibitory B kinase-β, and downstream inhibitory B degradation, p65 subunit of NF-kappa-B phosphorylation, and p65 nuclear translocation and DNA-binding activity. Similarly, andrographolide blocked p65 nuclear translocation and DNA-binding activity in the nuclear extracts from lung tissues of OVA-challenged mice.

Fertility Activity

Andrographis has confirmed anti-fertility as well as pregnancy-terminating effects. In India, where AP is used for common ailments such as diarrhea, fever, and other digestive disorders, the herb is recommended for only short-term treatment. This contraindication is attributable to the contraceptive nature of its chemical constitution. To determine the actual effects on fertility, studies were done in male rats. One study found that AP, given as dry leaf powder (105 mg. of powder/kg body weight) each day for 60 days, stopped spermatogenesis (development and maturation of sperm cells).[43] The author's observations suggested an anti-spermatogenic (sperm-production blocking) or anti-androgenic (blocking effects of androgens) ability of the plant. It should be noted that many herbal extracts have effects on reproductive functions and thus should not be used during pregnancy.

Additional studies in India reported anti-fertility effects on female mice.[44] When 2 grams per kilogram body weight of sun-dried Andrographis root powder were given to the animals every day for 6 weeks, none of the animals was pregnant after mating (five times) with proven fertile males that did not receive the treatment. The mice that did not receive the Andrographis had normal litters when bred with similar males. The researchers posit that Andrographis may act against fertility by preventing ovulation.

In studies of cultured human placental tissue, andrographolide sodium succinate was effective in inhibiting human progesterone production.[45] This hormone is necessary for a successful pregnancy. The form of Andrographis used was tissue specific—meaning that it affected only the tissue for which it was intended. It had no detrimental effects on other normal human tissue, even at the highest doses tested. The researchers concluded that the derivatives appeared to be promising as contraceptives.

Hepatoprotective Activity

In Ayurvedic medicine, 26 different formulations containing Andrographis have been used to treat liver disorders. The plant's four medicinal compounds were tested for a protective effect against liver toxicity produced in mice by giving them carbon tetrachloride (a cleaning solvent), alcohol, or other toxic chemicals.[46] These chemicals damage the liver by causing lipid peroxidation, a process in which free radicals produced by the chemical attack and destroy membranes surrounding liver cells. When Andrographis was given to animals 3 days in advance of the toxic chemicals, there was a significant protective effect in the liver. This effect was attributed to the anti-oxidant ability of Andrographis compounds.

In another study, Andrographolide produced a significant increase in bile flow.[47] Bile is produced in the liver and stored in the gallbladder and aids in digestion. When the chemical paracetamol was given to animals pre-treated with Andrographolide, the usual decrease in bile production seen with this chemical was prevented. In this case, andrographolide was more potent than silymarin.

Andrographolides are potent stimulators of gallbladder function. In animal experiments, those that received Andrographolides for 7 consecutive days showed an increase in bile flow, bile salts, and bile acids. These increases are beneficial and result in enhanced gallbladder function. Use of Andrographis, therefore, might decrease gallstone formation and also might aid in fat digestion. Andrographolides also prevented decreases in the amount of bile caused by acetaminophen toxicity.[48]

In an Indian study, 20 cases of infective hepatitis (hepatitis A) in men and women were treated with a decoction of Andrographolide equivalent to 40 g of the crude compound for more than 24 days. In all 20 patients, yellowing of the conjunctiva of the eye and of the urine returned to normal coloration. Of these patients, 90% regained their appetite and 83% had relief from general depression. Overall, 80% of the patients were considered cured and 20% were improved, based on biochemical tests and changes in symptoms.[49]

Central Nervous System Activity

Many compounds do not penetrate the blood–brain barrier. Andrographolide, however, does so and concentrates in the brain and particularly in the spinal cord.[50] Several studies have shown that AP products have a sedative effect. In mice given barbital as anesthesia, the animals became sedated more quickly and the anesthesia lasted longer. Also, less of the anesthesia was necessary if it was given along with Andrographis.[51] The studies indicate that these herbal products may act at the barbital receptors in the brain.

Respiratory Activity

Andrographolide has been used to treat tonsillitis, respiratory infections, and tuberculosis. In one study, the substance was used to treat 129 cases of acute tonsillitis. Of these patients, 65% responded to the therapy.[52] The same researchers used Andrographolide to treat 49 pneumonia patients, 35 of whom showed positive changes and 9 recovered completely.

Andrographolide was used to treat 111 patients with pneumonia and 20 with chronic bronchitis and lung infection. The overall effectiveness of treatment was 91%. Fever subsided within 3 days in 72% of the patients, and 40% of the patients had smaller areas of infection within one week.[53]

Tuberculosis usually is treated with the antibiotic Rifampin (Rifadin). When used alone, Rifampin therapy still results in 22.5% of patients' dying. In a study using an injectable solution of 2.5% andrographolide given to provide 50 to 80 mg/kg body weight per day for 2 months, the results were improved. Of 70 cases of tubercular meningitis, 30% of the patients were considered cured and the fatality rate was 8.6%.[54] The combination of Andrographolide plus rifampin resulted in a 2.6-fold decrease in fatality rates.

Additional Pharmacological Activity

Leptospirosis is a disease caused by the bacterium Leptospira interrogans. Infection with this organism results in fever, hemorrhagic lesions, central nervous system dysfunction, and jaundice. Several studies have reported efficacy in approximately 80% of patients treated with deoxyandrographolide, andrographolide, and neoandrographolide tablets.[55]

Acute pyelonephritis is an inflammation of the kidney caused by a local bacterial infection. In a study evaluating the effectiveness of Andrographolide in treating this disease, the herb was compared to nitrofurantoin, a standard clinical drug for pyelonephritis therapy. Andrographilide was found to be as effective as the standard drug, but with fewer side effects.[56]

Chorioepithelioma is a highly malignant tumor derived from the placenta. Hemorrhagic metastases develop relatively early in the course of the illness and frequently are found in the lungs, liver, brain, vagina, and various other pelvic organs. Andrographolide had a unique effect on these conditions. In one study, 60 patients with these conditions were treated with Andrographis and derived compounds. Of these patients, 41 had confirmed metastasis (spread of the cancer) of the lesions. Of the 41 patients, 12 patients treated with Andrographis alone recovered, and 4 women subsequently became pregnant (this condition usually results in difficulty in trying to get pregnant). Of the patients treated with other drugs in addition to herbal therapy, 47 did not experience a regrowth of the tumor during the time of the study.[57]

In a case study of a patient with an anal tumor, the results were reported as "satisfactory" when the tumor was treated with a decoction of Andrographis. In this therapy, a 500 ml decoction was prepared from 100 g of AP and 1000 ml water, filtering out residue and mixing the liquid with 10 ml of vinegar. When the temperature of the liquid below 40 degrees C., the anal tumor was treated in a sitz bath for 15 minutes twice daily.[58]

Additional diseases reported to be treated effectively with herbal combinations that include Andrographis are: Japanese B encephalitis, cervical erosion, pelvic infection,[59] otitis media purulence, cutaneous gangrene in infants,[60] vaginitis,[61] leprosy,[62] herpes,[63] chicken pox and mumps,[64] neurodermatitis, eczema, and burns.[65] When cobra venom was given to mice, Andrographis prolonged survival time and postponed the occurrence of respiratory failure caused by the venom.[66]

Dr. Sodhi's Experience

I have used Andrographis paniculata to treat liver diseases with much success. This herb in combination with other liver herbs has shown phenomenal liver regeneration. Hepatitis A, B, and C patients have shown remarkable recovery. In hepatitis A, symptoms often start to improve within one week. A combination of Andrographis with Tephrosia purpurea, Phyllanthus amarus, Swertia chirayita, calotropis Giganttea, Raphanus sativa, Beberis aristata, Terminalia arjuna, Belleric myrobalan, Terminalia chebula, Emblica officinalis, Solanum nignum, and Apple juice concentrate have prevented people from contracting hepatitis A. More than 3,000 patients who have traveled to Southeast Asia have not returned with hepatitis A and were treated with the above combination. I have used this treatment in lieu of vaccinations for my own travels to India and Thailand..

My 17-year-old niece visiting United States from India was diagnosed with hepatitis A. In less than a week after using combination of Andrographis with Tephrosia purpurea, Phyllanthus amarus, Swertia chirayita, calotropis Giganttea, Raphanus sativa, Beberis aristata, Terminalia arjuna, Belleric myrobalan, Terminalia chebula, Emblica officinalis, Solanum nignum, and Apple juice concentrate, her liver enzymes normalized. With other patients undergoing this regimen, hepatitis B has become negative, and the viral load of hepatitis C patients was kept below 300,000. I use this protocol with chronic inflammatory diseases such as RA, SLE, and fibromyalgia. I also have used Andrographis with a combination of other liver herbs for cancer patients.

Safety Profile

Rarely, people who use Andrographis experience dizziness and heart palpitations. As in the case with all herbal treatments, some individuals have an allergic reaction to Andrographis. Also, it has caused nausea if taken in larger doses. It is contraindicated in pregnancy as it has shown anti-fertility effects.

LD50 for ethanolic extract was 215 mg/kg when given orally, and 20 g/kg of raw herb when given orally.[67, 68] Overall, evidence to date indicates that andrographolides are naturally occurring compounds with low toxicity when used appropriately.

Dosage

Infusion or decoction: 20–40 ml tid juice of leaves and stem: 1-4 ml
Dried powder of whole plant:
Extract : 200 mg 2–3 times per day.

Ayurvedic Properties

Rasa: Tikta (bitter)
Guna: Laghu (light), ruksha (dry) Vipaka: Katu (pungent)
Veerya: Ushna (hot)
Dosha: Pacifies kapha and pitta

Notes

1. F. Sandberg, *Andrographidis herba Chuanxinlian: A review* (Gothenburg, Sweden: Swedish Herbal Institute, 1994). (Available in U.S. from the American Botanical Council)
2. A Sharma, L. Krishan, and S. S. Handa, "Standardization of the Indian crude drug Kalmegh by high pressure liquid chromatographic determination of andrographolide," *Phytochemical Analysis*, 1992, 3:129–131.
3. C. Weiming and L. Xiaotion, "Deoxyandrographolide 19ß-D-glucoside from the leaves of A. paniculata," *Planta Medica*, 1982, 15:245–246.
4. P. Siripong, B. Kongkathip, K. Preechanukool, P. Picha, K. Tunsuwan, and W. C. Taylor, "Cytotoxic diterpenoid constituents from *Andrographis paniculata*, Nees leaves," *J. Sci. Soc. Thailand*, 1992. 18(4):187–194.
5. Z. Y. Zheng, "Pharmacokinetic studies on 3H-andrographolide," *Chinese Herbal Med.*, 1982. 13(9):33–36.
6. M. S. Jean Barilla, "Andrographis paniculata: Can herbs fight common ailments, cancer, and chronic viral infections?" *A Keats Good Health Guide*, Keats Pub; illustrated edition (June 1999) pp17–20.
7. S. Yang, A. M. Evens, S. Prachand, A. T. Singh, S. Bhalla, K, David, and L.I Gordon, "Mitochondrial-mediated apoptosis in lymphoma cells by the diterpenoid lactone Andrographolide, the active component of Andrographis paniculata.," *Clin. Cancer Res.*, 2010 Oct 1;16(19):4755-68 .
8. H. P. Chao, C. D. Kuo, J. H. Chiu, and S. L Fu, "Andrographolide exhibits anti-invasive activity against colon cancer cells via inhibition of MMP2 activity," *Planta Med.* 2010 Nov; 76(16):1827-33.
9. V. Menon and S. Bhat, "Title of article," *Nat Prod Commun*, May 2010, 5(5):717–720.
10. Y. Tan, K. H. Chiow, D. Huang, and S. H. Wong," *Br J Pharmacol.*, April 2010, 159(7):1497–1510. (Epub, Feb. 19, 2010)
11. Mason and R. Roshan, "Increased tumor necrosis factor alpha (TNF-alpha) and natural killer cell (NK) function using an integrative approach in late stage cancers," *Immunol Invest.*, May 2002, 31(2):137–153.

12. K. Sheeja and G. Kuttan, "Effect of Andrographis paniculata as an adjuvant in combined chemoradio and whole body hyperthermia treatment—a preliminary study," *Immunopharmacol Immunotoxicol.*, 2008, 30(1):181–194.

13. A. Puri, R. Saxena, R. P. Saxena, and K. C. Saxena, "Immunostimulant agents from *Andrographis paniculata*," *J. Natural Products*, 1993, 56(7):995–999.

14. T. Matsuda, M. Kuroyanagi, S. Sugiyama, K. Umehara, A. Ueno, and K. Nishi, "Cell differentiation-inducing diterpenes from *Andrographis paniculata* Nees," *Chem. Pharm. Bull.* (Tokyo), 1994, 42(6):1216–1225.

15. S. Holt and L. Comac, *Miracle Herbs: How Herbs Combine with Modern Medicine to Treat Cancer, Heart Disease, AIDS, and More* (Caro Publishing Group, 1998).

16. Holt and Comac, Note 15.

17. L. Weibo, "Prospect for study on treatment of AIDS with traditional Chinese medicine," *J. Trad. Chinese Med.*, 1995, 15(1):3–9.

18. Matsuda et al., Note 14.

19. R. C. Saxena, R. Singh, P. Kumar, S. C. Yadav, M. P. Negi, V. S. Saxena, A. Joshu, V. Vijayabalaji, K. S. Goudar, K. Venkateshwarlu, and A. Amit, "A randomized double blind placebo controlled clinical evaluation of extract of Andrographis paniculata (KalmCold) in patients with uncomplicated upper respiratory tract infection," *Phytomedicine*, March 2010, 17(3-4):178–185.

20. Saxena et al., Note 19.

21. D. D. Caceres, J. L. Hancke, R. A. Burgos, and G. K. Wikman. Prevention of common colds with *Andrographis paniculata* dried extract: A pilot double-blind trial," *Phytomedicine*, 1997, 4(2):101–104.

22. R. A. Burgos and D. D. Caceres, "A double-blind study with a new mono drug: Kan-Jang: decrease of symptoms and enhancement of resistance in common colds." Research performed at the University of Chile, Departments of Pharmacology and School of Public Health, Santiago, Chile, and funded by the Swedish Herbal Institute, Aug. 1994.

23. W. L. Deng, "Preliminary studies on the pharmacology of the Andrographis product dihydroandrographolide sodium succinate," *Newsletters of Chinese Herbal Med.*, 1978, 8:26–28.

24. H. C. Madav, T. Tripathi, and S. K. Mishra, "Analgesic, antipyretic, and antiulcerogenic effects of andrographolide," *Indian J. Pharm. Sci.*, 1995, 57(3):121–125.

25. Madav et al., Note 24.

26. S. Vedavathy and K. N. Rao, "Antipyretic activity of six indigenous medicinal plants of Tirumala Hills, Andhra Pradesh, India," *Ethnopharmacology*, 1991, 33:193–196.

27. W. L Deng, "Outline of current clinical and pharmacological research on *Andrographis paniculata* in China," *Newsletters of Chinese Herbal Med.*, 1978, 10:27–31.

28. J. Yin and L. Guo, *Contemporary Traditional Chinese Medicine* (Beijing: Xie Yuan, 1993).

29. M. R. Sulaiman, Z. A. Zakaria, A. Abdul Rahman, A. S. Mohamad, M. N. Desa, J. Stanslas. S. Moin, and D. A. Israf, "Antinociceptive and antiedematogenic activities of andrographolide isolated from Andrographis paniculata in animal models," *Biol Res Nurs.*, Jan. 2010, 11(3):293–301.

30. P. Misra, N. L. Pal, P. Y. Guru, J. C. Katiyar, V. Srivastava, and J. S. Tandon, "Antimalarial activity of *Andrographis paniculata* (Kalmegh) against *Plasmodim berghei* NK 65 in *Mastomys natalensis*," *Int. J. Pharmacog.*, 1992, 30(4):263–274.

31. S. Gupta, M. A. Choudhry, J. N. S. Yadava, V. Srivastava, and J. S. Tandon, "Antidiarrheal activity of diterpenes of *Andrographis paniculata* (Kalmegh) against *Escherichia coli* enterotoxin in *in vivo* models," *Int. J. Crude Drug Res.*, 1990, 28(4):273–283.

32. Yin and Guo, Note 28.

33. Deng, Note 27.

34. Yin and Guo, Note 28.

35. D. Wang and H. Zhao, "Experimental studies on prevention of atherosclerotic arterial stenosis and restenosis after angioplasty with *Andrographis paniculata* Nees and fish oil," *J. of Tongji Medical University*, 1993, 13(4):193–198.

36. H. Zhao and W. Fang, "Protective effects of Andrographis paniculata Nees on post-infarction myocardium in experimental dogs," *J. of Tongji Medical University*, 1990, 10(4):212–217.

37. Zhao and Fang, Note 36.

38. L. Y. Huang, "The effects of andrographolides on experimental blood deficiency of cardiac muscle," *Chinese Herbal Med.*, 1987, 18(7):26–28.

39. Huang, Note 38.

40. Deng, Note 23.

41. S .Manez, J. J. Alcaraz, J. Paya, J. L. Rios, and J. L. Hancke, "Selected extracts from medicinal plants as anti-inflammatory agents," *Planta Med* 1990; 56(6): 656

42. Zhang Bao, Shouping Guan, Chang Cheng, Songlian Wu, Siew Heng Wong, Michael Kemeny D. Bernard P. L. Fred Wong W. S., "A novel antiinflammatory role for Andrographolode in asthma via inhibition of nuclear factor-kappaB pathway," *American Journal of Respiratory and Critical Care Medicine*, 2009, 179:657–665.

43. M. A. Akbarsha, B. Manivanan, K. S. Hamid, and B. Vijayan, "Antifertility effect of *Andrographis paniculata* (Nees) in male albino rat," *Indian Journal of Experimental Biology*, 1990, 28:421–426.

44. M. S. Zoha, A. H. Hussain, and S. A. Choudhury, "Antifertility effects of *Andrographis paniculata* in mice," *Bangladesh Med. Res. Council Bull.*," 1989, 15:34–37.

45. Yin and Guo, Note 28.

46. A. Kapil, I. B. Koul, S. K. Banerjee, and B. D. Gupta, "Antihepatotoxic effects of major diterpenoid constituents of *Andrographis paniculata. Biochemical Pharmacology*," 1993, 46(1):182–185.

47. B. Shukla, P. K. S. Visen, G.K. Patnaik, and B. N. Dhawan, "Choleretic effect of andrographolide in rats and guinea pigs," *Planta Med.*, 1992, 58:146–148.

48. Holt and Comac, Note 15.

49. G. N. Chturvedi, G. S. Tomar, S. K. Tiwari, and K. P. Singh, "Clinical studies on Kalmegh (*Andrographis paniculata* Nees) in infective hepatitis," *Journal of International Institute of Ayurveda*, 1983, 2:208–211.

50. Weibo, Note 17.

51. Deng, Note 23.

52. Author(s)?, "Second traditional Chinese medicine pharmaceutical factory in Shanghai test and manufacture of the water-soluble andrographolide injections," *Med. Industry*, 1976, 1:24–31.

53. Add info for study cited on page 20

54. Department of the Infectious Disease of the People's Hospital of Shantou Prefecture, "Clinical observation of seventy cases of tubercular meningitis treated with Andrographis and rifampin," *New Med.* 1976, 1:14–15.

55. Shanghai City Andrographis Research Group, "A study on water-soluble andrographolide," *Newsletters of Chinese Herbal Med.*, 1976, 3:10-18.

56. Department of Infectious Disease, Note 54.

57. Department of Gynecology and Obstetrics of the People's Hospital in Meixian Prefecture, "Summary of the effects of *Andrographis paniculata* on 60 cases of chorioepithelioma and malignant hydatidiform mole," *Chinese J. of Med.*, 1977, 12:755.

58. S. J. Hueng, "Treating anal tumor by washing using *Andrographis paniculata* extractions plus vinegar," *Chinese J. Anal. Intest. Dis.*, 1991, 11(2):40.

59. Yin and Guo, Note 28.

60. W. C. Qi, "Investigations of forty-five cases of infant cutaneous gangrene treated by Yi-Jian-Xi cream," *Traditional Chinese Med. in Fujian*, 1965, 4:32.

61. Lingtang Town Hospital of Gaoyou County, "Treating vaginitis using *Andrographis paniculata*," *Jiangshu Med.*, 1975, 6:45–46.

62. Field Hospital of the People's Liberation Army, "A summary of the clinical effects of *Andrographis paniculata* and andrographolide on 112 leprosy cases," *J. Protection and Cure of Dermal Diseases*, 1975, 2(31):158–164.

63. Q. Z. Huang, "Treating herpes using *Andrographis paniculata* products, *Guangxi Health*, 1974, 5:43.

64. Q. Z. Huang, "Treating herpes, chicken pox, mumps, and neurodermatitis using *Andrographis paniculata* products," *J. Barefoot Doctor Guangxi*, 1978, 9:21.

65. Cooperative Clinic of Zuoqiao, Sanca, Douchang, Jiangxi, "Treating burns using pumpkin pump plus Andrographis paniculata powder," *J. Barefoot Doctor*, 1975, 4:11.

66. T. K. Huang, *Handbook of compositions and pharmacology of traditional Chinese medicine* (Beijing: China Medical and Technology Press, 1994).

67. B. S. Aswal, D. S. Bhakuni, A. K. Goel, K. Kar, and B. N. Mehrotra, "Screening of Indian plants for biological activity," *Indian Journal of Experimental Biology*, 1984, 22:487.

68. W. K. Deng, R. J. Nie, and J. Y. Liu, "Comparison of pharmacological effect of andrographiloides," *Chin Pharm Bull.*, 1982, 17:195–198.

Additional Resources

A. Ala Abu-Ghafreh, H. Canatan, and I. E. Charles, "In vitro and In vivo anti-inflammatory effects of Andrographolide," *International Immunopharmacology*, March 2009, 9(3):313–318.

Y. Chung, "Andrographis paniculata," *Handbook of traditional Chinese medicine* (Guangzhou, 1979).

S. Y. Guo, D. Z. Li, W. S. Li, A. H. Fu, and L. F. Zhang, "Study of the toxicity of andrographolide in rabbits," *J. Beijing Med. Univ.*, 1988, 5:422–428.

K. Shreeja, C. Guruvayoorappan, and G. Kuttan, "Antiangiogenic activity of Andrographis paniculata extract and Andrographolide," *International Immunopharmacology*, Feb. 2007, 7(2):211–221.

K. Shreeja, et al., "Anti-oxidant and anti-inflammatory activities of the plant Andrographis paniculata Nees," *Immunopharmacology and Immunotoxicology*," 2006, 28(1):129–140.

Signal Transduction Companies, editorial, *Genetic Engineering News*, Jan. 1, 1996, 16(1).

P. B. Talukdar and S. Banerjee, "Studies on the stability of andrographolide, *Indian J.Chem.* 6:252–254.

W. Tang and G. Eisenbrandt, *Chinese Drugs of Plant Origin: Chemistry, Pharmacology, and Use in Traditional and Modern Medicine* (New York: Springer-Verlag, 1992).

Y. H. Wang, *The Pharmacology and Application of Traditional Chinese Medicine* (Beijing: People's Health Press, 1983).

Wen-Wan Chao, Yueh Hsiung Kuo, Wei-Chu Li, Bi-Fong Lin, "The production of nitric oxide and prostaglandin E2 in peritoneal macrophages is inhibited by Andrographis paniculata, Angellica and Morus alba ethyl acetate fractions," *Journal of Ethnopharmacology*, Feb. 25, 2009, 122(1): 68–75.

4

Asparagus racemosus

Introduction

Asparagus racemosus, or Shatavari, is a climbing plant that grows in low jungle areas throughout India. Shatavari is a cooling, calming, nourishing, and purifying herb, rich in Vitamin A, nutritious starches, and hormone analogues. This bittersweet herb is best known in Ayurveda as a female rejuvenative. Shatavari has been renowned for centuries in India for its therapeutic value in treating female reproductive disorders including infertility, decreased libido, threatened miscarriage, and cervical pH imbalance.

In India, Shatavari is considered to be women's equivalent of Ashwagandha, or "Indian ginseng." The name Shatavari is translated directly as "she who possesses 100 husbands." This herb tones, cleanses, nourishes, and strengthens the female reproductive organs and traditionally is used to treat premenstrual syndrome, amenorrhea, dysmenorrhea, leucorrhea, menopause, and pelvic inflammatory diseases such as endometriosis. Shatavari supports the health of deep tissues in the female reproductive system and is a blood builder, helping to reduce infertility, prepare the womb for conception, and prevent miscarriage. The herb also is effective as a post-partum tonic, helping to increase lactation and normalize the female reproductive system.

The benefits are not exclusive to women's health, however. This herb also is effective in treating male impotence and general sexual debility. Further, in traditional Ayurveda it is used to treat stomach ulcers, hyperacidity, and diarrhea. Decoctions of the herb have a soothing effect on dry, irritated membranes, making it useful for treating bronchitis and other respiratory ailments. Shatavari is classified in Ayurveda as a rasayana and is believed to bring into balance all of the body's fluids.[1] Ancient Ayurvedic texts recommend Shatavari as a remedy for nervous disorders, inflammation, liver disease, and certain infectious diseases.

Synonymous Names

Sanskrit: Shatavari
Hindi: Shatavari
English: Indian asparagus, Hundred roots, Asparagus roots
Chinese: Tian men dong

Habitat

Asparagus racemosus grows in low jungles areas throughout India.

Botanical Characteristics

Shatavari is a creeping variety of the plant genus Asparagus, characterized by a spreading root system. A climbing plant, it grows to a height of 2 meters, and bears many spiny branches. Its leaves are reduced to cladodes. Each Shatavari plant has many tuberous roots, which, when processed and dried, are used in medicinal preparations. The stem is pale gray or brown in color, and woody. The flowers are small, white, fragrant profusions, growing in simple or branched racemes.

More recent revisions in taxonomy have moved the genus Asparagus from the subfamily Asparagae in the family Liliaceae to the newly created family Asparagaceae. About 300 species of Asparagus are known to occur worldwide, including Asparagus officinalis (the common asparagus consumed as a vegetable), Asparagus sprengeri, and Asparagus acutifolius.[2]

Chemical Composition

Steroidal saponins and sapogenins are believed to account for the medicinal potency of Shatavari.[3] These chemicals include a unique group known as Shatavarins I-IV, ß-D-Glc-(1-4)-ß-D-Glc-(1-2) α-L-rha sarasapogenin, arasosapogenin.[4] Sterols and diosgenin also have been isolated from the roots of Shatavari.[5]

Additional chemical constituents include the alkaloid Asparagamine A, isolated from the plant's roots. Ripe fruits from Shatavari have yielded the flavonoids quercitin, rutin, hyperoside, cynidin 3-galactoside, and cynidin-3-glucohamnoside. Quercitin-3-glucuronide also has been isolated from the leaves of Shatavari.[6,7]

Pharmacological Activity

Ancient classical Ayurvedic literature ascribes many therapeutic attributes to the Shatavari root. The plant is described in Ayurvedic texts as bittersweet, emollient, cooling, galactogogic, aphrodisiac, diuretic, rejuvenative, carminative, stomachic, and antiseptic.[8] In addition, Shatavari root is recommended for treating nervous disorders, dyspepsia, diarrhea, dysentery, tumors, inflammation, hyperdipsia, neuropathy, hepatopathy, cough, bronchitis, hyperacidity, and certain infectious diseases.[9]

Uterotonic Activity

Animal studies have been conducted to affirm Shatavari's reputation as a uterine tonic. When extracts of Shatavari were tested in various animal tissues, Shatavari had a cholinergic action on guinea pig ileum. Ethyl acetate and acetone extracts of the root blocked spontaneous motility of the virgin rat's uterus.[10] The extracts also inhibited contractions that were chemically induced by spasmogens such as acetylcholine, barium chloride, and 5-hydroxytryptamine. The alcoholic extract was found to specifically block pitocin-induced contractions.

When powdered root extracts (including petroleum ether extract) of Shatavari were examined, however, no effect on uterine tissue was observed. This indicates the presence of a specific substance in the Shatavari alcoholic extract that specifically blocks pitocin-sensitive receptors but not other receptors in the uterus, confirming that Shatavari can be used as a uterine sedative.

A glycoside, Shatavarin I, isolated from Shatavari root, has been found to be responsible for the competitive block of oxytocin-induced contractions of rat, guinea pig, and rabbit uteri, in-vitro as well as in-vivo.[11]

Galactogogue Activity

The root extract of Shatavari is prescribed in Ayurveda to increase milk secretion during lactation.[12] In combination with other herbal substances, Shatavari has been demonstrated to increase milk production in females with deficient milk secretion.[13] Gradual decrease in milk secretion upon withdrawal of the herbs suggested that the increase in milk secretion was a result of herbal therapy only and not any psychological effect. In an another study, Shatavari, along with other herbal substances in the form of a commercial preparation, was reported to enhance milk output in women complaining of scanty breast milk on the fifth day after childbirth.[14]

Animal studies have confirmed the galatogogue effects of Shatavari. In one study, milk yield in buffaloes was increased significantly after administration of the herb.[15] When an alcoholic extract of Shatavari was administered to weaning rats, observations included increased weight of mammary glands, inhibited involution of lobulo-alveolar tissue, and maintenance of milk secretion.[16] The same extract in estrogen-primed rats led to well-developed lobulo-alveolar tissue and lactation. The increase in mammary gland weight and growth of the lobulo-alveolar tissue is theorized to be a result of the action of released corticoids and prolactin.[17] A significant increase in milk yield also was observed in guinea pigs and goats after administration of Shatavari, as well as increased growth of the mammary glands, alveolar tissues, and acini in guinea pigs.[18]

Gastrointestinal Activity

The powdered dried root of Asparagus racemosus often is prescribed in Ayurveda as a treatment for dyspepsia. Shatavari also has been mentioned for treating ulcerative disorders of the stomach, as well for duodenal ulcers. The juice of fresh root of Shatavari has been shown to have a definite curative effect for patients with duodenal ulcers.[19]

A clinical trial with human subjects confirmed the anti-ulcerogenic effects of Shatavari. In this study, 32 patients were given Shatavari root powder with a daily dose of 12 grams/day in four divided doses, for a period of 6 weeks. At the end of the study period, the majority of the study patients reported a significant reduction in symptoms. The study patients consistently reported a reduction in pain and burning sensations, along with a reduction of other symptoms related to duodenal ulcers. Because Shatavari does not have antacid and antisecretory properties, the observed reduction in acid secretion is believed to be a result of changes in gastric mucosa.[20]

Shatavari seemed to exert a direct healing activity on these patients' ulcers. The authors of this research postulated a number of possible mechanisms for this action, including the following:

1. Shatavari may prolong the lifespan of mucosal cells, increase the secretion and viscosity of mucus, and strengthen the mucosal barrier, thus reducing positive hydrogen diffusion back into the mucosa.

2. Shatavari may form a complex with mucus at the base of the ulcer, protecting it from the corrosive and proteolytic effects of acid-pepsin.

3. Shatavari may have cytoprotective action similar to that of prostaglandins.

Other possible mechanisms may be deactivation and binding of pepsin or of bile salts.

Oral administration of dry Shatavari root powder has been found to promote gastric emptying. The effectiveness is comparable to that of the synthetic dopamine antagonist metoclopromide.[21]

Animal studies further affirmed the anti-ulcer properties of Shatavari. In combination with the Ayurvedic herb Terminalia chebula, Shatavari protected gastric mucosa against pentagastrin- and carbachol-induced ulcers by significantly reducing both the severity of ulceration and the ulcer index. The decrease in volume and increased pH of the secretions in drug-treated rats suggested a reduced responsiveness of the gastric parietal cells to secretogogues and narcotizing agents.[22]

The fresh root juice of Shatavari produced similar results in cold stress and pyloric-ligation methods of inducing gastric ulcers in rats.[23] The results of this research suggest a reduction in acid and pepsin contents (aggressive factors) and an increase in mucin-bicarbonate secretions and the lifespan of the mucosal cells (defensive factors). This anti-ulcerogenic effect is believed to be a result of the regulation of the above two factors.[24]

Extracts of Shatavari root also have been shown to cause contractions in the smooth muscles of rabbit's duodenum, guinea pig's ileum, and rat's fundal strip without affecting peristaltic movement. These actions were similar to that of acetylcholine and were blocked by atropine, suggesting a cholinergic mechanism of action.[25] No effect was observed, however, on isolated rectus abdominus.

Immunomodulatory Activity

Intra-abdominal sepsis is a major cause of mortality following trauma and bowel surgery. In animal research, Shatavari provided protection against mixed bacterial abdominal sepsis induced by cecal ligation. Treatment with this herb also resulted in polymorphonuclear leucocytosis and prevented cyclophosphamide-induced neutropenia in rats.[26,27]

Oral administration of a decoction of powdered Shatavari root has been reported to produce neutrophilia, along with enhanced phagocytic activity of macrophages and polymorphs. The mortality rate of treated animals was reduced significantly, with a survival rate comparable to that of the group treated with a combination of metronidazole and gentamicin.

In an animal model of intraperitoneal adhesions, oral administration of a whole herb extract of Shatavari markedly reduced the number, character, and area of adhesions.[28] Additional research reported the revival of macrophage chemotaxis and interleukin-I and tumor necrosis factor-alpha production through the oral treatment of Shatavari root extract in ochratoxin A-treated mice.[29] And the alcoholic extract of Shatavari root enhanced both the humoral and the cell-mediated immunity of albino mice injected with the red blood cells of sheep as a particulate antigen.[30]

Effects of methanol and aqueous extracts of the tuberous roots of Chlorophytum arundinaceum, Asparagus adscendens, and Asparagus racemosus were examined in an experimental mouse model of stress, induced by swimming.[31] The extracts exerted an inhibitory effect on pro-inflammatory cytokines, namely interleukin 1beta and tumour necrosis factor alpha, and on the production of nitric oxide in mouse macrophage cells RAW 264.7 stimulated by lipopolysaccharide in-vitro. Similar inhibition was observed in the production of interleukin 2 in EL 4 lymphoma cells stimulated by concanavalin A. Also, corticosterone levels in serum and adrenal glands were measured. The findings suggest that these plants may be beneficial in the management of stress and inflammatory conditions.

Treatment with aqueous extract of Asparagus racemosus resulted in a significant increase of CD3(+) and CD4/CD8(+) percentages, suggesting its effect on T cell activation and delayed type hypersensitivity responses, suggesting activated lymphocyte activation.[32] The treated animals showed significant upregulation of Th1 (IL-2, IFN-g) and Th2 (IL-4) cytokine, suggesting its mixed Th1/Th2 adjuvant activity. Consistent with this finding is the higher antibody titres. Similarly, the extract was shown to exert an inhibitory effect on pro-inflammatory cytokines, namely interleukin 1beta and tumour necrosis factor alpha, and on the production of nitric oxide in mouse macrophage cells RAW 264.7

stimulated by lipopolysaccharide and concanavalin in-vitro.[33]

The immunoadjuvant potential of Asparagus racemosus aqueous root extract was evaluated in experimental animals immunized with diphtheria, tetanus, pertussis (DTP) vaccine. Oral administration of test material at 100 mg/kg per day dose for 15 days resulted in a significant increase (P = 0.0052) in antibody titers to Bordtella pertussis compared to control animals. The immunized animals (treated and untreated) were challenged with B. pertussis 18323 strain, and the animals were observed for 14 days. The treated animals did show a significant increase in antibody titers compared to the untreated animals after challenge (P = 0.002). After the brains of these animals were given live B. pertussis, the animals showed reduced mortality, degree of sickness, and less paralysis in those that subsequently were given aqueous extract of Asparagus racemosus. This may provide a basis for less vaccination, or even a decision not to vaccinate.[34]

Antihepatotoxic Activity

The alcoholic extract of Shatavari root has been shown to significantly reduce the enhanced levels of alanine transaminase, aspartate transaminase, and alkaline phosphatase in CC14-induced hepatic damage in rats,[35] indicating antihepatotoxic potential.

Anti-cancer Activity

An alcoholic extract of Shatavari's aerial parts demonstrated anti-cancer activity in a tissue culture study. This study, conducted on human epidermal carcinoma cells of the nasopharynx, suggests a potential anti-cancer role for the herb.[36]

A chloroform-methanol extract of fresh root of Shatavari has been reported to reduce the incidence of tumors in female rats. This action is believed to be mediated by the mammotropic and/or lactogenic influence of Shatavari on normal as well as estrogen-primed animals, which renders the mammary epithelium refractory to the carcinogen.[37] Sarsapogenin and Diosgenin derived steroidal constituents (1–12), isolated from Asparagus racemosus, have been shown to induce cell death and apoptosis of colon carcinoma cells.[38] An aqueous extract of the roots of Asparagus racemosus has revealed the potential to prevent hepatocarcinogenesis induced by treatment with diethylnitrosamine and DDT.[39]

Cardioprotective Activity

Alcoholic extracts of Shatavari root have been reported to produce positive inotropic and chronotropic effects on the heart of frogs at low doses and cardiac arrest at excessive doses. The extract produced hypotension in cats, which was blocked by atropine, indicating a cholinergic mechanism of action. The extract also produced congestion and complete stasis of blood flow in mesenteric vessels of mice and rats. With intravenous administration of the extract to rabbits, a slight increase in the bleeding time and no effect on clotting time were observed.[40]

Respiratory Activity

Higher doses of the alcoholic root extract of Shatavari were reported to cause a dilatory effect on the bronchial musculature of guinea pigs but failed to antagonize histamine-induced broncho-constriction. The extract also has been reported to produce depression of respiration in cats.[41]

Anti-bacterial activity

Shatavari has shown promise as an anti-bacterial agent. Laboratory studies have demonstrated the action of Shatavari roots against Escherichia coli, Shigella dysenteriae, Shigella sonnei, Shigella flexneri, and Staphylococcus aureus—bacteria associated with gastroenteritis, which can cause unpleasant symptoms such as vomiting and diarrhea. Shatavari root also was found to be effective against Vibrio cholerae (responsible for Asiatic or epidemic cholera), and Salmonella typhi (responsible for typhoid fever).[42]

Anti-fungal Activity

Extract of Asparagus racemosus roots and tubers was investigated against Candida albicans, Candida tropicalis, Candida krusei, Candida guillermondii, Candida parapsilosis, and Candida stellatoida, isolated from vaginal thrush patients. The extract of Asparagus racemosus showed a high degree of activity against all the Candida strains. The inhibitory effect of the extract against all the Candida tested was comparable to that of standard antibiotics used.[43]

Adaptogenic Activity

Animal studies have shown that Shatavari offers a protective effect against a variety of biological, physical, and chemical stressors. Aqueous extracts of the herb were administered orally to the research animals in a cisplatin model of alterations in gastrointestinal motility. The Shatavari extract exerted a normalizing effect, independent of the direction of pathological change. The extract reversed the effects of cisplatin on gastric emptying, and it normalized cisplatin-induced intestinal hypermotility.[44]

Neurological Activity

A study was undertaken to assess nootropic and anti-amnesic activities of Asparagus racemosus in rats.[45] The Morris water maze (MWM) and elevated plus maze (EPM) models were employed to evaluate learning and memory activity. Subsequently, the anti-amnestic activity was evaluated in scopolamine and sodium nitrite (NaNO(2))-induced amnestic models in rats. The rats pre-treated with Asparagus racemosus (50, 100 and 200mg/kg, p.o) for 7 days showed a significant decrease in escape latency in the MWM test, indicating nootropic activity. Asparagus racemosus also significantly reversed scopolamine and sodium nitrite-induced increase in transfer latency on EPM, indicating anti-amnesic activity. Further, Asparagus racemosus dose-dependently inhibited acetylcholinesterase enzyme in specific brain regions (prefrontal cortex, hippocampus, and hypothalamus). Thus, Asparagus racemosus showed nootropic and anti-amnesic activities in the models tested, and these effects probably will be mediated through augmentation of the cholinergic system because of its anti-cholinesterase activity.

Dr. Sodhi's Experience

When contemplating herbal treatment with Shatavari, the practitioner should consider the following:

- Is there an imbalance in female hormones?
- Is there concern about infertility?
- Are digestive symptoms present?
- Is libido low?
- Is there immune weakness?
- Is cancer present?
- Is milk production inadequate?
- Is aromatase inhibition desired?`

Shatavari is a notable herb for balancing female hormones. The literal meaning of the Sanskrit word for this plant combines the word Shat, meaning "100," with the word var, meaning "husbands," to describe its potential to increase women's sexual desire many fold. As an adaptogen, Shatavari is used to treat most female hormone imbalances, including both estrogen and progesterone dominance. It also is useful as a galactogogue, as it increases prolactin levels.

Also, Shatavari helps to calm gastrointestinal disturbances caused by problems with excessive acid production, such as gastritis and acid reflux. And it mitigates poor intestinal motility. Studies have shown that Shatavari improves both intestinal peristalsis and gastric emptying. Shatavari should be considered as a natural alternative to proton inhibitors. Because of its mucilaginous quality, it soothes and cools gastrointestinal irritation caused by excess pitta.

Case Histories

Osteoporosis with Low Estrogen

A 40-year old woman with osteoporosis and low estrogen came to our clinic seeking an alternative therapy to the synthetic hormones that her gynecologist had recommended. We advised certain dietary changes appropriate to her constitution and offered the following herbal protocol.

To balance hormones:

A combination of Dioscorea villosa (varhikand), Saraca indica (ashoka), and Terminalia arjuna (arjuna) extracts, in a proprietary blend of bamboo manna, coral powder, Cissus quadrangularis (hadjoda), and Cimicifuga racemosa, to be taken three times a day.

Combatition of Saraca indica, or Ashoka extract pyridoxine-5- phosphate, and Gota kola, Symplocos racemosus (lodh), bamboo manna, and aloe vera, also to be taken three times a day.

We also prescribed dietary supplements, including 1200 mg/day calcium, 600 mg/day magnesium fumarate, and a multivitamin containing 1000 IU Vitamin D. For dry vaginal tissues, we advised sesame oil applied daily to the internal vaginal walls.

After a few weeks, this patient's vaginal walls were healthier and less dry, and penetration was easier. After 3 months she had natural lubrication and her osteoporosis had converted to osteopenia. By the following year, her bone density was within normal ranges.

Hot flashes

A 53-year-old obese woman came to our clinic reporting hot flashes so severe that she awakened at night every hour, unable to sleep. She did not want to take hormones, either synthetic or botanical. We recommended the following treatment plan:

Exercise: Walking 45 minutes per day, to reduce hot flashes.

Dietary changes: We recommended that she get her consumption of soy products to no more than twice a week to avoid slowing her thyroid activity. She was instructed to eliminate red meat from her diet. We encouraged her to increase her intake of the following foods: beans, oatmeal, oat bran, flax meal, and wheat bran. We recommended 4 days of modified fasting with fruit and vegetable smoothies incorporating the following: apples, carrots, beets, and rice protein powder to flush the liver.

Protocols

For liver support: Tinospora cardifolia (guduchi), Picrorrhiza kurnoa (kutki), and Boerhaavia diffusa (purnarnava) in a proprietory blend of Phyllanthus amarus (bhumyamalaki), Swertia chirayita (kiraata), Calotropis gigantis (ark), Raphanus sativa (malaka), Berberis aristata (daaru Curcuma), Terminalia arjuna (arjun), Terminalia bellerica (bibhitaki), Terminalia chebula (haritaki), Emblica officinalis (amalaki), Solanum nigrum (kakmachi), and Andrographis paniculata and phyllanthus amarus (bhuunimb) extracts, to be taken three times a day

Shatavari 500 mg 2 capsules three times per day

A combination of Dioscorea villosa (varhikand), Saraca indica (ashoka), and Terminalia arjuna (arjuna) extracts, in a proprietary blend of bamboo manna, coral powder, Cissus quadrangularis (hadjoda), and Cimicifuga racemosa, to be taken three times a day.

This patient reported 1½ months later that she was sleeping well, her hot flashes reduced considerably and had lost 10 pounds.

For perimenopause and menopausal problems:

Shatavari extract 500–1000 mg two or three times a day

For low libido:

Shatavari as above, combined with Withania somnifera (ashwagandha) , Tribulus terrestris (gokhuru) extract, Shilajiit , saw palmetto 25 mg extract, Muira puma extract, Crocus sativus (Kumkuma), Emblica officinalis (amalaki), Piper longum (Pippli), Glycyrrhiza glabra (yastimadhu), Bacopa monniera (indriya brahmi), Sida cordifolia (bala), Mucuna pruriens (kapikachu), and Spilanthes acmella (akarkara) three times a day. The dose of the compound formulation also may be doubled.

For endometriosis:

Shatavari extract 500 mg one capsule three times per day

Combination of Saraca indica , of pyridoxine5-phosphate, Gota kola Symplocos racemosus (lodh), bamboo manna, and aloe vera one capsule three times per day

For aromatase inhibition in cancer and benign prostate hypertrophy:

When treating male and female cancers resulting from estrogen dominance, the following protocol can be followed:

As an anti-inflammatory:

Curcumin bound to MCT of coconut 1 teaspoon three times a day, with coconut milk

Anti-tumor:

Ashwgandha 500 mg three times a day,Proprietary Blend of Standardized extracts of Indian gooseberry, Catkins, Indian gallnut, long pepper, Indian pennywort, Cardamon, Nutmeg, Cinnamon, Bamboo manna, Sandalwood, Asparagus, Bael fruit, Tribulus terrestris, Terminalia chebula, Adhatoda vesica, Leptadenia reticulate, Aquilaria agallocha, Kush, Ashwagandha, Cyperus, Butterfly pea, Thatch grass, Turmeric, Indian trumpet flower, Caltrops, Gymnema auranticum, Spreading hogweed, Kudju, Uraria picta, Cashmere bark, Arni, Phaseolus tribolus, Desmodium, gangeticum, Castor root, Indian nightshade, clarified butter, dehydrated sugar cane and honey1 tablespoon three times a day; Shatavari extract 500 mg three times a day

For dysmenorrhea:

Shatavari extract 500 mg 1–2 capsules two or three times a day

For leaky gut syndrome:

Shatavari extract 500 mg 1–2 capsules two or three times a day, along with Bilva 1 teaspoon, three times a day in lukewarm water

For ulcerative colitis:

Shatavari extract 500 mg 1 capsule three times per day

Combination of Boswellia serrata extract, Bromolaine, Glucosamine Sulphate, Chondroitin Sulphate, curcumin and ginger extract 2 tablets three times per day

Probiotic 100 B: three times per day, best taken before 30 minutes before meals

Bilva: 1 teaspoon three times per day

Curcumin bound to MCT of coconut: 1 teaspoon three times per day, best taken in coconut milk

Pomegrante juice works well for any GI problem: ½ cup couple times per day

Pomegranate seed chutney: 1–2 teaspoons taken with every meal

Place all of the following ingredients in a blender and blend: 2 tablespoons dried pomegranate seeds that have been soaked overnight, one bunch of mint leaves, an inch of ginger fresh root, ¼ teaspoon black pepper, 1 teaspoon salt, one freshly squeezed lime or lemon

Ulcerative colitis is a serious disease. Its symptoms possibly can be reversed using dietary changes, but such changes may have to be continued for months, or perhaps for the rest of one's life, depending upon eating habits and lifestyle.

For insufficient milk production in breastfeeding:

Shatavari extract 500 mg 1–2 capsules two to three times a day, along with Ashwgandha extract 500mg 1–2 capsules three times a day.

For decreased capacity to exercise :

One hour prior to exercising: 2 capsules Shatavari along with 2 capsules Ashwgandha

For bacterial infections, including MRSA:

If the infection is acute, a physician should be contacted immediately. For treatment of repeat infections, and as an adjunct therapy to antibiotics, the following herbal protocol stopped the repeated MRSA infections:

- Shatavari extract 500 mg 1–2 capsules three times per day
- Pippli: 1 capsule three times per day
- Combination of Azadirachta indica (Neem), Emblica officinalis (Amla), Terminalia chebula (Haritaki), Terminalia bellerica, Tinospora cordifolia and Rubia cordifolia for support of immune system 2 capsules three times per day
- Curcumin bound to MCT of coconut: 1 teaspoon three times per day
- Probiotic 100 B: 1 capsule three times per day, taken 30 minute before meals

In addition to these supplements, all sugars and sweeteners should be eliminated, and water intake should be increased.

If low thyroid, the following extracts should be added, three times a day:

- Ashwgandha extract 500 mg 1 capsule three times per day
- Combination of Iodine, L-Tyrosine, Withania Somnifera, Bacopa Monnieri, Bauhinia Tomentosa, Commiphora Mukul, Piper Longum, Piper Nigrum, Zingiber Official, Crataeva Nurvula, Cinnamomum Zeylanicum & Cinnamomum Tamala, Elettaria Cardamomum 1 capsule twice per day

If kidney function is poor, add a kidney support formula such as combination of Didymocarpus pedicellat, Saxifraga ligulata, Tribulus terrestris, Ocimum sanctum, Shilajit, Arctostaphylos uva-ursi, Mimosa pudica (lajja, or lajwanti), Dolichos biflorus Cyperus rotundus, Crataeva religiosa and Achyranthus aspera (apamarg) , 1 tablet three times per day , to be added along with liver support , 1 tablet three times per day

SAFETY PROFILE

In Ayurveda, Shatavari has been described as absolutely safe for long-term use, even during pregnancy and lactation. Systemic administration of higher doses of all of the extracts did not produce any abnormalities in the behavior patterns of mice and rats.[45]

DOSAGE

The recommended dosage of Shatavari is 500 mg capsule taken twice a day after food or before food.

AYURVEDIC PROPERTIES

According to Ayurvedic practitioners, Shatavari produces a cooling effect. For this reason, it is particularly beneficial for ailments associated with excessive heat, such as fever and inflammatory conditions.

Shatavari is a sweet and bitter herb. It is pacifying to pitta and vata, and promotes kapha.

Rasa : Madhura (sweet), Tikta (bitter)
Guna: Guru (heavy), snigdha (unctuous)
Vipaka: Madhur (sweet)
Virya: Shita (cold)
Dosha: Pacifies Vata and Pitta

Notes

1. S. B. Rao, "Saponins (Sapogenins) from Indian medicinal plants: Part I, Sapogenins from Asparagus," *Indian J. Pharmacy*, 1952, 14:131–132.

2. H. A. Oketch-Rabah, "Phytochemical constituents of the Genus Asparagus and their biological activities," *Hamdard*, 1998, 41:33–43.

3. Y. U. Shao, O. Poobsasert, E. J. Kennelly, C. K. Chin, C. T. Ho, M. T. Huang, S. A. Garrison, and G. A. Cordell, "Steroidal saponins from Asparagus officinalis and their cytotoxic activity," *Planta Medica*, 1997, 63:258–262.

4. J. Singh and H. P. Tiwari, "Chemical examination of roots of Asparagus racemosus," *Journal of the Indian Chemical Society*, 1991, 68(7):427.

5. S. Ahmed and P. C. Jain, "Chemical examination of Asparagus racemosus," *Bulletin of Medico Ethnobotanical Research*, 1991, 12(3-4):157.

6. R. N. Chopra, I. C. Chopra, K. L. Handa, and L. D. Kapur, *Indigenous Drugs of India* (Calcutta, India: Academic Publishers, 1994), p. 496.

7. P. C. Sharma, M. B. Yelne, and T. J. Dennis, *Data Base on Medicinal Plants used in Ayurveda: Vol. I, Documentation & Publication Division* (Delhi: Central Council for Research in Ayurveda & Siddha, 2000), pp. 418–430.

8. Chopra et al, Note 6.

9. Sharma et al., Note 7.

10. M. H Jetmalani, P. B. Sabins, and B. B. Gaitonde, "A study on the pharmacology of various extracts of Shatavari- Asparagus racemosus (Willd)," *J Res Ind Med.*, 1967, 2:1–10.

11. J. Joshi and S. Dev, "Chemistry of Ayurvedic crude drugs: Part VIIIa-Shatavari-2: Structure elucidation of bioactive Shatavarin-I & other glycosidesb," *Indian J Chem*, 1988, 27B:12–16.

12. A. K. Nadkarni, *Indian Materia Medica*. Vol. I (Bombay: Popular Book Depot, 1954), pp.153–155.

13. G. V. Joglekar, R. H. Ahuj, and J. H. Balwani, "Galactogogue effect of Asparagus racemosus," *Indian Med J*, 1967, 61:165.

14. M. L. "Sholapurkar, "Lactare—for improving lactation," *Indian Practitioner*, 1986, 39:1023–1026.

15. A. B. Patel and U. K. Kanitkar, "Asparagus racemosus Willd. Form Bordi, as a galactogogue, in buffaloes," *Indian Vet J*, 1969, 46:718–721.

16. P. B. Sabins, B. B. Gaitonde, and M. Jetmalani, "Effect of alcoholic extract of Asparagus racemosus on mammary glands of rats," *Indian J Exp Biol.*, 1968, 6:55–57.

17. J. Meites, *Proceedings of the First International Pharmacology Meeting* (Vol I). (London: Pergamon Press, 1962), p. 151.

18. K. A. Narendranath, S. Mahalingam, V. Anuradha, and I. S. Rao, "Effect of herbal galactogogue (Lactare), a pharmacological and clinical observation," *Med Surg*, 1986, 26:19–22.

19. P. Kishore, P. N. Pandey, S. N. Pandey, and S. Dash, "Treatment of duodenal ulcer with Asparagus racemosus Linn," *J Res Indian Med Yog Homeo*, 1980, 15:409–415.

20. K. P. Singh and R. H. Singh, "Clinical trial on Satavari (Asparagus racemosus Willd.) in duodenal ulcer disease," *J. Res Ay Sid*, 1986, 7:91–100.

21. S. S. Dalvi, P. M. Nadkarni, and K. C. Gupta, "Effect of *Asparagus racemosus* (Shatavari) on gastric emptying time in normal healthy volunteers," *J Postgrad Med*, 1990, 36:91–94.

22. S. A. Dahanukar, S. G. Date, and S. M. Karandikar, "Cytoprotective effect of Terminalia chebula and Asparagus racemosus on gastric mucosa," *Indian Drugs*, 1983, 21:442.

23. B. De, R. N. Maiti, V. K. Joshi, V. K. Agrawal, and R. K. Goel, "Effect of some Sitavirya drugs on gastric secretion and ulceration," *Indian J Exp Biol*, 1997, 35:1084–1087.

24. R. K. Goel and S. K. Bhattacharya, "Gastroduodenal mucosal defense and mucosal protective agents," *Indian J Exp Biol*, 1991, 29:701–714.

25. Jetmalani, Sabins, and Gaitonde, Note 10.

26. S. Dahanukar, U. Thatte, N. Pai, P.B. Mose, and S. M. Karandikar, "Protective effect of Asparagus racemosus against induced abdominal sepsis," *Indian Drugs*, 1986, 24:125–128.

27. U. Thatte, S. Chhabria, S. M. Karandikar, and S. Dahanukar, "Immunotherapeutic modification of E. coli induced abdominal sepsis and mortality in mice by Indian medicinal plants," *Indian Drugs*, 1987, 25:95–97.

28. N. N. Regh, H. M. Nazareth, A. Isaac, S. M. Karandikar, and S. A. Dahanukar, "Immunotherapeutic modulation of intraperitoneal adhesions by Asparagus racemosus," *J Postgrad Med*, 1989, 35:199–203.

29. J. N. Dhuley, "Effect of some Indian herbs on macrophage functions in ochratoxin A treated mice," *J Ethnopharmacol*, 1997, 58:15–20.

30. S. Muruganadan, L. Garg, J. Lal, S. Chandra, and D. Kumar, " Studies on the immunostimulant and antihepatotoxic activities of Asparagus racemosus root extract," *J Med Arom Pl Sci*, 2000, 22:49–52.

31. A. S. Kanwar and K. K. Bhutani, "Effects of Chlorophytum arundinaceum, Asparagus adscendens and Asparagus racemosus on pro-inflammatory cytokine and corticosterone levels produced by stress, "*Phytother Res.*," June 17, 2010.

32. M. Gautam, S. Saha, S. Bani, A. Kaul, S. Mishra, D. Patil, N. K. Satti, K. A. Suri, S. Gairola, K. Suresh, S. Jadhav, G. N. Qazi, and B. Patwardhan, "Immunomodulatory activity of Asparagus racemosus on systemic Th1/Th2 immunity: implications for immunoadjuvant potential," *J Ethnopharmacol.*," Jan. 21, 2009, 121(2):241–247. (Epub Nov. 8, 2008)

33. A. S. Kanwar and K. K. Bhutani,. "Effects of Chlorophytum arundinaceum, Asparagus adscendens and Asparagus racemosus on pro-inflammatory cytokine and corticosterone levels produced by stress," *Phytother Res.*, June 17, 2010.

34. M. Gautam, S. Diwanay, S. Gairola, and Y. Shinde, "Immunoadjuvant potential of Asparagus racemosus aqueous extract in experimental system," *J Ethnopharmacol.*, April 2004, 91(2–3):251–255.

35. Muruganadan et al., Note 30.

36. Thatte et al., Note 27.

37. A. R. Rao, "Inhibitory action of Asparagus racemosus on DMBA-induced mammary carcinogoenesis in rats," *Int J Cancer*, 1981, 28:607–610.

38. K. K. Bhutani, A. T. Paul, W. Fayad, and S. Linder, "Apoptosis inducing activity of steroidal constituents from Solanum xanthocarpum and Asparagus racemosus," Aug. 17, 2010 , 10:789–793. (Epub Feb. 21, 2010)

39. A. Agrawal, M. Sharma, S. K. Rai, B. Singh, M. Tiwari, and R. M. Chandra, "The effect of the aqueous extract of the roots of Asparagus racemosus on hepatocarcinogenesis initiated by diethylnitrosamine," *Phytother Res.*, Sept. 2008, 22(9):1175–1182.

40. R. N. Roy, S. Bhagwager, S. R. Chavan, and N. K. Dutta, "Preliminary pharmacological studies on extracts of root of Asparagus racemosus (Satavari), Willd, N. O. Lilliaceae," *J Res Ind Med*, 1971, 6:132–138.

41. Roy et al., Note 40.

42. D. L. Boger, L. A. Mitscher, M. D. Mullican, S. D. Drake, and P. Kitos, "Antimicrobial and cytotoxic properties of 9, 10-dihydrophenanthrenes: structure-activity studies on juncusol," *Journal of Medicine Chemistry*, 1985, 28:1543–1547.

43. B. Uma, K. Prabhakar, and S. Rajendran, "Anticandidal activity of Asparagus racemosus," *Indian J Pharm Sci.* May 2009, 71(3):342–343.

44. Shao et al., Note 3.

45. R. K. Goel, T. Prabha, M. Mohan Kumar, M. Dorababu, M. Prakash, and G. Sing, "Teratogenicity of Asparagus racemosa wild root, a herbal medicine," *Indian Journal of Experimental Biology*, July 2006, pp 570-573.

❧ 5

Azadirachta indica

Introduction

Azadirachta indica, known in the common vernacular as Neem, has attracted much attention within the worldwide medical community because of its wide range of medicinal properties. Neem has been used extensively in Ayurvedic, homoeopathic, and folk medical traditions for thousands of years. A vast array of biologically active compounds have been isolated from this plant and studied in laboratory conditions for their pharmacological and insecticidal properties.

All parts of the Neem tree—its leaves, flowers, seeds, fruits, roots, and bark—are highly regarded in Ayurvedic medicine. The stem bark is an astringent, as are the root bark and young fruit. The flowers are used for dyspepsia, and the berries are purgative, emollient, and anthelmintic. Fresh Neem twigs often are used for cleaning the teeth. I used a Neem stick to brush my teeth as a young child and have never had any cavity or dental issues. The seed is a stimulant and is applied topically for rheumatism and skin diseases. The oils extracted from the leaves and seeds have antiseptic and insect repellent properties. The oils may be applied to boils, ulcers, and eczema.

Modern scientific research has validated the traditional uses of Neem for maintaining general health in India, but until recently have been virtually absent in the American market. Now, however, with scientific validation, products containing Neem are gaining popularity. Cultivation of the Neem tree also offers environmental advantages: the tree can grow in marginal soils, and every part can be used.

Research has confirmed the potency of Neem as an immunomodulatory, anti-inflammatory, anti-hyperglycemic, anti-ulcer, anti-malarial, anti-fungal, anti-bacterial, anti-viral, anti-oxidant, anti-mutagenic, and anti-carcinogenic remedy. In herbal preparations, Neem often is prescribed for contraception, skin problems, worm infestations, ulcers, gingivitis, fever, upset stomach, head lice, heart disease, and diabetes. It also is effective in treating arthritis, blood disorders, bronchitis, cough, diabetes, drowsiness, eczema, fever, jaundice, malaria, nausea, obesity, parasites, rheumatism, skin diseases, syphilis, and tumors.

Long valued for its insecticidal and insect repellent properties, Neem tree extract is a treatment for external parasites such as lice and mites. Research has addressed the effectiveness of Neem for controlling mosquito populations, with subsequent impact on mosquito-borne diseases such as malaria.

Synonymous Names

Botanical name: Azadirachta Indica
English: Neem tree, margosa tree
Sanskrit: Nimba

Hindi name: Neem, Nimb

Common Name: Bead Tree, Holy Tree, Margosa Tree

Habitat

The Neem tree is native to the Western Himalayas, growing in the warmer areas of India and Southeast Asia. It commonly is found in the forested areas of Andhra Pradesh, Tamil Nadu, and Karnataka. Neem also is cultivated in other tropical areas of Asia, as well as West Africa, the Caribbean, South America, Central America, Indonesia, and Australia.

Neem tolerates most types of soil, including dry, stony, and shallow soil with lateritic crusts, highly leached sands, and clays. Having an extensive and deep root system, the hardy Neem tree can grow and flourish even in marginal and leached soils.

Botanical Characteristics

The Neem tree is an adaptable, fast-growing evergreen tree that reaches heights between 21 and 60 feet (7 and 20 meters). Its dark brown to gray branches form a thick canopy, and the bark is moderately thick and longitudinally fissured. The leaves are compound and imparipinnate, arranged in alternating pairs with terminal leaflets. Each leaf is composed of up to 15 narrow lanceolate leaflets. The flowers are abundant, sweet-smelling white clusters that form in the leaf axils. Neem begins to produce its yellowish ovoid fruits after about 4 years and reaches full productive growth in about 10 years.

Chemical Composition

Chemical analysis has isolated the following active constituents from Neem:[1-15]

Limonoids

Azadirachtin, 3-deacetyl-3-cinnamoylazadirachtin, 1-tigloyl-3-acetyl-11-methoxyazadirachtin, 22,23-dihydro-23p-methoxyazadirachtin, nimbanal, 3-tigloylazadirachtol, 3-acetyl-salannol, nimbidiol, margocin, margocinin, margocilin, and others.

Terpenoids

Isoazadirolide, nimbocinolide, nimbonone, nibonolone, methylgrevillate, margosinone, margosinolone, nimosone, nimbosone, methyl nimbiol, methyl nimbionone, 13-acetyl-12-methoxy-8, 11,13-podocarpatriene, sugiol, 12,13-dimethoxy-8,11,13-podocarpatriene-3,7-dione, and gedunin have been isolated.

Neem oil has yielded salannin, 1,3-diacetyl salannin, deacetyl salannin, and salannol nimbidin, nimbidinin, and nimbinin. Analysis of Neem's root bark has revealed the presence of meliacin cinnamates, and analysis of the twigs has yielded isonimolide, isolimbolide, and isonimocinolide.

Polysaccharides

The following polysaccharides were identified in chemical analyses of Neem's fruit pulp: arabinogalatans and numerous other polysaccharides; G-IIa, G-IIIa, G-IIIb, GIIIDO$_2$IIa and GIIIDO$_2$'II. Other polysaccharides including CSP-II, -III, CSSP-I, -II, and -III have been isolated from Neem's stem bark.

Pharmacological Activity

Anti-diabetic activity

The clinical hypoglycemic effect of Azadirachta indica seeds was studied in Type-2 diabetes mellitus. Of these patients, 10 had no previous medication, 10 were taking oral hypoglycemic agents with a history of inadequate control, and 6 control subjects were given low (0.5 g tid) and high (2 g tid) doses of powdered part, aqueous extract, and alcoholic extract of Azadirachta indica for 14 days. On the 15th day, blood and urine samples for glucose were taken. Azadirachta indica was found to have significant hypoglycemic activity when taken in high doses and could be combined successfully with oral hypoglycemic agents in Type-2 diabetic patients whose diabetes was not controlled with oral hypoglycemic agents. [16]

Diabetic subjects in a clinical trial were given an aqueous Neem leaf extract. It was found that the insulin dosages could be reduced by 30%–50% without having a significant effect on blood glucose levels. [17]

Oral administration of a 10% aqueous Neem leaf extract to normo-glycemic animals at a dose of 200 mg/kg resulted in marked hypoglycemia. Intravenous administration of 0.15 mg/kg of a 50% aqueous leaf extract to dogs resulted in a significant decrease in blood glucose levels both in normoglycemic animals and in adrenaline-induced hyperglycemic animals. [18]

The anti-diabetic properties of Neem leaf and seed extracts were evaluated using normal and diabetic rabbits. The leaf and seed extracts both were found to have a marked hypoglycemic effect in the two groups of study animals. The effectiveness was similar to that of the drug glibenclamide (Glyburide). When the study animals were pre-treated with the extracts 2 weeks prior to the administration of alloxan, their blood glucose levels remained the same as the levels in the control diabetic animals. [19]

Oral treatment of diabetic rats with Allium sativum, Azadirachta indica, Momordica charantia, and Ocimum sanctum extracts (500 mg/kg of body weight) not only lowered the blood glucose level but also inhibited the formation of lipid peroxides, reactivated the anti-oxidant enzymes, and restored the levels of glutathione. [20] The herbal combination restored the mineral levels of copper, zinc, iron, magnesium, and selenium. The herbal extracts (50–500 microg) inhibited the generation of superoxide anions in both enzymatic and nonenzymatic in-vitro systems. These preparations also inhibited the ferrous-sodium ascorbate-induced formation of lipid peroxides in red blood cells. The in-vivo and in-vitro protective effects of the above-mentioned herbal preparation also were compared with that of glibenclamide. On the basis of these results, the combination of Allium sativum, Azadirachta indica, Momordica charantia, and Ocimum sanctum extracts not only possess hypoglycemic properties but also decrease the oxidative load in diabetes mellitus. Long-term use of such agents might aid in the prevention of diabetes-associated complications.

Anti-fungal activity

Neem leaf extract has shown anti-fungal potency against athlete's foot, ringworm, candida, and scabies. Neem oil and its aqueous solution also is an excellent remedy against the fungal strains that cause jock itch and nail infections.

Aspergillus flavus is a common fungus that poses significant problems, especially in elderly patients. Laboratory research using a leaf extract of Neem showed significant inhibition of aflatoxin synthesis and fungal spore infections resulting from Aspergillus flavus. [21]

Growth of Candida albicans populations and replication of the polio virus also were inhibited by the Neem fraction. Neem enhanced the survival rate of mice with systemic candidiasis and reduced the rate of fungal colony formation in affected mice. These factors demonstrate a potent, broad-spectrum, anti-microbial activity.

Scabies treatment

Neem is included in multi-herbal preparations to heal scabies infections. In one study, Neem was used in the form of a paste for treating scabies in 814 people. In 97% of these cases, relief was obtained within 3 to 15 days of treatment.[22]

Anti-viral activity

In-vitro and in-vivo studies were conducted to evaluate the inhibitory potential of a pure Neem compound and an aqueous Neem extract on the replication of dengue virus type-2.[23] In-vitro, the anti-viral activity of aqueous Neem leaf extract, measured in cloned larval cells of Aedes albopictus employing the virus inhibition assay, was evidenced in a dose-dependent manner. The aqueous extract of Neem leaves at its maximum non-toxic concentration of 1897 mg/ml completely inhibited the virus. The authors of the previous study conducted another in-vivo investigation. Neem leaf extract at a maximum non-toxic concentration of 120–130 mg/ml resulted in inhibition of virus replication, as confirmed by the absence of dengue-related clinical symptoms in suckling mice. By comparison, pure Neem oil did not reveal any inhibition of dengue virus type-2 replication in either in-vitro or in-vivo systems.

The anti-viral and virucidal effect of a methanolic extract fraction of Neem leaves was studied to determine its activity and the possible mechanism of action against the Coxsackie B group of viruses.[24] Neem inhibited plaque formation in six antigenic types of Coxsackie virus B at a concentration of 1000 micrograms/ml in-vitro.

Virus inactivation, yield reduction, and the effect of time on additional assays suggested that Neem was most effective against Coxsackie virus B-4 early in its replicative cycle. This evidence suggests that Neem's rich chemical constitution of flavonoids, triterpenoids, and their glycosides give the herb anti-viral potency against the coxsackie B group of viruses in-vitro.

Neem leaf extract at a concentration of 3-4 mg/ml inhibited plaque formation by the chickungunya and measles viruses, along with an overall reduction in virus volume.[25]

Anti-bacterial activity

The anti-bacterial effectiveness of a mouthwash containing Neem was tested against salivary streptococcus mutans and lactobacillus over a period of 2 months. The effectiveness of Neem in reversing incipient carious lesions also was assessed. Streptococcus mutans was inhibited by Neem mouthwash, with or without alcohol as well as chlorhexidine, and lactobacillus growth was inhibited by chlorhexidine alone. These initial data seem to prove the effectiveness of Neem in inhibiting streptocuccus mutans and reversing incipient carious lesions. Longer-term clinical trials will be of value to fully establish Neem's activity against common oral bacterial strains.[26, 27]

The anti-bacterial activity of Neem seed oil was observed in-vitro against 14 strains of pathogenic bacteria using the tube dilution method. This activity was determined to be significant, independent of temperature and energy. Most of the pathogens were killed more rapidly at 39.2 F (4ºC) than at 98.6 F (37ºC). Neem's anti-bacterial action seems to be attributable mainly to the inhibition of cell membrane synthesis (see Note 13). Neem seed oil was shown to have significant anti-bacterial efficacy against Bacillus subtilis, Salmonella typhosa, and Salmonella paratyphi.

A spermicidal fraction prepared from Neem oil, NIM-76, was investigated for its antimicrobial action against several bacterial and fungal strains, as well as the polio virus. NIM-76 showed a stronger activity than whole Neem oil, and inhibited the growth of pathogens, including Escherichia coli and Klebsiella pneumoniae, which were not affected by the whole oil.[28]

Analgesic activity

The analgesic potency of an aqueous Neem extract was demonstrated in mice, using an experimental pain model. In the glacial acetic acid-induced writhing test, Neem extract reduced both the incidence and the number of writhes in a dose-dependent manner. It also enhanced tail withdrawal latencies in the tail flick test for pain at similar dosages.[29]

Anti-atherosclerotic activity

In an examination of the anti-atherosclerotic properties of Neem leaf extract in rats, Neem decreased serum cholesterol significantly without changing serum protein, blood urea, and uric acid levels.[30]

Anti-pyretic activity

In Ayurveda, Neem is considered to be a powerful blood purifier and detoxifier. An animal study using rabbits evaluated the anti-pyretic effect of a 75% methanolic extract of Neem leaves and bark. When the extract was administered at a dose of 400 mg/kg, significant anti-pyretic activity was observed. The hexane, chloroform, 90% ethanol, and water-soluble fractions of the Neem extracts also were anti-pyretic at dosages of 150 mg/kg.[31]

Anti-ulcerogenic activity

When aqueous extracts of Neem leaf at doses of 10, 40, or 160 mg leaf/kg body weight were given to rats exposed to 2 hours of cold-restraint stress, a reduction in the severity of ulcers was observed, along with a decrease in damage to gastric mucosa from ethanolic ulcer induction. Neem prevented the degradation of mast cells, increasing the volume of gastric mucus in the stressed animals.[32]

In another study, Neem exhibited a strong protective effect on gastric lesions in rats, including those induced by acetylsalicylic acid, stress, serotonin, and indomethacin. Neem also offered protective value against histamine or cysteamine induced duodenal lesions in guinea pigs and rats. Rats and dogs showed improved healing of acetic acid-induced chronic gastric lesions after receiving oral doses of Neem extract.[33]

Anxiolytic activity

A behavioral examination of rats was conducted to determine the anxiolytic activity of Neem leaf extract. When a single dose of the extract was given 45 minutes before both maze and open-field behavioral tests, a significant anxiolytic effect was observed. Low doses of Neem produced an effect comparable to that of diazepam. At higher doses, however, Neem did not seem to have a corresponding effect.[34]

Central nervous system activity

In a research study as tested by an open-field paradigm and Morris' water maze, a propensity toward anxiety and disturbances of learning/memory were observed in animals subjected to hypoperfusion for 2 weeks. Azadirachta indica (500 mg/kg/day x 15 days) significantly reduced these hypoperfusion-induced functional disturbances. Reactive changes in brain histology such as gliosis, perivascular lymphocytic infiltration, recruitment of macrophages and cellular edema following long-term hypoperfusion were also attenuated effectively by Azadirachta indica. The study provides experimental evidence for possible neuroprotective potentiality of Azadirachta indica.[35]

Hepatoprotective activity

The effect of aqueous Neem leaf extract was evaluated in paracetamol-induced hepatotoxicity in rats. Liver necrosis was produced by administering a single dose of paracetamol. The liver damage was evidenced by elevated levels of serum aspartate aminotransferase, alanine aminotransferase, gamma glutamyl transpeptidase (gamma-GT), and by histopathological observations of liver sections. Aqueous Neem leaf extract significantly reduced all of the elevated enzyme levels. Paracetamol-induced liver necrosis also was reduced, as observed macroscopically and histopathologically.[36]

Anti-inflammatory activity

Polysaccharides isolated from the stem bark of Neem have exhibited significant anti-inflammatory activity. Nimbidin, the crude bitter principle from Neem seed oil consisting of a mixture of limonoids, exhibited a dose-dependent inhibition of carrageenan-induced edema. Doses of 40 and 80 mg/kg also produced significant inhibition of both kaolin-induced edema and formaldehyde-induced arthritis. Inhibition of croton oil-induced granuloma formation was also observed. When administered orally, a methanolic extract of the bark and leaves of Neem inhibited laboratory (carrageenan)-induced swelling (edema) in rat tissues, as did sodium nimbate. Formaldehyde induced arthritis in rats was also inhibited by 20 mg/kg sodium nimbate.[37,38]

Anti-fertility activity

Neem has been shown in many studies to block fertility. Female Wistar rats of proven fertility were given single doses of Neem oil via an intrauterine route. The control animals received the same volume of peanut oil. All the control animals became pregnant and delivered normal litters. The rats treated with Neem oil remained infertile for variable periods ranging from 107 to 180 days even after repeated matings with males of proven fertility. The block in fertility was shown to be reversible, as half of the animals regained fertility and delivered normal litters by 5 months after treatment, without any apparent teratogenic effects.[39] Unilateral administration of Neem oil in the uterus blocked pregnancy only on the side of application, whereas the contralateral side of the uterus treated with peanut oil had normally developing fetuses. No sign of implantation or fetal resorption was noted in the treated side. The ovaries on both sides had 4–6 corpora lutea, indicating that the treatment had no effect on ovarian function. The Neem-treated animals showed significant leukocytic infiltration in the uterine epithelium between days 3 and 5 post-coitum. These results suggest that the intrauterine application of Neem oil appears to induce a pre-implantation block in fertility.

Neem was tested to determine its potential as a self-administered, orally delivered method for termination of early pregnancy.[40] Purified Neem extracts containing immunomodulatory-stimulating cells and macrophages were tested on rats, baboons, and monkeys. The onset of pregnancy was confirmed by surgery and counting of implants on day 7 in rats, and by chorionic gonadotropin and progesterone assays in the primates. Termination was defined as complete resorption on day 15 in rats and by bleeding and decline of chorionic gonadotrophin and progesterone in baboons. Pregnancy was terminated successfully both in rodents and in primates with no significant side-effects. Fertility was regained in both species after one or two irregular cycles. The animals' offspring had normal developmental landmarks and mothered normal litters. The active principle in Neem was partially fractionated by activity-guided purification.

A cascade of events is believed to be involved in Neem's anti-fertility activity. In primates, an early observation is a decrease in progesterone. In the above study, a transient increase in CD4 and CD8 cells was noted in the spleen at 96 hours, and in CD8 cells in mesenteric lymph nodes. The treatment caused an elevation of both immunoreactive and bioactive TNF-alpha and gamma-interferon in serum, mesenteric lymph nodes, and fetoplacental tissue. This study indicates that Neem does have the potential for termination of pregnancy.

A study was designed to investigate the effect of methanolic extract of Neem leaves on the histology of the ovary and also on serum levels of FSH and LH in female Wistar rats. Eighteen (18) rats weighing 110g–150g were used, randomly divided into three groups (A, B, and C) of six rats each: Group A served as the control, receiving distilled water equivalent in volume to the test extract. Group B was treated with 200mg/kg of the methanolic extract of Neem leaves. Group C received 400mg/kg of the methanolic extract of Neem leaves. Administration was by gavage and lasted 14 days. The histological sections of the experimental groups revealed no histopathological features. No statistically significant difference was observed in the serum levels of FSH in the treated groups. Serum levels of LH, however, were reduced significantly compared to the control. This study indicates that extract of Neem leaves may affect fertility adversely by reducing serum levels of LH and, subsequently, the release of ova during ovulation.[41]

When an ethanol extract of Neem flower was administered to male rats, a marked decrease in the weight of testes and epididymis was observed, and spermatogenesis was arrested. The motility and density of sperm also were reduced significantly.[42] Androgen levels and spermatogenesis also were observed to be decreased significantly, as measured by reduced testicular weight, as well as reductions in protein, sialic acid, and glycogen content.

Administration of Neem seed extract also was shown to cause degenerative changes in ovarian follicles, as well as degeneration of endometrial epithelium, disorganization of uterine glands, and breakage and deterioration of luminal epithelium.[43] No changes in hormonal parameters were observed.

An active fraction of the hexane extract of the Neem seed resulted in a long-term, reversible, anti-fertility effect after a single intrauterine administration in female rats of proven fertility. The mechanism of action appears to involve the intervention of local cell-mediated immunity in the reproductive system.[44]

Anti-tumor and immune modulating activity

A study was designed to investigate the effects of aqueous Azadirachta indica leaf extract (AAILE) on serum glycoprotein contents and the incidence rate of tumors in the colon of rats subjected to dimethylhydrazine (DMH) treatment.[45] Forty rats were divided equally and randomly into four groups: Group I (normal control), Group II (DMH-treated), Group III (AAILE), and Group IV (DMH + AAILE treated). Group II and IV animals were injected subcutaneously with DMH (30 mg/kg b.wt.) every week for two durations of 10 and 20 weeks. AAILE was given orally three times a week on alternate days (100 mg/kg b.wt.) to animals belonging to Groups III and IV. Blood samples were drawn from all the animals by ocular vein puncture every month to estimate total sialic acid (TSA) and lipid bound sialic acid (LSA), which served as markers for the cancer. No incidence of tumor was recorded in the animals given DMH treatment for 10 weeks. DMH treatment for 20 weeks, however, showed a 100% incidence of tumor. Animals treated with DMH for both time durations showed a significant increase in the levels of TSA in comparison to the normal control, which decreased significantly following AAILE supplementation, however. There was no significant difference between LSA levels of DMH treated animals and normal controls. Azadirachta indica-treated animals showed the reversal of tumors.

The anti-tumor effects of Neem were observed in a laboratory study on Sarcoma-180 ascites tumor cells in mice. This activity was believed to be a result of action of the polysaccharides gia and gib, isolated from Neem's stem bark.[46]

In another study, Neem leaf preparation (NLP) was found to activate natural killer (NK) cells

(CD56(+)CD3(-)) to enhance their cytotoxic ability towards tumor cells and stimulate the release of interleukin-12 (IL-12) from macrophages of healthy individuals and head-and-neck squamous cell carcinoma patients.[47] NLP upregulated cytotoxic (CD16(+) and CD56(dim)) NK cells, and the cytotoxicity of NK-sensitive K562 cells by NLP stimulated peripheral blood, mononuclear cells decreased significantly after IL-12 neutralization. This NK-mediated cytotoxicity was manifested by upregulation of IL-12-dependent intracellular expression of the perforin-granzyme B system.

Moreover, in this study, NK cytotoxic function was abolished after the use of concanamycin A, a perforin inhibitor, but not by brefeldin A, a Fas inhibitor, which confirmed participation of the perforin-granzyme B system. In addition, NLP upregulated the expression of CD40 in CD14(+) monocytes and CD40L in CD56(+) lymphocytes. Neutralization of CD40 and CD40L in NLP-stimulated peripheral blood mononuclear cells culture resulted in significant downregulation of IL-12 release and cytotoxicity of NK cells. This demonstrates the role of a CD40–CD40L interaction in the observed functions. Signals involved in the NLP-induced release of IL-12, and thereby induction of NK cell cytotoxicity, are mediated by activating the p38MAPK pathway but not through the ERK1/2 signaling pathway. Overall, the results suggest that NLP effects NK cellular cytotoxicity by CD40-CD40L-mediated endogenous production of IL-12, which critically controls perforin-dependent tumor cell cytotoxicity.

In another study, Azadirachta indica demonstrated augmentation of the CD3-CD56+ natural killer (NK) and CD8+CD56 T-cell-mediated tumor cell cytotoxicity by Neem leaf glycoprotein (NLGP).[48] These NK and T cells were isolated from the peripheral blood of head and neck squamous cell carcinoma patients with a state of immunosuppression. NLGP induces TCR alpha beta-associated cytotoxic T lymphocyte (CTL) reaction to kill oral cancer (KB) cells. This CTL reaction is assisted by NLGP-mediated upregulation of CD28 on T cells and HLA-ABC, CD80/86 on monocytes. CTL-mediated killing of KB cells and NK-cell-mediated killing of K562 (erythroleukemic) cells are associated with activation of these cells by NLGP. This activation is evidenced by increased expression of early activation marker CD69 with altered expression of CD45RO/CD45RA. NLGP is a strong inducer of IFNgamma from both T and NK cells; however, IFNgamma regulates the T-cell-mediated cytotoxicity only without affecting NK-cell-mediated one.

The reason for this differential regulation may lie within upregulated expression of IFNgamma-receptor on T-cell surface, not on NK cells. The NLGP-induced cytotoxicity is dependent on upregulated perforin/granzyme B expression in killer cells, which again is IFNgamma-dependent in T cells and independent in NK cells. Although FasL expression is increased by NLGP, it may not be truly linked with the cytotoxic functions, as brefeldin A could not block NLGP-mediated cytotoxicity such as concanamycin A, a perforin inhibitor. Based on these results, it was concluded that NLGP might be effective to recover the suppressed cytotoxic functions of NK and T cells from patients having head and neck squamous cell carcinoma.

To find an effective, nontoxic, dendritic cell (DC)-maturating agent for human use, CD14(+) monocytes were differentiated with GMCSF/IL-4 and matured with Neem leaf glycoprotein (NLGP).[49] NLGP matured DCs (NLGP-DCs) showed upregulated expression of CD83, CD80, CD86, CD40 and MHCs. This action was compared to lipopolysacchride (LPS).

NLGP-DCs secrete a high amount of IL-12p70 with low IL-10. NLGP upregulates the expression of crucial transcription factor ikaros, indicating maturation toward the DC1 phenotype. In this study, increased expression of CD28 and CD40L on T cells following co-culture with NLGP-DCs was observed as promoting DC-T interactions. As a result, T cells secrete a large amount of IFN gamma with low IL-4 and generate an anti-tumor type 1 immune microenvironment. Such NLGP-DCs present carcinoembryonic antigen (CEA) effectively to T cells to increase T cell-mediated cytotoxicity of CEA(+) tumor cells in-vitro and in-vivo. With the emergence of NLGP as a promising DC-maturating agent, NLGP-DCs also can be used as a candidate vaccine for antigen-specific cancer immunotherapy.

Neem leaf glycoprotein (NLGP)-mediated immune activation and associated immune polarization was studied.[50] NLGP-induced activation was reflected in upregulation of the early activation marker CD69 on lymphocytes, monocytes, and dendritic cells. Activation also was denoted by CD45RO enhancement, with a decrease in CD45RA phenotype and CD62L (L-selectin). NLGP-activated T cells secreted a greater amount of the signature T-helper (Th)1 cytokines interferon-gamma and a lesser amount of the Th2 cytokine interleukin (IL)-4. Similar type 1 directness was also observed in antigen-presenting monocytes and dendritic cells by upregulation of IL-12, tumor necrosis factor-alpha and downregulation of IL-10.

Creating the type 1 microenvironment also is assisted by NLGP-induced downregulation of FoxP3(+) T-Reg cells. A type 1-specific transcription factor, T-bet, is upregulated in circulating immune cells after their stimulation with NLGP. In creating the type 1 immune network, increased phosphorylation of STAT1 and STAT4 with decreased phosphorylation of STAT3 might have significance. The conclusion is that NLGP may be effective in maintaining normal immune homeostasis by upregulating the type 1 response in immunosuppressed hosts, which may play a significant role in induction of the host protective antitumor functions.

Involvement of the nitric oxide (NO) release in carcinoembryonic antigen-pulsed macrophages with Neem leaf glycoprotein (CEAM phi NLGP) vaccination and its relationship to vaccine-induced type 1 immune response were studied.[51] Vaccination with CEAM phi NLGP resulted in macrophage activation, as evidenced by its increased number and expression of the CD69 marker. Activated macrophages demonstrated upregulation in synthesis of IL-12 and downregulation in IL-10, along with excess IFN gamma production in splenic cells, as evidenced from the mRNA analysis. Induction of this type 1 immunity was confirmed by expression of type 1 specific transcription factor T-bet and enhancement of the intracellular glutathione content. The vaccination also induced greater nitric oxide (NO) production from macrophages. Dependence of the induced type 1 immune response on the NO release and vice versa was studied by in-vitro neutralization of IFN gamma/IL-12 and in-vivo inhibition of NO production by methylene blue. The results clearly demonstrated the interdependence of two anti-tumor immune functions: NO production and generation of type 1 immune response. Understanding the mechanism of this NO-related immune modulation would have great impact in proposing CEAM phi NLGP vaccination in the clinic for treating CEA+ tumors.

A study investigated the combination of chemopreventive efficacy of Azadirachta indica (AI) and Ocimum sanctum (OS) against N-methyl-N'-nitro-N-nitrosoguanidine (MNNG)-induced gastric carcinogenesis, based on changes in oxidant–antioxidant status, cell proliferation, apoptosis, and angiogenesis.[52] Male Wistar rats were assigned to four groups: Rats in groups 1 and 2 received MNNG (150 mg/kg body weight intragastric (i.g.) three times with a gap of 2 weeks in between the treatment. The Group 2 rats additionally received ethanolic AI (100 mg/kg body weight i.g.) and OS (150 mg/kg body weight i.g.) leaf extract three times per week for 26 weeks. The Group 3 rats were given AI and OS leaf extract alone Group 4 served as the control.

To biomonitor chemoprevention, the following were used: lipid and protein oxidation and status of the anti-oxidants, superoxide dismutases. catalase, reduced glutathione (GSH), and GSH-dependent enzymes, together with markers of proliferation (proliferating cell nuclear antigen [PCNA], glutathione S-transferase-Pi [GST-P]), invasion (cytokeratin [CK]), angiogenesis (vascular endothelial growth factor [VEGF]), and apoptosis (Bcl-2, Bax, cytochrome C and caspase-3).

As a result, the rats that had been administered MNNG developed forestomach carcinomas that displayed low lipid and protein oxidation coupled to enhanced anti-oxidant activities, and overexpression of PCNA, GST-P, CK, VEGF and Bcl-2 with downregulation of Bax, cytochrome C, and caspase-3. Co-administration of AI and OS extract suppressed MNNG-induced gastric carcinomas accompanied by modulation of the oxidant-antioxidant status, inhibition of cell proliferation and angiogenesis, and induction of apoptosis. Results of this study suggest that chemoprevention by AI and OS in combination may be mediated by their anti-oxidant, antiangiogenic, antiproliferative, and apoptosis inducing properties.

A study was carried out to investigate the ability of Neem leaf preparation (NLP) to protect against apoptosis of circulating blood cells induced by cisplatin and 5-fluorouracil (cis + 5-FU) in carcinoma-bearing mice.[53] In comparison to the untreated control, during cis + 5-FU therapy, significant downregulation of leukocyte apoptosis was noted in mice that had been pre-treated with NLP or granulocyte colony stimulating factor (GCSF) during cis + 5-FU therapy. The enhanced cytotoxicity may be associated with the NLP-induced increase of the cytotoxic T and NK cell pool. The authors of this study concluded that the efficacy of NLP is comparable to GCSF in its ability to protect against leukocyte apoptosis induced by cis + 5-FU. NLP would be a better choice of treatment because GCSF is tumor-promoting, angiogenic, and expensive.

O6-alkylguanines are potent mutagenic, pro-carcinogenic, and cytotoxic lesions induced by exogenous and endogenous alkylating agents. Facilitated elimination of these lesions by increasing the activity of O6-methylguanine-DNA methyltransferase (MGMT) is likely to be a beneficial chemoprevention strategy, but this has not been examined.

Because marginal enhancement of this protein may be adequate for genomic protection, the researchers studied alterations in MGMT activity and expression in human peripheral blood lymphocytes and cancer cell lines induced by water-soluble and alcohol-soluble constituents of several plants with established anti-oxidant and medicinal properties.[54] Both the ethanolic and the aqueous extracts from Neem (Azadirachta indica), holy basil (Ocimum sanctum), winter cherry (Withania somnifera), and oregano (Origanum majorana) increased the levels of MGMT protein and its demethylation activity in a time-dependent manner with a maximum three-fold increase after 72 hours following treatment. The extracts from gooseberry (Emblica officinalis), common basil (Ocimum basilicum), and spearmint (Mentha viridis) were relatively less efficient in raising MGMT levels. Increased levels of MGMT mRNA accounted, at least in part, for increased activity of the DNA repair protein. The herbal treatments also increased glutathione S-transferase-pi (GSTP1) expression, albeit to a lesser extent than MGMT. These data provide the first evidence for upregulation of human MGMT by plant constituents and raise the possibility of rational dietary approaches for attenuating alkylation-induced carcinogenesis. Further, they reveal the putative anti-oxidant responsiveness of the MGMT gene in human cells.

The immunomodulatory effects of Neem oil were studied in mice.[55] The animals were treated intraperitoneally with Neem oil. The control animals received the emulsifying agent with or without peanut oil. Peritoneal lavage, collected on subsequent days, showed a maximum number of leukocytic cells on day 3 after the treatments. The peritoneal macrophages exhibited enhanced phagocytic activity and expression of MHC class-II antigens. The Neem oil treatment also induced the production of gamma interferon. The spleen cells of the Neem-treated animals showed a significantly higher lymphocyte proliferative response than that of the controls to an in-vitro challenge with either Con A or tetanus toxoid. Pre-treatment with Neem oil, however, did not augment the anti-Tetanus Toxoid (TT) antibody response.

The results of this study indicate that Neem oil acts as a non-specific immunostimulant, and that it selectively activates the cell-mediated immune mechanisms to elicit an enhanced response to subsequent mitogenic or antigenic challenges. The aqueous extracts of Neem's bark, leaves, and seeds caused increases in phagocytic activity and induced the expression of antigens on macrophages, indicating an enhancement of antigenic potency, stimulated lymphocyte proliferative response of splenocytes to mitogens, and selectively activated T-cell response. Significant inhibition in the intracellular multiplication of chlamydia and on the cytopathic effect of herpes were observed when mouse spleen cells were treated with Neem extracts. These results indicate that Neem has powerful immunomodulatory effects.

Cardioprotective activity

Administration of Neem leaf extract resulted in potent and dose-dependent hypotension in rabbits and guinea pigs. The extract also acted against irregular heart rhythms in rabbits when dysrhythmia was induced by Ouabain (g-strophanthin, a poisonous cardiac glycoside). The researchers theorized that this action may have an effect on vascular smooth muscle, resulting in vasodilation.[56]

Insecticidal activity

An insecticide containing Neem extract was tested against mosquito larvae in a study conducted in Iran under both laboratory and field conditions.[57] The anti-mosquito LC50 and LC90 values for the active principle, Neemarin, were 0.35 and 1.81 mg/L for Anopheles stephensi, the main local malaria vector, and 0.69 and 3.18 mg/L for Culex quinquefasciatus. Mortality in the pupal stage was significantly higher than in the other stages. In field trials with recommended dosages of 1 and 2 litre (L)/hectare, the mortality of Anopheles spp. larvae also was higher than the Culex spp. The main action of the compound seemed to be to prevent adult emergence and increase pupal mortality. The maximum time of efficacy was 7 days at the highest concentration (2 L/hectare).

In another study, wood scrapings were soaked in various concentrations of Neem oil diluted with acetone. Control of Anopheles stephensi and Aedes aegypti mosquitoes breeding in water storage overhead tanks was achieved with the application of the wood scrapings for a period of 45 days.[58]

The repellent properties of several plant substances, including Neem, were evaluated for their effectiveness against mosquitoes and compared with a synthetic repellent. In this investigation, Neem was found to be as effective as a personal insect repellent.[59]

A field study was carried out to evaluate the mosquito repellent action of Neem oil in tribal forested villages of District Mandla, India. Various concentrations of Neem oil mixed in coconut oil were applied to the exposed body parts of human volunteers. The results revealed a protection rate from the bites of anopheline mosquitoes of 81%–91% during the 12-hour period of observation. Thus, Neem oil, as an indigenous product, offers a practical solution for controlling mosquito populations and associated diseases.[60]

The repellent action of Neem oil was evaluated on mosquitoes in two villages near Delhi, India. Kerosene lamps containing Neem oil were burned in the living rooms of houses, and mosquitoes resting on walls or attracted to human volunteers were collected inside the rooms. Neem oil mixed in kerosene reduced the bite rates of human volunteers, as well as the number of mosquitoes resting on walls in the rooms. Protection was observed to be more pronounced against nopheles than against Culex. This 1% Neem oil-kerosene mixture may provide economical personal protection against mosquito bites.[61]

When applied to the exposed body parts of human volunteers, a repellent containing 2% Neem oil provided complete protection from the bites of all anopheline mosquito species for 12 hours. Neem oil is considered safe for external use, making it an ideal protection against malaria.[62]

In addition to its effectiveness against mosquitoes, Neem offers insecticidal potency against a number of other pest species. In India, Neem has been used as an insecticide for centuries. In tropical areas of the world where Neem grows, wreaths of its leaves are placed on doors and Neem trees are planted near houses to repel insects and other pests. Various Neem products are used in organic farming to protect crops from insect pests.

Neem seed kernel extract induced histological and histochemical alterations in the ovaries of Caryedon gangara.[63] This action was evaluated by observing oogenesis in normally maturing females reared on tamarind seed compared to those treated with Neem kernel extract. Degenerative changes in the yolk deposition of oocytes in the treated females and disturbances in the post-vitellogenic follicles were noted.

The effects of the chemicals azadirachtin, salannin, nimbin, and 6-desacetylnimbin, isolated from Neem seed kernels, have been studied on ecdysone 20-monooxygenase activity using various preparations of Drosophila melanogaster, Aedes aegypti, and Manduca sexta. In this study, the preparations were incubated with radio-labeled ecdysone and with increasing concentrations of the compounds. Neem was found to inhibit the ecdysone 20-monooxygenase (E-20-M) in all three insect species in a dose-dependent manner.[64]

In another study, aqueous and ethanolic extracts of Neem seeds, flowers, and leaves disrupted the growth and development of tobacco caterpillar larvae and Sodoptera litura at concentrations of 0.25%, 0.5%, and 1.0%. Among the abnormalities observed in the treated larvae were reductions in their size and weight. Neem seed kernel extract was found to have the highest activity, followed by that of the leaf, seed coat, and flower.[65]

Ethnoveterinary Usage

Neem bark serves as a treatment for wounds, diarrhea, ticks, and lice in poultry. The leaves are used to treat abscesses and are applied after castration and also are effective against bleeding, udder infections, fever, foot rot, and lice in ruminants. The seeds are used to remove ticks in ruminants, and the bark, seeds, leaves, and roots are insect repellents.[66,67] All parts of the Neem plant, as well as the gum and the oil, are effective against worms, wounds in the mouth, glossitis, E. coli bacillosis, swelling of the liver, jaundice, bloody dysentery, and intestinal wounds. Neem also is a remedy for constipation, indigestion, respiratory and throat disorders, asthma, pleuropneumonia, and swelling of mucous membranes in the respiratory tract and lungs. Neem is used to treat skin disorders including ringworm, alopecia, eczema, urticaria, scabies, ticks, and lice in animals. Other indications include metritis, orchitis, tetanus, stoppage of urination, swelling of the kidney, mastitis, otitis, abscess in the ear, cattle plague and rheumatism.

Dr. Sodhi's Experience

When determining whether to prescribe Neem, the practitioner should consider the following:

- Is the skin affected?
- Is an infection present (fungal, bacterial, spirochete, viral)?
- Is there any dysglycemia?
- Is contracting malaria a concern?
- Are natural ways to prevent insect bites or intestinal parasites preferred?
- Are natural contraceptives desirable?
- Adjunct to chemotherapy and vaccination therapy in cancer

My experience has shown Neem to be a quintessential herb for treating a wide variety of skin conditions. It can be used for skin disorders, including nonspecific rashes and dermatitis, fungal and bacterial infections, psoriasis, eczema, herpes simplex, and herpes zoster. In addition, I have had considerable success in prescribing Neem as a malaria prophylactic and as a contraceptive. Neem is an antimicrobial agent as well, effective against fungal, bacterial, and spirochete infections such as Lyme disease. Last but not least, Neem can reduce blood sugar levels, often in combination with other blood-sugar modulating Ayurvedic herbs such as Momordica charantia (Karveellak) and Gymnema sylvestre (Shardunika).

Case Histories

Eczema

A 30-year-old male came to my clinic from Dubai with a serious case of eczema covering his entire body. This patient had been treated with steroids several times. Each time, he had recovered only to have the eczema reappear 3 weeks after finishing the steroid treatment. I began this patient's treatment with allergy and blood testing. The results showed that his liver was inflamed and that he was highly allergic to wheat and dairy. His personal life also was pitta-aggravating and stressful, as his wife's family often fought with his family and he had frequent conflicts with his father. I prescribed an anti-pitta diet that excluded all nightshades and oranges and offered the following herbal protocol:

Skin support: A combination of Neem, Emblica officinalis (amalaki), Terminalia chebula (haritaki), Terminalia bellerica (bahera), Tinospora cordifolia (guduchi), and Rubia cordifolia (manjistha) one capsule three times per day

Liver support: One tablet three times per day—a combination of Tinospora cardifolia (guduchi), Picrorrhiza kurnoa (kutki), and Boerhaavia diffusa (purnarnava) extracts, in a proprietory blend of Phyllanthus amarus (bhumyamalaki), Swertia chirayita (kiraata), Calotropis gigantis (ark), Raphanus sativa (malaka), Berberis aristata (daaruCurcuma), Terminalia arjuna (arjun), Terminalia bellerica (bibhitaki), Terminalia chebula (haritaki), Emblica officinalis (amalaki), Solanum nigrum (kakmachi), Andrographis paniculata (bhuunimb))

Digestive support: Triphala: Emblica officianalis (amalaki), Terminalia bellerica (bahera/bibhitaki), Terminalia chebula (haritaki) one capsule three times per day

Immune support: One capsule three times per day, compound formula containing Emblica officinalis (amalaki), Ocinum sanctum (tulsi), Terminalia bellerica (bibhihtaki/ bahera), with Tinospora cordifolia (guduchi) and Glycyrrhiza glabra (mulathi), Terminalia chebula (haritaki) and Adhatoda vasica (vasaka) one capsule three times per day

- Anti-inflammatory: One teaspoon three times per day of medium chain triglyceride bound curcuminoids, a highly bio-available compound
- Finally, Ashwagandha: One capsule three times per day—as anti-inflammatory, stress adaptogen, and immune balancer

All herbal supplements were to be taken with meals. In addition, the patient was given a probiotic supplement of 100 B organisms twice daily. I also prescribed lifestyle changes including pitta-pacifying yoga postures and breathing exercises.

Three weeks later, his skin had cleared, and he subsequently decided to leave Dubai and come to the United States to distance himself from his family tensions. He divorced his wife because she would not accompany him, and he since has remarried and continues to live in the United States. He has had no recurrences of the eczema despite the continuing (long-distance) conflicts with his father.

Lyme disease

In an interesting case involving Lyme disease, a 45-year-old man called my clinic in a state of desperation. He was a health food store owner who was familiar with our herbal company because he had purchased our products for his store. He reported that he had undergone three or four courses of antibiotics for his Lyme disease with no signs of improvement. His body was swollen, he had widespread body aches, and he was extremely fatigued. We prescribed the following herbal protocol, although he refused to make any lifestyle or dietary changes:

- A combination of Neem in a proprietary blend of Emblica officinalis (amalaki), Terminalia chebula (haritaki), Terminalia bellerica (bahera), Tinospora cordifolia (guduchi), and Rubia cordifolia (manjistha): 2 capsules three times per day
- A combination of Boswelliay-a serrata, Zingiber officinale, Withania somnifera and Curcuma longa: Two capsules three times per day
- For Liver support: A combination of Tinospora cardifolia (guduchi), Picrorrhiza kurnoa (kutki), and Boerhaavia diffusa (purnarnava) extracts, in a proprietary blend of Phyllanthus amarus (bhumyamalaki), Swertia chirata (chirayita), Calotropis gigantis (ark), Raphanus sativa (malaka), Berberis aristata (daaru Curcuma), Terminalia arjuna (arjun), Terminalia bellerica (bibhitaki), Terminalia chebula (haritaki), Emblica officinalis (amalaki), Solanum nigrum (kakmachi), Andrographis paniculata (bhuunimb)): One tablet three times per day
- A medium chain triglyceride bound curcuminoids (a highly bio-available compound): One teaspoon three times per day as anti-inflammatory protocol
- Ashwgandha: two capsules three times per day

In addition, he was prescribed Probiotic 100 B, one capsule three times per day and Triphala, one capsule three times per day After 1½ months of treatment, this patient's symptoms were completely resolved.

Methicillin-resistant staphylococcus aureus (MRSA)

Several cases of MRSA have been treated successfully at our clinic. Patients who were getting repeated shots of antibiotic when put on our following protocol had no recurrence of MRSA:

- A combination of Neem in a proprietary blend of Emblica officinalis (amalaki), Terminalia chebula (haritaki), Terminalia bellerica (bahera), Tinospora cordifolia (guduchi), and Rubia cordifolia (manjistha): Two capsules three times per day

A medium chain triglyceride bound curcuminoids (a highly bio-available compound): One teaspoon three times per day with yogurt or coconut milk.

Probiotic 100B: One capsule three times a day.

Along with this protocol patients were given following dietary recommendations: NO refined or natural sugars, a diet rich in organic animal protein, beans, vegetables, and whole grains

Patients were also advised to do brisk walking for 30 minutes, yoga, and Pranayama breathing.

Chicken pox

On a family trip to Hawaii, our younger son got chicken pox and we were evicted from the hotel as a result. A friend, Dr Arthor Brownstein, came to my rescue. He hosted us and also helped me find Neem leaves in Hawaii. A mud pack with Neem leaves was applied to my son twice a day for one hour each. After two days of applying the mud pack, all chicken pox lesions dried up and crusted. We were able to fly back to Seattle on the third day.

On a similar note, foot-and-mouth disease of animals is a pox virus similar to the chicken pox virus. Millions of animals have been incarcerated in Europe, where a similar virus is easily treated in India by farmers who make decoctions of Neem leaves and feed it to animals. Animal hooves also are washed with same decoction. Within 2 to 3 days, the animals are back to normal. A similar decoction is given to animals as a prophylactic measure.

Sample Herbal Protocols

For skin infections: 1000 mg of Neem extract should be taken internally three times a day, in a base of Emblica officinalis (amalaki), Terminalia chebula (haritaki), Terminalia bellerica (bahera/bibhitaki), Tinospora cordifolia (guduchi), and Rubia cordifolia (manjistha). In addition, 500–1000 mg of Curcumin longum (Curcuma) extract and 100 billion organism probiotic capsules (or powder) should be taken twice daily. At least once a day, add 1000 mg of Neem extract to a tub of warm water along with one cup of Epsom salts, and soak the affected areas.

For herpes simplex and herpes zoster: 1500 mg Neem extract should be taken three times a day. As an external application, Neem soothes nerve endings and helps with pain. It also can be added to the bath, as above.

Eczema: In infants, eczema usually clears up when internal probiotics (100B capsule spread out over the course of a day) are given, along with daily baths in tepid water containing 500 mg of Neem extract. A nursing mother's diet also should be modified to eliminate inflammatory foods such as nightshades and oranges, as well as processed foods. Whole grains, vegetables, and fruits should be emphasized as long as the mother is nursing.

In cases of eczema in older children, Neem can be used with curcumin, along with an anti-allergic immune modulating formulation such as that noted in the eczema case above. The dosage of each should be adjusted for the child's size and age.

Tropical diseases: Neem is effective as a malaria prophylaxis and insect repellent, both to deter external insect bites and to protect against internal parasitic infestations, especially amoeba and Giardia. As a repellent, 500 mg of Neem extract three times a day should be taken for 10 days before entering the infested area. The same protocol should be followed for the duration of exposure, and for 10 additional days after leaving the area. Neem spray also can be applied externally and does not cause neurological damage, as is the case with some topical insect repellents.

Diabetes: To treat diabetes, Neem extract 500 mg, 1–3 capsules should be given three times a day, with appropriate dietary changes and daily exercise. For blood sugar control, Neem works best in combination with other formulation such as Gymnema and Shilajeet mumiyo.

Bacterial vaginitis: For bacterial vaginitis, the patient should insert one capsule of Neem into the vagina as high as possible and remain in a supine position for 15 to 20 minutes. At night, before bed, the patient may insert a probiotic capsule containing 100B live organisms. This protocol should be continued for 7–10 days unless the infection is chronic, in which case the treatment may have to be continued for several weeks or months. To increase the effectiveness of the herb, moisture should be added prior to inserting the capsules by injecting water into the vagina with an ear-cleaning bulb or empty syringe.

Hepatitis B, C and HIV: In treating hepatitis B and C, as well as HIV infections, the following should be given: a combination of Neem, Emblica officinalis (amalaki), Terminalia chebula (haritaki), Terminalia bellerica (bahera), Tinospora cordifolia (guduchi), and Rubia cordifolia (manjistha), in combination with liver and immune modulating formulas such as a combination of Tinospora cardifolia (guduchi), Picrorrhiza kurnoa (kutki), and Boerhaavia diffusa (purnarnava) extracts, in a proprietary blend of Phyllanthus amarus (bhumyamalaki), Swertia chirayita (kiraata), Calotropis gigantis (ark), Raphanus sativa (malaka), Berberis aristata (daaruCurcuma), Terminalia arjuna (arjun), Terminalia bellerica (bibhitaki), Terminalia chebula (haritaki), Emblica officinalis (amalaki), Solanum nigrum (kakmachi), Andrographis paniculata (bhuunimb) 1-2 tablets three times per day and a compound formula containing each Emblica officinalis (amalaki), Ocinum sanctum (tulsi), Terminalia bellerica (bibhihtaki/bahera), with Tinospora cordifolia (guduchi), and Glycyrrhiza glabra (mulathi), Terminalia chebula (haritaki) and Adhatoda vasica (vasaka) one capsule three times per day

Safety Profile

Neem has a low toxicity profile and a longstanding history of human use. No toxicity has been observed with moderate use, although toxic effects have been observed in the liver and kidneys of laboratory animals after administration of concentrated aqueous suspensions of fresh and dried leaves. Severe poisoning in infants and small children characterized by vomiting, loose stools, drowsiness, metabolic acidosis, anemia, polymorphonuclear leukocytosis, seizures, loss of consciousness, coma, cerebral edema, Reye's syndrome-like symptoms and death have been reported to occur within hours after ingestion of Neem oil.[68,69,70] Neem oil should be used only for topical application. Also, Neem should not be used in early pregnancy and in infertility issues. Neem should not be taken on an empty stomach because of its effects on blood sugar. Caution has to be taken while on oral hypoglycemic drugs and insulin, as it has hypoglycemic effects.

Dosage

Infusion: 10–20 ml
Powder: 1–2 g
Extract: 250 mg two times per day

Ayurvedic Properties

Rasa: Tikta (bitter), kashaya (astringent)
Guna: Laghu (light)
Vipaka: Katu (pungent)
Veerya: Shita (cold)
Dosha: Balances kapha and pitta

Notes

1. S. R. Rojatkar, V. S. Bhat, M. M. Kulkarni, V. S. Joshi, and B. A. Nagasampagi, "Tetranortriterpenoids from Azadirachta indica," *Phytochemistry*, 1989, 28(1):203.

2. P. L. Majumdar, D. C. Maiti, W. Kraus, and M. Bokel, "Nimbidiol, a modified diterpenoid of the root bark of Azadirachta indica," *Phytochemistry*, 1987, 26(11):3021.

3. I. Ara, B. S. Siddiqui, S. Faizi, and S Siddiqui, "Tricyclic diterpenoids from the root bark of Azadirachta indica," *Phytochemistry*, 1990, 29(3):911.

4. S. Siddiqui, B. S. Siddiqui, S. Faizi, and T. Mahmood, "Isoazadiorolide, a new tetratriterpenoid from Azadirachta indica A. Juss (Meliaceae)," *Heterocycles*, 1986, 24(11):3163.

5. S. Siddiqui, B. S. Siddiqui, T. Mahmood, and S. Faizi, "Tetranortriterpenoids from Azadirachta indica A. Juss (Meliaceae)," *Heterocycles*, 1989 29(1):87.

6. I. Ara, B. S. Siddiqui, S. Faizi, and S. Siddiqui, "Diterpenoids from the stem bark of Azadirachta indica," *Phytochemistry*, 1989, 28(4):1177.

7. I. Ara, B. S. Siddiqui, S. Faizi, and S. Siddiqui, "Margosinone and margosinolone, two new polyacetate derivatives from Azadirachta indica," *Fitoterapia*, 1989, 60(6):519.

8. I. Ara, B. S. Siddiqui, S. Faizi, and S. Siddiqui, "Tricyclic diterpenoids from the stem bark of Azadirachta indica," *Journal of Natural Products*, 1989, 51(6):1054.

9. S. A. Khalid, H. Duddeck, and M. Gonzalez-Sherra, "Isolation and characterization of an antimalarial agent from the neem tree Azadirachta indica" *Journal of Natural Products*, 1989, 52(5):922.

10. D. N. Tewari, *Monograph on Neem* (Dehradun, India: International Book Distributors, 1992).

11. I. Ara, B. S. Siddiqui, S. Faizi, and S. Siddiqui, "Isolation of meliacin cinnamates from the root bark of Azadirachta indica, A. Juss (Meliaceae)," *Heterocycles*, 1989, 29(4):729.

12. S. Siddiqui, T. Mahmood, B. S. Siddiqui, and S. Faizi, "Isonimolide and isolimbolide, two new tetranortriterpenoids from the twigs of Azadirachta indica A. Juss (Meliaceae)," *Heterocycles*, 1987, 26(7):1827.

13. P. P. Singh, A. Y. Junnarkar, G. P. Thomas, R. M. Tripathi, and R. K. Varma, "A pharmacological study of Azadirachta indica," *Fitoterapia*, 1990, 61(2): 164.

14. A. K. Sen, A. K. Das, and N. Banerji, "A water soluble arabinogalactan from the fruit pulp of Azadirachta indica," *Indian Journal of Chemistry*, 1993, 328:862.

15. Y. Kurokawa, T. Takeda, and Y. Ogihara, "Further studies on the structure of polysaccharides from the bark of Melia azadirachta," *Shoyakugaku Zasshi*, 1990, 44(1):29.

16. A. Waheed, G. A. Miana, and S. I. Ahmad, "Clinical investigation of hypoglycemic effect of seeds of Azadirachta-inidca in type-2 (NIDDM) diabetes mellitus," *Pak J Pharm Sci.*, Oct. 2006, 19(4):322–325.

17. R. Shukla S. Singh, and C. R. Bhandari, "Preliminary clinical trials on antidiabetic actions of Azadirachta indica," *Medicine, Surgery*, 1973; 13:11–12.

18. K. Murthy, Rao D. Satyanarayana, Rao D. Narayana, Rao D. Krishna, and L. B. Murthy, "Gopalakrishna. A preliminary study on hypoglycemic and antihyperglycemic effects of Azadirachta indica," *Indian Journal of Pharmacology*, 1978, 10(3):247–250.

19. P. Khosla, S. Bhanwra, J. Singh, S. Seth, and R. K. Srivastava, "A study of hypoglycaemic effects of Azadirachta indica (Neem) in normal and alloxan-diabetic rabbits," *Indian Journal of Physiology and Pharmacology*, 2000, 44(1):69.

20. A. Chandra. A. A. Mahdi, R. K. Singh, F. Mahdi, and R. Chander, "Effect of Indian herbal hypoglycemic agents on anti-oxidant capacity and trace elements content in diabetic rats," *J Med Food*, Sept. 2008, 11(3):506–512.

21. H.J. Zeringue and D. Bhatnagar, "Inhibition of aflatoxin production in Aspergilhis flavus infected cotton balls after treatment with neem (Azadirachta indica) leaf extracts," *J. Am. Oil Chem. Soc.*, 1990, 67(4):215.

22. V. Charles and S. X. Charles, "The use and efficacy of Azadirachta indica ADR ('Neem') and Curcuma longa ('Turmeric') in scabies. A pilot study, Medical and Cancer Research and Treatment Centre, Nagercoil, India," *Trop Geogr Med.*, Jan. 1992, 44(1–2):178–181.

23. M. M. Parida, C. Upadhyay, G. Pandya, and A. M. Jana, "Inhibitory potential of neem (Azadirachta indica Juss) leaves on dengue virus type-2 replication, Division of Virology, Defence Research and Development Establishment, Gwalior 474 002, MP, India," *J Ethnopharmacol*, Feb. 2002, 79(2):273–278.

24. L. Badam, S. P. Joshi, and S. S. Bedekar, " 'In vitro' anti-viral activity of neem (Azadirachta indica. A. Juss) leaf extract against group B coxsackieviruses, National Institute of Virology, Pune, India," *J Commun Dis.*, June 1999, 31(2):79–90.

25. D. K. Luscombe and S. A. Taha, "Pharmacological studies on the leaves of Azadirachta indica extract on Chikungunya and measles virus," *Journal of Pharmacy and Pharmacology*, 1974.

26. P. M. Raveendra, D. A. Leelavathi, and N. Udapa, "Evaluation of antiplaque activity of Azadirachta indica leaf extract gel—a 6 week clinical study," *Journal of Ethnopharmacology*, 90(1), Jan. 2004:99–103.

27. A. Vanka, S. Tandon, S. R. Rao, N. Udupa, and P. Ramkumar, "The effect of indigenous Neem Azadirachta indica [correction of (Adirachta indica)] mouth wash on Streptococcus mutans and lactobacilli growth," *Indian J Dent Res.*, July–Sept., 2001,12(3):133–144.

28. M. Sai Ram, G. Ilavazhagan, S. K. Sharma, S. A. Dhanraj, B. Suresh, M. M. Parida, A. M. Jana, K. Devendra, and W. Selvamurthy, "Anti-microbial activity of a new vaginal contraceptive NIM-76 from neem oil (Azadirachta indica)," *J Ethnopharmacol.*, Aug. 2000, 71(3):377–382.

29. N. Khanna, M. Goswami, P. Sen, and A. Ray, "Antinociceptive action of Azadirachta indica (neem) in mice: Possible mechanisms involved," *Indian Journal of Experimental Biology*, 1995, 33:848.

30. R. R. Chattopadhyay, S. K. Sarkar, S. Ganguly, and R. N. Banerjee, "Active effects of Azadirachta indica on some biochemical constituents of blood in rats," *Science and Culture*, 1992, 58(1 & 2):39.

31. S. G. Khattak, S. N. Gilani, and M. Ikram, "Antipyretic studies on some indigenous Pakistani medicinal plants," *Journal of Ethnopharmacology*, 1985, 14:45.

32. G. P. Garg, S. K. Nigam, and C. W. Ogle, "The gastric antiulcer effects of the leaves of the Neem tree," *Planta Medica*, 1993, 59:215.

33. K. P. Bhargava, M. B. Gupta, G. P. Gupta, and C. R. Mitra, "Anti-inflammatory activity of saponins and other natural products," *Indian Journal of Medical Research*, 1970, 58:724.

34. A. K. Jaiswal, S. K. Bhattacharya, and S. B. Acharya, "Anxiolytic activity of Azadirachta indica leaf extract in rats," *Indian Journal of Experimental Biology*, 1994, 32(7):489.

35. S. Yanpallewar, S. Rai, M. Kumar, S. Chauhan, and S. B. Acharya, "Neuroprotective effect of Azadirachta indica on cerebral post-ischemic reperfusion and hypoperfusion in rats," *Life Sci.*, Feb 4, 2005, 76(12):1325–1338.

36. R. R. Chattopadhyay, S. K. Sarkar, S. Ganguly, R. N. Banerjee, T. K. Basu, and A. Mukherjee, "Hepatoprotective activity of Azadirachta indica leaves on paracetamol induced hepatic damage in rats," *Indian Journal of Experimental Biology*, 1992, 30(8):738.

37. T. Fujiwara, E. Sugishita, and T. Takeda, et al., "Further studies on the structure of polysaccharides from the bark oiMelia azadirachta," *Chemical and Pharmaceutical Bulletin*, 1984, 32:1385.

38. N. R. Pillai and G. Santhakumari, "Antiarthritic and anti-inflammatory actions of nimbidin," *Planta Medica*, 1981, 43:59

39. S. N. Upadhyay, C. Kaushica, and G. P. Talwar, *Antifertility Effects of Neem (Azadirachta indica) Oil by Single Intrauterine Administration: A Novel Method for Contraception* (New Delhi, India: National Institute of Immunology).

40. G. P. Talwar, S. Shah, S. Mukherjee, and R. Chabra, "Induced termination of pregnancy by purified extracts of Azadirachta Indica (Neem): Mechanisms involved," *International Am J Reprod Immunol.*, June 1997, 37(6):485–491.

41. L. L. Owolabi, S. C. Gbotolorun, A. O. Akpantah, M. O. Ekong, M. A. Eluwa, and T. B. Ekanem, "Effect of methanolic extract of Neem leaf (Azadirachta indica) on ovarian histology and hormonal milleu," *Nig Q J Hosp Med.*, Oct.–Dec. 2008, 18(4):194–197.

42. A. Purohit, V. S. Joshi, and V. P. Dixit, "Contraceptive efficacy of Azadirachta indica (flower and bark) in male rats, a biochemical and sperm dynamics analysis," *Journal of Bioscience*, 1990, 7(4):129.

43. A. O. Prakash, A. Mishra, and R. Mathur, "Studies on the reproductive toxicity due to the extract of Azadirachta indica (seeds) in adult cyclic female rats," *Indian Drugs*, 1991, 28(4):163.

44. S. Garg, G. P. Talwar, and S. N. Upadhyay, "Immunocontraceptive activity guided fractionation and characterization of active constituents of neem (Azadirachta indica) seed extracts," *Journal of Ethnopharmacology*, 1998, 60(3):235.

45. A. Ramzanighara, F. Ezzatighadi. D. V. Rai, and D. K. Dhawan, "Effect of Neem (Azadirchta indica) on serum glycoprotein contents of rats administered 1,2 dimethylhydrazine," *Toxicol Mech Methods*, May 2009, 19(4):298–301.

46. T. Fujiwara, T. Takeda, Y. Ogihara, M. Shimizu, T. Nomura, and Y. Tomita, "Studies on the structure of polysaccharides from the bark of Melia azadirachta," *Chemical and Pharmaceutical Bulletin*, 1982, 30:4025.

47. A. Bose and R. Baral, "Natural killer cell mediated cytotoxicity of tumor cells initiated by neem leaf preparation is associated with CD40-CD40L-mediated endogenous production of interleukin-12," *Hum Immunol.*, Oct. 2007, 68(10):823–831.

48. A. Bose, K. Chakraborty, K. Sarkar, S. Goswami, T. Chakraborty, S. Pal, and R. Baral, "Neem leaf glycoprotein induces perforin-mediated tumor cell killing by T and NK cells through differential regulation of IFNgamma signaling," *J Immunother.*, Jan. 2009, 32(1):42–53.

49. S. Goswami, A. Bose, K. Sarkar, S. Roy, T. Chakraborty, U. Sanyal, and R. Baral, "Neem leaf glycoprotein matures myeloid derived dendritic cells and optimizes anti-tumor T cell functions," *Vaccine*. Feb. 3, 2010, 28(5):1241–1252.

50. A. Bose, K. Chakraborty, K. Sarkar, S. Goswami, E. Haque, T. Chakraborty, D. Ghosh, S. Roy, S. Laskar, and R. Baral, "Neem leaf glycoprotein directs T-bet-associated type 1 immune commitment," *Hum Immunol.*, Jan. 2009, 70(1):6–15.

51. K. Sarkar, A. Bose, E. Haque, K. Chakraborty, T. Chakraborty, S. Goswami, D. Ghosh, and R. Baral, "Induction of type 1 cytokines during neem leaf glycoprotein assisted carcinoembryonic antigen vaccination is associated with nitric oxide production," *Int Immunopharmacol.*," June 2009, 9(6):753–760.

52. P. Manikandan, P. Vidjaya Letchoumy, D. Prathiba, and S. Nagini, "Combinatorial chemopreventive effect of Azadirachta indica and Ocimum sanctum on oxidant-anti-oxidant status, cell proliferation, apoptosis and angiogenesis in a rat forestomach carcinogenesis model," *Singapore Med J.*, Oct. 2008, 49(10):814–822.

53. D. Ghosh, A. Bose, E. Haque, and R. Baral, "Neem (Azadirachta indica) leaf preparation prevents leukocyte apoptosis mediated by cisplatin plus 5-fluorouracil treatment in Swiss mice," *Chemotherapy*, 2009, 55(3):137–144.

54. S. K. Niture, U. S. Rao, and K. S. Srivenugopal, "Chemopreventative strategies targeting the MGMT repair protein: Augmented expression in human lymphocytes and tumor cells by ethanolic and aqueous extracts of several Indian medicinal plants," *Int J Oncol.*, Nov. 2006, 29(5):1269–1278.

55. S. N. Upadhyay, S. Dhawan, S. Garg, and G. P. Talwar, *Immunomodulatory Effects of Neem (Azadirachta indica) Oil* (New Delhi, India: National Institute of Immunology).

56. E. B. Thompson and C. C. Anderson, "Cardiovascular effects of Azadirachta indica extract," *Journal of Pharmaceutical Science*, 1978, 67, 1476.

57. H. Vatandoost and V. M. Vaziri, Larvicidal *Activity of a Neem Tree Extract (Neemarin) Against Mosquito Larvae in the Islamic Republic of Iran* (Tehran, Iran: University of Medical Science, School of Public Health and Institute of Health Research).

58. B. N. Nagpal, A. Srivastava, and V. P. Sharma, "Control of mosquito breeding using wood scrapings treated with neem oil, Malaria Research Centre, Delhi, India," *Indian J Malariol.*, June 1995, 32(2):64–69.

59. N. G. Das, D. R. Nath, I. Baruah, P. K. Talukdar, and S. C. Das, "Field evaluation of herbal mosquito repellents," *J Commun Dis.*, Dec. 1999, 31(4):241–245.

60. A. K. Mishra, N. Singh, and V. P. Sharma, "Use of neem oil as a mosquito repellent in tribal villages of mandla district, madhya pradesh. Malaria Research Centre (Field Station), Medical College Building, Jabalpur, India," *Indian J Malariol.*, Sept. 1995, 32(3):99–103.

61. V. P. Sharma and M. A. Ansari, "Personal protection from mosquitoes (Diptera: Culicidae) by burning neem oil in kerosene, Malaria Research Centre (ICMR), Delhi, India.," *J Med Entomol.*, May 1994, 31(3):505–507.

62. V. P. Sharma, M. A. Ansari, and R. K. Razdan, "Mosquito repellent action of neem (Azadirachta indica) oil, Malaria Research Centre, Delhi, India.," *J Am Mosq Control Assoc.*, Sept. 1993, 9(3):359–360.

63. B. Sufia and N. B. Chatterjee, "Histological and histochemical alteration induced by extract of neem, Azadirachta indica, kernels in the ovaries of Caryedon gangara (Caleoptera: Bruchidae)" *International Journal of Toxicology, Occupational and Environmental Health*, 1991, 1(1):247.

64. M. J. Mitchell, S. L. Smith, S. Johnson, and E. D. Morgan, "Effects of the neem tree compounds azadirachtin, salanin, nimbin and 6-desacetylnimbin on ecdysone 20-monooxygenase activity," *Archives of Insect Biochemistry and Physiology*, 1997, 35(1-2):199.

65. S. T. Prabhu and R. P. Singh, "Insect-growth regulatory activity of different parts of neem (Azadirachta indica Juss.) against tobacco caterpillar, Sodoptera litura (E)," World Neem Conference, Bangalore, India, 1993.

66. International Institute of Rural Reconstruction, *Ethnoveterinary Medicine in Asia. An Information Kit on Traditional Animal Health Care Practices, Part I, General Information* (Silang, Philippines: IIRR, 1994).

67. M. K. Jha, *Folk Veterinary Medicine of Bihar—A Research Project* (Anand, Gujrat: NDDB, 1992).

68. D. Sinniah and G. Baskaran, "Margosa oil poisoning as a cause of Reye's syndrome," *Lancet*, 1981, 1:487–489.

69. R. Sinniah, D. Sinniah, L. S. Chia, and G. Baskaran, "Animal model of margosa oil ingestion with Reye-like syndrome: Pathogenesis of microvesicular fatty liver," *J. Pathol*, 1989, 159:255–264.

70. S. M, Lai, K. W. Lim, and H. K. Cheng, "Margosa oil poisoning as a cause of toxic encephalopathy," *Singapore Med J*, 1990, 31:463–465.

Bacopa monnieri

Introduction

Bacopa monnieri, also referred to as water hyssop and Brahmi, has been used in the Ayurvedic system of medicine for centuries. This inconspicuous, creeping herb is renowned as a brain tonic, because of its reputation for enhancing memory, learning and concentration. Bacopa also provides relief from anxiety and epileptic disorders.

Bacopa forms the basis for a number of important Ayurvedic herbal preparations, including Brahmighritam and Brahmirasayanam. Ancient texts dating back as far as the sixth century BC record the use of Brahmi to promote mental function and treat mental disease. Brahmi remains an important herb in Ayurvedic medicine. It is also an important component of Chinese herbal medicine.

In Ayurveda, Brahmi is classified as astringent, bitter and coolant. It is a potent nervine, cardiotonic and diuretic, and improves respiratory function in cases of bronchoconstriction, asthma and hoarseness. Brahmi's fresh juice may be applied externally to relieve the pain of inflamed joints.

Current medical research has focused on Bacopa's effects on memory, learning and concentration. The results of such research have tended to support the traditional claims. Additional research has investigated Brahmi's potential as a safe herbal therapy for conditions including anxiety, epilepsy, bronchitis, asthma, IBS, and gastric ulcers. The herb's anti-oxidant properties offer protection from free radical damage in heart disease and certain cancers. All parts of Bacopa monierri have medicinal value.[1,2,3]

Names

English: Water hyssop, Thyme-leaved gratiola
Hindi: Brahmi
Sanskrit: Barambhi, nirabarhmi

Habitat

Brahmi is a low-growing herb which grows easily in moist and damp areas such as stream beds. In tropical regions, Brahmi grows naturally in wet soil, shallow water and marshes. It is native to India and Southeast Asia. Brahmi is found growing up to an altitude of 4000 feet (1320 meters). Brahmi is easily cultivated if adequate water is available. It's flowers and fruit appear in summer.

Botanical description

A member of the Scrophulariaccae family, this small, creeping herb is much-branched, with small leaves and light purple flowers. Bacopa's soft, sessile leaves are succulent, reniform and spatulate, measuring about 2.5 mm in length. The plant's stem has soft, ascending branches, and is about 10-30 cm long and 1-2 mm thick.

Brahmi's flowers are blue or white in color, and grow on peduncles that are usually longer than the leaves. The fruits are ovoid, with acute capsules included in a persistent calyx.

CHEMICAL COMPOSITION

The active constituents of Brahmi include alkaloids, saponins, and sterols.[4,5,6,7,8,9,10] Many of these principles, including the alkaloids brahmine and herpestin, and the saponins d-mannitol and harsaponin, acid A, and monnierin, were isolated in India over 40 years ago. Other active constituents have since been identified, including betulic acid, stigmastarol, beta-sitosterol, as well as numerous bacosides and bacopasaponins. The constituents believed to be responsible for Brahmi's cognitive effects are bacosides A and B.

Specific chemical analysis of the herb has identified the following:

Saponins and triterpenes – Bacosides and bacopasaponins, based on the bacogenins A_1-A_5, are the most prominent. These include bacosides A, B and C, with bacoside A constituting about 2.5-3%. Ebelin lactone is an acid hydrolysis byproduct of Bacoside A, yielding jujubogenin on degradation. Bacopasaponin D (a pseudojujubogenin glycoside), the bacopasaponins E and F (based on jujubogenin), hersaponin and monnierin have also been identified, along with the triterpenes betulic acid, bacosine, p-sitosterol, stigmastanol and stigmasterol.

Alkaloids – The aerial parts of Brahmi contain the alkaloids Brahmine and herpestine.

Flavonoids – A variety of flavonoids have been identified from Brahmi, including glucuronyl-7-apigenin and glucuronyl-7-luteolin, along with luteolin-7-glucoside and luteolin.

PHARMACOLOGICAL ACTIVITY

Cognitive activity

Since Brahmi's primary therapeutic use is to enhance cognitive function, the majority of research on the plant has attempted to determine the mechanisms of these effects. Studies have included clinical trials using human subjects. The acute and chronic effects of Brahmi on cognitive function have been studied in children as well as adults. In adults, it appears that Brahmi must be administered chronically in order to obtain cognitive-enhancing effects.

Significant cognitive-enhancing benefits were demonstrated when Brahmi extracts were administered regularly over a span of time. In a randomized, double-blind, placebo-controlled trial effect of Bacopa was investigated on hundred and thirty six patients. Out of one hundred and thirty-six (136) subjects that volunteered; 103 met entry criteria, 98 commenced, and 81 completed the trial. Bacopa significantly improved verbal learning, memory acquisition, and delayed recall as measured by audio verbal and visual memory performance by the Rey Auditory Verbal Learning Test (AVLT), the Rey-Osterrieth Complex Figure Test (CFT), and the Reitan Trail Making Test (TMT). Subjective memory performance was measured by the Memory Complaint Questionnaire (MAC-Q).[11]

In another study, Forty-six healthy volunteers (ages 18-60) were randomly and evenly divided into treatment and placebo groups. The same battery of cognitive tests were administered at baseline, five, and 12 weeks after the initiation of treatment. At the end of the 12-week study, the subjects receiving Brahmi showed significant improvements in verbal learning, memory consolidation, and speed of early information processing as compared to the placebo group. These effects were not observed at baseline or at five weeks. The study authors theorized that Brahmi's cognitive effects may be the result of the herb's anti-oxidant properties and/or its cholinergic effects.[12]

The same researchers undertook another study to further evaluate the cognitive effects of Brahmi extracts were evaluated in healthy human subjects in a double-blind, placebo-controlled, independent group trial design. The randomly selected subjects received 300 mg Brahmi extract or a placebo. The patients who received the Brahmi extract showed improvements in speed of visual information processing, learning rate, and memory consolidation as compared to the placebo. These results reached a maximum after 12 weeks of treatment.

Brahmi has also been found to enhance cognitive function in children. In a double-blind, randomized, placebo-controlled trial, 36 children with diagnosed attention-deficit/hyperactivity disorder were studied over a 16-week period. Nineteen of the children received an extract of Brahmi at a dosage of 50 mg twice daily for 12 weeks, and 17 were given a placebo. The mean age of the children in the two groups was 8.3 years and 9.3 years, respectively.

The children were evaluated using numerous cognitive function tests at baseline, four, eight, 12 and 16 weeks. A significant benefit was observed in Bacopa-treated subjects at 12 weeks as evidenced by improvement on sentence repetition, logical memory, and paired associate learning tasks. Evaluation showed these improvements were maintained at 16 weeks (after four weeks' placebo administration).[13]

One hundred and seven healthy participants were recruited for this double-blind placebo-controlled independent group design investigation. Sixty-two participants completed the study with 80% treatment compliance. Neuropsychological testing using the Cognitive Drug Research cognitive assessment system was conducted at baseline and after 90 days of treatment with a extract of Bacopa monnieri (2 x 150 mg) or placebo. The Bacopa monnieri product significantly improved performance on the 'Working Memory' factor, more specifically spatial working memory accuracy. The number of false positives recorded in the Rapid visual information processing task was also reduced for the Bacopa monnieri group following the treatment period.[14]

In a double-blind, placebo-controlled trial of 38 healthy volunteers (ages 18-60), subjects were given a single dose of 300 mg Bacopa monnieri extract or a placebo. The patients were examined two hours after receiving the extract, to determine the herb's maximum pharmacodynamic effect. Acute doses of the extract resulted in no significant changes in cognitive function when compared to baseline values. Parameters measured included attention, working and short-term memory, verbal learning, decision making, memory consolidation, executive processes, planning and problem solving, speed of information processing, and motor responsiveness.[15]

Brahmi's enhancing effect on learning has been demonstrated in animal studies. An aqueous suspension of an alcoholic extract of the herb was administered to rats for three or more days, according to a variety of schedules. The animals treated with Bacopa showed improved acquisition, improved retention and delayed extinction. Treated animals showed a shorter reaction time than the controls in conditioned flight reaction. This measurement was confirmed by the continuous avoidance response assessment.[16] Treatment with Brahmi also produced an improvement in learning capability as confirmed by a maze-learning experimental method.[17]

Animal studies have revealed the mechanisms of Brahmi's effect on cognitive function. The triterpenoid saponins and their bacosides have been determined to be responsible for Bacopa's ability to enhance nerve impulse transmission. The bacosides repair damaged neurons by enhancing kinase activity and neuronal synthesis, and by restorating synaptic activity and ultimately nerve impulse transmission.[18]

In a study using rats, Brahmi exerted a positive effect on passive-avoidance tasks, maximal electro-shock seizures and locomotor activity by improving cognitive effect. When Brahmi was given in combination with phenytoin (PHT) for two weeks, cognitive impairment caused by PHT was significantly reversed by the herbal extract. The study animals showed improvements in both memory acquisition and retention.[59] These results suggest that Brahmi offers an important contribution to the restoration of cognitive function, possibly in conjunction with the application of growth factors.[19]

Animals treated with Brahmi extract showed significant improvement in a series of tests which measured visual-motor and perceptual ability as well as memory span. The tests were administered at baseline and at the end of treatment. Significant improvements were noted in strengthened exploratory drive (as measured by maze learning), perceptual images of patterns, and increased perceptual organization and reasoning ability (as measured by reaction time).[20]

Loss of cholinergic neuronal activity in the hippocampus is a primary characteristic of Alzheimer's disease.[21] Animal study results have shown bacosides to have anti-oxidant activity in the hippocampus, frontal cortex, and striatum.[22] Animal research has shown that Brahmi extracts modulate the expression of important enzymes involved in generation and scavenging of reactive oxygen in the brain.[23] In vitro research has determined that Brahmi exerts a protective effect against DNA damage in astrocytes[24] and human fibroblasts.[25]

Anti-amnesic activity

Benzodiazepines are known to produce amnesia by involvement of GABAergic system and by interference of long term potentiation (LTP). A study was done to evaluate effect of Bacopa monnieri on downstream molecules of LTP after diazepam induced amnesia in mice. Morris water maze scale was used to evaluate the effect of Bacopa monnieri after screening for muscle coordination by rota rod. The index of acquisition and retrieval was recorded as escape latency time (ELT). Behavioral results showed that Bacopa monnieri (120 mg kg(-1) oral) significantly reversed diazepam (1.75 mg kg(-1) i.p.) induced amnesia in Morris water maze task. The molecular studies revealed that diazepam upregulated mitogen activated protein kinase (MAP kinase), phosphorylated cAMP-response element-binding protein (pCREB) and inducible nitric oxide synthase (iNOS), while it down regulated nitrite, nitrate, total nitrite, cAMP response element binding protein (CREB) expression, phosphodiesterase, cyclic adenosine monophosphate (cAMP) without affecting calmodulin levels. Bacopa monnieri suppressed the diazepam induced upregulation of MAP kinase, pCREB and iNOS and attenuated the downregulation of nitrite. It did not affect the cAMP, PDE, nitrate, total nitrite, total CREB level. These behavioral findings displayed the reversal of diazepam-induced amnesia by Bacopa monnieri.[26]

A follow up to the Benzodiazepam study was done now using Scopolamine, an anticholinergic drug. Scopolamine is reported to produce amnesia by interference of long term potentiation and has been used for discerning the efficacy of various antiamnesic drugs. The intoxication with anticholinergics and benzodiazepines tend to produce neurodegeneration which cause memory deficits. Study was done to evaluate how scopolamine affects downstream signaling molecules of long term potentiation and if Bacopa monnieri can modulate the scopolamine induced amnesia. Morris water maze scale was used to test the amnesic effect of scopolamine and its reversal by Bacopa monnieri. Rota-rod test was used to screen muscle coordination activity of mice before water maze investigations were carried out.

The results showed that scopolamine down regulated protein kinase C and iNOS without affecting cAMP, protein kinase A, calmodulin, MAP kinase, nitrite, CREB and pCREB. Bacopa monnieri reversed the scopolamine induced amnesia by significantly improving calmodulin and by partially attenuating protein kinase C and pCREB. These observations suggest involvement of calmodulin in evoking antiamnesic effects of Bacopa monnieri.[27]

PSAPP mice expressing the "Swedish" amyloid precursor protein and M146L presenilin-1 mutations are a well-characterized model for spontaneous amyloid plaque formation. To evaluate the effect of Bacopa monnieri extract (BME) on amyloid (Abeta) pathology in PSAPP mice, two doses of BME (40 or 160 mg/kg/day) were administered starting at 2 months of age for either 2 or 8 months. The data suggested that Bacopa monnieri extract lowers A beta 1-40 and 1-42 levels in cortex by as much as 60%, and reverses Y-maze performance and open field hyper locomotion behavioral changes present in PSAPP mice. The data suggest that Bacopa monnieri extract has potential application in Alzheimer's disease therapeutics.[28]

Anti-anxiety and anti-depressant activity

A study was done to evaluate effects of Bacopa monnieri whole plant standardized dry extract on cognitive function and affect and its safety and tolerability in healthy elderly study participants. The study was a randomized, double-blind, placebo controlled clinical trial with a placebo run-in of 6 weeks and a treatment period of 12 weeks. Volunteers were recruited from the community to a clinic in Portland, Oregon by public notification. Fifty-four (54) participants, 65 years or older (mean 73.5 years), without clinical signs of dementia, were recruited and randomized to Bacopa or placebo. Forty-eight (48) completed the study with 24 in each group. Standardized Bacopa monnieri extract 300 mg/day or a similar placebo tablet orally for 12 weeks. The primary outcome variable was the delayed recall score from the Rey Auditory Verbal Learning Test (AVLT). Other cognitive measures were the Stroop Task assessing the ability to ignore irrelevant information, the Divided Attention Task (DAT), and the Wechsler Adult Intelligence Scale (WAIS) letter digit test of immediate working memory. Affective measures were the State-Trait Anxiety Inventory, Center for Epidemiologic Studies Depression scale (CESD)-10 depression scale, and the Profile of Mood States. Vital signs were also monitored. Controlling for baseline cognitive deficit using the Blessed Orientation-Memory-Concentration test, Bacopa participants had enhanced AVLT delayed word recall memory scores relative to placebo. Stroop results were similarly significant, with the Bacopa group improving and the placebo group unchanged. CESD-10 depression scores, combined state plus trait anxiety scores, and heart rate decreased over time for the Bacopa group but increased for the placebo group. No effects were found on the DAT, WAIS digit task, mood, or blood pressure. The dose was well tolerated with few adverse events (Bacopa n = 9, placebo n = 10), primarily stomach upset.[29]

A one-month, limited clinical trial of 35 patients with diagnosed anxiety neurosis demonstrated that administration of Brahmi syrup (30 ml. daily in two divided doses, equivalent to 12 g dry crude extract of Bacopa) resulted in a significant decrease in anxiety symptoms, level of anxiety, level of disability, and mental fatigue, and an increase in immediate memory span. Other changes noted were increased body weight, decreased respiration rate, and decreased systolic blood pressure.[30]

Research using a rat model of clinical anxiety demonstrated a Bacopa extract of 25-percent bacoside A exerted anxiolytic activity comparable to Lorazepam, a common benzodiazepine anxiolytic drug. Importantly, the Bacopa extract did not induce amnesia, a side effect associated with Lorazepam, but instead had a memory-enhancing effect.[31]

Anti-epileptic activity

Although Brahmi is indicated as an anti-epileptic in Ayurveda, animal research shows anticonvulsant activity only at high doses over extended periods of time. Research in India showed that hersaponin (an active constituent) protected study animals against seizures.[32] In an additional study, Brahmi extracts given for 15 days demonstrated anticonvulsant activity. However, when Brahmi was administered acutely at lower doses, anticonvulsant activity was not observed.[33]

Anti-oxidant properties

In research on the frontal cortex, striatal and hippocampal regions of rat's brains, Brahmi was shown to exert anti-oxidant activity.[34] This action was believed to be the result of the herb's alteration of superoxide dismutase, catalase and glutathione peroxidase levels. Brahmi's anti-oxidant activity was comparable to Deprenyl.

This study also revealed that Brahmi induced a dose-related action in all brain regions, while Deprenyl acted only on the frontal cortex and striatum. The effect was considered to be the result of an increase in oxidative free radical scavenging. Brahmi's alcoholic extract was found to protect against ferrous sulphate and cumene hydroperoxide induced experimental lipid peroxidation, at levels equivalent to the anti-oxidants EDTA and vitamin E. These effects extended to hepatic glutathione content and were found to be dose dependent.[35]

Bronchodilatory activity

Animal studies have demonstrated that Brahmi extracts exert a relaxant effect on chemically-induced bronchoconstriction, probably by inhibiting calcium influx across cell membranes. An earlier in vitro study demonstrated Brahmi's broncho-vasodilatory activity on rabbit and guinea pig tracheas, pulmonary arteries, and aortas.[36]

A subsequent study confirmed these results. Methanolic sub-fractions of Brahmi extracts were given to anesthetized rats prior to induction of bronchoconstriction with carbachol, an acetylcholine analogue. Nearly all of the Brahmi sub-fractions inhibited carbachol-induced bronchoconstriction, hypotension, and bradycardia in this animal model.[37,38]

An in vitro study also demonstrated the potent mast cell-stabilizing activity of Brahmi's methanol extract. This action was comparable to disodium cromoglycate, a commonly allergy medication.[39] These studies indicate the potential of Brahmi in bronchoconstrictive and allergic conditions.

Gastrointestinal activity

A variety of study models, including clinical trials, have investigated Brahmi's gastroprotective effects.

In a double-blind, randomized, placebo-controlled trial of 169 patients with Irritable Bowel Syndrome (IBS), the effectiveness of an Ayurvedic preparation containing Brahmi and Bael fruit with a standard drug therapy consisting of clidinium bromide, chlordiazepoxide, and psyllium.

The subjects were divided into five sub-groups based on the type of IBS they experienced, and were randomly assigned to standard drug treatment, botanical treatment, or placebo three times daily. Although this study's results revealed standard drug therapy to be superior to the Ayurvedic preparation in most cases, patients with IBS characterized by diarrhea experienced greater improvement with the herbal therapy. The Ayurvedic therapy was superior to the placebo in all parameters examined.[40]

Animal and in vitro studies suggest that Brahmi may have a protective and curative effect against gastric ulcers. The prophylactic and healing properties of a Brahmi extract standardized for bacoside A were evaluated for their effects in five gastric ulcer models in mice. At a dose of 20 mg/kg given over a period of ten days, the extract healed penetrating ulcers induced by acetic acid, strengthened the mucosal barrier, and decreased mucosal exfoliation. The extract also alleviated stress-induced ulcers, as observed by a significant reduction in lipid peroxidation in gastric mucosa. Possible explanations for this action include Brahmi's anti-oxidant properties and its ability to balance SOD and catalase levels.[41]

In vitro studies [42] have demonstrated Brahmi's direct spasmolytic activity on intestinal smooth muscle tissue, by inhibiting calcium influx across cell membrane channels. These results suggest a potential therapeutic role for Brahmi in treating conditions characterized by intestinal spasms, such as IBS.

Another in vitro study demonstrated Brahmi extract's anti-microbial activity against Helicobacter pylori, a bacteria associated with chronic gastric ulcers. When the extract was incubated with human colonic mucosal cells infected with Helicobacter pylori, an accumulation of prostaglandin E and prostacyclin, prostaglandins which are known to be protective for gastric mucosa, was observed.[43]

Cardioprotective activity

Brahmi is often mentioned in Ayurvedic texts as a cardiotonic, however, few studies have been conducted to support this claim. In research using rabbit aortas and pulmonary arteries, Brahmi extract exerted a vasodilatory effect on calcium chloride-induced contraction in both types of tissue. It is believed that Brahmi exerted this effect by interfering with calcium channel flux in the experimental tissue cells. Bacopa also stabilized mast cells in vitro, exerted anti-inflammatory activity by inhibiting prostaglandin synthesis and lysosomal membrane stabilization.[44]

Thyroid regulatory activity

High doses of Brahmi extract (200 mg/kg) increased levels of the thyroid hormone T4 by 41% when given orally to mice. The thyroid hormone T3 was not stimulated, suggesting that Brahmi extract may directly stimulate synthesis and/or release of T4 at the glandular level, while not affecting conversion of T4 to T3. While this study indicates that Brahmi extract stimulates thyroid function, the doses given to create this effect were very high. The typical 200-400 mg daily dose of Brahmi given to humans may not produce the same effect.[45]

Wound healing activity

Methanolic extract of Bacopa monnieri and its isolated constituent Bacoside-A were screened for wound healing activity. Bacoside-A was screened for wound healing activity by excision, incision and dead space wound on Swiss albino rats. Significant wound healing activity was observed in both extract and the Bacoside-A treated groups. The SDS-PAGE caseinolytic zymogram analysis of inhibition of matrix metalloproteases (MMPs) enzyme from the excision wound by Bacoside-A, an isolated constituent, was done with the concentrations 100 and 200 micromg/ml. In Bacoside-A treated groups, epithelialization of the excision wound was faster with a high rate (18.30 +/- 0.01 days) of wound contraction. The tensile strength of the incision wound was increased (538.47 +/- 0.14 g) in the Bacoside-A treated group. In the dead space wound model, the weight of the granuloma was also increased (89.15 +/- 0.08 g). The histological examination of the granuloma tissue of the Bacoside-A treated group showed increased cross-linking of collagen fibers and absence of monocytes. The wound healing activity of Bacoside-A was more effective in various wound models compared to the standard skin ointment Nitrofurazone.[46]

Anti-arthritic

Study investigated the therapeutic efficacy of Bacopa monnieri in treating rheumatoid arthritis using a type II collagen-induced arthritis rat model. Arthritis was induced in male Wistar rats by immunization with bovine type II collagen in complete Freund's adjuvant. Bacopa monnieri extract (BME) was administered after the development of arthritis from day 14 onwards. The total duration of experiment was 60 days. Paw swelling, arthritic index, inflammatory mediators such as cyclooxygenase, lipoxygenase, myeloperoxidase and serum anti-collagen IgG and IgM levels were analyzed in control and experimental rats. Arthritic induction significantly increased paw edema and other classical signs of arthritis coupled to upregulation of inflammatory mediators such as cyclooxygenase, lipoxygenase, neutrophil infiltration and increased anti-collagen IgM and IgG levels in serum. BME significantly inhibited the footpad swelling and arthritic symptoms. BME was effective in inhibiting cyclooxygenase and lipoxygenase activities in arthritic rats. Decreased neutrophil infiltration was evident from decreased myeloperoxidase activity and histopathological data where an improvement in joint architecture was also observed. Serum anti-collagen IgM and IgG levels were consistently decreased. Thus the study demonstrates the potential anti-arthritic effect of Bacopa monnieri for treating arthritis which might confer its anti-rheumatic activity.[47]

Anti-withdrawal effect and Anti-toxicity activity

Animal and in vitro studies indicate that Brahmi extract may have a protective effect against certain drugs and their side effects. An in vitro study using guinea pig ileum isolates studied the effect of Brahmi extract on drug-induced morphine withdrawal. When tissue isolates were treated with a Brahmi extract at a concentration of 1,000 pg/ml prior to injection of morphine, the treatment significantly reduced the associated withdrawal effects.[48] This effect may be due to the anticholinergic and calcium antagonistic activities reported in other studies.(Dar A, Channa S et al)

Further research examined the effects of an alcoholic Brahmi extract on morphine-induced hepatoxicity in rats, as measured by lipid peroxide accumulation and anti-oxidant enzyme levels. When Brahmi was administered along with morphine in rat hepatic tissue, lipid peroxidation was inhibited, and anti-oxidant enzymes and glutathione levels were increased in rat hepatic tissue, when compared to morphine alone. These results suggest that Brahmi exerts a protective effect on the hepatic anti-oxidant status in morphine-treated rats.[49] Similar research reported the same type of effect on the mitochondrial enzyme activity in the brains of morphine treated rats.[50]

Morphine intoxicated rats received 10-160 mg/kg body weight of morphine hydrochloride intraperitoneally for 21 days. Bacopa monnieri Extract (BME) pretreated rats were administered with BME (40 mg/kg) orally once a day 2 h before the injection of morphine for 21 days. Pretreatment with Bacopa monnieri Extract has shown to possess a significant protective effect against morphine-induced liver and kidney functions in terms of serum glutamate oxaloacetate transaminase, serum glutamate pyruvate transaminase, alkaline phosphatase, lactate dehydrogenases and gamma-glutamyl transferase activities and urea, creatinine and uric acid level respectively. Histopathological changes of liver and kidney were also in accordance with the biochemical findings. The results of this study indicate that Bacopa monnieri extract exerted a protection against morphine-induced liver and kidney toxicity.[51]

Some anti-epileptic drugs, such as phenytoin, can result in cognitive impairment.[52] When Brahmi extract was given along with this drug to mice, cognitive impairment was significantly reversed, as evidenced by improved memory acquisition and retention.[53]

Anti-cancer activity

In vitro research demonstrated that various fractions of Brahmi extract exert cytotoxic activity against sarcoma-180 cells. This action may be due to inhibition of DNA replication in the cancerous cell line.[54]

Ethnoveterinary usage

Brahmi's leaves are used in tribal veterinary medicine, particularly in the treatment of epilepsy.[55]

Dr. Sodhi's Experience

When considering treatment with Brahmi, the following questions should be asked by the practitioner:

- Is there damage to or weakness of connective tissue and/or collagen?
- Is mental weakness present?
- Has the skin been damaged? Are there wounds or burns?
- Is the disorder auto-immune?

Brahmi is an immune-modulating herb that also strengthens collagen. Because of these properties, it provides excellent therapy for all auto-immune disease affecting tissues containing collagen, such as rheumatoid arthritis, lupus, lichen sclerosis, and scleroderma. Brahmi supports the skin and is used for wound and burn healing, both internally and externally. Brahmi is also used as a brain tonic. Ironically, its leaves look like tiny brains.

Herbal Protocols

Scleroderma

For collagen support and immune modulation – Combination of Brahmi extract, Ginkgo biloba, Convolvulus pluricaulis (Shankhapushpi) extract, Withania Somnifera (Ashwagandha) and Gotu kola 2-3 capsules three times a day.

For inflammation and immune modulation

A medium chain triglyceride bound curcuminoids which is a very bio-available compound one teaspoon twice a day.

Boswellia serrata (Salai) extract, 300 mg, with Zingiber officinale (yastimadhu) and Withania somnifera (Ashwagandha) extracts, 100 mg each, three times a day.

Commiphora mukul (Guggul) extract, 300 mg, in a formulation with 80 mg of Triphala, consisting of equal parts Emblica officinalis (Amalaki), Terminalia bellerica (Bibhitaki), Terminalia chebula (Haritaki), and 25 mg Guggulu whole herb, three times a day.

For liver support

Tinospora cardifolia (Guduchi), Picrorrhiza kurnoa (Kutki), and Boerhaavia diffusa (Purnarnava) extracts, Phyllanthus amarus (Bhumyamalaki), Swertia chirayita (Kiraata), Calotropis gigantis (ark), Raphanus sativa (malaka), Berberis aristata (daaru Curcuma), Terminalia arjuna (arjun), Terminalia bellerica (bibhitaki), Terminalia chebula (haritaki), Emblica officinalis (amalaki), Solanum nigrum (kakmachi), and Andrographis paniculata (bhuunimb).

Lupus protocol

For Lupus patients, the following Salai protocol should be used: Boswellia serrata (salai) extract, Zingiber officinale and Withania somnifera each, and Curcuma longa (Curcuma) extract and (Ashwagandha) extracts 2-3 times per day.

When treating Lupus, Brahmi should be added to the above protocol for connective tissue repair.

Safety profile

Therapeutic doses of Brahmi are not associated with any known side effects. The herb has been used safely in Ayurvedic medicine for hundreds of years. A double-blind, placebo-controlled clinical trial of healthy male volunteers investigated the safety of pharmacological doses of isolated bacosides over a four-week period. Concentrated bacosides given in single (20-30 mg) and multiple (100-200 mg) daily doses were well-tolerated, and no adverse effects were reported.[Singh HK]

Drug Interactions

Brahmi has been observed in animal models to decrease the toxicity of morphine[Sumathhy T] and phenytoin.[Vohora D] It has also been shown, although inconsistently, to have a slight sedative effect, so caution is advised when using the herb in combination with other known sedatives. Since Brahmi appears to stimulate T4 activity in animals at very high doses, Brahmi may alter the activity of thyroid stimulating drugs or inhibit the effect of thyroid suppressant drugs.

Dosage

Traditional daily doses of Brahmi are 5-10 g of non-standardized power, 8-16 ml of infusion, and 30 ml daily of syrup.

Dosages of a 1:2 fluid extract are: 5-12 ml. per day for adults and 2.5-6 ml. per day for children ages 6-12.

For Brahmi extracts standardized to 20% bacosides A and G, the dosage is 200-400 mg daily in divided doses for adults, and 100-200 mg daily for children.

Ayurvedic properties

Rasa: Tikta (bitter)
Guna: Laghu (light), snigdha (unctuous)
Veerya: Ushna (hot)
Vipaka: Katu (pungent)
Dosha: Pacifies kapha and vata

Notes

1. Chopra RN, Indigenous Drugs of India, 2nd ed. Calcutta India: U.N. Dhur and Sons: 1958:341.

2. Nadkarni KM. The Indian Materia Medica. Columbia, MO: South Asia Books; 1988:624-625.

3. Bone K. Clinical Applications of Ayurvedic and Chinese Herbs: Monographs for the Western Herbal Practitioner. Warwick, Queensland: Phytotherapy Press; 1996.

4. Kapoor LD: CRC Handbook of Ayurvedic Medicinal Plants. Boca Raton, FL: CRC Press Inc; 1990;61.

5. Chakravarty AK, Garai S, Masuda K, et al. Bacopasides III-V: Three new triterpenoid glycosides from Bacopa monniera. Chem Pharm Bull (Tokyo) 2003;51:215-217.

6. Hou CC, Lin SJ, Cheng JT, Hsu FL. Bacopaside III, bacopasaponin G. and bacopasides A, B, and C from Bacopa monniera. J Nat Prod 2002;65:1759-1763.

7. Mahato SB, Garai S, Chakravarty AK. Bacopasaponins E and F: two jujubogenin bisdesmosides from Bacopa monniera. Phytochemistry 2000;53:711-714.

8. Chakravarty AK, Sarkar T, Masuda K, et al. Bacopaside I and II: two pseudojujubogenin glycosides from Bacopa monniera. Phytochemistry 2001;58:553-556.

9. Chatterjee N. Rastogi RP. Dhar ML 1963 Chemical examination of Bacopa monnieri, I. Isolation of chemical constituents. Indian Journal of Chemistry 1:212

10. Proliac A, Chabaud A. Raynaud J 1991 Two O-glucuronyl flavones in the stems and leaves of Bacopa monnieri L. (Scrofulariaceae). Pharmaceutica Acta Helvetica 66(5-6}:153

11. Morgan A, Stevens J. Does Bacopa monnieri improve memory performance in older persons? Results of a randomized, placebo-controlled, double-blind trial. J Altern Complement Med. 2010 Jul;16(7):753-9.

12. Stough C, Lloyd J, Clarke J, Downey LA, Hutchison CW, Rodgers T, Nathan PJ. The chronic effects of an extract of Bacopa monniera (Brahmi) on cognitive function in healthy human subjects. Psychopharmacology (Berl). 2001 Aug;156(4):481-4.

13. Negi KS, Singh YD, Kushwaha KP, et al. Clinical evaluation of memory enhancing properties of Memory Plus in children with attention deficit hyperactivity disorder. Ind J Psychiatry 2000;42:Supplement.

14. Stough C, Downey LA, Lloyd J, Silber B, Redman S, Hutchison C, Wesnes K, Nathan PJ. Examining the nootropic effects of a special extract of Bacopa monniera on human cognitive functioning: 90 day double-blind placebo-controlled randomized trial. Phytother Res. 2008 Dec;22(12):1629-34.

15. Nathan, P. J., Clarke, J., Lloyd, J., Hutchison, C. W., Downey, L. and Stough, C. (2001), The acute effects of an extract of Bacopa monniera (Brahmi) on cognitive function in healthy normal subjects. Human Psychopharmacology: Clinical and Experimental, 16: 345–351.

16. Singh HK. Dhawan BN 1982 Effect of Bacopa monniera Linn. (Brahmi) extract on avoidance responses in rat. *Journal of Ethnopharmacology* 5{2):205

17. Dey CD, Bose S, Mitra S 1976 Effect of some centrally active phyto products on maze learning of albino rats. Indian Journal of Physiology and Allied Sciences 30(3):88

18. Singh HK, Dhawan BN. Neuropschopharmacological effects of the Ayurvedic nootropic Bacopa monniera Linn. (Brahmi) Indian J Pharmacol 1997;29:S359-S365.

19. Kidd PM 1999 A review of nutrients and botanicals in the integrative management of cognitive dysfunction. Alternative Medicine Review 4:3:144.

20. Sharma R, Chaturvedi C, Tewari PV. Efficacy of Bacopa monnieri in revitalizing intellectual functions in children.

21. Enz A, Amstutz R, Boddeke H, et al Brain selective inhibition of acetylcholinesterase: a novel approach to therapy for Alzheimer's disease. Prog Brain Res 1993;98:431-438.

22. Amar Jyoti, Deepak Sharma. Neuroprotective role of Bacopa monniera extract against aluminium-induced oxidative stress in the hippocampampus of rat brain. NeuroToxicology; Vol 27(4); Jul 2006; pp 451-457.

23. Chowdhuri DK, Parmar D, Kakkar P, et al. Antistress effects of bacosides of Bacopa monnieri; modulation of Hsp 70 expression, superoxide dismutase and cytochrome P450 activity in rat brain. Phytother Res 2002;16:639-645.

24. Russo A, Borrielli F, Campisi A et al. Nitric oxide-related toxicity in cultured astrocytes; effect of Bacopa monniera. Life Sci 2003;73:1517-1526.

25. Russo A, Izzo A, Borrelli F, et al. Free radical scavenging capacity and protective effect of Bacopa monniera L. on DNA damage. Phytotherapy Res 2003;17:870-875.

26. Saraf MK, Prabhakar S, Pandhi P, Anand A. Bacopa monniera ameliorates amnesic effects of diazepam qualifying behavioral-molecular partitioning. Neuroscience. 2008 Aug 13;155(2):476-84.

27. Saraf MK, Anand A, Prabhakar S. Scopolamine induced amnesia is reversed by Bacopa monniera through participation of kinase-CREB pathway. Neurochem Res. 2010 Feb;35(2):279-87.

28. Holcomb LA, Dhanasekaran M, Hitt AR, Young KA, Riggs M, Manyam BV. Bacopa monniera extract reduces amyloid levels in PSAPP mice. J Alzheimers Dis. 2006 Aug;9(3):243-51.

29. Calabrese C, Gregory WL, Leo M, Kraemer D, Bone K, Oken B. Effects of a standardized Bacopa monnieri extract on cognitive performance, anxiety, and depression in the elderly: a randomized, double-blind, placebo-controlled trial. J Altern Complement Med. 2008 Jul;14(6):707-13.

30. Singh RH, Singh L. Studies on the anti-anxiety effect of the Medyha Rasayana drug, Brahmi (Bacopa monniera Wettst.) – Part I. J Rest Ayur Siddha 1980;1:133-148.

31. S.K. Bhattacharya1, S. Ghosal. Anxiolytic activity of a standardized extract of Bacopa monniera: an experimental study. Phytomedicine Volume 5, Issue 2, April 1998, Pages 77–82

32. Ganguly DK, Malhotra CL. Some behavioral effects of an active fraction from Herpestis monniera, Linn. (Brahmi). Ind J Med Res 1967;55:473-482.

33. Martis G, Rao A. Neuropharmacological activity of Herpestis monniera. Fitoteropia 1992;63:399-404.

34. Bhattacharya SK, Bhattacharya A, Kumar A, Ghosal S 2000 Anti-oxidant activity of Bacopa monniera in rat frontal cortex, striatum and hippocampus. Phyto therapy Research 14(3): 174-179.

35. Tripathi YB, Chaurasia S, Tripathi E, Upadhyay A, Dubey GP 1996 Batopa monniera Linn, as an anti-oxidant: mechanism of action. Indian Journal of Experimental Biology 34(6):523

36. Dar A, Channa S. Relaxant effect of ethanol extract of Bacopa monniera on trachea, pulmonary artery and aorta from rabbit and guinea pig. Phytother Res 1997;11:323-325

37. Channa S, Dar A, Yaqoob M, et al. Bronchovasodilatory activity of fractions and pure constitutients isolated from Bacopa monniera. J Ethnopharmacology 2003;86:27-35

38. Dar A, Channa S 1997 Bronchodilatory and cardiovascular effects of an ethanol extract of Bacopa monniera in anesthetized rats. Phytomedicine 4(4):319

39. Samiulla DS, Prashanth D, Amit A, Mast cell stabilizing activity of Bacopa monnieri. Fitoterapia 2001;72:284-285.

40. Yadav SK, Jain AK, Triphathi SN, Gupta JP, Irritable bowel syndrome: therapeutic evaluation of indigenous drugs. Indian J Med Res 1989;90:496-503.

41. Sairam K, Rao CV, Babu MD, Goel RK, Prophylactic and curative effects of Bacopa monniera in gastric ulcer models. Phytomedicine 2001;8:423-430.

42. Dar A, Channa S. Calcium antagonistic activity of Bacopa monniera on vascular and intestinal smooth muscles of rabbit and guinea pig. J Ethnopharmacol 1999;66:167-174.

43. Goel RK, Sairam K, Babu MD, et al. In vitro evaluation of Bacop monniera on anti-Helicobacter pylori activity and accumulation of prostaglandins. Phytomedicine 2003;10:523-527.

44. Jain P, Khanna NK, Trehan TN, et al. Antiinflammatory effects of an Ayurvedic preparation., Brahmi Rasayan, in rodents. Indian J Exp Biol 1994;32:633-636.

45. Kar A, Panda S, Bharti S. Relative efficacy of three medicinal plant extracts in the alteration of thyroid hormone concentrations in male mice. J Ethnopharmacol 2002;82:75-81.

46. Sharath R, Harish BG, Krishna V, Sathyanarayana BN, Swamy HM. Wound healing and protease inhibition activity of Bacoside-A, isolated from Bacopa monnieri wettest. Phytother Res. 2010 Aug;24(8):1217-22.

47. Viji V, Kavitha SK, Helen A. Bacopa monniera (L.) wettst inhibits type ii collagen-induced arthritis in rats. Phytother Res. 2010 Mar 22.

48. Sumathi T, Nayeem M Balakrishna K, et al. Alcoholic extract of Bacopa monniera reduces the in vitro effects of morphine withdrawal in guinea pig ileum. J Ethnopharmacol 2002;82:75-81.

49. Sumathhy T, Subramanian S, Govindasamy S, et al. Protective role of Bacopa monniera on morphine-induced hepatotoxicity in rats. Phytotherapy Res 2002:15;643-645.

50. Sumathy T, Govindasamy S, Balakrishna K, Veluchamy G. Protective role of Baope monniera on morphine-induced brain mitochondrial enzyme activity in rats. Fiterapia 2002;73:381-385.

51. Sumathi T, Niranjali Devaraj S. Effect of Bacopa monniera on liver and kidney toxicity in chronic use of opioids. Phytomedicine. 2009 Oct;16(10):897-903.

52. Smith DB. Cognitive effects of anti-epileptic drugs. Adv Neurol 1991;55:197-212.

53. Vohora D, Pal SN Pillai KK. Protection from phenytoin-induced cognitive deficit by Bacopa monniera, a reputed Indian nootropic plant. J Ethnopharmacol 2000;71:383-390.

54. Elangovan V, Govindasamy S, Ramamoorthy N, Balasubramaanian K. In vitro studies on the anticancer activity of Bacopa monnieri. Fitoterapia 1995;66:211-215.

55. Jha MK1992 Folk veterinary medicine of Bihar-a research project. NDDB, Anand, Gujrat.

7

Berberis aristata

Introduction

Berberis aristata, known in Ayurveda as Daruhaldi, is a spiny shrub commonly found on the slopes of the sub-Himalayas. The root bark of Daruhaldi forms the base for the Ayurvedic preparation Rasaunt, a bitter tincture that is highly effective in treating skin disorders. In addition to the root bark, all the other parts of Daruhaldi have medicinal value.

Rasaunt most often is used as a wash for topical treatment of skin ulcers and sores, acne, and hemorrhoids. To make the preparation, the roots and lower parts of Daruhaldi's stem are boiled in water and strained. The remaining water is allowed to evaporate, leaving a semi-solid mass of cylindrical pieces with a faint odor and a bitter taste.

A versatile preparation, Rasaunt either may be diluted with water to form a medicinal wash for the uses named above, or mixed with alum or ghee (clarified butter) to make an ointment. In this form, Rasaunt is used topically for treating eye disorders, and for external inflammation, including swollen glands.

Daruhaldi also may be taken internally in the form of a bitter tonic, which has stomachic, cholagogue, antiperiodic, and alterative properties. The sweet, juicy fruits are given to children as a cooling laxative. Daruhaldi extract, sweetened with honey, is used to treat liver aliments and jaundice. Because of its anti-inflammatory properties, Daruhaldi is useful in treating rheumatism.

Synonymous Names

English: Indian barberry, tree turmeric
Hindi: Daruhaldi
Sanskrit: Daru Curcuma

Habitat

The Daruhaldi shrub grows wild in the sub-Himalayan tract at altitudes ranging from 3000 feet to 7500 feet (850 to 2,500 meters). It also grows in Ceylon, and is cultivated in many other areas.

Botanical Characteristics

Daruhaldi is an erect, spiny shrub that reaches a height of 9–18 feet (3-6 meters). The yellowish brown bark peels away easily from the stem in long strips. The inner wood is hard and yellow. The spines growing along Daruhaldi's stem are actually modified leaves, which have three branches and are about 1.5 cm long.

The deep green leaves grow in clusters of five to eight. They are elliptical in shape and have toothed margins, measuring about 5 cm long and 2 cm wide. The plant's yellow flowers grow on stalks and measure about 12 mm in diameter when they are fully opened. The purple fruits are plum-shaped, measuring about 7 mm long. Each fruit contains 2 to 5 seeds, ranging in color from yellow to pink.

Daruhaldi flowers from early March until the end of April and bears fruit from mid-May throughout June. The fruit stays on the shrub for quite a long time after becoming ripe, but falls off soon after the rainy season begins.

Chemical Composition

The chief active constituent of Berberis aristata is the bitter alkaloid berberine. Also present are various tannins, resins, gums, starches, and other alkaloids.[1, 2, 3,4,5,6]

Alkaloids

Daruhaldi's root and stem bark contain high concentrations of the alkaloids berberine, berbamine, aromaline, karachine, palmatine, oxyacanthine, oxyberberine, taxilamine, and jatrorrhizine. The chitrianines A, B, and C, and dihydropalmatine-N-oxide also have been isolated from Daruhaldi's roots.

Flavonoids and polyphenolics

Daruhaldi's roots and flowers contain quercetin and 3-O-diglucoside, quercitrin, rutin, and dihydrokaempferol. The flowers contain caffeic and chlorogenic acids.

Fatty acids, hydrocarbons, and phytosterols

Stearic palmitic, linoleic and oleic acids, n-triacontane and n-triacontanol, and beta-sitosterol are present in the root.

Pharmacological Activity

Anti-diarrheal activity

The anti-diarrheal value of Daruhaldi's alkaloid berberine has been studied in clinical research with human subjects affected by cholera.[7] Berberine was found to relieve diarrhea in both bacteriologically positive and negative patients. Mortality rate, volume, and duration of the diarrhea were all reduced, and berberine produced effects that were superior to the drug chloramphenicol.[8]

A randomized, double-blind, clinical trial was conducted to assess the effectiveness of berberine in treating acute watery diarrhea. The study patients were given berberine, tetracycline, or a combination of the two. The patients who were given tetracycline or tetracycline with berberine experienced considerably reduced volume and frequency of diarrheal stools and duration of diarrhea. Less intravenous and oral rehydration fluids were needed.[9]

In another study, however, patients given berberine alone did not experience significant improvement in diarrhea symptoms. But further analysis showed a reduction in stool volume, as well as concentrations of cyclic adenosine monophosphate levels in the stool. After a 24-hour period, patients in all of the study groups showed a decreased level of cholerae organisms in stools.[10]

Animal studies also have confirmed the anti-diarrheal properties of Daruhaldi. When herbal extracts were given to study animals in the early stages of cholera, significant reductions in mortality were observed. Berberine also protected rats from amoebic infection in both short-term and long-term study groups.

Anti-amoebic activity

Berberine's anti-amoebic activity was observed in Entamoeba histolytica, Giardia lamblia, and Trichomonas vaginalis cultures. Berberine sulphate inhibited the growth of all cultures, as well as induced morphological changes.[11] When Entamoeba histolytica was exposed to berberine, a clumping of chromatin was observed in the cell nuclei, and the formation of autophagic vacuoles and aggregates of small vacuoles in the cytoplasm were observed. In Giardia lamblia treated with berberine, an irregularly shaped vacuole appeared in the cytoplasm, which enlarged gradually during the cell culture. In addition, the trophozoites became swollen and deposits of glycogen were seen in the cytoplasm. Soon after exposure of Trichomonas vaginalis to berberine, autophagic vacuoles increased in numbers.

Anti-fungal activity

Santonin and berberine, isolated from Berberis aristata rhizomes, were evaluated for their capacity to impair spore germination in various types of fungal strains. Both alkaloids showed effectiveness against most of the fungi tested. When the two chemicals were mixed, the effectiveness was synergistically increased.[12]

Hepatoprotective activity

An aqueous-methanol extract prepared from Daruhaldi fruits was investigated for its protective action against liver damage caused by acetaminophen. Before administration of the extract, the study animals given a toxic dose of 1 g/kg of acetaminophen experienced a 100% mortality rate. When the animals were pre-treated with the extract, death rates were decreased by 10%. In addition, post-treatment with Daruhaldi was shown to decrease hepatic damage.[13, 14]

In additional animal investigations, Daruhaldi increased the length of sleep periods induced by pentobarbital, and also increased strychnine-induced lethality in mice. These results suggest that Daruhaldi inhibits microsomal drug-metabolizing enzymes.[15]

Anti-inflammatory activity

Inflammation by cholera toxin was inhibited by berberine in a dose-dependent manner. This action was most effective when injections were given at the inflammation site. By contrast, the drugs hydrocortisone and cyproheptadine did not inhibit this type of inflammation.[16]

Anti-chlamydial activity

The activity of the preparation Rasaunt was tested for its effectiveness against ten strains of Chlamydia psittaci. Rasaunt was compared with penicillin, tetracycline, oxytetracycline, and sodium sulphadiazine, in experiments using 7-day-old embryonated hens' eggs. The Chlamydia strains were isolated from domestic animals under a variety of clinical conditions. These experiments demonstrated that Rasaunt had considerable antichlamydial activity at doses of 0.5 mg per embryo.[17]

Anti-leishmanial activity

In-vitro studies have shown berberine to have leishmanicidal properties against the promastigote form of Leishmania donovani. At a concentration of 1 ug/ml, berberine inhibited the growth of promastigotes by 50%, and at concentrations of 5 ug/ml, complete inhibition was observed. A concentration of 10 ug/ml of berberine significantly inhibited endogenous respiration of the organism, as well as glucose oxidation. The mechanism for this action is believed to be inhibition of nucleic acid and protein synthesis.[18]

In a study using hamsters, berberine markedly diminished the parasitic load of L. donovani infection. berberine also proved to be less toxic than pentamidine in both eight-day and long-term study models. Treatment with berberine rapidly improved the hematological profile of infected animals. In in-vitro cell cultures, the extract inhibited the multiplication of amastigotes in macrophage cultures as well as their transformation to promastigotes in a cell-free culture.[19]

The anti-leishmanial activity of berberine is believed to be the result of an inhibitory action on macromolecular biosynthesis and a decrease in deoxyglucose uptake. This probably is attributed to interaction with the DNA of the L. donovani promastigotes.

Anti-platelet activity

Berberine's anti-platelet activity was observed in platelet-rich plasma prepared from the blood of normal human volunteers. The alkaloid inhibited collagen-induced platelet aggregation in a dose dependent manner. This research also indicated that berberine selectively inhibits platelet aggregation by interfering with the collagen-mediated adhesion process, because the substance did not inhibit aggregation mediated by activation of thromboxane A_2, an increase in calcium influx, or stimulation of G-protein linked pathways.[20]

Anti-bacterial activity

The effects of both a berberine chloride solution and a Berberis tincture on large bacterial cultures were studied in-vitro. The tincture was found to be more effective than the solution in inhibiting bacterial growth, probably because of its higher concentration of Berberine.[21]

The anti-bacterial properties of berberine also were evaluated for their application in veterinary medicine. For this research, a berberine hydrochloride solution was tested along with four standard intra-uterine preparations in 21 cows with second-degree endometritis. Five applications of each preparation were given on alternate days over a 9-day period. A cure rate of 81% was observed for a combination of oxytetracycline, oleandomycin, neomycin, prednisolone, and chlorpheniramine maleate, 67% for tetracycline, 57% for Lugol's solution, 52% for the berberine hydrochloride solution, and 33% for chlortetracycline.[22]

The antimicrobial activities of hydroalcoholic extracts of four Berberis species—Berberis aristata, Berberis asiatica, Berberis chitria, and Berberis lyceum—were investigated for their action against eleven bacterial and eight fungal strains. Berberis aristata root extract significantly inhibited the growth of Bacillus cereus, Escherichia coli, Staphylococcus aureus, and Aspergillus flavus. Daruhaldi's stem extract was effective against Bacillus cereus and Streptococcus pneumoniae.[23]

Ophthalmic activity

Rasaunt, the Ayurvedic preparation made from Daruhaldi's root bark, has been used for centuries as an ophthalmic tincture. Laboratory investigation of this application has showed that both the ethanolic and the aqueous extracts of Daruhaldi root were effective in treating eye infections and conjunctivitis. Research was carried out to investigate the anti-inflammatory effect of topical application of Curcuma longa (C. longa) and Berberis aristata (B. aristata) aqueous extracts on experimental uveitis in the rabbit. Anterior uveitis was induced in rabbits by intravitreal injection of lipopolysaccharide from Escherichia coli after pre-treatment with C. longa and B. aristata aqueous extracts. Subsequently, the anti-inflammatory activity of C. longa and B. aristata was evaluated by grading the clinical signs and histopathologic changes and estimating the inflammatory cell count, protein, and TNF-alpha levels in the aqueous humor. The anterior segment inflammation in the control group was significantly higher than in both the extract-treated groups, as observed by clinical and histopathologic grading.[24]

Anti-depressant-like activity

A study was designed to explore the anti-depressant activity and its possible mechanism of action.[25]

The involvement of L-arginine-nitric oxide (NO)-cyclic guanosine monophosphate (cGMP) signaling pathway in the anti-depressant action of berberine chloride was investigated. The anti-depressant activity was assessed in forced-swim and tail-suspension tests. Total immobility period was recorded during a 6-minute test. Berberine (5-20 mg/kg, i.p.) produced a reduction in the immobility period in both tests. When berberine (5 mg/kg, i.p.) was co-administered with other anti-depressant drugs, it enhanced the anti-immobility effect of subeffective doses of imipramine (2 mg/kg, i.p.), desipramine (5 mg/kg, i.p.), tranylcypromine (4 mg/kg, i.p.), fluoxetine (5 mg/kg, i.p.), venlafaxine (2 mg/kg, i.p.) or bupropion (10 mg/kg, i.p.) in forced-swim test. However, berberine did not modify the effects of mianserin (32 mg/kg, i.p.) or trazodone (2 mg/kg, i.p.)—the two atypical anti-depressant drugs.

The neurochemical analysis revealed that berberine (5 mg/kg, i.p.) increased the levels of norepinephrine, serotonin, or dopamine in the mouse whole brain. The anti-depressant-like effect of berberine (5 mg/kg, i.p.) in forced-swim test was prevented by pre-treatment with L-arginine (750 mg/kg, i.p.) [substrate for nitric oxide synthase (NOS)]. Pre-treatment of mice with 7-nitroindazole (25 mg/kg, i.p.) [a specific neuronal nitric oxide synthase (nNOS) inhibitor] produced potentiation of the action of subeffective dose of berberine (2 mg/kg, i.p.). In addition, treatment of mice with methylene blue (10 mg/kg, i.p.) [direct inhibitor of both nitric oxide synthase (NOS) and soluble guanylate cyclase (sGC)] potentiated the effect of berberine (2 mg/kg, i.p.) in the forced-swim test. Further, reduction in the immobility period elicited by berberine (5 mg/kg, i.p.) was inhibited by pre-treatment with sildenafil (5 mg/kg, i.p.) [phosphodiesterase 5 inhibitor]. The various modulators and their combination with berberine did not produce any changes in locomotor activity.

The above findings demonstrated that berberine exerted an anti-depressant-like effect in various behavioral paradigms of despair, possibly by modulating brain biogenic amines (norepinephrine, serotonin, or dopamine) and, further, the anti-depressant-like effect of berberine in the forced-swim test involved an interaction with the L-arginine-NO-cGMP pathway.

The same researchers gave additional commentary and further elucidation about the above mentioned research.[26] Evidence has demonstrated that berberine possesses central nervous system action, particularly the ability to inhibit monoamine oxidase-A, an enzyme involved in the degradation of norepinephrine and serotonin (5-HT). With this background, the study was carried out to elucidate the anti-depressant-like effect of berberine chloride in different behavioral paradigms of despair. Berberine (5, 10, 20 mg/kg, i.p.) inhibited the immobility period in mice in both forced swim and tail-suspension tests; however, the effect was not dose-dependent. Berberine (5 and 10 mg/kg, i.p.) also reversed the reserpine-induced behavioral despair. Berberine (5 mg/kg, i.p.) enhanced the anti-immobility effect of subeffective doses of various typical but not atypical anti-depressant drugs in the forced swim test. Following its acute administration in mice, berberine (5 mg/kg, i.p.) resulted in increased levels of norepinephrine (31%), serotonin (47%), and dopamine (31%) in the whole brain. Chronic administration of berberine (5 mg/kg, i.p.) for 15 days significantly increased the levels of norepinephrine and (29%), serotonin (19%), as well as dopamine (52%) but at higher dose (10 mg/kg, i.p.), there was no change in the norepinephrine (12%) levels but a significant increase in the serotonin (53%) and dopamine (31%) levels was found. The anti-depressant-like effect of berberine (5 mg/kg, i.p.) in the forced swim test was prevented by pre-treatment with L-arginine (750 mg/kg, i.p.) or sildenafil (5 mg/kg, i.p.). To the contrary, pre-treatment of mice with 7-nitroindazole (7-NI)

(25 mg/kg, i.p.) or methylene blue (10 mg/kg, i.p.) potentiated the effect of berberine (2 mg/kg, i.p.) in the forced swim test. Pre-treatment of mice with (+)-pentazocine (2.5 mg/kg, i.p.), a high-affinity sigma-1 receptor agonist, produced synergism with subeffective dose of berberine (2 mg/kg, i.p.). Pre-treatment with various sigma receptor antagonists viz. progesterone (10 mg/kg, s.c.), rimcazole (5 mg/kg, i.p.), and N-[2-(3,4-dichlorophenyl) ethyl]-N-methyl-2-(dimethylamino) ethylamine (BD1047; 1 mg/kg, i.p.) reversed the anti-immobility effects of berberine (5 mg/kg, i.p.).

Berberine at a lower dose did not affect the locomotor activity and barbiturate-induced sleep time. It produced mild hypothermic action in rats and displayed an analgesic effect in mice. Taken together, these findings demonstrate that berberine exerted anti-depressant-like effect in various behavioral paradigms of despair possibly by modulating brain biogenic amines (norepinephrine, serotonin, and dopamine). Further, nitric oxide pathway and/or sigma receptors are involved in mediating its anti-depressant-like activity in mouse forced swim test.

Anti-hyperglycemic activity

The anti-hyperglycemic activity of root of Berberis aristata in alloxan-induced diabetic rats was studied.[27] Five groups of albino Wistar rats were used (n = 6). The two doses of 71.42 and 100 mg/kg body weight ethanol extract of B. aristata were selected for their anti-diabetic activity. Blood glucose levels were estimated in all the groups by the commercial kit (Span diagnostic Pvt. Ltd, Surat) on the 1st, 5th, 10th, and 20th day of treatment with Berberis aristata. Serum cholesterol, triglycerides, HDL, liver glycogen, and body weight were estimated on the 20th day of treatment in all the groups as compared to the diabetic control group. The different extracts of root of B. aristata were also tested for glucose tolerance in normal fasted rats. The ethanol extract of root of B. aristata 71.42 and 100 mg/kg body weight showed a significant ($P<0.01$) reduction of the serum glucose level in the alloxan-induced diabetic rats at the 15th day, compared to the diabetic control group. The cholesterol and triglycerides level was increased significantly ($P<0.01$) in the diabetic animals compared to the normal control group. The level of cholesterol and triglyceride was reduced significantly ($P<0.01$) when compared to the diabetic control group. The level of HDL cholesterol was significantly ($P<0.05$) increased in the extract-treated group when compared to diabetic control group. In the oral glucose tolerance test, the ethanol extract of Berberis aristata increased glucose tolerance. Thus, the ethanol extract of Berberis aristata shows promise to develop a standardized phytomedicine for diabetes mellitus.

Ethnoveterinary Usage

Daruhaldi's roots, stem, and fruits are used to treat diarrhea, kidney stones, and enhance the chance of pregnancy in ruminants. The leaves and stem are used for eye disease of ruminants and swine.[28,29]

Dr. Sodhi's Experience

Practitioners should consider the following questions when considering treatment with Daruhaldi:

- Is the liver involved?
- Is there gall bladder congestion, or a need to stimulate bile production?
- Are there parasites, or are parasites likely present?

Daruhaldi is more effective for cleansing the gall bladder than any other herb that is used for liver support. Daruhaldi's cholerectic action purges the liver and increases bile flow. It is especially useful for treating gall bladder sludge, a common disorder that occurs after juice fasts or crash diets such as those using apple cider vinegar. In this case, surplus fat that has accumulated must be removed from the body quickly. Gall bladder sludge has to be addressed quickly to prevent the formation of stones. In homeopathic medicine, Daruhaldi is used to treat gall stones.

Also, Daruhaldi is used in treating intestinal parasites. It has been shown to be effective against protozoa and spirochetes, including Lyme disease and amoebic infections. Its fruit is edible and is eaten traditionally in India to cleanse the blood.

Case History

Gall stones

A 39-year-old overweight woman came into my clinic with gall bladder sludge and multiple small gall stones. She had used crash dieting in the past, even though she had been warned that this could cause gall stones. She was unwilling to do panchakarma, an Ayurvedic detoxification program that often is effective in these circumstances. I did not want to do a liver flush, as the small stones present might get stuck in the Sphincter of Oddi. Allergy testing showed that the patient had positive responses to beef, lamb, pork, dairy, and wheat. We put her on the following herbal protocol, in addition to eliminating certain foods from her diet.

Liver support

Tinospora cardifolia (guduchi), Picrorrhiza kurnoa (kutki), and Boerhaavia diffusa (purnarnava) extracts in a proprietary blend of Phyllanthus amarus (bhumyamalaki), Swertia chirayita (kiraata), Calotropis gigantis (ark), Raphanus sativa (malaka), Berberis aristata (daaru Curcuma), Terminalia arjuna (arjun), Terminalia bellerica (bibhitaki), Terminalia chebula (haritaki), Emblica officinalis (amalaki), Solanum nigrum (kakmachi), Andrographis paniculata (bhuunimb) extracts: three times a day: Bile salts, 50-100 mg extract

Dietary oil was limited to olive oil, which has the strongest cholerectic effect and does not turn into stones as ghee might in cases of gall bladder sludge. The patient's dietary fiber was increased with a kapha-balancing diet.

A follow-up appointment was scheduled for the patient after 6 weeks of treatment, and she was instructed to report to the emergency room if she experienced any pain. She called a few times with an upset stomach, so we added Zingiber officinale tea to her protocol and traced her discomfort back to foods that she wasn't supposed to be eating. After 6 weeks, another ultrasound showed that her gall bladder was clear, and we did not have to do a liver flush. The patient lost 5 pounds during the herbal treatment. She was able to maintain the diet and lost another 30 lbs, stabilizing at 150 pounds.

Protocols

- Weaning : To wean a 2-to-3 year-old child who does not want to stop nursing, mix Daruhaldi extract with water and apply directly to the breast. Because it is a blood cleanser, it will be good for the child, but because of the bitter taste, the child will stop nursing.

- Conjunctivitis: Dissolve one gram of raw Daruhaldi in 200 cc distilled water with a bit of Santalum album (Chandana). Rose water also could be used. After straining through cheesecloth, apply the solution as eye drops. The infection should clear up in 2 to 3 days.

- Vaginal infections (bacteria, trichomoniasis, candida): In the morning, insert one capsule of a probiotic containing 100 billion mixed organisms as deeply into the vagina as possible. In the evening, insert one capsule containing Azadirachta indica (neem), Embelia ribes (vidang), Piper longum (Pippli), Aegle marmelos (bilva), Momordica charantia (karela), Berberis aristata (daaruhaldi), Holarrhena antidysenterica (kutaj), and Ocimum santum (tulsi). Continue this protocol for 7–10 days. After a few days rest, use a vaginal swab test to make sure that the infective organisms are no longer present.

Boils and skin ulcers: The same decoction that is used as a treatment for conjunctivitis may be made into a paste, with or without the addition of 300 mg. Neem (Azadirachta indica) in a blend of Emblica officinalis (amalaki), Terminalia chebula (haritaki), Terminalia bellerica (bahera), Tinospora cordifolia (guduchi), and Rubia cordifolia (manjistha). Apply this decoction directly onto the boil or ulcer. It will be absorbed locally, and the inflammation will decrease as phagocytosis decreases and pus production stops. The most common source of boils and skin ulcers is Staphylococcus aureus, which is extremely painful. It often occurs in the groin, usually in babies, children, and females, possibly from protein deficiency. With this topical treatment, the boils will fall off easily, and discomfort is relieved in just one day.

Ayurvedic Properties

Rasa: Tikta (bitter), kashaya (astringent)
Guna: Laghu (light), ruksha (rough)
Veerya: Ushna (hot)
Vipaka: Katu (pungent)
Dosha: Balances kapha and vata and purges excess pitta.

Safety Profile

The lethal dose for berberine sulphate in mice is 25 mg/kg. For a 50% ethanolic extract of the roots a lethal dose has been reported as 200 mg/kg.[30]

Dosage

Decoction: 5–10 ml
Powdered root: 1–3 g
Extract: 100 – 300 mg/day

Notes

1. A. K. Chauhan and M. P. Dobhal, "Characterization of a new alkaloid from the roots of Berberis chitria," *Pharmazie*, 1989, 44(7):S10.

2. R. Sivakumar and A. G. Ramachandran Nair, "Polyphenolic constituents of the flowers of Berberis aristata," *Journal of the Indian Chemical Society*, 1991, 68:531.

3. A. Rahman and A. A. Ansari, "Alkaloids of Berberis aristata: Isolation of aromoline and oxyberberine," *Journal of the Chemical Society of Pakistan*, 1983, 5(4):283.

4. G. Blasko, N. Murugesan, A. J. Freyer, M. Sharma, A. A. Ansari, and A. Rahman, "Karachine: An unusual protoberberine alkaloid," *Journal of the American Chemistry Society*, 1982, 104:20–39.

5. G. Blasko and M. Sharma, "Taxilamine, a pseudobenzyl isoquinoline alkaloid," *Heterocycles*, 1982, 19(2):257.

6. F. A. and A. Shoeb, "Isoquinoline derived alkaloids from Berberis chitria," *Phytochemistry*, 1985, 24(3):633.

7. N. K. Dutta and M. V. Panse, "Usefulness of berberine (an alkaloid from Berberis aristata) in the treatment of cholera (experimental)," *Indian Journal of Medical Research*, 50:732.

8. S. C. Lahiri and N. K. Dutta, "Berberine and chloramphenicol in the treatment of cholera and severe diarrhea," *Journal of the Indian Medical Association*, 1967 48:1.

9. U. Khin-Maung, M. Khin, W. Nyunt-Nyunt, and U. Tin-U, "Clinical trial of high-dose berberine and tetracycline in cholera," *J Diarrhoeal Dis Res.*, Sept. 1987, 5(3):184–187.

10. U. Khin-Maung, M. Khin, W. Nyunt-Nyunt, A. Kyaw, and U. Tin, "Clinical trial of berberine in acute watery diarrhea," *British Medical Journal*, 1985, 291:1601.

11. Y. Kaneda, M. Torii, T. Tanka, and M. Aikawa, "In vitro effects of berberine sulfate on the growth and structure of Entamoeba histolytka, Giardia lamblia and Trichomonas vaginalis," *Annals of Tropical Medicine and Parasitology*, 1991 85(4):417.

12. B. Singh, J. S. Srivastava, R. L. Khosa, and U. P., Singh, "Individual and combined effects of berberine and santonin on spore germination of some fungi," *Folia Microbiol (Praha)*, 2001, 46(2):137–142.

13. A. H. Gilani and K. H. Janbaz, "Preventive and curative effects of Berberis aristata fruit extract on paracetamol and CC14-induced hepatotoxicity," *Phytotherapy Research*, 1995, 9:489.

14. A. H. Gilani and K. H. Janbaz, "Prevention of acetaminophen-induced liver damage by Berberis aristata leaves," *Biochemistry Society Transactions*, 1992, 20(4):347S.

15. K. H. Janbaz and A. H. Gilani, "Studies on preventive and curative effects of berberine on chemical induced hepatotoxicity in rodents," *Fitoterapia*, 2000, 71:25.

16. M. H. Akhter, M. Sabir, and N. K. Bhide, "Antiinflammatory effect of berberine in rats injected locally with cholera toxin," *Indian Journal of Medical Research*, 1977, 65(1): 133.

17. V. D. Purohit, R. K. P Gupta, and R. N. S. Khanna, "In vivo studies on anti-chlamydial activity of some antibiotics and an indigenous drug (Berberis aristata) against Chlamydiapsittaci isolates, Haryana Agriculture University," *Journal of Research*, 1988, 18(4):253.

18. S. K. Ghosh, M. M. Rakshit, and D. K. Ghosh, "Effect of berberine chloride on Leishmania donovani," *Indian Journal of Medical Research*, 1983, 78:407.

19. A. K. Ghosh, F. K. Bhattacharya, and D. K. Ghosh, "Leishmania donovani: amastigote inhibition and mode of action of berberine," *Experimental Parasitology*, 1985, 60(3):404.

20. Y. B. Tripathi and S. D. Shukla Berberis aristata inhibits PAF-induced aggregation of rabbit platelets," *Phytotherapy Research*, 1996, 10:628–630.

21. M. P. Dobhal and P. C. Joshi, "In-vitro antimicrobial efficacy of Berberis chitria," *Fitoterapia*, 1992, 63(1):69.

22. S. Pepeljnjak and J. Petricic, "Anti-microbial effect of berberine and tinctura Berberidis," *Pharmazie*, 1992 47:307.

23. M. L. Dhar, M. M. Dhar, B. N. Dhawan, B. N. Mehrotra, and C. Ray, "Screening of Indian plants for medicinal activity," *Indian Journal of Experimental Biology*, 1968, 6:237.

24. S. K. Gupta, R. Agarwal, S. Srivastava, P. Agarwal, S. S. Agrawal, R. Saxena, and N. Galpalli, "The anti-inflammatory effects of Curcuma longa and Berberis aristata in endotoxin-induced uveitis in rabbits," *Invest Ophthalmol Vis Sci.*, Sept. 2008, 49(9):4036-4040.

25. S. K. Kulkarni and A. Dhir, "Possible involvement of L-arginine-nitric oxide (NO)-cyclic guanosine monophosphate (cGMP) signaling pathway in the anti-depressant activity of berberine chloride," *Eur J Pharmacol.*, Aug. 2007,13;569(1–2):77–83.

26. S. K. Kulkarni and A. Dhir, "On the mechanism of anti-depressant-like action of berberine chloride," *Eur J Pharmacol.*, July 28, 2008, 589(1-3):163–172.

27. B. C. Semwal, J. Gupta, S. Singh, Y. Kumar, and M. Giri, "Antihyperglycemic activity of root of Berberis aristata D.C. in alloxan-induced diabetic rats," *Int J Green Pharm*, 2009, 3:259–262.

28. M. K. Jha, *Folk Veterinary Medicine of Bihar—a Research Project* (Anand, Gujrat: NDDB, 1992).

29. International Institute of Rural Reconstruction, *Ethnoveterinary Medicine in Asia. An Information Kit on Traditional Animal Health Care Practices* (Silang, Philippines: IIRR, 1994).

30. M. Blumenthal, *The Complete German Commission E monographs. Therapeutic Guide to Herbal Medicines* (Austin, Texas:American Botanical Council, 1998).

8

Boerhaavia diffusa

Introduction

The Sanskrit name for the creeping herb Boerhaavia diffusa is Punarnava, which literally means "one which renews the body." In Ayurvedic tradition, Punarnava is a rejuvenative herb, restoring youthful energy to the body.

Although Punarnava's roots are the primary source of its medicinal properties, other parts of the plant are useful as well. Because it is a potent diuretic, Punarnava increases urinary output, boosting filtration, flushing the kidneys, and reducing excess body fluids. Punarnava is useful in any condition characterized by fluid retention, including congestive heart failure, renal disease, anasarca (generalized body swelling) and rheumatic disorders.[1]

The fresh juice extracted from Punarnava's roots forms the base for external preparations, which can be used to reduce swelling, cure skin infections, and treat eye ailments such as night blindness and conjunctivitis. It also is used to treat anemia, loss of appetite, jaundice, and obesity.

Synonymous Names

English: Spreading hogweed, pigweed
Hindi: Gadahpurna, Lal Punarnava, Beshakapore
Sanskrit: Punarnava

Habitat

Punarnava thrives in sandy soil, growing wild in waste areas and roadsides throughout India, to an altitude of 6,000 feet (2000 meters).

Botanical Characteristics

Punarnava is a many-branched, creeping herb with a stout, woody stem that spreads over the ground. Its ovate leaves are thick, growing in pairs in each leaf-node, one smaller than the other. The leaves are smooth and white on their lower surface, and rough and green above.

Punarnava flowers and bears fruit during the rainy season. The plant's small, red flowers grow in short clusters on long stalks. The oblong fruit is ridged, glandular, and one-seeded.

Chemical Constituents

Punarvavoside, a unique anti-fibrinolytic agent, has been isolated from Punarnava's root extract.[2] Other chemical constituents include alkaloids, sterols and steroidal compounds including sitosterol and its ester, and palmitic, tetracosanoic, hexacosanoic, stearic, and arachidic acids. Ecdysone, triacontanol, and sitosterol also have been identified.

Other chemical constituents include:[3-8]

Rotenoids: Punarnava's roots contain the rotenoidsboeravinone A, B, C2, D, and F.

Lignans: Liriodendrin and syringaresinol mono-B-D-glucoside have been isolated from Punarnava using methanol extraction.

Xanthones: The benzene extract of Punarnava yielded boerhavine, a dihydroisofuranoxanthone.

Pharmacological Activity

Diuretic activity

Punarnava's diuretic activity, long understood in Ayurveda, has been confirmed in clinical studies. When patients with nephrotic syndrome were given the herb, a diuretic effect comparable to the drug furosemide was observed. In addition, urinary protein excretion was reduced and serum protein levels were increased.

After a month of treatment with Punarnava, the same patients exhibited increased immunoglobulins and immune complexes. Punarnava root harvested during the rainy season showed maximum diuretic activity when compared with plants harvested during dry seasons.[9]

Boerhaavia diffusa treatment inhibited deposition of calcium oxalate crystal and renal cell damage in animal studies. Oxalate excretion significantly increased in hyperoxaluric animals compared to the control, and also reduced BUN and creatinine levels.

Hepatoprotective activity

Root extracts from Punarnava are used in Ayurveda to treat hepatic disorders, and animal research has confirmed this use. One study examined the effects of powdered and aqueous extracts of Punarnava roots on blood serum levels in thioacetamide intoxicated mice.[10]

Research sought to determine whether seasonal differences, root thickness, or form of administration altered Punarnava's hepatoprotective effects.[11] An aqueous extract (2 ml/kg) of Punarnava roots ranging from 1–3 cm in diameter, harvested during the summer months, offered protection for several serum parameters, including GOT, GPT, ACP, and ALP. The extract did not protect against GLDH or bilirubin. The powdered form of Punarnava also offered some hepatoprotective effect, although not as significant as the aqueous extract.

Additional research showed that the chloroform and methanolic extracts of Punarnava roots also exhibited hepatoprotective activity, and oral administration of an ethanolic extract of the whole plant showed activity against carbon tetrachloride-induced hepatotoxicity in rats and mice. A strong cholerectic action was observed, resulting in increased bile production. Toxicity studies showed oral doses up to 2 g/kg in mice to be safe.[12]

In the acetaminophen-induced liver damage model, aqueous and ethanolic extracts decreased the activities of alkaline phosphatase, lactate dehydrogenase, alanine aminotransferase, aspartate aminotransferase, and the level of bilirubin in the serum that were elevated by acetaminophen.[13]

Inhibition of bone resorption

Punarnava's methanolic extract, as well as its flavonoids eupalitin-3-O-B D-galactopyranosyl-(1-2)-B-D-glucopyrano-side and eupalitin-3-O-B-D-galactopyranoside, significantly inhibited bone resorption.[14]

Anti-stress activity

In research on the brains of rats, Punarnava has been shown to have anti-stress activity. The level of the chemical GABA in brain tissue is a useful indicator of stress. Treatment with Punarnava extract caused differential effects on GABA levels in various regions of the brains of rats under stress.[15]

Radioprotective activity

The radioprotective effects of an aqueous ethanolic extract of Punarnava were studied in mice.[16] The study animals were sublethally irradiated with a single radiation dose of 600 rads, and then treated intraperitoneally with 20 mg/kg of Punarnava extract. Bone marrow and intestinal tissues, those most susceptible to radiation damage, were protected by the administration of Punarnava. When the animals were exposed to radiation and treated with Punarnava, the total white blood cell count was lowered on the third day and reached an almost normal level by the ninth day. Serum and liver alkaline phosphatase levels, which were increased after radiation exposure, were reduced in the treated animals. The study animals that received the Punarnava treatment also showed reductions in lipid peroxidation levels in both liver and serum when compared to the untreated animals. DNA isolated from the bone marrow of mice exposed to gamma radiation showed heavy damage, which was reduced by treatment with Punarnava. These results confirm the radioprotective effect of Punarnava extract.[16]

Anti-cancer activity

Methanol extract of Boerhaavia diffusa showed anti-proliferative and anti-estrogenic properties against MCF-7 breast cancer cell lines. Methanolic extract of Boerhaavia diffusa competitively bound to the estrogen receptors, and Boerhaavia reduced the mRNA expression of the pS2 estrogen-responsive gene, indicating anti-estrogenic action. Boerhaavia arrested cell cycle growth at the G0–G1 phase. These results demonstrate that Boerhaavia diffusa possesses anti-proliferative, and ante-estrogenic properties and suggest that it may have therapeutic potential in estrogen-dependent breast cancers.[17]

Alkaloid Punarnavine isolated from the plant Boerhaavia diffusa showed anti-metastatic activity against B16F-10 melanoma cells in C57BL/6 mice. Administration of Punarnavine (40 mg/kg body weight) prophylactically (95.25%), simultaneously (93.9%), and 10 days after tumor inoculation (80.1%) could inhibit the metastatic colony formation of melanoma in lungs. The survival rate of the metastatic tumor-bearing animals compared to the control animals was increased significantly by the administration of Punarnavine. Biochemical and histopathological parameters also improved in the treated animals. Punarnavine administration down regulated the expression of MMP-2, MMP-9 (matrix metalloproteinase), ERK-1, ERK-2 (ERK—extracellular-signal-regulated kinase) and vascular endothelial growth factor (VEGF) in the lung tissue of metastasis-induced animals.[18]

Boerhaavia diffusa enhanced natural killer (NK) cell activity, antibody-dependent cellular cytotoxicity, antibody-dependent complement-mediated cytotoxicity, and the activity was observed in the treated group much earlier than in the metastatic tumor-bearing control. Production of the cytokine IL-2 was enhanced significantly by administration of Boerhaavia diffusa compared to the untreated metastatic tumor-bearing control. Levels of granulocyte macrophage colony-stimulating factor receptor (GM-CSF) and pro-inflammatory cytokines such as IL-1beta, IL-6, and TNF-alpha were lowered significantly by Boerhaavia diffusa administration compared to the metastatic control.[19]

Ethanolic extract of Boerhaavia diffusa inhibited human cervical cancer cells inducing apoptosis, as evident from DNA fragmentation and caspase-9 activation.[20]

Anti-fibrinolytic activity

Punarnava root extract administered to monkeys fitted with intrauterine devices (IUDs) produced a reduction in the amount and duration of menstrual flow and menstrual iron loss.[21] These findings indicate Punarnava's anti-fibrinolytic and anti-inflammatory action, substantiating its use in IUD-induced menorrhagia. The chemical punarnavoside has been identified as an anti-fibrinolytic agent.

Dr. Sodhi's Experience

An herbal protocol using Punarnava should be considered under the following conditions:

- Is a kidney condition present?
- Is there kidney failure?
- Is there heart congestion?
- Is vasodilation desirable?
- Is there liver degeneration or cirrhosis?
- Is there edema?
- Is nephrotic syndrome present?
- Is inflammation present, especially in the kidneys, heart, or liver?

The literal meaning of Punarnava in Sanskrit is "new" (nava) and "again" (punar), so Punarnava refers to something that makes one "new again." Punarnava acts primarily in the liver and kidneys. It also is an excellent remedy for eye conditions. And Punarnava is an effective abortifacient.

I found Punarnava to be effective for regenerating kidney cells and in treating kidney failure. As a liver stimulant, Punarnava helps to repair liver damage caused by alcoholic cirrhosis and drug toxicity. It also is a valuable anti-inflammatory. Because of its diuretic effect, I have used Punarnava with success to treat congestive heart failure. When my patients with high blood pressure don't respond to conventional treatments, I add Punarnava to their regimen. Punarnava also is an effective bronchodilator and has a long history of being used for respiratory problems in Ayurveda.

Safety Profile

Punarnava is considered safe if used under appropriate medical supervision. The lethal dosage of a 50% ethanolic extract of Punarnava's root was found to be 1000 mg/kg body weight in adult rats.

Dosage

Root juice: 9–12 g
Leaf juice: 12–25 g
Root powder: 8–15 g
Extract: 100 - 200 mg TID

Ayurvedic Properties

In Ayurveda, Punarnava is considered the best rejuvenative herb for the urinary system. In Ayurvedic texts, two varieties of Punarnava, white and red, are mentioned. A third blue variety is also cited in Raja Nighantu. The white variety of Punarnava is pungent, bitter, and astringent in taste, pungent in post-digestive effect, and has cold potency. The white variety of Punarnava is considered to pacify all three doshas. The red variety alleviates pitta dosha but aggravates vata dosha. Punarnava possesses light and dry attributes.

Rasa: Madhur (sweet), tikta (bitter), kashaya (astringent)
Guna: Laghu (light), ruksha (dry)
Vipaka: Madhur (sweet)
Veerya: Ushna (hot)
Dosha: Pacifies the tridosha

Ayurvedic Preparations

Sesame oil compounded with Punarnava is used in Ayurveda along with enemas to treat vata ascites and flatulence. In large doses, Punarnava is a purgative. In smaller doses, Punarnava stimulates the appetite and works as a mild laxative. Kapha anemia is treated effectively by Punarnava combined with ghee. Cardiac asthma is curbed effectively by the popular formulation punarnavasava.

Notes

1. International Institute of Rural Reconstruction, *Ethnoveterinary Medicine in Asia: An Information Kit on Traditional Animal Health Care Practices. Part I, General Information* (Silang, Philippines, IIRR, 1994).

2. G. K. Jain and N. M. Khanna, "Punarnavoside: A new antifibrinolytic agent from Boerhaavia diffusa Linn," *Indian Journal of Chemistry*, 1989, 28(B):163–166.

3. N. Lami, S. Kadota, Y. Tezuka, and T. Kikuchi, "Constituents of the roots *of Boerhaavia diffiisa* L. II Structure and stereochemistry of a new rotenoid, boeravinone C2," *Chemical and Pharmaceutical Bulletin*, 1990, 38(6):1558.

4. G. K. Jain and N. M. Khanna, "Punarnavoside, a new antifibrinolytic agent from *Boerhaavia diffusa* Linn.," *Indian Journal of Chemistry*, 1989, 28B(2):163.

5. S. Kadota, N. Lami, Y. Tezuka, and T. Kikuchi, "Constituents of the roots *of Boerhaavia diffusa* L. I. Examination of sterols and structures of new rotenoids boeravinones A and B," *Chemical and Pharmaceutical Bulletin,*" 1989, 37(12):3214.

6. N. Lami, S. Kadota, T. Kikuchi, and Y. Momose, "Constituents of the roots *of Boerhaavia diffusa* L. III. Identification of Ca^{2*} channel antagonistic compound from the methanol extract," *Chemical and Pharmaceutical Bulletin*, 1991, 39(6):1551.

7. N. Lami, S. Kadota, and T. Kikuchi, "Constituents of the roots of *Boerhaavia diffusa* L. IV. Isolation and structure determination of boeravinones D, E and F," *Chemical and Pharmaceutical Bulletin*, 1991, 39(7):1863.

8. B. Ahmed and Chung-PingYu, "Boerhavine, a dihydroisofuranoxanthone from *Boerhaavia diffusa, Phytochemistry*, 1992, 31(12):4382–4384.

9. A. S. Mishra, J. Vermaand, and N. Kumari, "Studies on medicinal properties of Convolvulus pluricaulis and Boerhaavia diffusa," *Biojournal*, 1995, 6(1/2):31.

10. S. K. Pareta, K. C. Patra, P. M. Mazumder, and D. Sasmal, "Aqueous extract of Boerhaavia diffusa root ameliorates ethylene glycol-induced hyperoxaluric oxidative stress and renal injury in rat kidney," *Pharm Biol.*, Dec. 2011, 49(12):1224–1233.

11. A. K. Rawat, S. Mehotra, S. C. Tripathi, and U. Shome, "Hepatoprotective activity of Boerhaavia diffusa L. roots—a popular Indian ethnomedicine," *J Ethnopharmacol.*, March 1997, 56(1):61–66.

12. B. K. Chandan, A. K. Sharma, and K. K. Annand, "Boerhaavia diffusa: A study of its hepatoprotective activity," *Journal of Ethnopharmacology*, 1991, 31(3):299–307.

13. M. T. Olaleye, A. C. Akinmoladun, A. A. Ogunboye, and A. A. Akindahunsi, "Anti-oxidant activity and hepatoprotective property of leaf extracts of Boerhaavia diffusa Linn against acetaminophen-induced liver damage in rats," *Food Chem Toxicol.*, Aug.–Sept., 2010, 48(8–9):2200–2205.

14. J. Li, H. Li, S. Kadota, T. Namba, T. Miyahara, and U. G. Khan, "Effects on cultured neonatal mouse calvaria of the flavonoids isolated from Boerhaavia repens," *Journal of Natural Products*, 1996, 59(11):1015.

15. K. Sharma, K. V. Pasha, and P. C. Dandiya, *Effect of Boerhaavia diffusa Linn on GABA Levels of the Brain During Stress* (New Delhi, India: Conference on Pharmacology and Symposium on Herbal Drugs 1991).

16. K. A. Manu, "Studies on the protective effects of Boerhaavia diffusa L. against gamma radiation—Induced damage in mice integrative cancer therapies," 2007, 6(4), 381–388.

17. S. Sreeja and S. Sreeja, "An in vitro study on antiproliferative and antiestrogenic effects of Boerhaavia diffusa L. extracts," *J Ethnopharmacol.* Nov.12, 2009, 126(2):221–225.

18. K. A. Manu and G. Kuttan, "Anti-metastatic potential of Punarnavine, an alkaloid from Boerhaavia diffusa Linnl," *Immunobiolog,* 2009, 214(4):245–255.

19. K. A. Manu and G. Kuttan, "Boerhaavia diffusa stimulates cell-mediated immune response by upregulating IL-2 and downregulating the pro-inflammatory cytokines and GM-CSF in B16F-10 metastatic melanoma bearing mice," *J Exp Ther Oncol.*, 2008, 7(1):17–29.

20. R. Srivastava, D. Saluja, B. S. Dwarakanath, and M. Chopra, "Inhibition of human cervical cancer cell growth by ethanolic extract of boerhaavia diffusa Linn. (Punarnava) root," *Evid Based Complement Alternat Med.*, 2011, Article ID 427031, 13 pages, 2011. doi:10.1093/ecam/nep223

21. M. Barthwal and K. Srivastava, "Management of IUD-associated menorrhagia in female rhesus monkeys (Macaca mulatta)," *Adv Contracept.*, March 1991, 7(1):67–76.

Boswellia serrata

Introduction

Boswellia serrata, or Salai, is one of Ayurveda's most potent anti-inflammatory herbs.[1] On its own or in combination with other herbs, Boswellia is used both externally and internally to treat rheumatoid arthritis, back pain, fibrositis, and osteoarthritis. Clinical trials and animal studies with Boswellia have confirmed its anti-inflammatory and pain relieving effects.

Boswellia is a moderately large, branching tree that grows throughout India, North Africa, and the Middle East. Boswellia's medicinal properties are found primarily in the thick, gummy sap that lies under its bark. This resin, uncovered when the bark is peeled away in strips, is sometimes referred to as Indian frankincense. Extracts of Boswellia's resin have been used for centuries in Ayurveda for their astringent, stimulant, expectorant, and antiseptic properties.

As an anti-arthritis and anti-inflammatory agent, Boswellia offers promise as an alternative to conventional treatment with non-steroidal anti-inflammatory drugs (NSAIDs). Unlike these drugs, which include Ibuprofen, Vioxx, and Celebrex, Boswellia does not irritate the sensitive lining of the digestive tract. Research indicates that Boswellia also may provide an alternative to dangerous steroids such as prednisolone. Human efficacy, comparative, and pharmacokinetic studies have confirmed the safety and effectiveness of Boswellia as an anti-inflammatory agent.

The chemical constituents responsible for Boswellia's anti-inflammatory activity have been isolated and are called boswellic acids. These acids have been shown to reduce inflammation by reducing the infiltration of white blood cells into damaged tissues. Boswellic acids also improve blood flow to the joints, and block the chemical reactions that lead to inflammation in intestinal disorders such as Crohn's disease and ulcerative colitis.

Synonymous Names

English: Indian olibanum tree
Hindi: Shallaki, Salai
Sanskrit: Sallaki
Other names include Susrava, Gajabhakshya, Subaha, Surabhi, Maheruna, Kunduruki, and Vallaki.

Habitat

Boswellia grows natively in dry areas of central India, the Deccan peninsula, and the eastern states. It is also widespread in northern Africa and the Middle East.

BOTANICAL CHARACTERISTICS

Boswellia is a deciduous tree that grows to an average height of 12–15 feet (4–5 meters), with a trunk girth of 3–5 feet (1–1.5 meters). Its opposite, sessile leaves vary in shape from lanceolate to obtuse and have a serrate margin and a rounded base. Boswellia blossoms from January to March, bearing cream colored flowers on long racemes. The triangular fruit is about 3 cm in diameter.

Boswellia's fragrant bark is reddish-green in color. To extract the gum resin, long cuts are made in the tree's bark, which then is peeled away in strips, revealing the gummy sap underneath.

CHEMICAL COMPOSITION

Boswellia's gum resin is made up of volatile oils, terpenoids, and sugars. Its active chemical constituents are a group of triterpenes identified as boswellic acids (BA). These include four pentacyclic triterpene acids along with their derivatives.[5,6] Boswellia's volatile oil contains the alcohols anisaldehyde, oc-pinene, alpha-phellandrene and sesquiterpene. Sugars present in Boswellia's gum resin include arabinose, galactose, xylose, galacturonic acid, and digitoxose. Analysis of the leaves has shown the presence of D-fructose, D-lactose, D-glucose, L-sorbose, raffinose, rhamnose, and D-galactose. The following are sources of information about the chemical composition of Boswellia serrata:[2,3,4,5,6,7]

PHARMACOLOGICAL ACTIVITY

Anti-arthritis activity

The effectiveness of Boswellia in treating osteoarthritis was demonstrated in a 2008 clinical study. The 90-day, double-blind, randomized, placebo controlled study was conducted to evaluate the effectiveness and safety of Boswellia extract, an anti-arthritis drug based on Boswellia's essential extract.[8] The 75 osteoarthritis patients who participated in the study received either 100 mg or 250 mg of Boswellia extract or a placebo daily for 90 days. Each patient's pain level and physical function were evaluated at days 7, 30, 60, and 90. Blood tests were conducted to monitor levels of cartilage degrading enzymes. A battery of biochemical parameters was also measured to evaluate the drug's safety. Of the 75 original study participants, 70 completed the 90-day study. The patients receiving both dosages of Boswellia extract showed significantly improved pain scores and functional ability. Interestingly, these benefits were recorded in the treatment group receiving the 250 mg dose as early as 7 days after beginning treatment. Significant reductions in cartilage degrading enzyme levels also were observed in patients receiving Boswellia.

Results of this study show that Boswellia's extract reduces pain and improves physical function in osteoarthritis patients. The extract's anti-arthritis activity may be attributed to reductions in both pro-inflammatory modulators and enzymatic degradation of cartilage. The safety of treatment with Boswellia also was confirmed by this study.

Another clinical study measured the effect of Boswellia on the symptoms of arthritis patients.[9] The study group consisted of 175 men and women who had suffered from arthritis for one to 6 years, and 70% were bedridden. The study measured the effects of Boswellia extract on parameters including joint stiffness in the morning, loss of grip strength, general pain, and difficulty performing routine jobs. Of these patients, 67% showed significant improvement and 30% showed some improvement after receiving treatment with Boswellia.

A standardized Ayurvedic herbal formulation consisting of Withania somnifera, Boswellia serrata, Zingiber officinale, and Curcuma longa was studied to evaluate the efficacy and safety of patients with symptomatic osteoarthritis (OA) of the knees. Ninety patients were screened for osteoarthritis according to American College of Rheumatology criteria to enroll into a randomized, double-blind, placebo-controlled, parallel efficacy, single-center, 32-week drug trial.[10] Concurrent analgesics, non-steroidal anti-inflammatory drugs, and steroids in any form were not allowed. Lifestyle and dietary restrictions, per routine Ayurveda practices, were not imposed. To measure efficacy, the pain visual analogue scale (VAS) (maximum pain in each knee recorded by the patient during the preceding 48 hours) and modified WOMAC (Western Ontario McMaster University OA Index, Likert scale, version 3.0) were used. Routine laboratory testing was done primarily to monitor drug safety. Of the patients, 45 were treated with the Boswellia preparation and 45 were in the placebo group. The Boswellia-treated group showed significant reduction in pain ($P < 0.05$). Similarly, improvement in the WOMAC scores at week 16 and week 32 also were significantly superior ($P < 0.01$). Both groups reported mild adverse events without any significant difference. None reported drug-related toxicity.

Laboratory models have demonstrated the mechanism of Boswellia's anti-arthritic activity. In these experiments, Boswellic acids inhibited leukotriene synthesis via 5-lipoxygenase without affecting either 12-lipoxygenase or cyclooxygenase. No subsequent impairment in the peroxidation of arachidonic acid by iron and ascorbate was observed. These results indicate that boswellic acids are specific, non-redox inhibitors of leukotriene synthesis, and probably interact directly with 5-lipoxygenase or block its translocation.[11]

Boswellia frereana extract was studied in cartilage degeneration and to determine its potential as a therapy for treating osteoarthritis.[12] Cartilage degradation was induced in-vitro by treating interleukin-1alpha (IL-1alpha) over a 28-day period, in the presence or absence of Boswellia frereana. Boswellia frereana inhibited breakdown of the collagenous matrix. Boswellia frereana reduced MMP9 and MMP13 mRNA levels, inhibited MMP9 expression and activation, and significantly reduced the production of nitrite (stable end product of nitric oxide), prostaglandin E2, and cycloxygenase-2. Epilupeol was identified as the principal constituent of Boswellia frereana. Boswellia frereana prevents collagen degradation and inhibits the production of pro-inflammatory mediators and MMPs.

Anti-inflammatory activity

In animal studies, boswellic acids have been shown to reduce inflammation in several ways: They deter inflammatory white cells from infiltrating damaged tissue. They improve blood flow to the joints. They also block chemical reactions that set the stage for inflammation to occur in chronic intestinal disorders such as Crohn's disease and ulcerative colitis.[13]

Boswellic acids (BA), a natural mixture isolated from oleo gum resin of Boswellia serrata, is composed of four major pentacyclic triterpene acids: beta-boswellic acid (the most abundant), 3-acteyl-beta-boswellic acid, 11-keto-beta-boswellic acid, and 3-acetyl-11-keto-beta-boswellic acid. Boswellic acids (BA) are anti-inflammatory, immunomodulatory, anti-tumor, anti-asthmatic, and in Crohn's disease by inhibiting pro-inflammatory mediators in the body. Specifically, leukotriene's via inhibition of 5-lipoxygenase, the key enzyme of leukotriene synthesis, is the scientifically proven mechanism for its anti-inflammatory and anti-arthritic activity. Boswellic acid has proven to be as effective with topical application as with the systemic route through different acute and chronic models of inflammation; e.g., arachidonic acid and croton oil-induced mouse ear edema, carrageenan-induced rats paw edema, and adjuvant induced arthritis in rats. The most evident action is the inhibition of 5-lipoxygenase, cytokines (interleukins and TNF-alpha), and the complement system are also involved. Leukocyte elastase and oxygen radicals are believed to be the targets of Boswellia's action.[14,15]

An oral administration of boswellic acids significantly reduced lysosomal protease cathepsin G activities (inflammation model) in human blood ex-vivo versus the placebo. Boswellic acids inhibited chemoinvasion but not chemotaxis of challenged neutrophils, and suppressed Ca(2+) mobilization in human platelets induced by the lysosomal protease cathepsin G released from activated neutrophils.[16]

The effect of acetyl-11-keto-beta-boswellic acid (isolate of boswellic acid), a natural inhibitor of the pro-inflammatory transcription factor NF-kappaB, was studied for the development of atherosclerotic lesions in apolipoprotein E-deficient mice. Atherosclerotic lesions were induced by a weekly injection of lipopolysaccharides in apolipoprotein E-deficient mice.[17] Lipopolysaccharides alone increased the size of atherosclerotic lesions by approximately 100%, and treatment with acetyl-11-keto-beta-boswellic acid significantly reduced the size of lesions by approximately 50%. Acetyl-11-keto-beta-boswellic acid treatment led to a significant downregulation of several NF-kappaB-dependent genes such as MCP-1, MCP-3, IL-1alpha, MIP-2, VEGF, and TF. It also potently inhibited the IkappaB kinase (IKK) activity immuno-precipitated from lipopolysaccharides-stimulated mouse macrophages and mononuclear cells, leading to decreased phosphorylation of IkappaB alpha and inhibition of p65/NF-kappaB activation. But it did not affect the plasma concentrations of triglycerides, total cholesterol, antioxidized LDL antibodies, and various subsets of lymphocyte-derived cytokines. This inhibition of NF-kappaB activity by boswellic acids can represent classical treatments for chronic inflammatory diseases such as atherosclerosis.

A study was conducted to understand the molecular basis for the effect of gum resin of Boswellia serrata containing boswellic acids, which inhibit leukotriene biosynthesis.[18] TNF alpha represents one of the most widely recognized mediators of inflammation. One mechanism by which TNF alpha causes inflammation is to potently induce the expression of adhesion molecules such as Vascular Cell Adhesion Molecule-1 (VCAM-1). The genetic basis of the anti-inflammatory effects of boswellic acid was studied in a system of TNF alpha-induced gene expression in human microvascular endothelial cells. First, a whole genome screen for TNF alpha-inducible genes in human microvascular cells (HMEC) was done. TNF alpha induced 522 genes and down regulated 141 genes. Of the 522 genes induced by TNF alpha in HMEC, 113 genes were clearly sensitive to boswellic acid treatment. These genes were related directly to inflammation, cell adhesion, and proteolysis. Boswellic acid prevented the TNF alpha-induced expression of matrix metalloproteinase and also prevented the inducible expression of mediators of apoptosis. TNF alpha-inducible expression of Vascular Cell Adhesion Molecule-1(VCAM-1) and Intercellular Adhesion Molecule-1 (ICAM-1) were sensitive to boswellic acids. The TNF alpha-induced VCAM-1 gene expression was completely prevented by boswellic acids. [This exciting research is a testimonial to the wonderful results achieved in my clinical practice, using a combination of boswellic acids to treat chronic and acute inflammatory diseases.]

Gastrointestinal activity (inflammatory bowel diseases)

Juvenile Crohn's disease patients are in a constant catabolic state, resulting in poor weight gain and growth failure. Anti-inflammatory, immunomodulatory, and monoclonal antibody drugs, as well as growth hormone, frequently fail to achieve sustained remission or reverse growth failure. An uncontrolled prospective case study was undertaken in six moderate-to-severe Crohn's disease patients. Dairy products, certain grains and carrageenan containing foods were eliminated. The patients were asked to follow a dairy-free, gluten free, carrageenan-free diet and were given 3 grams of protein/kg/day along with fish peptides, bovine colostrum, Boswellia serrata, Curcuma, and a multivitamin. Lactobacillus, a probiotic, was administered twice weekly. Recombinant human growth hormone was administered daily.[19]

Within 2 months after starting this treatment, all six patients went into remission, with discontinuation of all pharmacological drugs. Three patients remained in sustained remission for 4 to 8 years. One patient with severe disease had a recurrence of Crohn's disease symptoms after being in complete remission for 18 months; one patient was in remission for 3 years but symptoms recurred when she became less compliant to the nutraceutical approach; and one patient who had been recently treated remained in remission after 6 months. Of the six patients, two already had achieved normal growth before the start of treatment with the addition of growth hormone, and the four growing patients had good-to-excellent growth response. We at Ayurvedic and naturopathic Clinic have achieved similar results in our clinical practice in almost all Crohn's disease patients. Currently, no effective preventive measures or medical therapies are available for intestinal fibrosis. The only viable option is to do surgery in fibrostenotic enteropathies such as Crohn's disease.

Combined oral administration of Boswellia and Scutellaria extracts significantly improved the course and macroscopic findings of 2,4,5-trinitrobenzene-induced chronic colitis assessed by disease activity index, colon weight, length, adhesions, strictures, dilatation, thickness, edema, ulcerations, and extension of damage. The histological severity of the colonic fibrosis also was notably improved by the treatment. This antifibrotic mechanism of action seems to be mediated by the inhibition of TGF-beta1/Smad3 pathway.[20]

Patients with chronic diarrhea and histologically proven collagenous colitis were randomized to receive either oral Boswellia serrata extract 400 mg three times daily for 6 weeks or a placebo. A complete colonoscopy and histology were performed before and after treatment. Clinical symptoms and quality of life were assessed by standardized questionnaires and SF-36 (a multi-purpose, short-form health survey with only 36 questions). The primary endpoint was the percentage of patients with clinical remission after 6 weeks (stool frequency <or=3 soft/solid stools per day on average during the last week). Patients of the placebo group with persistent diarrhea received open-label Boswellia serrata extract therapy for 6 more weeks. Patients receiving the Boswellia serrata extract showed higher remission than those in the placebo group.[21]

A semisynthetic form of acetyl-11-keto-beta-boswellic acid showed protection in experimental murine colitis induced by dextran sodium sulfate The responses observed with acetyl-11-keto-beta-boswellic acid were comparable to corticosteroids.[22]

The use of non-steroidal anti-inflammatory drugs (NSAIDs) is associated with several side effects, of which ulceration is the most common. Boswellic acid is a powerful anti-inflammatory that does not cause ulcer production and protects the mucosa of intestines. An activity evaluation was done with the following universally accepted animal models: pyloric ligation, ethanol-HCl, acetylsalicylic acid, indomethacin, and cold-restrained stress induced ulceration in rats. Boswellic acid possess a dose-dependent, anti-ulcer effect against different experimental models. This study showed different degrees of inhibition of the ulcer score toward different ulcerogenic agents. The ulcer score against various ulcer-inducing agents—pyloric ligation, ethanol/HCl, (acute and chronic) acetylsalicylic acid, indomethacin, and cold-restrained stress—was inhibited by 39%, 38%, 51%, 31%, 37%, and 42%, respectively, at 250 mg/kg. Boswellic acid might have increased the gastric mucosal resistance and local synthesis of cytoprotective prostaglandins while inhibiting the leukotriene synthesis.[23]

Anti-asthmatic activity

Boswellia's anti-asthma properties have been demonstrated in clinical research. In a double-blind, placebo-controlled study, 40 asthmatic patients, ranging in age from 18 to 75 years, were given a 300 mg preparation of Boswellia's gum resin three times each day for 6 weeks. Of the patients studied, 70% showed a reduction in asthma attacks as a result of treatment with Boswellia. The herbal treatment also was associated with improvement in biochemical parameters, including a decrease in eosinophil count and ESR in these patients.[24]

A meta-analysis was done using various herbal preparations for asthma-related respiratory diseases. Multiple database searches identified randomized placebo-controlled trials where possible data were combined for meta-analysis. The primary outcome measures were lung function, exacerbations and reduction in corticosteroid use. The secondary outcome measures were symptoms and symptom scores, use of reliever medications, changes in rates of consultation, and adverse effects. An analysis of twenty six studies on various lung pathologies have revealed that use of Boswellia, Mai-Men-Dong-Tang, Pycnogenol, Jia-Wei-Si-Jun-Zi-Tang and Tylophora indica improved lung function, and reduced daily oral steroid dosage.[25]

Immunomodulatory activity

Both the delayed hypersensitivity reaction and the primary humoral response to sheep erythrocytes were inhibited by a single dose (50–200 mg/kg) of boswellic acids given to laboratory mice. At lower doses, the secondary response was enhanced appreciably. When boswellic acids were given orally to the animals over a 3-week period, total body weight, leucocyte counts, and humoral antibody levels were all increased.[26] Acetyl-11-keto-β-boswellic acid exhibited the most potent anti-bacterial activity and was further evaluated in time kill studies, mutation prevention frequency, post-antibiotic effect, and a biofilm susceptibility assay against oral cavity pathogens.[27] Acetyl-11-keto-β-boswellic acid exhibited concentration-dependent killing of Streptococcus mutans and also stopped the formation of biofilms generated by Streptococcus mutans and Actinomyces viscosus. Acetyl-11-keto-β-boswellic acid can be an excellent mouthwash for mouth cavity diseases.

Anti-tumor activity

Boswellia extract has shown potential anti-carcinogen activity, inducing apoptosis in human cervical carcinoma cells. Increased levels of stress proteins have been observed in carcinoma cells treated with the extract. Boswellia also appeared to strengthen the activity of calpain, a calcium-binding protein. Boswellia may be a valuable therapeutic agent in human cervical carcinoma. Boswellia increased the lifespan of mice with Ehrlich ascites carcinoma by 25%, and decreased S-180 tumors, also by 24%. Boswellic acids also inhibited the synthesis of DNA, RNA, and protein in human leukemia cells in a dose-dependent manner.[28]

Activation of the serine/threonine kinase (Akt) is associated with the aggressive clinical behavior of prostate cancer. In human prostate cancer, cell lines LNCaP and PC-3 express predominantly Akt1 and Akt2. Boswellic acids inhibited the phosphorylation of cellular Akt and the Akt signaling pathways, including glycogen synthase kinase-3beta and BAD phosphorylation, nuclear accumulation of p65, the androgen receptor, beta-catenin, and c-Myc (regulator gene that codes for a transcription factor). These events created apoptosis in prostate cancer but not in nontumorigenic cells. The tirucallic acid derivatives inhibited proliferation and induced apoptosis in tumors xenografted onto chick chorioallantoic membranes and decreased the growth of pre-established prostate tumors in nude mice without overt systemic toxicity.[29]

The mechanism of acetyl-keto-beta-boswellic acid (AKBA) in LNCaP and PC-3 human prostate cancer cells induced apoptosis in both cell lines at concentrations above 10 microg/mL. AKBA induced apoptosis was correlated with the activation of caspase-3 and caspase-8, as well as with poly (ADP) ribose polymerase (PARP) cleavage. AKBA induced apoptosis in prostate cancer cells through a DR5-mediated pathway, which probably involves the induced expression of CAAT/enhancer binding protein homologous protein (CHOP).[30] Other studies suggest that AKBA is a novel inhibitor of STAT3 activation.[31]

An interesting study was done at the Department of Community and Preventive Medicine, New York Medical College.[32] Researchers applied one-minute downward pressure on the tip of any one of the front three teeth (1st incisor, 2nd incisor, and canine) at the right and left sides of the upper and lower jaw, by a wooden toothpick. This procedure led to temporary disappearance of headache, toothache, chest pain, abdominal pain, and backache, often with improved memory and concentration.

Because these beneficial changes resembled the effects of giving one optimal dose of DHEA, the increase in DHEA was measured. This mechanical stimulation of one of these front teeth increased abnormally reduced DHEA levels and normal cell telomeres from markedly reduced values to near normal values, and improved acetylcholine in the hippocampus. Large organ representation areas for the adrenal gland and hippocampus may exist at these front teeth.

This method can be used for emergency pain control and can explain the beneficial effect of bruxism and tooth brushing through the increase of DHEA levels and activities of the hippocampus by increasing acetylcholine. Increasing the normal cell telomere to an optimally high level resulted in the disappearance of pain and improvement or significant reduction of malignant tumors. Repeated daily press needle stimulation increased telomere and DHEA, which eliminated the pain, and the effects lasted 0.5 to 11 months. Adding Boswellia serrata or Astragalus not only increased the telomeres and eliminated pain and improved cancer parameters but also reduced the size of the Astrocytoma grade I by 10% to 20% and the glioblastoma by 15% to 90% in less than 2 to 6 months.

Multiple brain metastases in breast cancer patients represent a life-threatening condition with limited success following standard therapies. Multiple brain metastases were reversed successfully using Boswellia serrata in a breast cancer patient who had not shown improvement after standard therapy. This suggests a potential new area of therapy for breast cancer patients with brain metastases, which may be useful as an adjuvant to our standard therapy.[33]

Currently, the Cleveland clinic has been actively recruiting patients to evaluate Boswellia serrata and standard treatment or standard treatment alone in treating patients who have undergone surgery and radiation therapy for newly diagnosed or recurrent high-grade glioma. More information can be found from the clinical trials website: http://clinicaltrials.gov/ct2/show/NCT00243022

In a randomized, placebo-controlled, double blind study in Germany, patients who were irradiated for brain tumors were given Boswellia serrata with great success in reducing brain swelling.[34] Patients often suffer from cerebral edema and usually are treated with dexamethasone, which has various side-effects. Forty-four patients with primary or secondary malignant cerebral tumors were assigned randomly to radiotherapy plus either Boswellia serrata (4200 mg/day) or a placebo. MRI, toxicity, cognitive function, quality of life, and the need for dexamethasone were assessed. A reduction of cerebral edema of >75% was found in 60% of the patients receiving Boswellia serrata and in 26% of the patients receiving the placebo. There were no severe adverse events in either group, though six patients in the Boswellia group reported minor gastrointestinal discomfort. Boswellia serrata did not have a significant impact on quality of life or cognitive function.

Neuronal activity

Increasing evidence implicates impairment of axonal integrity in mechanisms underlying neurodegenerative disorders. Beta-boswellic acid enhanced axonal length, neurite branching, and tubulin polymerization dynamics in hippocampal cells.[35]

Incensoleacetate, isolated from Boswellia, inhibited hippocampal neurodegeneration and exerted a beneficial effect on functional outcome in a mouse model of closed head injury. The result was reduced neurological severity scores and improved cognitive ability in an object recognition test, suggesting a novel neuroprotective mechanism.[36]

Dermatological activity

A cream containing 0.5% boswellic acid was tested in treating clinical manifestations of photoaging of facial skin with a randomized, double-blind, placebo-controlled, split-face study. Fifteen female volunteers applied the creams with or without boswellic acids on a half side of the face once daily for 30 days. In comparison to the placebo, significant improvements of the Dover's global score were seen for photoaging, tactile roughness, and fine lines. Also, with noninvasive diagnostic techniques, an increase of elasticity, a decrease of sebum excretion, and a change of echographic parameters were observed with topical boswellic acid cream in contrast to the placebo.[37]

Analgesic activity

Animal studies have shown that Boswellia's gum resin has sedative and analgesic properties. A study was done to examine the effects of aroma hand massage on pain, state anxiety, and depression in hospice patients with terminal cancer. This study followed a nonequivalent control group pretest–posttest design. The subjects were 58 hospice patients with terminal cancer who were hospitalized. Of these, 28 were assigned to the aroma hand massage, and 30 were assigned to the control group with a general oil hand massage. The aroma hand massage was done on each hand for 5 minutes for 7 days with blended oil—a mixture of bergamot, lavender, and frankincense in a ratio of 1:1:1, which was diluted 1.5% with 50 ml. sweet almond oil. The control group received general-oil hand massage, using only sweet almond carrier oil on each hand for 5 minutes for 7 days. The aroma hand massage experimental group showed more significant differences than the control group in pain score changes ($t=-3.52$, $p=.001$) and depression ($t=-8.99$, $p=.000$).[38]

Anti-fungal activity

Boswellia's essential oil showed significant anti-fungal activity against the plant pathogen Phytophthora parasitica; however, it exhibited weak anti-fungal action against human pathogens.[39]

Cholesterol-lowering activity

Treatment with Boswellia extract reduced cholesterol biosynthesis in both in-vivo and in-vitro experiments.[40]

Dr. Sodhi's Experience

Herbal treatment with Boswellia may be indicated under the following conditions:

- Is inflammation of any type present?
- Are there problems with joints and/or cartilage?
- Does the patient have fibrosis?
- Is Crohn's disease or ulcerative colitis present?
- Do you want to modulate the immune system and reduce inflammation at the same time?
- Is cancer present?

Whenever I am presented with a case involving inflammation, Boswellia is the first herb that comes to my mind. I have used it with great success for inflammatory conditions involving the skin, joints, brain, intestines, and respiratory tract. Boswellia reduces inflammation by blocking leukotriene pathways, so it can be used for inflammatory conditions associated with increased leukotriene synthesis, including skin rashes, lung inflammation, asthma, bronchitis, joint pain, and ulcerative colitis.

Boswellia shrinks inflamed tissues by improving blood supply to the affected area, and enhancing the repair of damaged blood vessels. Because it is a resin, however, additional oils must given along with Boswellia to facilitate the herb's crossing the blood–brain barrier. The different anti-inflammatory herbs used in Ayurveda exert their effects via different mechanisms, so they often are used together to increase their anti-inflammatory power synergistically. Boswellia's effects are enhanced when it is combined with Zingiber officinale (shunthi), Curcuma longum (Curcuma), and in modern Ayurveda, bromelain.

Boswellia also can be helpful in the treatment of cancer, as inflammation is considered by many to be one of its underlying causes. Thus, Boswellia's anti-inflammatory activity makes it useful as an adjunct therapy during chemotherapy. Centella asiatica (brahmi), Curcuma longum (Curcuma), Withania somnifera (ashwagandha), and Boswellia enhance the absorption of chemotherapeutic drugs while reducing their side-effects. Further, Boswellia is one of only a few herbs that can cross the blood–brain barrier—more if taken with a fat. This property makes the herb potentially useful in the treatment of brain tumors and inflammation.

Case Histories

Fibrosis

A 62-year-old man with extensive fibrosis in his back came into our clinic for a naturopathic manipulation. After the manipulation, he experienced more flexibility but was still extremely sore, so I prescribed the following typical Boswellia formulation at a double dose:

Boswellia serrata (Boswellia) extract, 300 mg, with Zingiber officinale (shunthi) and Withania somnifera (ashwagandha) extracts, 100 mg each, and Curcuma longum (Curcuma) extract, 50 mg, in a base of bromelain 1600 GDU glucosamine sulphate and chondroitin sulphate.

By the evening his soreness was considerably improved, and by the next day he was fine.

Shoulder pain with popping

A 24-year-old woman visited our clinic complaining of shoulder pain, constriction, and a popping sound in her shoulder when she moved her arm. I prescribed the Boswellia formulation as described above, also at a double dose, plus 1000 mg fish oil three times a day, and an additional dose of Curcuma longum (Curcuma), 500 mg, also three times a day. Within 2 days the patient's shoulder pain was gone and her arm moved freely.

Rheumatoid arthritis

A 39-year-old woman with rheumatoid arthritis came to our clinic in frustration, after having been treated with several rheumatoid modifying prescription medications. At the time of her visit, she was taking prednisone, enbrel, chloroquine, and ibuprofen. She was experiencing gastrointestinal side-effects such as gastritis, gastric ulcers, and a lack of appetite. She had been told that there was no connection between her rheumatoid arthritis and her diet, so she was extremely surprised when I told her that there were definite associations.

We began her treatment with an anti-inflammatory diet, eliminating oranges, wheat, dairy, peanuts, and nightshades, and emphasizing pitta-pacifying foods. In addition, we prescribed sesame oil retention enemas consisting of 10–15 ml warm sesame oil. She also underwent a course of panchakarma detoxification treatments.

Within 2 weeks, she began to notice a significant change in her rheumatoid arthritis symptoms. In 4 months she was completely off prednisone, and her ESR and RA factors, which had remained unchanged on prednisone, began to drop.

Juvenile rheumatoid arthritis

In this interesting case, a 12-year-old boy had been diagnosed with rheumatoid arthritis as a young child. At that time, he was given prednisone, which generally is the first line of treatment in childhood onset rheumatoid arthritis. The boy's parents brought him to our clinic in hopes of finding an alternative treatment to prednisone.

When we explored the patient's medical history, we learned that he had first experienced inflammatory symptoms when he received his first hepatitis B vaccine. At that time, he ran a fever and his entire body became swollen. These symptoms lasted 7 to 8 days. This event was classified as a "minor vaccination reaction," and he was given the second hepatitis B vaccine on schedule. After the second injection, the reaction was more severe; however, he still continued to receive the hepatitis B protocol and was given prednisone for each subsequent reaction.

After the course of hepatitis B vaccine, the boy was considered to be in remission. Six months later, however, the swelling occurred again, but this time the symptoms were not linked to a vaccination. At this point, the family brought him to see me. We gave him homeopathic doses of Thuja to neutralize the vaccination, and put him on the anti-inflammatory diet described in the case above. In addition, we gave him the following anti-inflammatory supplements: the Boswellia formulation described above, along with curcumonoids at a dose of 500 mg three times a day, 1000 mg fish oil supplements three times daily, and probiotics.

We also gave the patient's parents a combination oil composed of Commiphora mukul (guggul) and Boswellia and instructed them to use the warmed oil as part of a daily anti-inflammatory massage. And was prescribed soaking in a bath containing 2 cups of Epsom salts once a week. After 3 weeks of this treatment, almost all of the swelling was gone, and in 9 months his RA factor was back to normal. He now is 22 years old and is a basketball player. He has experienced no further symptoms.

Polymyalgia rheumatica

A 58-year-old female accountant was referred to our clinic by a rheumatologist because of her blood pressure, RA factor, and blood sugar were rising with long-term prednisone treatment. By the time she was referred to our clinic, this patient was ready to make a real commitment to improving her health. She decided to take 3 months off work so she could focus on her deteriorating health. When we began treatment, she was taking 20 mg of prednisone each day. We put her on the Boswellia protocol described in the cases above, and after one week she was able to reduce her prednisone dose to 15 mg.

We also began a panchakarma detoxification series using a compound herbal formula containing Boswellia, guggulu (Commiphora mukul), ashwagandha (Withania somnfera), and nirgundi (Vitex nirgunda) using local cedar needles, Texas bicotta, castor leaves, and nettles, wrapped in a tight ball in a cotton cloth and then rubbed on marma points with the heated compound oil formulation.

After these treatments, she felt so much better that she reduced her prednisone by another 5 mg to 10 mg per day. She continued to receive panchakarma treatments three times a week and was able to reduce her prednisone another 5 mg.

When she reached a 5 mg daily dose of prednisone, she began to run into trouble. Her joints began to swell, her adrenal glands began to over-function, and she began to experience energy crashes, fatigue, vertigo when standing, blackness in front of her eyes, intense sugar cravings, and emotional labiality. These symptoms were the result of withdrawal from synthetic corticosteroids and her body's attempts to resume endogenous corticosteroid production.

At this point, we added the following to her daily herbal regimen:

- Glyzyrrhiza glabra (yastimadhu) extract, 1/8 teaspoon in the morning only, to extend the half-life of the corticosteroids she was taking exogenously and producing endogenously.

- Lotus seeds, which contain steroid compounds similar to prednisone, prepared by soaking 10 to 12 dried seeds overnight and eating them in the morning.

With this additional protocol, she was able to stabilize at a daily dose of 5 mg of prednisone. We kept her on this new supplementation program, together with the original protocol, for another 3 weeks, without making any other changes. During week 4, she began to further reduce her prednisone gradually by shaving off more progressively each day. On day one, she took off one shaving; day two, two shavings; and day three, three shavings. She was able to tolerate this gradual reduction well, and 6 weeks later she was able to stop the prednisone completely. We still see this patient at our clinic, and she has had no further symptoms of polymyalgia rheumatica. She is still taking a maintenance dose of 300 mg Boswellia formulation, plus 500 mg Curcuma and 1000 mg fish oil, each taken once a day.

Psoriatic arthritis

A 54-year-old woman with psoriatic arthritis and psoriasis all over her body came to my clinic for treatment. At that time she was taking 10 mg prednisone, 100 units of Enbrel, and 7.5 mg of methotrexate. We gave her the Boswellia protocol and decided to have her withdraw from one medication at a time. We began with prednisone, and after one month had her reduce her dose to 7.5 mg.

She also began a panchakarma detoxification series, and her skin began to peel off. Two weeks later we reduced her dose of prednisone to 5 mg, and in another 2 weeks, to 2.5 mg. The 2-week intervals provided sufficient time for the adrenal glands to adjust and increase their endogenous production of corticosteroids to replace the synthetic ones that were being withdrawn. At 2.5 mg of prednisone, she began to experience an exacerbation of symptoms, so we added Glycyrrhiza glabra (yastimadhu) extract.

At this point we began working on reducing the methotrexate, to 5 mg from 7.5 mg the first month, then to 2.5 mg a month later. Although prednisone usually can be reduced at 2-week intervals, methotrexate takes longer; usually, at least a month between dose reductions is required. When the patient was doing well on 2.5 mg of prednisone and 2.5 mg of methotrexate, we had her begin to reduce the Enbrel, cutting back by 5 units each week. After 9 months, the patient had withdrawn from all her medications by reducing them every day as described above.

At the end of the treatment plan, the patient's skin was as clear as a baby's skin. She remains a patient at our clinic, now coming in for help with menopausal symptoms. She is on a maintenance protocol of all supplements at single doses taken twice a day, and if any symptoms recur, such as a rash, she doubles the dosage until the symptoms subside.

Crohn's disease

A 28-year-old man with Crohn's colitis came to my clinic for treatment. He was taking both sulfasalazine and prednisone for the disorder. I prescribed an herbal protocol consisting of 600 mg Boswellia three times a day, Curcuma longum (Curcuma) extract 500 mg three times a day with an oil or fat, probiotics (100 billion organisms once a day on an empty stomach), and Asparagus racemosus, (Shatavari) 500 mg three times a day for intestinal health, motility, and inflammation.

After 6 weeks of this treatment, the patient's symptoms started to improve. Nine months later, all of his ulcers were completely healed—unusual in Crohn's disease. He did not have to undergo any detoxification (panchakarma) treatments.

Ulcerative colitis

A 17-year-old girl from Pennsylvania came to our clinic weighing 85 pounds at 5 feet 5 inches tall. She had been diagnosed with ulcerative colitis when she was younger and had experienced many exacerbations, each of which was treated with either prednisone or sulfasalazine. We started her on the Boswellia herbal protocol, along with food allergy testing, which showed that she was sensitive to wheat and gluten, as well as nightshades (peppers, potatoes, tomatoes, eggplant), oranges, and dairy products. The patient started to improve with this protocol, and within 5 months she weighed to 130 pounds. She did not undergo any detoxification treatments. She continues on a maintenance dose of the same herbs and supplements.

Another teenaged patient, a boy, had been seen in our clinic first at age 11, when we treated him with success for ulcerative colitis using the Boswellia protocol. At age 17, he began having problems again because he went off his diet and supplements in order to do things with other children his age.

Unfortunately, in cases of ulcerative colitis, once an exacerbation begins, the protocol must be started all over again. Some patients have a tendency to relax their dietary and lifestyle guidelines when they feel better, but the sensitivities that caused the disorder originally are still present and will resurface if they do not remain vigilant.

Glioblastoma

A 40-year-old Greek male came to clinic with stage four Glioblastoma the size of a grapefruit. He had been diagnosed at the University of Washington Medical School, where he was told that nothing could be done for him. We put him on a ketogenic diet with liberal use of coconut oil, coconut milk, coconut, and ghee. He went through Panch Karma detox treatment and was given the following protocol:

- A medium chain triglyceride bound to Curcuminoids (a highly bio-available compound), one teaspoon twice a day dissolved in rice milk or coconut milk.

- A combination of extracts of Boswellia serrata, Zingiber officinale, Withania somnifera (Ashwagandha), bromelain, glucosamine sulphate, and chondroitin sulphate, three times a day.

- A combination of Commiphora mukul (guggul) extract and Triphala, consisting of equal parts Emblica officinalis (amalaki), Terminalia bellerica (bibhitaki), and Terminalia chebula (haritaki) three times a day.

- A combination of extracts of Bacopa monnieri, Centella asiatica, Ginkgo biloba, Convolvulus pluricaulis (shankhapushpi) and Withania Somnifera (Ashwagandha), three times a day.

Withania somnifera, 500 mg three times per day.

He was instructed to do alternate nostril breathing for 15 minutes twice a day along with yoga and was instructed to walk in nature for 45–60 minutes per day. Following treatment for one year, the MRI showed that his tumor had shrunk from the size of a grapefruit to the size of a walnut. Then he was operated on at University of Washington Medical School. He had some coordination issues resulting from surgery complications and has since moved back to Greece.

Protocols

Rheumatoid and psoriatic arthritis:

Diet: The following foods should be completely avoided: oranges, wheat dairy, peanuts, and nightshades. A constitutional pitta-pacifying diet should be maintained.

Exercise: Yoga is important, especially suukshma pranayam (joint breathing exercises), coordinating deep breathing with small joint rotation, flexion, extension of all joints, including the head/neck, shoulders, elbows, wrist, hands, hips, knees, and ankles. This is vital if the patient can't do regular exercise or walk. Micro-movements help to remove immune complexes that block normal joint function in arthritis patients and, in turn, reduce inflammation.

The following therapies are also useful:

Swimming in arthritis pools, preferably those that are not sanitized with chlorine;

epsom salt baths and/or hot tubs at home. The patient can do exercises in the tub, inhaling with the mouth closed and exhaling with mouth open while exercising the joints.

Herbal therapy:

Boswellia protocol: Boswellia serrata (Boswellia) extract, 300 mg, with Zingiber officinale (yastimadhu) and Withania somnifera (Ashwagandha) extracts, 100 mg each, and Curcuma longum (Curcuma) extract, 50 mg, in a base of bromelain 1600 GDU glucosamine sulphate and chondroitin sulphate. This formulation should be given at a double dose, twice daily.

Encephalitis:

Encephalitis is an inflammation of the brain caused by a bacterial or viral infection, so Boswellia must be administered in an oil base to ensure its transport across the blood–brain barrier. The Boswellia formulation may be taken with fish oils, ghee, coconut oil, and/or olive oil. A combination of oils ensures that the body gets a broad spectrum of the oils, which can aid in reducing inflammation.

Crohn's disease and ulcerative colitis:

Restorative and meditative yoga and breathing exercises appropriate to the patient's constitution, in addition to regular aerobic exercise such as walking, strengthen internal resilience and improve the body's response to stress.

Herbal therapy:

600 mg Boswellia (the formulation described above) three times a day, along with Curcuma longum (Curcuma) extract 500 mg three times a day, with an oil or fat.

probiotics, 100 billion organisms once a day, on an empty stomach.

For intestinal health, motility and inflammation, Asparagus racemosus (shataavari):

500 mg three times a day.

For additional dietary support:

pomegranate (or pomegranate juice if the whole fruit not available); dried seeds can be purchased at Indian markets and soaked overnight. Fresh mint, salt, and a little lemon, blended together to make a chutney which soothes the gastrointestinal system.

Bronchial asthma:

Boswellia is especially useful in cases of bronchial asthma if the eosinophil count is elevated, because the herb blocks leukotriene synthesis. Recovery usually takes about 2 months.

Herbal therapy:

For inflammation and immune modulation: Boswellia formulation (above), three times a day.

For respiratory support: Tylophora asthmatica (antraapaachak) extract, 150 mg in a blend with Piper longum, Emblica officinalis, and Zingiber officinale extract, three times a day.

For immune support: 400 mg each Emblica officinalis (amalaki), Ocimum sanctum (tulsi), Terminalia bellerica (bibhitaki/bahera), with Tinospora cordifolia (guduchi) and Glycyrrhiza glabra (shunthi), 200 mg. each, plus Terminalia chebula (haritaki) and Adhatoda vasica (vasaka), 100 mg each, three times a day.

Allergic dermatitis with pruritis (pitta dominance):

Boswellia formulation 300–600 mg three times a day, with Curcuma longum (Curcuma), 500 mg three times a day, with oil or fat. If the rash is from a fungal infection or blood congestion (i.e., blood-borne disease rather than pitta dominance), use Neem (Azadirachta indica).

Because it is a resin, Boswellia absorption is increased significantly if it is taken with an oil. Good transport vehicles are olive, hemp seed, Neem (Azadirachta indica), coconut, and walnut oils, as well as ghee and fish oil. It also is well absorbed with pomegranate juice. Taking Boswellia with food further enhances its activity.

Safety Profile

Boswellia has been well tolerated in most studies; however, some people experience stomach discomfort, including nausea, acid reflux (heartburn), a feeling of fullness, stomach pain, or diarrhea. Irritation of the skin has been reported from a multi-herb product containing Boswellia. Care should be taken not to exceed the recommended dosage.

Dosage

Gum resin: 2–3 g
Oil: 1–1.5 ml
Bark decoction: 56–112 ml
Standardized extract for 50% boswellic acid 300 mg three times per day

Ayurvedic Properties

Rasa: Kashaya (astringent), tikta (bitter), madhur (sweet)
Guna: Laghu (light), ruksha (dry)
Veerya: Ushna (hot)
Vipaka: Katu (pungent)
Dosha: Balances kapha and pitta

Notes

1. M. K Jha, *Folk Veterinary Medicine of Bihar—A Research Project* (Anand, Gujrat: NDDB, 1992).

2. Sharma S, Thawani V, Hingorani L. Pharmacokinetic study of 11-Keto beta-Boswellic acid, *Phytomedicine*, Feb. 2004, 11(2–3):255–260.

3. B. Mahajan, S.C. Taneja, V.K. Sethi, and K.L. Dhar, "Two triterpenoids from Boswellia serratagum resin," *Phytochemistry*, 1995, 39(2):453–455.

4. J.C.E. Simpson and N.E. Williams, "The triterpene group. Part I. B-Boswellic acid, "*Journal of the Chemical Society*, 1938, 686. [Is 686 the page number? If so, we need volume and issue, as in #3.]

5. R.A. Sharma and K.C. Varma, "Studies on Gum Obtained from Boswellia serrata Roxb. *Indian Drugs*, 1980, 17:225.

6. V.M. Bhuchar, A.K. Agrawal, and S.K. Sharma, "Constituents of gum obtained from Boswellia serrataexudate," *Indian Journal of Technology*, 1982, 20(1):38.

7. M.L. Gangwal and D.K. Vardhan, "Carbohydrate contents of Boswellia serrata," *Asian Journal of Chemistry*, 1995, 7(3):677.

8. K. Sengupta, K.V. Alluri, A.R. Satish, S. Mishra, T. Golakoti, K.V. Sarma, D. Dey, and S.P. Raychaudhuri, "A double blind, randomized, placebo controlled study of the efficacy and safety of 5-Loxin(R) for treatment of osteoarthritis of the knee," *Arthritis Res Ther.*, July 30, 2008, 10(4):R85.

9. N. Kimmatkar, V. Thawani, L. Hingorani, and R. Khiyani, "Efficacy and tolerability of Boswellia serrata extract in treatment of osteoarthritis of knee: A randomized double blind placebo controlled trial." *Phytomedicine*, Jan. 2003, 10(1):3–7.

10. A. Chopra, P. Lavin, B. Patwardhan, and D.A. Chitre, "32-week randomized, placebo-controlled clinical evaluation of RA-11, an Ayurvedic drug, on osteoarthritis of the knees," *J Clin Rheumatol.*, Oct. 2004, 10(5):236–245.

11. H.P.T. Ammon, H. Safayhi, T. Mack, and J. Sabieraj, "Mechanism of anti-inflammatory actions of Curcuma and boswellic acids," *Journal of Ethnopharmacology*, 1993, 38(2,3): 13.

12. E.J. Blain, A.Y. Ali, and V.C. Duance, "Boswellia frereana (frankincense) suppresses cytokine-induced matrix metalloproteinase expression and production of pro-inflammatory molecules in articular cartilage," *Phytother Res.*, June 2010, 24(6):905–912.

13. M. Abdel-Tawab, O. Werz, and M. Schubert-Zsilavecz, "Boswellia serrata: An overall assessment of in vitro, preclinical, pharmacokinetic and clinical data," *Clin Pharmacokinet.*, June 2011, 50(6):349–369.

14. G.B. Singh, S. Singh, S. Bani, and A. Kaul, *Boswellic Acids— A New Class of Anti-inflammatory Drugs with a Novel Mode of Action*, International Seminar on Traditional Medicine, Calcutta, India, November 7–9, 1992.

15. G.B. Singh and C.K. Atal, "Pharmacology of an extract of Boswellia guggalex–Boswellia serrata, a new non-steroidal anti-inflammatory agent," *Agents and Actions*, 1986, 18:407.

16. L. Tausch A. Henkel, U. Siemoneit, D. Poeckel, N. Kather, L. Franke, B. Hofmann, G. Schneider, C. Angioni, G. Geisslinger, C. Skarke, W. Holtmeier, T. Beckhaus, M. Karas, J. Jauch, and O. Werz, "Identification of human cathepsin G as a functional target of boswellic acids from the anti-inflammatory remedy frankincense," *J Immunol.*, Sept. 2009, 183(5):3433–3442.

17. C. Cuaz-Pérolin, L. Billiet, E. Baugé, C. Copin, D. Scott-Algara, F. Genze, B. Büchele, T. Syrovets, T. Simmet, and M. Rouis, "Antiinflammatory and antiatherogenic effects of the NF-kappaB inhibitor acetyl-11-keto-beta-boswellic acid in LPS-challenged ApoE-/- mice," *Arterioscler Thromb Vasc Biol.*, Feb. 2008, 28(2):272–277.

18. S. Roy, S. Khanna, H. Shah, C. Rink, C. Phillips, H. Preuss, G.V. Subbaraju, G. Trimurtulu, A.V. Krishnaraju, M. Bagchi, D. Bagchi, and C.K. Sen, "Human genome screen to identify the genetic basis of the anti-inflammatory effects of Boswellia in microvascular endothelial cells," *DNA Cell Biol.*, April 2005, 24(4):244–255.

19. A.E. Slonim, M. Grovit, and L. Bulone, "Effect of exclusion diet with nutraceutical therapy in juvenile Crohn's disease," *J Am Coll Nutr.*, June 2009, 28(3):277–285.

20. G. Latella, R. Sferra, A. Vetuschi, G. Zanninelli, A. D'Angelo, V. Catitti, R. Caprilli, and E. Gaudio, "Prevention of colonic fibrosis by Boswellia and Scutellaria extracts in rats with colitis induced by 2,4,5-trinitrobenzene sulphonic acid," *Eur J Clin Invest.*, June 2008, 38(6):410–420.

21. A. Madisch, S. Miehlke, O. Eichele, J. Mrwa, B. Bethke, E. Kuhlisch, E. Bästlein, G. Wilhelms, A. Morgner, B. Wigginghaus, and M. Stolte, "Boswellia serrata extract for the treatment of collagenous colitis: A double-blind, randomized, placebo-controlled, multicenter trial," *Int J Colorectal Dis,.* Dec. 2007, 22(12):1445–1451.

22. C. Anthoni, M.G. Laukoetter, E. Rijcken, T. Vowinkel, R. Mennigen, S. Müller, N. Senninger, J. Russell, J. Jauch, J. Bergmann, D.N. Granger, and C.F. Krieglstein, "Mechanisms underlying the anti-inflammatory actions of boswellic acid derivatives in experimental colitis," *Am J Physiol Gastrointest Liver Physiol.*, June 2006, 290(6):G1131–1137.

23. S. Singh, A. Khajuria, S.C. Taneja, R.K. Khajuria, J. Singh, R.K. Johri, and G.N. Qazi, "The gastric ulcer protective effect of boswellic acids, a leukotriene inhibitor from Boswellia serrata, in rats," *Phytomedicine*, June 2008, 15(6–7):408–415.

24. I. Gupta, V. Gupta, A. Pariha, et al., "Effects of Boswellia serratagum resin in patients with bronchial asthma: Results of a double-blind, placebo-controlled, 6 week clinical study," *European Journal of Medical Research*, 1998, 3(11):511.

25. C.E. Clark, E. Arnold, T.J. Lasserson, and T. Wu, "Herbal interventions for chronic asthma in adults and children: A systematic review and meta-analysis," *Prim Care Respir J.*, July 18, 2010.

26. M.L. Sharma, A. Kaul, A. Khajuria, S. Singh, and G.B. Singh, "Immunomodulatory activity of Boswellic acids (pentacyclictriterpene acids) from Boswellia serrata," *Phytotherapy Research*, 1996, 10(2):107.

27. A.F. Raja, F. Ali, I..A. Khan, A.S. Shawl, and D.S. Arora, "Acetyl-11-keto-β-boswellic acid (AKBA); targeting oral cavity pathogens," *BMC Res Notes*, Oct. 13, 2011, 4:406.

28. Y. Shao, C.T. Ho, C.K. Chin, V. Badmaev, and M.T. Huang, "Inhibitory activity of boswellic acids from Boswellia serrata against human leukemia HL-60 cells in culture," *Planta Medica*, 1998, 64(4):328.

29. A.C. Estrada, T. Syrovets, K. Pitterle, O. Lunov, B. Büchele, J. Schimana-Pfeifer, T. Schmidt, S.A. Morad, and T. Simmet, "Tirucallic acids are novel pleckstrin homology domain-dependent Akt inhibitors inducing apoptosis in prostate cancer cells," *Mol Pharmacol.*, March 2010, 77(3):378–387.

30. M. Lu, L. Xia, H. Hua, and Y. Jing, "Acetyl-keto-beta-boswellic acid induces apoptosis through a death receptor 5-mediated pathway in prostate cancer cells," *Cancer Res.*, Feb 15, 2008, 68(4):1180–1186.

31. A.B. Kunnumakkara, A.S.Nair, B. Sung, M.K. Pandey, and B.B. Aggarwal, "Boswellic acid blocks signal transducers and activators of transcription 3 signaling, proliferation, and survival of multiple myeloma via the protein tyrosine phosphatase SHP-1," *Mol Cancer Res.*, Jan. 2009, 7(1):118–128.

32. Y. Omura, N. Horiuchi, M.K. Jones, D.P. Lu, Y. Shimotsuura, H. Duvvi, A. Pallos, M. Ohki, and A. Suetsugu, "Temporary anti-cancer & anti-pain effects of mechanical stimulation of any one of 3 front teeth (1st incisor, 2nd incisor, & canine) of right & left side of upper & lower jaws and their possible mechanism, & relatively long term disappearance of pain & cancer parameters by one optimal dose of DHEA, Astragalus, Boswellia serrata, often with press needle stimulation of True ST. 36," *Acupunct Electrother Res.* 2009, 34(3–4):175–203.

33. Zirbel R; Fernando RC; Tuschen-Burger E; Sahinbas H Afrikanischer Weihrauch, Boswellia carterii: Therapieeinsatz bei chronisch-entzundlichen und allergischen Erkrankungen und in der komplementaren Onkologie. Jan 1, 2004; 53(6): 356-63

34. S. Kirste, M. Treier, S.J. Wehrle, G. Becker, M. Abdel-Tawab, K. Gerbeth, M.J. Hug, B. Lubrich, A.L. Grosu, and F. Momm, "Boswellia serrata acts on cerebral edema in patients irradiated for brain tumors: a prospective, randomized, placebo-controlled, double-blind pilot trial," *Cancer*, Aug. 15, 2011, 117(16):3788–3795.

35. O. Karima, G. Riazi, R. Yousefi, and A.A. Movahedi, "The enhancement effect of beta-boswellic acid on hippocampal neurites outgrowth and branching (an in vitro study)," *Neurol Sci.*, June 2010, 31(3):315–320.

36. A. Moussaieff, N.A. Shein, J. Tsenter, S. Grigoriadis, C. Simeonidou, A.G. Alexandrovich, V. Trembovler, Y. Ben-Neriah, M.L. Schmitz, B.L. Fiebich, E. Munoz, R. Mechoulam, and E. Shohami, "Incensole acetate: a novel neuroprotective agent isolated from Boswelliacarterii," *J Cereb Blood Flow Metab..* July 2008, 28(7):1341–1352.

37. P. Calzavara-Pinton, C. Zane, E. Facchinetti, R. Capezzera, and A. Pedretti,"Topical boswellic acids for treatment of photoaged skin," *Dermatol Ther.*, Jan–Feb, 2010, 23 (Suppl 1):S28–32.

38. S.Y. Chang, "Effects of aroma hand massage on pain, state anxiety and depression in hospice patients with terminal cancer," *Taehan Kanho Hakhoe Chi.* [check for word breaks] – this is fine and is correct Aug. 2008, 38(4):493–502.

39. M.L. Gangwal and D.K. Vardhan, "Antifungal activity of essential oil of Boswellia serrata," *Asian Journal of Chemistry*, 1995, 7(3):675.

40. U. Zutshi, P.G. Rao, S. Kaur, G.B. Singh, S. Singh, and C.K. Atal, "Mechanism of cholesterol lowering effects of Boswellia guggulsx. Boswellia serrata Roxb," *Indian Journal of Pharmacology*, 1986, 18(3):182.

10

Centella asiatica

Introduction

Centella asiatica has been referred to as "one of the miracle elixirs of life." This creeping plant, commonly called Gotu kola, is known in Ayurvedic tradition as a rasayana, or rejuvenative tonic. Its range of medicinal uses is exceptional. According to folklore, one ancient Chinese herbalist lived more than 200 years of age as a result of using Gotu kola.

Gotu kola is highly valued for its effectiveness in treating a variety of skin disorders, including leprosy. It provides healing action for wounds and psoriasis. Gotu kola is believed to have a refreshing effect on the mind and is used to treat depression. European herbalists use the herb to treat the conditions that underlie connective tissue swelling in disorders such as scleroderma, psoriatic arthritis, and rheumatoid arthritis.

Modern research has confirmed many of the traditional uses of Gotu kola, and has suggested interesting new uses as well. Gotu kola offers potential for treating high blood pressure and pooling of blood in the veins, known as venous insufficiency. Gotu kola traditionally is used as an herbal therapy for syphilis, ulcers, epilepsy, bronchitis, asthma, and hepatitis.

Synonymous Names

English: Indian pennywort, Gotu Kola
Hindi: Brahmi
Sanskrit: Mandukparni
Other names include: Centella, Centella asiatica, Hydrocotyle, Indian pennywort, Luei gong gen, Marsh pennywort, Asiatic Pennywort, Luei Gong Gen, Takip-kohol, Antanan, Pegagan, Pegaga, vallaarai, Kula kud, and Bai Bua Bok.

Habitat

Gotu kola is found in India, Sri Lanka, Southeast Asia, China, Madagascar, South Africa, the southeastern United States, Mexico, Venezuela, and Columbia. It grows in moist habitats along ditches and in low wet areas, up to an altitude of 7500 feet (2500 meters).

Botanical Characteristics

Gotu kola is an herbaceous, perennial creeper that thrives in and around water. The herb's pink to pale violet flowers appear during August and September. Gotu kola has the faint aroma of tobacco and a slightly bitter taste.

The leaves are small, green, and fan-shaped, and measure about 2–5 cm in diameter. The long petioles, which arise from the stem nodes, grow in rosettes. The stems are slender, prostrate, often reddish-colored, and interconnect one plant with another.

The flowers range from white to pink or pale violet. The fruit is small and oval, consisting of two to five seeds enclosed within a thick, hard pericarp. The rootstock consists of rhizomes that grow down vertically. They are cream-colored and covered with root hairs. The leaves and stems of the Gotu kola plant are used for medicinal purposes. Gotu kola is easily cultivated and matures within 3 months. The whole plant, including the roots, is harvested manually.

Chemical Composition

Gotu kola's triterpenoids asiatic acid, 6-hydroxy asiatic acid, madecassic acid, betulinic acid, thankunic acid, and isothankunic acid, with their glycosides, make up as much as 8% of its chemical constitution. Its major saponins are asiaticoside, asiaticoside A, asiaticoside B, madecassoside, braminoside, brahmoside, brahminoside, thankuniside and isothankuniside.

Essential oil: Essential oil comprises about 0.1 % of the aerial parts of the Gotu kola plant. Up to about 80% of the oil consists of sesquiterpenoids, of which β-caryophyllene, cc-humulene and germacrene-D, elemene and bicycloelemene, and trans-farnesene are the most abundant.

Flavone derivatives: Quercetin and kaempferol glycosides and astragalin have been found.

Phytosterols: Stigmasterol, sitosterol.

Amino acids: Gotu kola's leaves contain the amino acids alanine, arginine, aspartic acid, glutamic acid, glycine, histidine, isoleucine, leucine, lysine, methionine, phenylalanine, proline, threonine, and tryptophan.

Pharmacological Activity

Gotu kola has a revitalizing effect on the brain and nervous system and is believed to increase attention span and concentration, counteracting the effects of aging.[5,6] The plant is valued as a adaptogen.[7] It has anti-bacterial, anti-viral, anti-ulcerogenic stimulant and diuretic properties. Gotu kola also is effective in treating venous insufficiency and is used in some areas for opium detoxification.

Wound-healing activity

Gotu kola's triterpenoids have been shown to facilitate wound healing in animals.[8] These active principles strengthen skin, enhance anti-oxidant concentration, and increase blood supply to inflamed tissues. Because of these properties, Gotu kola is used externally for burns, psoriasis, prevention of post-surgery scar formation, episiotomy recovery, and external fistulas. In traditional medicines, Gotu kola is used to treat leprosy.

In one animal study that confirmed Gotu kola's wound-healing capacity, the wound chambers were treated with an extract of the herb, and the active components asiatic acid, madecassic acid, and asiaticoside were evaluated. The wound chambers treated with the extract showed an increase in total protein, DNA, collagen, dry weight, and uronic acid. The enhancement of wound-healing capability caused by Gotu kola was believed to be the result of an increase in collagen matrix within the wound.[9]

When treated with Gotu kola, maturation of scars is stimulated by the production of type I collagen. The treatment also results in a marked decrease in inflammatory reaction and myofibroblast production.[10]

Cartilage destruction is one of the primary features in osteoarthritis. In a zymosan-induced acute arthritis model, standardized Centella asiatica fraction inhibited proteoglycan depletion without modulating joint swelling and inflammatory cell infiltration. Cartilage protective activity might be induced at least partially by the inhibition of nitric oxide production.[11]

Diabetes is largely understood to delay wound healing. To assess Gotu kola's capacity to assist healing in the presence of diabetes, a topical solution of asiaticoside extracted from Gotu kola was applied to punch wounds in experimental animals. The extract increased hydroxyproline content, tensile strength, collagen content, and epithelialization, significantly facilitating the healing process.[12] Gotu kola extract also protected skin against radiation injury.[13]

Centella asiatica cream and hyaluronic acid were used for improving the appearance of stretch marks (striae rubra). The women participants with bilateral stretch marks applied the cream twice daily for 12 weeks to the randomized left or right, outer aspect of the thigh. No treatment was administered to the contralateral side. The participants were evaluated at weeks 2, 4, 8, and 12. The primary efficacy endpoints included color, texture, softness, and overall appearance of the stretch marks by the participant and the investigator at week 12. The treated thigh demonstrated a statistically significant difference in the mean change in participant and investigator evaluations in overall appearance, texture, color, and softness compared to the untreated thigh at week 12. No adverse events occurred during the study.[14]

Stasis sore of the lower limbs is a typical chronic venous insufficiency complication, and its treatment is still a widely controversial issue. The common therapies do not show complete efficacy. A multicentric clinical trial was conducted at the Plastic and Reconstructive Surgery of "Sapienza" University of Rome.[15] Idrastin (a combination of Aesculus hippocastanum, Vitis vinifera, Ruscus aculeatus, allantoin, and Centella asiatica and hyaluronic acid) lymph-draining cream was used in patients with stasis ulcers of the lower limbs. The 80 patients enrolled were split into two groups of 40 patients: Group A was treated by only elastocompressive therapy, and group B by elastocompressive therapy and Idrastin. The multicentric analysis considered the following parameters: local pain, perilesional flogosis, granulation tissue, and healing time. In group B, where the combination of herbs was added: the pain stopped in 72 hours; inflammation disappeared in one week; tissue granulation growth stopped in one week; and the lesions healed in 4 weeks. These results were statistically and significantly different from elastocompressive therapy.

Asiaticoside, a major triterpenoid saponin component isolated from Centella asiatica, has been studied with septic lung injury induced by cecal ligation and puncture in mice. The mice pre-treated with asiaticoside showed significantly decreased cecal ligation and puncture induced mortality, lung pathological damage, the infiltration of mononuclear, polymorphonuclear (PMN) leucocytes, and total proteins. The mechanisms might be related to upregulation of PPAR-gamma (peroxisome proliferator-activated receptors) expression to some extent, which inhibits mitogen activated protein kinases (MAPKs) and the NF-kappaB pathway.[16]

The madecassoside triterpenoid component of Centella asiatica showed cardioprotective effects from lipopolysaccharide (LPS) induced injury to the heart. It inhibited LPS-stimulated TNF-alpha production by blocking ERK1/2, p38 and NF-kappaB pathways in cardiomyocytes.[17]

Similar results were obtained in a liver injury model of mice. They showed remarkable hepatoprotective results by the same mechanism—inhibition of TNF-alpha and MAPKs.[18]

Centella asiatica aqueous extract at low concentrations could be useful to promote corneal epithelium wound healing.[19]

Anti-ulcerogenic activity

Gotu kola has been shown to have anti-ulcerogenic properties. The plant's fresh juice was studied to determine its effect on laboratory-induced gastric ulcers in rats. The juice was tested on ulcers induced by ethanol, aspirin, cold restraint stress, and pyloric ligation. Oral doses of 200 and 600 mg/kg were given twice daily for 5 days. At the end of the study period, significant protection was shown against ulcers induced by all four ulcerogenic agents, and the results were comparable to those elicited by sucralfate (SF, 250 mg/kg, p.o., BD×5 days). Gotu kola's action is believed to be a result primarily of its capacity to strengthen mucosal defense factors.[20,21]

Animal studies showed that Centella asiatica extracts inhibited gastric ulceration induced by cold and restraint stress in rats. The antiulcer activity was compared to famotidine (H_2-antagonist) and sodium valproate (antiepleptic or anti-seizure). Both the drugs and the herb extract showed a dose dependent reduction of gastric ulceration.[22]

Immunomodulatory activity

Laboratory studies using mice examined the effect of Gotu kola extract on immune function. An alcoholic extract of the plant stimulated the reticuloendothelial system in mice. An in-vitro study using the aqueous extract of Gotu kola also showed therapeutic action on classic and alternative immunomodulatory pathways.[23,24]

Anti-arthritic activity

The aqueous extract of Centella asiatica revealed significant antinociceptive activity in mice subjected to acetic acid induced writhing and the hot-plate method, similar to aspirin but less potent than morphine and significant anti-inflammatory activity comparable to mefenamic acid. These results suggest that the aqueous Centella extract possess antinociceptive and anti-inflammatory activities that justify the traditional use of this plant in treating inflammatory conditions and rheumatism.[25,26]

The anti-rheumatoid arthritic effect of madecassoside in type II collagen-induced arthritis in mice was studied to investigate the therapeutic potential and underlying mechanisms of madecassoside. Madecassoside (10, 20, and 40 mg/kg), orally administered from the day of the antigen challenge for 20 consecutive days, dose-dependently alleviated the severity of the disease based on the reduced clinical scores, and elevated the body weights of the mice. Also, a histopathological examination indicated that madecassoside alleviated infiltration of inflammatory cells and synovial hyperplasia, and provided protection against joint destruction. Madecassoside reduced the serum level of anti-type II collagen IgG, suppressed the delayed type hypersensitivity against type II collagen and moderately suppressed proliferation of lymphocytes from popliteal lymph nodes. Centella asiatica has clinical uses in rheumatoid arthritis, and the underlying mechanisms of action may be mainly through regulation of the abnormal humoral and cellular immunity, as well as protection from joint destruction.[27]

Anti-tubercular activity

Another interesting use of Gotu kola is seen in its effectiveness against tuberculosis. This effect was studied on guinea pigs that had been infected with tubercle bacillus 15 days previously. The animals were injected with a 4% solution of hydroxyasiaticoside extracted from Gotu kola. The extract was shown to reduce the quantity of tubercular lesions in the lungs, liver, nerve cells, and spleen of the infected animals. The extract also decreased the spleen volume of the treated animals. These results demonstrate the anti-tubercular activity of Gotu kola.[28]

Cardiotonic and venous insufficiency activity

Clinical trials have affirmed the effectiveness of Gotu kola in treating venous insufficiency and varicose veins. These conditions are characterized by pooling of blood in the legs and leakage of fluid from the veins resulting from the loss of elasticity. An ultrasound examination of patients with varicose veins showed improvement in vascular tone after treatment with Gotu kola.[29,30]

In a study of patients with post phlebetic syndrome, they showed a greater number of circulating endothelial cells compared to the normal subjects. During a 3-week treatment with Centella asiatica triterpenic fraction (CATF), the patients who received 90 mg CATF daily in three divided dosages showed a statistically significant decrease in circulating endothelial cells, thereby protecting the integrity of the vascular intima.[31]

Ninety-four patients suffering from venous insufficiency of the lower limbs were divided into three groups, treated with (1) titrated extracts of Centella asiatica (TECA), (2) a combination of asiatic acid (30%), madecasic acids (30%), and asiaticoside (40%) (120 mg/day, 60 mg/day) or (3) a placebo for 2 months. A significant difference (p less than 0.05) in favor of TECA was shown for the symptoms of heaviness in the lower limbs and edema, as well as for the overall evaluation by the patient. The venous sufficiency improved in the TECA groups but was aggravated in the placebo group.[32]

Fifty-two patients with venous hypertension (pressure greater than 42 mmHg) were divided into three groups. Group A (20 patients) was treated with Total Triterpenic fraction of Centella Asiatica (TTFCA) 60 mg tid; Group B (20 patients) was treated with 30 mg tid; Group C (12 patients) was treated with placebo; and Group D (10 normal subjects) was treated with TTFCA 60 mg tid in an open study. After 4 weeks of treatment, significant improvements were observed in a dose-dependent manner in the parameters tested, such as filtration rate, ankle edema, and ankle circumference. No significant changes were observed in the placebo and the control subjects treated with TTFCA.[33]

Eighty-seven patients with chronic venous hypertensive microangiopathy were administered TTFCA for 60 days. The microcirculatory effects of two dosages (30 mg bid and 60 mg bid) versus the placebo were assessed in a double-blind study. The microcirculatory parameters—peri-malleolar skin flux at rest (RF) and transcutaneous PO_2 and PCO_2—improved as a result. The microcirculatory parameters were improved, as compared to the placebo, in a dose-dependent manner; the higher the dose, the more improved were the symptoms.[34]

The microcirculatory parameters and vascular permeability improved in all the patients (10 normal subjects, 22 patients with moderate, superficial venous hypertension, 12 patients with postphlebitic limbs and severe venous hypertension) as measured by laser Doppler flowmetry.[35]

A combination of ascorbic acid, quercetin, gotu kola extract (10% asiatic acid), and green tea extract (40% epigallocatechin gallate) was studied in atherosclerosis model cell lines. The combination revealed a reduction of monocyte adhesion to the endothelium. This may offer the prospect of new treatment for ischemic heart disease.[36]

Centella asiatica resulted in interesting findings in lipid metabolism in an oxidative stress model of rats. Centella asiatica powder significantly ($P < 0.05$) lowered serum low-density lipoprotein compared to that of the control rats, and significantly increased ($P < 0.05$) level of high-density lipoprotein and lowered triglyceride level compared to the rats that were fed only the normal diet. However, the cholesterol level of rats fed both Centella asiatica extract and powder was found to be significantly ($P < 0.05$) higher than that of the control rats. Interestingly, consumption of Centella significantly decreased the body and liver weights of the rats, and no histological changes were noticed.[37]

Gotu kola has a cardiotonic effect—reducing blood pressure by improving venous insufficiency. In my clinical experience, patients with heart disease and high blood pressure who took Gotu kola experienced a significant reduction in diastolic blood pressure.

Anti-anxiety and insomnia activity

Gotu kola's triterpenoids are reported to decrease anxiety and increase mental function. Patients who took Gotu kola were less likely to be startled by a sudden noise (a potential indicator of anxiety) than those who took a placebo.[38]

Brahmoside and brahminoside constituents of Centella are sleep-promoting, and the anxiolytic activity is considered to be caused in part by binding to cholecystokinin receptors (CCK_B), a group of G protein-coupled receptors that bind the peptide hormones cholesystokinin or gastrin and were thought to play a potential role in modulation of anxiety, nociception, memory, and hunger in animals and humans.[39]

The effectiveness of Gotu kola in treating anxiety and insomnia also have been demonstrated in animal research. The alcoholic extract, when given orally to rats and mice treated with phenobarbitone, significantly prolonged sleeping time. The herb also significantly reduced the duration of convulsions in rats when given electroshock treatment. In a behavioral test, Gotu kola reduced the length of the immobility phase, indicating sedative, antidepressive, and analgesic actions.[40]

In another study, 500 mg of 70% hydro-ethanolic extract of Centella asiatica was given twice a day after meals to a total of 33 (18 male and 15 female) patients with generalized anxiety disorder. Hamilton's Brief Psychiatric Rating Scale was used to screen the subjects. They were investigated thoroughly using the standard questionnaires based on the psychological rating scale at baseline (day 0), mid-term (day 30), and final (day 60). The scale also includes a number of direct queries about current levels of experienced stress. Centella extract significantly ($p<0.01$) decreased anxiety related disorders and also significantly ($p<0.01$) reduced stress phenomenon and its correlated depression. All of the patients improved their willingness for adjustment and cognition ($p<0.01$).[41]

Anti-depressant properties

The anti-depressant action of Centella asiatica was compared to imipramine (Tofranil). Triterpenes of Centella reduced the immobility time and ameliorated the imbalance of amino acid levels, confirming the anti-depressant activity.[42] Another study showed it to decrease corticosterone and increase the contents of 5-hydroxytryptamine, dopamine, and norepinephrine and their metabolites 5- hydroxyindoleacetic acid (5-HIAA), 3-methoxy-4-hydroxyphenyl glycol (MHPG) in the rat brain.[43]

In a study conducted with 60 subjects in an age group of 65 years and older, using Mini Mental State Examination (MMSE) scoring, activities of daily living and the Yesavage geriatric depression scale were evaluated. MMSE scoring improved significantly after administration of Centella asiatica for 6 months in the elderly subjects with mild cognitive impairment at a dosage of 500 mg twice a day. Improvements were observed in depression, hypertension, peripheral neuritis, insomnia, loss of appetite, and constipation. This indicates that Centella is an ideal remedy for age-related cognitive decline in elderly people.[44]

Inflammatory bowel disease

Colitis was induced in rats by intracolonic instillation of dinitrobenzene sulphonic acid. Centella asiatica extract was administered orally (0.2 or 2 mg/kg) daily. Four days after administration of dinitrobenzene sulphonic acid, treatment with Centella asiatica extract significantly reduced the incidence of diarrhea and the loss of body weight. This was associated with a significant reduction in colonic tissue myeloperoxidase activity. Centella extract reduced NF-kappaB activation, inducible nitric oxide synthase, nitrotyrosine, poly(ADP-ribose) polymerase (PARP), matrix metalloproteinase-9 (MMP-9), and –MMP-2 activity in the colon and reduced the upregulation of Intercellular Adhesion Molecule 1 (ICAM-1) and the expression of P-Selectin, suggesting a beneficial effect for treating inflammatory bowel disease.[45]

Cognitive and neuroprotective properties

Centella asiatica used as a brain and nervous system tonic is shown to increase attention span and concentration.[46] And fresh juice of Centella asiatica has been shown to increase dendritic length and dendritic branching points along the length of dendrites, making Centella an excellent choice to treat stress, neurodegenerative diseases, and memory loss.[47] A study demonstrated cognitive-enhancing and anti-oxidant properties of Centella in normal rats. The rats treated with Centella showed a dose dependent increase in cognitive behavior in passive avoidance and elevated plus-maze paradigms in streptozocin-induced cognitive impairment. A significant decrease in malondialdehyde and an increase in glutathione and catalase levels were observed in rats treated with 200 and 300 mg/kg of Centella. Alzheimer's disease is considered to be an oxidative stress-induced disease. Streptozocin-induced cognitive impairment in animals is similar to Alzheimer's disease in humans.[48]

A cell line expressing amyloid beta 1-42 (A beta) in the neuroblastoma cell line, and an embryonic cortical primary cell culture showed an increased phosphorylation of cyclic AMP response element binding (CREB) protein in both cell lines. The effects were thought to be a result of extracellular signal-regulated kinase- ribosomal S6 kinase (ERK/SRK) signaling pathways.[49]

Oral administration of methanol extract of Centella, 50 mg/kg/day for 14 days, significantly increased the anti-oxidant enzymes including superoxide dismutase (SOD), catalase, and glutathione peroxidase (GSHPx) in lymphoma-bearing mice.[50]

Asiatic acid derivatives have been shown to exert significant neuroprotective effects on cultured cortical cells by increasing the cellular oxidative defense mechanisms and thereby protecting neurons from the oxidative damage caused by exposure to excess glutamate.[51]

Another study demonstrated the protective effects of asiaticoside derivatives against beta-amyloid neurotoxicity when tested on B103 cell cultures and hippocampal slices. Of 28 of the asiaticoside derivatives' three components, asiatic acid showed a strong inhibition of beta-amyloid- and free radical-induced cell death in B103 cell cultures and hippocampal slices. All of these findings suggest that Centella can have a beneficial role in reversing neurodegenerative diseases including Alzheimer's disease.[52]

PSAPP mice are characterized as the model for amyloid plaque formation. Centella asiatica extract was given to PSAPP mice at doses of 2.5 mg/kg and 5.00 mg/kg. Significant decreases in amyloid beta 1-40 and 1-42 were detectable by ELISA following an 8-month treatment with 2.5 mg/kg of Centella extract, and a reduction in Congo Red-stained fibrillar amyloid plaques was detected with the 5.0 mg/kg dose. Centella impacted the amyloid cascade altering amyloid beta pathology in the brains of PSAPP mice and modulated components of the oxidative stress response that has been implicated in the neurodegenerative changes of Alzheimer's disease.[53]

In Parkinson's disease model rats, 1-methyl-4-phenyl-1,2,3,6-tetrahydropyridine (MPTP) was used to induce neurotoxicity in the aged Sprague Dawley rats. Centella asiatica extract was effective in protecting the brain against neurodegenerative changes.[54]

A fungal toxin, 3-nitropropionic acid (3-NPA), is highly neurotoxic and creates a pathology similar to Huntington's disease. In the experimental animals, an aqueous extract of Centella asiatica abolished oxidative stress and protein oxidation in cytosol and mitochondria of brain by 3-NPA and offered neuroprotection.[55]

The neuroprotective effect of asiatic acid was studied in a mouse model of permanent cerebral ischemia. The asiatic acid significantly reduced the infarct volume by 60% at day 1 and by 26% at day 7 post-ischemia, and improved the neurological outcome at 24-hour post-ischemia. The asiatic acid reduced blood–brain barrier permeability and mitochondrial injury.[56]

Centella asiatica has been shown to completely reverse 3-nitropropionic-acid (3-NPA), a neurotoxin induced brain damage in mice.

Depletion of glutathione levels, total thiols, anti-oxidant enzymes and cholinergic enzymes in brain were predominantly restored to normalcy with Centella asiatica extract given prophylactically.[57]

Anti-seizure activity

Hexane, chloroform, ethyl acetate, and butanol extract of Centella asiatica have had anti-seizure and neuroprotective effects in pentylenetetrazol (PTZ)-induced epilepsy in experimental rats. This effect was not present in the aqueous extract of Centella.[58]

Similar results were found in another study, which saw recovery of the levels of acetylcholine and acetylcholinesterase in PTZ-induced seizures.[59]

Lead is a neurotoxic heavy metal, and children in the developmental stage are particularly susceptible to the toxic effects of lead exposure. Epidemiological investigations have established the relationship between chronic lead exposure and cognitive impairments in young children. Aqueous extracts of C. asiatica to lead-exposed rats showed a significant increase in the weight of reproductive organs, reduction in lead-induced oxidative stress in the tissues, and improvement in selected reproductive parameters.[60]

Similar results were obtained in mice exposed to arsenic, where aqueous extract of Centella provided protection.[61] Exposure to arsenic significantly depleted delta-aminolevulinic acid dehydratase (ALAD) activity, reduced glutathione (GSH) level and superoxide dismutase (SOD,) and increased thiobarbituric acid reactive substance (TBARS) activity in the red blood cells. The results included significant depletion of ALAD activity, GSH level, glutathione peroxidase (GPx), SOD, and catalase (CAT) activities, and an increase in TBARS levels in liver tissues. There was a significant depletion of SOD, CAT, and GPx activities in the kidneys and increased TBARS levels in the kidneys and brain, accompanied by increased arsenic concentration in the blood and soft tissues. Centella asiatica provided significant protection against ALAD, GSH, and TBARS levels, particularly at doses of 200 and 500 mg. Centella asiatica also provided significant recovery in the inhibited liver ALAD and G6PD activities. But the concentration of arsenic did not change in blood and soft tissues. This is because Centella is given for only 5 days, whereas the mice were exposed to arsenic for 5 weeks.

Physical performance

Eighty healthy, elderly volunteers—4 males and 76 females (mean age 65.05 ± 3.56 years)—were recruited to participate in the study and were assigned randomly to receive either a placebo or the standardized extract of Centella asiatica at doses of 250, 500, and 750 mg once daily for 90 days. The subjects were evaluated to establish baseline data of physical performance using the 30-s chair stand test, hand grip test and 6-minute walk test. The health-related quality of life was assessed using SF-36. These assessments were repeated every month throughout the 3-month experimental period. After 2 months of treatment, Centella asiatica at doses of 500 and 750 mg per day increased lower extremity strength assessed via the 30-s chair stand test. In addition, the higher doses could improve the life satisfaction subscale within the physical function subscale. The conclusion is that Centella can increase vigor and strength in healthy elderly people.[62]

Anti-microbial and anti-viral activity

Asiaticoside has shown anti-microbial activity against Pseudomonas pyocyaneus and Trichoderma mentagrophytes.[63] And Gotu kola's alcoholic extract has been found to have anti-viral activity against the Herpes simplex type II virus.[64]

Anti-fertility activity

Centella asiatica has exhibited anti-spermatogenic and anti-fertility effects on reproductive system of the male rats. The Centella-treated groups showed some degeneration of spermatogenic cells and reduction of spermatozoa in the lumen of the seminiferous tubules. The serum testosterone level was reduced in all treatments, with decreased sperm motility and sperm count. Treatment with medium (200 mg/kg) and high (300mg/kg) doses showed the most significant reduction (p less than 0.05) in the sperm count. In human doses, this translates to 14–21 grams per day of the Centella extract. In therapeutic doses it has not shown any side effects.[65]

Anti-cancer activity

The triterpenoid compound asiatic acid derived from Centella asiatica has displayed cytotoxic activity on fibroblast cells and several other cell lines. Asiatic acid markedly inhibited cancer cell proliferation. Apoptosis of SW480 human colon cancer cells was induced by asiatic acid through DNA fragmentation and nuclear chromatin condensation. Asiatic acid-induced caspase-9 activity, caspase-3, and poly(ADP-ribose) polymerase (PARP) cleavage, resulting in irreversible apoptotic death in the tumor cells.[66]

Radioprotection

Even at low levels, radiation is known to cause behavioral disturbances such as taste aversion and decreased performance and learning. Centella asiatica (aqueous extract) was tested and compared with ondansetron, a standard antiemetic drug. A dose of 2 Gy radiation indicated significant body weight loss and induced taste aversion. The Centella-fed animals showed less radiation-induced body weight loss and disturbance in taste aversion. Ondansetron elicited a higher degree of protection from taste aversion than Centella on the first post-irradiation day, but on the second post-irradiation day, both were equally effective. The Centella-treated animals showed consistent improvement in taste aversion, whereas the results from the ondansetron-treated animals were inconsistent.[67]

Centella also was tested for its radioprotective properties at a sublethal dose (8 Gy) of Co 60 gamma radiation. A 100 mg/kg dose significantly increased the survival time and weight loss in mice.[68]

Dermatological activity

A randomized double-blind study was carried out on photoaged skin of 20 female volunteers to investigate the effects of topically applied 5% vitamin C and 0.1% madecassoside on the clinical, biophysical, and structural skin properties. Two-thirds of the subjects showed an improvement. After 6 months of treatment, they showed significant improvement in the clinical score for deep and superficial wrinkles, suppleness, elasticity, firmness, roughness, and skin hydration. Histologically, improvements were noticed in the papillary dermis with the reappearance of a normally structured elastic fiber network.[69]

In another study, a cosmetic cream consisting of ethanolic extracts of Glycyrriza glabra, Curcuma longa, seeds of Psorolea corlifolia, Cassia tora, Areca catechu, Punica granatum, fruits of Embelica officinale, leaves of Centella asiatica, Cinnamon zeylanicum, and fresh gel of aloe vera was used with 18 subjects (6 males and 12 females) for 6 weeks on the back of the volar forearm. This was done to evaluate viscoelastic properties in terms of extensibility via a suction measurement, firmness using laboratory fabricated instruments such as ball bouncing and skin hydration using electric (resistance) measurement methods. The formulation showed an increase in percentage extensibility, firmness, and improved skin hydration, and was found to be more effective than the control product.[70]

Similar results were obtained in an open clinical trial of herbal cream containing boswellic acid, Sylibin, and Centella asiatica extracts. Significant improvement was noted in the extensibility and firmness of the skin.[71]

Centella asiatica preparations have been shown to decrease the stretch marks (striae gravidarum) that many women develop during pregnancy. In a placebo-controlled study of 100 pregnant women, a cream compound containing Centella asiatica extract, vitamin E (alpha tocopherol), and collagen-elastin hydrolysates was compared to the placebo. The compounded cream was associated with fewer women developing stretch marks than in the placebo.[72]

Topical applications of Centella preparations have been beneficial in decreasing scarring as seen during wound healing. This treatment appears to stimulate and mature the scar by producing type I collagen, which results in decreased inflammation and myofibroblast production.[73]

Erectile dysfunction

A combination of five herbal extracts—Panax quinquelotius (Ginseng), Eurycoma longifolia (Tongkat Ali), Epimedium grandiflorum (Horny goat weed), Centella asiatica (Gotu Kola), and flower pollen extracts— enhanced erectile function in male rats. This combination at 7.5 mg/kg produced a higher penile erection index than sildenafil at doses of 0.36 mg/kg but similar to 0.71mg/kg of sildenafil.[74]

Anti-allergic and anti-purutic activity

Centella asiatica extract showed anti-allergic and anti-pruritic actions. The results were comparable to ketotofen fumarate and chlorpheniramine in-vitro using the sheep serum method.[75]

Ethnoveterinary Usage

The whole Gotu kola plant is used to treat jaundice, contagious abortion, foot and mouth disease, colic, and swelling of the respiratory tract in ruminants.[76]

Dr. Sodhi's Experiences

When considering treatment with Gotu kola, the following questions should be asked by the practitioner:

- Is there collagen tissue weakness?
- Is venous insufficiency present?
- Do you need help wound healing?
- Is there auto-immune disease present?
- Is there cognitive decline present?
- Do you need to protect nervous system from heavy metals?
- Is there diabetic neuropathy present?

I have seen remarkable results in patients of Systemic Lupus Erythematous (SLE), in which patients have gone into complete remission in 9 months with a combination of Centella asiatica, Boswellia serrata, Bacopa monnieri, and curcumin. For any disease in which a person needs to strengthen collagen, Centella will be helpful. Similar protocols have been successful in reversing scleroderma and Lichen planus. I have used a similar protocol along with Terminalia arjuna and Potaba for fibrosis of the lung.

Centella, in combination with curcumin, is amazing in removing stretch marks.

Centella also gives excellent results in treating venous insufficiency, spider veins, and hemorrhoids.

Safety Profile

In therapeutic doses, Centella has no side effects or toxicity. Contact dermatitis has been reported on a few occasions using topical preparations, although I have not seen these side effects in my clinical practice.

High doses of Gotu kola may cause skin irritation with external use, headache, stomach upset, nausea, dizziness, and drowsiness. Pregnant women should take lower doses.

Dosage

Dried leaves: 1000 mg to 4000 mg per day
Standardized extract: 60 mg/day two times per day
Fresh leaves: 1–2 per day taken empty stomach daily

Ayurvedic properties

Guna: Laghu (light)
Rasa: Tikta (bitter), kashaya (astringent)
Veerya: Shita (cold)
Vipaka: Katu (pungent)
Dosha: Balances kapha and pitta

Notes

1. A.S. Ramaswamy, S.M. Periyasamy, and N.K. Basu, "Pharmacological studies on Centella asiatica", *Journal of Research and Education in Indian Medicine*, 1970, 4:160.

2. C.A. Newall, L.A. Anderson, and J.D. Phillipson, *Herbal Medicines* (London: Pharmaceutical Press, 1996).

3. K.C. Wong and G.L. Tan, "Essential oil of Centella asiatica (L.), Urb. Sch.," *Journal of Essential Oil Research*, 1994, 6(3):307.

4. B. Singh and R.P. Rastogi, "A reinvestigation of the triterpenes of Centella asiatica," *Phytochemistry*, 1969, 8:917.

5. B. Brinkhause, M. Lindner, et al, "Chemical, pharmacological and clinical profile of the East Asian medical plant Centella asiatica," *Phytomedicine*, Oct. 2000, 7(5):427–448.

6. M. Subathra, S. Shila, M.A. Devi, and C. Panneerselvam, "Emerging role of Centella asiatica in improving age-related neurological anti-oxidant status," *Exp Gerontol.*, 2005, 40(8–9):707–715.

7. D. Winston and S. Maimes, "Adaptogens: Herbs for strength, stamina, and stress relief," *Journal,* month, 2007, pp. 226-227. This is a book here is the link for it http://www.amazon.com/Adaptogens-Strength-Stamina-Stress-Relief/dp/1594771588#_

8. E.X. Maquart, F. Chastang, A. Simeon, P. Birembaut, P. Cillery, and Y. Wegrowski, "Triterpenes from Centella asiatica stimulate extracellular matrix accumulation in rat experimental wounds," *European Journal of Dermatology*, 1999, 9(4):289.

9. A. Shukla, A.M. Rasik, G.K. Jain, R. Shankar, D.K. Kulshreshtha, and B.N., Dhawan, "In vitro and in vivo wound healing activity of asiaticoside isolated from Centella asiatica," *Journal of Ethnopharmacology*, 1999, 65(1):1.

10. A.D. Widgerow and L.A. Chait, "New innovations in scar management," *Aesthetic Plastic Surgery,* 24(3): 227–234.

11. A. Hartog, H.F. Smit, P.M. van der Kraan, M.A. Hoijer, and J. Garssen, "In vitro and in vivo modulation of cartilage degradation by a standardized Centella asiatica fraction," *Exp Biol Med* June 2009, 234(6):617–623.

12. A. Shukla, A.M. Rasik, and B.N. Dhawan, "Asiaticoside-induced elevation of anti-oxidant levels in healing wounds," *Phytotherapy Research*, 1999 13(1):50.

13. Y-J Chen, Y-S Dai, and B-F Chen et al., "The effect of tetrandrine and extracts of Centella asiatica on acute radiation dermatitis in rats, "Biological and Pharmaceutical Bulletin," 1999 22(7):703.

14. Z.D. Draelos, M.H. Gold, M. Kaur, B. Olayinka, S.L. Grundy, E.J. Pappert, and B. Hardas, "Evaluation of an onion extract, Centella asiatica, and hyaluronic acid cream in the appearance of striae rubra," *Skinmed*, Mar–Apr 2010, 8(2):80–86.

15. S. Chiummariello, F. De Gado, C. Monarca, M. Ruggiero, B. Carlesimo, N. Scuderi, and C. Alfano, "Multicentric study on a topical compound with lymph-draining action in the treatment of the phlebostatic ulcer of the inferior limbs," *G Chir.*, Nov–Dec, 2009, 30(11–12):497–501.

16. L.N. Zhang, J.J. Zheng, L. Zhang, X. Gong, H. Huang. C.D. Wang, B. Wang, M.J. Wu, X.H. Li, W.J. Sun, Y.J. Liu, and J.Y. Wan, "Protective effects of asiaticoside on septic lung injury in mice," *Exp Toxicol Pathol*, May 12, 2010.

17. W. Cao, X.Q. Li, X.N. Zhang, Y. Hou, A.G. Zeng, Y.H. Xie, and S.W. Wang, "Madecassoside suppresses LPS-induced TNF-alpha production in cardiomyocytes through inhibition of ERK, p38, and NF-kappaB activity," *Int Immunopharmacol.*, July 2010, 10(7):723–729.

18. L. Zhang, H.Z. Li, X. Gong, F.L. Luo, B. Wang, N. Hu, C.D. Wang, Z. Zhang, and J.Y. Wan, "Protective effects of Asiaticoside on acute liver injury induced by lipopolysaccharide/D-galactosamine in mice," *Phytomedicine*, Aug. 2010, 17(10):811–819.

19. R.B. Idrus, S.R. Chowdhury, N.A. Manan, O.S. Fong, M.I. Adenan, and A.B. Saim, "Aqueous extract of Centella asiatica promotes corneal epithelium wound healing in vitro," *J Ethnopharmacol.*, Jan 24, 2012.

20. K. Sairam, C.Y. Rao, and R.K. Goel, Effect of Centella asiatica Linn, on physical and chemical factors of induced gastric ulceration and secretion in rats," Indian Journal of Experimental Biology, 2001, 39(2):137.

21. C.L. Cheng and M.W.L. Koo, "Effects of' Centella asiatica on ethanol-induced gastric mucosal lesions in rats," *Life Sciences*, 2000, 67(21):2647. Is this right OR 26–47. ? It is right 2647

22. T.K. Chatterjee, A. Chakraborty, M. Pathak, and G.C. Sengupta, "Effects of plant extract Centella asiatica (Linn.) on cold restraint stress ulcer in rats," *Indian J Exp Biol.*, 1992, 30:889–891.

23. F.J. DiCarlo, L.J. Haynes, N.J. Silver, and G.H. Phillips, "Reticuloendothelial system stimulants of botanical origin," *Journal of the Reticuloendothelial Society*, 1964, 1:224.

24. R.P. Labadie, J.M. Nat, J.M Simons, et al., "Ethnopharmacognostic approach to the search for immunomodulators of plant origin," *Planta Medica*, 1989, 55:339.

25. M.N. Somchit, M.R. Sulaiman, A. Zuraini, L.N. Samsuddin, N. Somchit, D.A. Israf, et al., "Antinociceptive and antiinflammatory effects of Centella asiatica," *Indian J Pharmacol.*, 2004, 36:377–380.

26. C.A. Newall, L.A. Anderson, and J.D. Phillipson, Hydrocotyle. *Herbal Medicines A Guide for Health Care Professionals* (London: Pharmaceutical Press, 1996), pp. 170–172.

27. M. Liu, Y. Dai, X. Yao, Y. Li, Y. Luo, Y. Xia, and Z. Gong, "Anti-rheumatoid arthritic effect of madecassoside on type II collagen-induced arthritis in mice." *Int Immunopharmacol.*, Nov. 2008, 8(11):1561–1566.

28. P. Boiteau, M. Dureuil, and A. Rakoto-Ratsimamanga, "Antitubercular properties of hydroxyasiaticoside (a water-soluble derivative of asiaticoside from Centella asiatica extracts)," *Comptes Rendus de l'Academie des Sciences* (Paris, Serie D), 1949, 228:1165.

29. A. Cataldo, V. Gasbarro, et al, "Effectiveness of the combination of Alpha tocopherol, Rutin, Melilotus, and Centella asiatica in the treatment of patients with chronic venous insufficiency," *Minerva Cardioangiol*, April 2001, 49(2):159–163.

30. M.R. Arpaia, R. Ferrone, and M. Amitrano, "Effects of Centella asiatica extract on mucopolysaccharide metabolism in subjects with varicose veins," *International Journal of Clinical Pharmacology Research*, 1990, 10(4):229.

31. G.P. Montecchio, A. Samaden, S. Carbone, M. Vigotti, S. Siragusa, and F. Piovella, "Centella asiatica triterpenic fraction (CATTF) reduces the number of circulating endothelial cells in subjects with post phlebetic syndrome," *Haematologica*, 1991, 76:256–259.

32. J.P. Pointel, H. Boccalon, M. Cloarec, C. Ledevehat, and M. Joubert, "Titrated extract of Centella asiatica (TECA) in the treatment of venous insufficiency of the lower limbs," *Angiology*, 1987, 38:46–50.

33. G.V. Belcaro, A. Rulo, and R. Grimaldi, "Capillary filtration and ankle edema in patients with venous hypertension treated with TTFCA," *Angiology*, 1990, 41:12–18.

34. M.R. Cesarone, G. Laurora, M.T. Sanctis, L. Incandela, R. Grimaldi, C. Marelli, et al., "The microcirculatory activity of Centella asiatica in venous insufficiency: A double-blind study. *Minerva Cardioangiol.* 1994, 42:299–304.

35. G.V. Belcaro, R. Grimaldi, and G. Guidi, "Improvement of capillary permeability in patients with venous hypertension after treatment with TTFCA," *Angiology*, 1990, 41:533–540.

36. V. Ivanov, S. Ivanova, T. Kalinovsky, A. Niedzwiecki, and M. Rath, "Plant-derived micronutrients suppress monocyte adhesion to cultured human aortic endothelial cell layer by modulating its extracellular matrix composition," *J Cardiovasc Pharmacol.*, July 2008, 52(1):55–65.

37. M. Hussin, A.A. Hamid, S. Mohamad, N. Saari, F. Bakar, and S.P. Dek, "Modulation of lipid metabolism by Centella asiatica in oxidative stress rats," *J Food Sci.*, March 2009, 74(2):H72–78.

38. J. Bradwejn, Y. Zhou, et al., "A double-blind, placebo-controlled study on the effects of Gotu kola (Centella asiatica) on acoustic startle response in healthy subjects," *J Clin Psychopharmacol*, Dec. 2000, 20(6):680–684.

39. A.S. Ramaswamy, S.M. Pariyaswami, and N. Basu, "Pharmacological studies on Centella asiatica Linn., *Indian J Med Res.*, 1970, 4:160–164.

40. M. R. Sakina and P.C. Dandiya, "A psychoneuropharmacological profile of Centella asiatica extract," *Fitoterapia*, 1990, 61:291.

41. U. Jana, T.K. Sur, L.N. Maity, P.K. Debnath, and D. Bhattacharyya, "A clinical study on the management of generalized anxiety disorder with Centella asiatica," *Nepal Med Coll J.*, March 2010, 12(1):8–11.

42. Y. Chen, T. Han, L. Qin, Y. Rui, and H. Zheng, "Effect of total triterpenes from Centella asiatica on the depression behaviour and concentration of amino acid in forced swimming mice," *Zhong Yao Cai*, 2003, 26:870–873.

43. Y. Chen, T. Han, Y. Rui, M. Yin, L. Qin, and H. Zheng, "Effects of total triterpenes of Centella asiatica on the corticosterone levels in serum and contents of monoamine in depression rat brain.," *Zhong Yao Cai*, 2005, 28:492–496.

44. S. Tiwari, A. Singh, K. Patwardhan, S. Gehlot, and I.S. Gambhir, "Effect of Centella asiatica on mild cognitive impairment (MCI) and other common age-related clinical problems," *Digest J Nanomat Biostruct.*, 2008, 3:215–220.`

45. R. di Paola, E. Esposito, E. Mazzon, R. Caminiti, R.D. Toso, G. Pressi, and S. Cozzocrea S. 3,5-Dicaffeoyl-4-malonylquinic acid reduced oxidative stress and inflammation in a experimental model of inflammatory bowel disease," *Free Radic Res.*, Jan. 2010, 44(1):74–89.

46. B. Brinkhaus, M. Lindner, D. Schuppan, and E.G.Hahn, "Chemical, pharmacological and clinical profile of the East Asian medical plant Centella asiatica," *Phytomedicine.* 2000, 7:427–448.

47. Rao K.G. Mohanda, Rao S. Muddanna, and Rao S, Gurumadhva, "Enhancement of amygdaloid neuronal dendritic arborization by fresh leaf juice of Centella asiatica (Linn) during growth spurt period in rats," *Evid Based Complement Alternat Med.*, June 2009, 6(2):203–210. E-pub Aug. 13, 2007.

48. M.H. Kumar Veerendra and Y.K. Gupta, "Effect of Centella asiatica on cognition and oxidative stress in an intracerebroventricular streptozotocin model of Alzheimer's disease in rats," *Clin Exp Pharmacol Physiol.*, 2003, 30:336–342.

49. Y. Xu, Z. Cao, I. Khan, and Y. Luo, "Gotu kola (Centella asiatica) extract enhances phosphorylation of cyclic AMP response element binding protein in neuroblastoma cells expressing amyloid beta peptide," *J Alzheimers Dis.*, 2008, 13:341–349.

50. G. Jayashree, G. Kurup Muraleedhara, S. Sudarslal, and V.B. Jacob, "Anti-oxidant activity of Centella asiatica on lymphoma-bearing mice," *Fitoterapia*, 2003, 74:431–434.

51. M.K. Lee, S.R. Kim, S.H. Sung, D. Lim, H. Kim, H. Choi, et al. "Asiatic acid derivatives protect cultured cortical neurons from glutamate-induced excitotoxicity," *Res Commun Mol Pathol Pharmacol.*, 2000, 108:75–86.

52. I. Mook-Jung, J.E. Shin, S.H. Yun, K. Huh, J.IY. Koh, H.K. Park, et al., "Protective effects of asiaticoside derivatives against beta-amyloid neurotoxicity," *J Neurosci Res.*, 1999, 8:417–425.

53. M. Dhanasekaran, L.A. Holcomb, A.R. Hitt, B. Tharakan, J.W. Porter, K.A. Young, and B.V. Manyam, "Centella asiatica extract selectively decreases amyloid beta levels in hippocampus of Alzheimer's disease animal model," *Phytother Res.*, Jan. 2009, 23(1):14–19.

54. N. Haleagrahara and K. Ponnusamy, "Neuroprotective effect of Centella asiatica extract (CAE) on experimentally induced parkinsonism in aged Sprague-Dawley rats," *J Toxicol Sci.*, 2010, 35(1):41–47.

55. G.K. Shinomol and initial? Muralidhara, "Prophylactic neuroprotective property of Centella asiatica against 3-nitropropionic acid induced oxidative stress and mitochondrial dysfunctions in brain regions of prepubertal mice," *Neurotoxicology*, Nov. 2008, 29(6):948–957. Please see this http://journals.ohiolink.edu/ejc/article.cgi?issn=0161813x&issue=v29i0006&article=948_pnpocaibropm

56. R.G. Krishnamurthy. M.C. Senut, D. Zemke, J. Min, M. B. Frenkel, E.J. Greenberg, S.W. Yu, N. Ahn, J. Goudreau, M. Kassab, K.S. Panickar, and A. Majid, "Asiatic acid, a pentacyclic triterpene from Centella asiatica, is neuroprotective in a mouse model of focal cerebral ischemia," *J Neurosci Res.*, Aug. 15, 2009, 15, 87(11):2541–2550.

57. G.K. Shinomol, H. Ravikumar, and initial there is no mention of his initial anywhere Muralidhara, "Prophylaxis with Centella asiatica confers protection to prepubertal mice against 3-nitropropionic-acid-induced oxidative stress in brain," *Phytother Res.*, June 2010, 24(6):885–892.

58. W. Rajendra, "The antiepileptic effect of Centella asiatica on the activities of Na/K, Mg and Ca-ATPases in rat brain during pentylenetetrazol-induced epilepsy," *Indian J Pharmacol.*, April 2010, 42(2):82–86.

59. G. Visweswari, K.S. Prasad, P.S. Chetan, V. Lokanatha, and W. Rajendra, "Evaluation of the anticonvulsant effect of Centella asiatica (gotu kola) in pentylenetetrazol-induced seizures with respect to cholinergic neurotransmission," *Epilepsy Behav.*, March 2010, 17(3):332–335.

60. S.B. Sainath, R. Meena, Ch. Supriya, K.P. Reddy, and P.S. Reddy, "Protective role of Centella asiatica on lead-induced oxidative stress and suppressed reproductive health in male rats," *Environ Toxicol Pharmacol.*, Sept. 2011, 32(2):146–154.

61. S.J. Flora and R. Gupta, "Beneficial effects of Centella asiatica aqueous extract against arsenic-induced oxidative stress and essential metal status in rats," *Phytother Res.*, Oct. 2007, 21(10):980–988.

62. L. Mato, J. Wattanathorn, S. Muchimapura, T. Tongun, N. Piyawatkul, K. Yimtae, P. Thanawirattananit, and B. Sripanidkulchai, "Centella asiatica improves physical performance and health-related quality of life in healthy elderly volunteer evid based complement," *Alternat Med.* Oct. 30. 2009.

63. W. Tschesche and G. Wulff, "Uber die antimikrobielle Wirksamkeit von Saponinen," *Zeitschrift fur Naturforschung*, 1965, 20b:543.

64. M.S. Zheng, "An experimental study of the anti-HSV-II action of 500 herbal drugs," *Journal of Traditional Chinese Medicine*, 1989, 9:113.

65. I. Yunianto, S. Das, and M. Mat Noor, "Antispermatogenic and antifertility effect of Pegaga (Centella asiatica L) on the testis of male Sprague-Dawley rats," *Clin Ter.*, May–June, 2010, 161(3):235–259.

66. X.L. Tang, X.Y. Yang, H.J. Jung, S.Y. Kim, S. Y.Jung , D.Y.Choi, W.C. Park, and H. Park, "Asiatic acid induces colon cancer cell growth inhibition and apoptosis through mitochondrial death cascade," *Biol Pharm Bull.*, Aug. 2009, 32(8):1399–1405.

67. V. Shobi and H.C. Goel, "Protection against radiation-induced conditioned taste aversion by Centella asiatica," *Physiol Behav.* 2001, 73:19–23.

68. J. Sharma and R. Sharma, "Radioprotection of Swiss albino mouse by Centella asiatica extract," *Phytother. Res.* 2002, 16:785–786.

69. M. Haftek, S. Mac-Mary, M.A. Le Bitoux, P. Creidi, S. Seité, A. Rougier, and P. Humbert , "Clinical, biometric and structural evaluation of the long-term effects of a topical treatment with ascorbic acid and madecassoside in photoaged human skin," *Exp Dermatol.*, Nov. 2008, 17(11):946–952.

70. M.S. Ahshawat, S. Saraf, and S. Saraf, "Preparation and characterization of herbal creams for improvement of skin viscoelastic properties," *Int J Cosmet Sci.*, June 2008, 30(3):183–193.

71. L. Martelli, E. Berardesca, and M. Martelli, "Topical formulation of a new plant extract complex with refirming properties. Clinical and non-invasive evaluation in a double-blind trial," *Int J Cosmet Sci.*, June 2000, 22(3):201–216.

72. G.L. Young and D. Jewell, "Collaboration creams for preventing stretch marks in pregnancy (Review), and "Creams for preventing stretch marks in pregnancy (Review), *The Cochrane Collaboration* (New York John Wiley and Sons Ltd, 2005), pp. 1–7.

73. A.D. Widgerow, L.A. Chait, R. Stals, and P.J. Stals, "New innovations in scar management," *Aesthetic Plast Surg.* 2000, 24:227–234.

74. N. Qinna, H. Taha, K.A. Matalka, and A.A. Badwan, "A new herbal combination, Etana, for enhancing erectile function: An efficacy and safety study in animals," *Int J Impot Res.* Sept–Oct, 2009, 21(5):315–320.

75. M. George, L. Joseph, and initial? Ramaswamy, "Anti-allergic, anti-pruritic, and anti-inflammatory activities of Centella asiatica extracts," *Afr J Tradit Complement Altern Med.*, July 3, 2009, 6(4):554–559. NO initials please see the link. It is not even mentioned in the pubmed http://www.ncbi.nlm.nih.gov/pmc/articles/PMC2816466/

76. M.K. Jha, *The Folk Veterinary System of Bihar—A Research Survey* (Anand, Gujrat: NDDB, 1992).

11

Cedrus deodara

Introduction

Cedrus deodara is a magnificent tree that can reach a tremendous height and breadth. Like most cedars, Cedrus deodara grows in a pyramidal shape, with graceful, tiered branches. The tree may live to a great age, and as it ages, the lower branches may begin to dip toward the ground, creating a striking silhouette. Cedrus deodara needles are the longest of any cedar, measuring from 1½ to 2 inches in length.

The primary pharmacological activity of Cedrus deodara is found in its oil. The oil has antiseptic qualities, making it useful in treating skin diseases, sores, wounds, and ulcers. Other important uses include the oil's capacity to ease headache, lower fever, relieve diarrhea, and soothe urogenital diseases. The heartwood of Cedrus deodara has anti-inflammatory, sedative, cardiotonic, and laxative properties. The tree's leaves are bitter and acrid to the taste and have anti-inflammatory properties.[1]

The aromatic inner wood of Cedrus deodara is used in making incense, and the essential oil is used in aromatherapy and as an insect repellant. The oil also has anti-fungal properties and encourages sweating and urination. In Ayurveda, the tree is reputed to increase digestive function, detoxify the body, soothe coughing, and cure skin disorders including eczema and psoriasis.

Synonymous Names

English: Himalayan cedar
Hindi: Deodar
Sanskrit: Devadaru
Devdar, Deodar cedar, Devadaram, Devataram, Devadaru, Devadarus, Devdar

Habitat

Deodara grows throughout the western Himalayas, extending from Kashmir to Garhwal, and reaching altitudes up to 3,000 meters above sea level. The tree is native to western Afghanistan, northern Pakistan, north-central India, southwestern Tibet, and western Nepal.[2]

The tree grows best in well-drained, sandy, loamy, and clay soils but also can grow in acid, alkaline, or neutral soils. It is not shade-tolerant. Although the tree is hardy and able to sustain high winds, it cannot tolerate atmospheric pollution.

Botanical Characteristics

Cedrus deodara is a majestic evergreen conifer. The tree reaches heights of 85 meters, with a trunk girth up to 3 meters. The ascending, spreading branches form a graceful, thick canopy, with a conic crown and drooping branchlets. The yellowish-brown heartwood is rich in oil and strongly scented, and the thick, furrowed bark covering it is dark and rough.

The evergreen leaves grow in dense clusters of dark green needles at the end of long shoots. The needles measure 2–4 cm in length and have a silver sheen. Deodar's solitary cones grow at the ends of its branchlets. The tree's female cones are barrel shaped, measuring 7–13 cm long and 5–9 cm wide. When mature, these cones disintegrate and release triangular, winged seeds. Its male cones are 4–6 cm long and shed their pollen in autumn.

Chemical Composition

The heartwood of Cedrus deodara yields about 2.1 % of essential oil,[3] consisting mainly of the sesquiterpene hydrocarbons oc-himachalene, 3-himachalene, and other isomers including 8-himachalene, with p-methyl acetophenone, p-methyl-Δ^4-tetrahydroacetophenone, atlantone, and himachalol.

Additional constituents include:
  Hydrocarbons
    The petroleum ether extract of the bark oil yields saturated, straight-chain and branched-chain hydrocarbons (C_U-C_{20}).
  Flavonoids

Deodara's stem bark contains deodarin (3', 4', 5,7-tetrahydroxy-8-C-ethyldihydroflavonoi), taxifolin and quercetin.[5]

Pharmacological Activity

Anti-cancer activity

An ethanolic extract of Cedrus deodara was shown to have cytotoxic activity against carcinomas of the nasopharynx when examined using tissue cultures.[6] A lignan mixture, isolated from the stem wood of Cedrus deodara, was studied for its in-vitro cytotoxicity against human cancer cell lines. The extract showed significant dose-dependent effects against cancer cell lines from breast, cervix, neuroblastoma, colon, liver, and prostate tissues.[7] These results indicate that Cedrus deodara has cytotoxic potential against human cancer cell lines. The extract has the ability to induce tumor regression in-vivo, as well as inducing apoptosis, as indicated by annexin V positive cells, induction of intracellular caspases, DNA fragmentation, and DNA cell cycle analysis.[8]

Anti-spasmolytic activity

Cedrus deodara's alkaloid himacholol has been identified as an anti-spasmolytic. When tested on smooth muscle tissue samples including pig ileum, rabbit jejunum, rat uterus, and guinea pig seminal vesicle, himacholol had anti-spasmolytic activity comparable to the chemical papaverine.[9]

An in-vivo investigation of the effect of himacholol on intestinal tissue in cats showed anti-spasmolytic activity equal to papaverine, but with a faster onset of action. Himachalol had no spasmolytic effect in bronchial muscle tissue in guinea pigs but was 3.3 times more potent than papaverine in antagonizing epinephrine-induced contractions in the guinea pig seminal vesicle.[10]

Anti-oxidant activity

Fractionation and purification processes were used to determine Cedrus deodara's anti-oxidant properties. Three compounds with potent anti-oxidant activity were isolated in significant yields and identified by spectroscopic methods.[11]

Anti-inflammatory activity

Cedrus deodara's volatile oil was studied for its anti-inflammatory and analgesic activity at doses of 50 and 100 mg/kg body weight. The oil significantly inhibited carrageenan-induced rat paw edema and both chronic phases of inflammation in adjuvant arthritic rats at both doses. The oil also was found to possess analgesic activity in acetic acid-induced writhing and hot plate reaction tests in mice.[12]

Anti-fungal activity

The essential oil of Cedrus deodara is an effective antifungal treatment for phycomycotic diseases affecting humans and animals.[13, 14] Aspergillus is an increasingly common fungal infection in patients with compromised immune systems, and existing anti-fungal treatments carry negative side effects. Treatment with himacholol provided substantial protection against invasive aspergillosis in mice. A combination therapy including himacholol proved to be a better regimen than standard treatments, as evidenced by enhanced survival rates of infected mice.[15]

Ethnoveterinary Usage

The wood and bark of Cedrus deodara are used in veterinary medicine to treat dysentery, skin diseases and ulcers.[16] The oil protects against mange in buffaloes, calves, goats and camels, and is used to treat sore hooves in cattle. The tree's heartwood oil has been shown to cure scabies infections.[17, 18]

Safety Profile

No adverse side effects have been observed from internal ingestion or external application of Cedrus deodara.[4 19 See note 5]

Dosage

Powdered wood: 3–6 g Decoction: 28–56 ml Oil: 0.5–3 ml

Ayurvedic Properties

Rasa: Tikta (bitter)
Guna: Laghu (light) ,snigdha (unctuous)
Veerya: Ushna (hot)
Vipaka: Katu (pungent)
Dosha: Pacifies vata and kapha

Notes

1. U.A. Shinde, A.S. Phadke, A.M. Nair, A.A. Mungantiwar, V.J. Dikshit, and M.N. Saraf, "Studies on the anti-inflammatory and analgesic activity of Cedrus deodara (Roxb.) Loud. wood oil, *J Ethnopharmacol.*, April, 1999, 65(1):21–27.

2. A. Farjon, Pinaceae, *Drawings and Descriptions of the Genera* (City: Koeltz scientific books, 1990).

3. M.C. Nigam, A. Ahmad, and L.N. Misra, "Composition of the essential oil of Cedrus deodara,*Indian Perfumer*," 1990, 34(4):278.

4. S.C. Bisarya, "Allohimachalol, a new type of sesquiterpenoid," *Tetrahedron*, 1964, 29:3761.

5. S.K. Tandan, S. Singh, S. Gupta, S. Chandra, and L. Jawahar, "Subacute dermal toxicity study of Cedrus deodara wood essential oil," *Indian Veterinary Journal*, 1989, 66(11):1088.

6. M.L. Dhar, M.M. Dhar, B.N. Dhawan B. N. Mehrotra, and C. Ray, "Screening of Indian plants for biological activity, Part I, *Indian Journal of Experimental Biology*, 1968, 6:232.

7. S.K. Singh, M. Shanmugavel, H. Kampasi, R. Singh, D.M. Mondhe, J.M. Rao, M.K. Adwankar, A.K. Saxena, and G.N. Qazi, "Chemically standardized isolates from Cedrus deodara stem wood having anticancer activity," *Planta Med.*, June 2007, 73(6):519–526. Epub May 2007.

8. Singh et al., Note 7.

9. J. Lal, K. Sambasivarao, S. Chandra, R.C. Naithani, S.K. Chattopadhyay, and M. Sabir, "Spasmolytic constituents of Cedrus deodara (Roxb.) Loud: pharmacological evaluation of himachalol." *Indian Veterinary Journal*, 1976, 53(7):543.

10. K. Kar, V.N. Puri, G.K. Patnaik, R.N. Sur, B.N. Dhawan, D.K. Kulshrestha, and R.P. Rastogi, "Spasmolytic constituents of Cedrus deodara (Roxb.) Loud: pharmacological evaluation of himachalol." *J Pharm Sci.*, Feb. 1975, 64(2):258–262.

11. A.K. Tiwari, P.V. Srinivas, S.P. Kumar, and J.M. Rao, "Free radical scavenging active components from Cedrus deodara." *J Agric Food Chem.*, Oct. 2001, 49(10):4642.

12. Shinde et al., Note 1.

13. H.V. Mall, A. Asthana, N.K. Dubey, and S.N. Dixit, "Toxicity of cedarwood oil against some dermatophytes," *Indian Drugs*, 1985, 22(6):296.

14. A. Dixit and S.N. Dixit, "A promising antifungal agent," *Indian Perfumer*, 1982, 26(2–4):216.

15. L. Chowdhry, Z.K. Khan, and D.K. Kulshrestha, "Comparative in vitro and in vivo evaluation of himachalol in murine invasive aspergillosis, *Indian J Exp Biol.*, July 1997, 35(7):727–734.

16. International Institute of Rural Reconstruction, "Ethnoveterinary medicine in Asia. An information kit on traditional animal health care practices. Part I, General information" (Silang, Philippines: IIRR, 1994).

17. Tandan et al., Note 5.

18. K. Kar, V.N. Puri, G.K., Patnaik, et al., "Studies on comparative efficacy of Cedrus deodara oil, benzyl benzoate and tetraethylthiuram monosulphide against sarcoptic mange in sheep," *Journal of Pharmaceutical Science*, 1975, 64(2):258.

19. P.K. Agrawal, S.K. Agarwal, R.P. Rastogi, and B.G. Osterdahal, "Dihydroflavanonols from Cedrus deodara (a 13C NMR Study1)," *Planta Med.*, Sept. 1981, 43(9):82- ?

Additional Resources

Gupta SC, Yadav SC, Jawahar L, Chandra R, Lal J 1988 Molluscicidal activity of *Cedrus deodara* (wood essential oil) against *Lytnnaea auricularia rufescens* Grey: laboratory and field evaluations. Journal of Veterinary Parasitology 2(2):109.

Kumar A, Dutta, GP 1987 Indigenous plant oils as larvicidal agent against *Anopheks stephensi* mosquitoes. Current Science 56(18):959.

Singh D, Rao SM, Tripathi AK1984 Cedarwood oil as a potential insecticidal agent against mosquitoes. Naturwissenschaften 71(5):265.

Chandra S, Prasad MC, Tandon SK, Gupta S Jawahar L 1989 Evaluation of a formulation of *Cedrus deodara* wood essential oil on blood urea nitrogen and blood glucose level and on skin irritation. Indian Veterinary Journal 66:30.

Sharma PR, Shanmugavel M, Saxena AK, Qazi GN. Induction of apoptosis by a synergistic lignin composition from Cedrus deodara in human cancr cells. Phytotherapy Research 2008 Dec; 22(12):1587-94.

Chandra S, Sambasivarao K, Raviprakash V, Lal J, Sabir M.Vascular permeability-increasing action of Cedrus deodara wood oil. Indian Vet J. 1978 Dec;55(12):963.

Pandey G.S. (Ed.) 1998 Indian materia medica. Chaukhambha Bharati Academy, Gokul Bhawan, Varanasi.

Cissus quadrangularis

Introduction

Cissus quadrangularis is a rambling shrub that is native to the hotter parts of India and Ceylon. It has been used in Ayurvedic medicine since ancient times as a general tonic and analgesic, but its most highly valued property is as a bone healer. To treat fractures and associated swelling, a paste made from the stem of Cissus is applied directly over the injury.

The entire Cissus plant is of medicinal value and is considered to be an alterative, anthelmintic, aphrodisiac, and anti-asthmatic. It is useful in treating gastrointestinal disorders such as colic and dyspepsia. Cissus also is an important Siddha medicine. Traditional practitioners burn the plant to ash before using it in various ways.

The leaves and stem of Cissus frequently are eaten with curry in southern India.

Preliminary research studies have revealed that Cissus may have the potential to act in the management of metabolic syndrome, particularly weight loss and central obesity.[1]

Synonymous Names

English: Bone setter
Hindi: Hadjora
Sanskrit: Asthisanhari, Asthishrinkhla

Habitat

Cissus quadrangularis grows natively in hot, dry regions of India, such as the Deccan peninsula. It also is found on the lower slopes of the Western Ghats and is widespread across drier areas of Arabia and Africa.

Botanical Characteristics

A low-growing shrub, Cissus quadrangularis has a characteristic four-sided stem. This is a climbing plant, often found growing over lower-growing vegetation. The thick stem is glabrous and fleshy, with constrictions at its nodes. Its alternate, simple leaves also are thick, and ovate, with serrated margins. The leaves measure about 8 cm long and 6 cm wide. Numerous tendrils grow out of the plant's nodes.

Cissus quadrangularis' small flowers occur in umbellate cymes opposite the leaves. The flower has a lobed, cup-shaped calyx and greenish-yellow petals with red tips. The fruit consists of small, round berries.

Chemical Composition

Following is the chemical composition of Cissus quadrangularis:[2,3,4,5]

The stem has revealed unique stilbene derivatives, termed quadrangularins A, B, and C. The alkaloids resveratrol, piceatannol, pallidol, and parthenocissin also are found in the stem.

Other lipids and phytosterols identified in the plant are:

4-Hydroxy-2-methyltricos-2-en-22-one, 9-methyl-octadec-9-ene, heptadecyl octadecanoate, icosanyl icosanoate, 31-methyltritriacontan-1-ol, 7-hydroxy-20-oxo-docosanyl cyclohexane and 31-methyltriacontanoic acid, 7-oxoonocer-8-ene-3-21-diol, onocer-7-ene-3-21-diol, onocer-7-ene-3-21-diol, α-amyrin, α-amyrone taraxeryl acetate, friedelan-3-one, taraxerol, P-sitosterol, and isopentacosanoic acid.

Cissus quadrangularis is rich in vitamin C and beta-carotene. Analyses have showed that Cissus contains ascorbic acid at a concentration of 479 mg, and carotene, 267 units per 100 grams of freshly prepared paste, in addition to calcium oxalate.

Pharmacological Activity
Bone-Healing Activity

Cissus quadrangularis has been studied extensively to verify its bone-healing properties. Clinical trials and animal studies have shown that treatment with Cissus facilitates the remodeling process of the healing bone, speeding the restoration of bone tensile strength. Cissus has shortened fracture healing time between 33% and 55%. The effect of Cissus has been observed in bones weakened by cortisol; when Cissus extracts were given, the cortisol-induced weakening was halted and the healing process began.

Animal studies have allowed more insight into the process by which Cissus promotes bone healing. In one such study, a phytosterol fraction isolated from Cissus demonstrated significant bone-healing activity in experimental bone fractures of the right humerus of young rats. When Cissus extract was injected daily for 6 weeks, increases in total body weight and substantially improved bone healing rates were observed. The researchers concluded that Cissus acts by enhancing regeneration of connective tissue and mineralization.[6]

Further animal studies using radioactive tagging and micro-autoradiography of various tissues indicate Cissus stimulate bone healing via the anterior pituitary and adrenal glands. Radioactive analysis showed that the sterol fraction of the herb stimulated the osteogenic cells at the fracture site after metabolism in the liver.[7,8]

Cissus also improved the healing rate of experimental fractures of dog femurs. Bone ossification rates in treated animals were significantly faster than in the untreated animals. After 3 weeks of treatment, the callus in the untreated animals contained cartilaginous tissue with only a few thin and sparse bony trabeculae, whereas the treated animals had considerably advanced ossification, and the callus consisted of a network of bony trabeculae. After 6 weeks, ossification was complete and remodeling was advanced in the treated animals in comparison to the untreated animals, in which ossification was still in progress.[9]

An aqueous extract of Cissus, applied topically or given by injection, hastened the healing of fractures as measured by a reduction in convalescence time. The extract improved the strengthening of bones as much as 90% over a 6-week period and had an influence on both the organic and the mineral phases of fracture healing.[10] Calcium-45 uptake studies also demonstrated speedier completion of the calcification process, suggesting that Cissus may be useful not only in building up bones but in improving functional efficiency as well. An extract of the plant was found to neutralize the anti-anabolic effect of cortisone in healing of fractures, possibly because of its high vitamin C content.[11]

Further research indicates that Cissus acts as a glucocorticoid antagonist.[12] Anabolic/androgenic compounds are well known to act as antagonists to the glucocorticoid receptor as well as to promote bone growth and fracture healing, so it has been postulated that Cissus possesses anabolic and/or androgenic properties.

Although the increased rate of bone healing may be of great significance to patients with chronic diseases such as osteoporosis,[13] the anti-glucocorticoid properties of Cissus are likely of much more interest to the average body builder or athlete, because endogenous glucocorticoids, particularly cortisol, catabolize not only bone but muscle tissue as well. Numerous studies have suggested that glucocorticoids, including the body's endogenous hormone cortisol, activate pathways that degrade not only bone but skeletal muscle tissue as well.

A published report documented exactly how glucocorticoids induce muscle breakdown. The report explains that these substances activate the ubiquitin-proteasome pathway of proteolysis,[14] a mechanism that removes damaged and non-functional proteins. When the body is under stress from disease, trauma, or excessive training, normal tissue is broken down as well. By exerting an anabolic, anti-glucocorticoid effect, Cissus helps to preserve muscle tissue during times of physical and emotional stress. The possibility also exists that Cissus may improve the healing rate of connective tissue in general, including tendons. If this claim is backed up by additional research, Cissus may have great benefit to body builders and athletes.

Cissus has shown to increase to levels of IGF-I, IGF-II and IGF binding protein-3 in human osteoblast cells.[15]

Periodontal Regeneration

Twenty patients with periodontal disease were given either bovine-derived hydroxyapatite combined with Cissus quadrangularis or bovine-derived hydroxyapatite alone after scaling and root planing. Baseline and 6-month surgical measurements were taken, and appropriate statistical analysis was performed. Favorable clinical results for both hard and soft tissue measurements were obtained for both groups when compared to baseline ($p < 0.001$). Composite graft material with Cissus showed a trend toward better performance in periodontal regenerative therapy.[16]

Anti-Osteoporosis

Postmenopausal osteoporosis and its related fractures have become a global health issue. Postmenopausal osteoporosis, the most frequent metabolic bone disease, is characterized by rapid loss of mineralized bone tissue. Hormone replacement therapy is not desirable to many women because of its side-effects. Cissus quadrangularis is effective in healing fractures. A petroleum–ether extract of Cissus quadrangularis was studied on an osteoporotic rat model developed by ovariectomy. Cissus reduced bone loss by reducing osteoclastic activity and encouraged osteoblastic activity. Weight of the femur increased. The biological activity of Cissus quadrangularis on bone was attributed to its phytogenic steroids.[17] When a friedelin-rich fraction of Cissus quadrangularis was given to ovariectomized mice, the mice showed improved sexual behavioral parameters, vaginal cornification, increased uterine weight, and elevated levels of serum estrogen.[18]

In another study, petroleum ether extract of Cissus quadrangularis enhanced the differentiation of marrow mesenchymal stem cells into alkaline phosphatase-positive osteoblasts, and increased extracellular matrix calcification. Cells grown in osteogenic media containing Cissus quadrangularis exhibited higher proliferation, differentiation, and calcification rates than did control cells, verifying its use in Ayurvedic medicine for bone healing.[19]

Another study showed upregulation of osteoblastic activity by enhancing alkaline phosphatase activity and the mineralization process, mediated by p38 mitogen-activated protein kinase (MAPK)-dependent pathway.[20]

Anti-Inflammatory and Analgesic Activity

Cissus quadrangularis possesses analgesic properties comparable to aspirin and anti-inflammatory drugs such as ibuprofen. Cissus is an ingredient in the Ayurvedic preparation, Laksha Guggulu, which has proven to be highly effective in relieving pain, reducing swelling, and promoting healing of simple fractures, as well as in curing various disorders associated with fractures.

Thirty patients with osteoarthritis of the knee joint were given Laksha Guggulu, a preparation of Cissus with other herbs. The patients were divided into three groups: Group A was treated with Laksha Guggulu taken orally; Group B was treated with medicated oil massage, and knee joint traction; and Group C was treated with Laksha Guggulu, medicated oil massage and knee joint traction. Progress was measured by joint pain, edema, tenderness, restriction of joint movement, stiffness, local crepitation, and walking distance. Significant results were obtained on pain in joint movement, restriction in joint movement, joint stiffness, and local crepitation in nearly all the groups, with best result in group C.[21]

The mechanism of action was elaborated in this study, in which an ethyl acetate extract of Cissus quadrangularis potently inhibited lipopolysaccharide-induced nitric oxide (NO) production in macrophage cells in a dose-dependent manner. The mRNA, protein expressions of inducible nitric oxide synthase and p65 NF-κB nuclear translocation were suppressed. Also it induced heme oxygenase-1 gene expression at the protein and mRNA levels in a dose-dependent and time-dependent manner.[22]

Anti-Obesity Activity

Once considered a problem unique to developed countries, obesity and obesity-related complications (such as metabolic syndrome) are rapidly spreading around the globe. A number of clinical studies have been undertaken to investigate the usefulness of Cissus quadrangularis in the management of metabolic syndrome, particularly for weight loss and central obesity.[23]

In a randomized, double-blind, placebo-controlled study, 123 overweight and obese persons were treated with Cissus for 8 weeks while consuming a normal diet or a calorie-controlled diet. At the end of the trial period, significant reductions in weight and central obesity, as well as in fasting blood glucose, total cholesterol, LDL-cholesterol, triglycerides, and C-reactive protein levels were observed in the participants who received the formulation, regardless of diet. These results suggest that Cissus may be useful in managing weight loss and metabolic syndrome.[18] A combination of Cissus quadrangularis /Irvingia gabonensis even produced more profound effects than Cissus alone.[24]

Another double-blind placebo controlled design, initially involved 168 overweight and obese persons (38.7% males; 61.3% females; ages 19–54), of whom 153 completed the study. All the participants received two daily doses of 300 mg of Cissus quadrangularis extract and were encouraged to maintain their normal levels of physical activity. Anthropometric measurements and blood sampling were done at the beginning and the end of the study period.

Significant ($p < 0.001$) reductions in plasma TBARS were seen, along with significant reductions in weight, body fat, total cholesterol, LDL-cholesterol, triglycerides, and fasting blood glucose levels. These changes were accompanied by a significant increase in HDL-cholesterol levels, plasma serotonin, and creatinine. The increases in plasma serotonin and creatinine were hypothesized to be a mechanism of controlling appetite and promoting lean muscle mass by Cissus quadrangularis.[25]

Anti-Ulcer Properties

Cissus quadrangularis extract had healing effects on gastric ulcers, through modulation of polyamines and proliferating cell nuclear antigen in rats.[26] Administration of acetic acid was accompanied by reduced proliferating cell nuclear antigen. Administration of Cissus quadrangularis protected the stomach by reducing the ulcer area in a dose-dependent manner. Cissus significantly increased the (3)H-thymidine, putrescine, spermine, and spermidine in ulcerated rats. Gastroprotection was rendered in the ulcerated area by increased expression of transforming growth factor-alpha (TGF-α). It also reversed changes in gastric mucosa of the ulcerated rats with significant elevation in mitochondrial tricarboxylic acid cycle enzymes and proliferating cell nuclear antigen levels.

Cissus quadrangularis also has shown antisecretory and cytoprotective properties.[26]

In a number of studies, Cissus quadrangularis has had protective action against NSAID-induced ulcers in animals. Pre-treatment with Cissus reversed aspirin-induced damage to tumor necrosis factor-alpha (TNF-alpha), interleukin-1beta (IL-1beta), microvascular permeability, activity of nitric oxide synthase-2 (NOS-2), mitochondrial anti-oxidants, lipid peroxidation, and DNA damage.[27]

Ethnoveterinary Usage

Cissus quadrangularis is fed to cattle as a galactogogue to induce the flow of milk. The whole plant is used in cases of fractures, sprains, rheumatism, irregular growth of teeth, broken horns, anthrax, hematuria, elephantiasis, dislocation of hip, various wounds, and cracked tail.[28]

Dr. Sodhi's Experience

Herbal treatment with Cissus may be indicated when the following conditions are present:

- Is there any problem with bones?
- Are there fractures?
- Is any bone loss or osteopenia/osteoporosis present?
- Are there peri-menopause or menopausal issues?
- Are there issues with syndrome-X?
- Is weight loss needed?

Cissus is an excellent bone-healer. My grandmother, who was also a physician, treated many bone fractures using Cissus. She put a small piece of the plant's stem in milk (to enhance absorption) and had the patient drink the mixture. This enhanced healing of the fracture and sped recovery time. Curcumin longum (Curcuma) is also a bone-healer and can be used together with Cissus. I have found that when the two herbs are used together, fractures heal in as little as 3 to 4 weeks. I also have used Cissus to treat osteopenia and osteoporosis.

Case Histories

Osteoporosis

A 42 year-old woman who came to our clinic was experiencing early menopause along with osteoporosis. She was taking the drug Fosamax but had refused hormone therapy. After one year of Fosamax, she had experienced no improvement in her osteoporosis symptoms. We prescribed the following herbal protocol for this patient:

For bone and hormonal support:

A blend of Asparagus racemosus, Dioscorea villosa (varhikand), Saraca indica (ashok), and Terminalia arjuna (arjuna), bamboo manna, coral powder, Cissus quadrangularis (hadjoda), and Cimicifuga racemosa: three times per day.

Curcuma longum, 500 mg extract: three times a day.

In addition, we prescribed the following supplements daily:

calcium, 1200 mg,

magnesium fumate, 600 mg, and

a multivitamin with 1000 IU of Vitamin D.

We monitored this patient at 3-month intervals. The first thing she noticed was that her bone pain was gone and she could walk without any pain. Her menopausal symptoms also were improved. Six months after she began her therapy, we did a bone scan, which indicated that her bone density had improved significantly. One year later, her bone density reading was back within the osteopenic range, and after 2 years, it was normal. She is staying on this protocol permanently. Her vaginal dryness is gone. Twenty years later she is a yoga teacher and teaching people a healthy living style.

Safety Profile

Safety studies in rats showed no toxic effects at dosages of Cissus quadrangularis extract as high as 2500 mg/kg of body weight after 90 days. No mutagenicity, chromosomal aberration, or genotoxicity was noted. The plant's fresh juice may irritate the skin and cause itching.[29]

Dosage

Decoction of dried stalks: 10–30 ml juice; 10–20 ml

Powder: 2.5 g

The typical recommended daily dosage of Cissus extract is between 100 mg and 500 mg, depending on the concentration of the extract and the severity of symptoms. For the powder of the dried plant, Ayurvedic texts recommend a dosage of 3 to 6 grams of raw herb powder to accelerate fracture healing.

Ayurvedic Properties

Guna: Laghu (light), Ruksha: (dry)
Rasa: Madhur (sweet)
Veerya: Ushna (hot)
Vipaka: Amla (sour)
Dosha: Pacifies vata and pitta

Notes

1. Julius Oben, Dieudonne Kuat, Gabriel Agbor, Claudia Momo, Xavio Talla "The use of a Cissus quadrangularis formulation in the management of weight loss and metabolism," *Lipids in Health and Disease*, 2006, 5:24.

2. S.A. Adesanya, R. Nia, M.T. Martin, N. Boukamcha, A. Montagnac, and M. Paies, "Stilbene derivatives from Cissus quadrangularis," *Journal of Natural Products*, 1999, 62(12):1694.

3. K.N. Udupa, G. Prasad, and S.P. Sen, "The effect of phytogenic anabolic steroids of Cissus quadrangularis in the acceleration of fracture repair," *Life Sciences*, 1965, 4(3):317.

4. M.M. Gupta and R.K. Verma, "Lipid constituents of Cissus quadrangularis," *Phytochemistry*, 1991, 30(3):875.

5. K.N. Chidambara Murthy, A. Vanitha, M. Mahadeva Swamy, and G.A. Ravishankar, "Anti-oxidant and antimicrobial activity of Cissus quadrangularis L." *J Med Food*, Summer 2003, 6(2):99–105.

6. B.K. Potu, M.S. Rao, N.G. Kutty, K.M. Bhat, M.R. Chamallamud, and S.R. Nayak, "Petroleum ether extract of Cissus quadrangularis (LINN) stimulates the growth of fetal bone during intra uterine developmental period: A morphometric analysis," *Clinics* (Sao Paulo), Dec. 2008, 63(6):815–820.

7. G.C. Prasad, S.C. Chatterjee, and K.N. Udupa, "Effect of phytogenic steroid of Cissus quadrangularis on endocrine glands after fracture," *Journal of Research in Indian Medicine*, 1970, 4(2):132.

8. G.C. Prasad and K.N. Udupa, "Pathways and site of action of phytogenic steroids from Cissus quadrangularis," *Journal of Research in Indian Medicine*, 1972 7:29.

9. S.S. Chopra, M.R. Patel, and R. Awadhiya, "Studies on Cissus quadrangularis in experimental fracture repair: A histopathological study," *Indian Journal of Medical Research*, 1976, 64(9): 136.

10. K.N. Udupa and G.C. Prasad, "Biochemical and Ca45 studies on the effect of Cissus quadrangularis in fracture healing," *Indian Journal of Medical Research*, 1964, 52(5):480.

11. G.C. Prasad and K.N. Udupa, "Effect of Cissus quadrangularis on the healing of cortisone-treated fracture," *Indian Journal of Medical Research*, 1963, 51:667–676.

12. S.S. Chopra, M.R. Patel, L.P. Gupta, and I.C. Datta, "Studies on Cissus quadrangularis in experimental fracture repair: Effect on chemical parameters in blood," *Indian J Med Res.*, June 1975, 63(6):824–828.

13. A. Shirwaikar, S. Khan, and S. Malini, "Antiosteoporotic [verify or change]This is what is mentioned in the citation in pubmed. I cannot and should not change it effect of ethanol extract of Cissus quadrangularis Linn. on ovariectomized rat," *J Ethnopharmacol.*, Dec. 2003, 89(2–3):245–250.

14. L. Combaret, D. Taillandier, D. Dardevet, D. Bechet, C. Ralliere, A. Claustre, J. Grizard, and D. Attaix, "Glucocorticoids regulate mRNA levels for subunits of the 19 S regulatory complex of the 26 S proteasome in fast-twitch skeletal muscles," *Biochem J.*, Feb 2004, 15, 378 (Pt 1):239–246.

15. S. Muthusami, I. Ramachandran, S. Krishnamoorthy, R. Govindan, and S. Narasimhan, "Cissus quadrangularis augments IGF system components in human osteoblast like SaOS-2 cells," *Growth Horm IGF Res.*, Dec. 2011, 21(6):343–348.

16. A. Jain, J. Dixit, and D. Prakash. "Modulatory effects of Cissus quadrangularis on periodontal regeneration by bovine-derived hydroxyapatite in intrabony defects: exploratory clinical trial," *J Int Acad Periodontol.*, April 2008, 10(2):59–65.

17. B.K. Potu, M.S. Rao, G.K. Nampurath, M.R. Chamallamudi, K. Prasad, S.R. Nayak, P.K. Dharmavarapu, V. Kedage, and K.M. Bha, "Evidence-based assessment of antiosteoporotic activity of petroleum-ether extract of Cissus quadrangularis Linn. on ovariectomy-induced osteoporosis," *Ups J Med Sci.* 2009, 114(3):140–148.

18. U.M. Aswar, S. Bhaskaran, V. Mohan, and S.L. Bodhankar, "Estrogenic activity of friedelin rich fraction (IND-HE) separated from Cissus quadrangularis and its effect on female sexual function," *Pharmacognosy Res.*, May 2010, 2(3):138–145.

19. B.K. Potu, K.M. Bhat, M.S. Rao, G.K. Nampurath, M.R. Chamallamudi. S.R. Nayak, and M.S. Muttigi, "Petroleum ether extract of Cissus quadrangularis (Linn.) enhances bone marrow mesenchymal stem cell proliferation and facilitates osteoblastogenesis," *Clinics (Sao Paulo)*, 2009, 64(10):993–998.

20. D. Parisuthiman, W. Singhatanadgit, T. Dechatiwongse, and S. Koontongkaew, "Cissus quadrangularis extract enhances biomineralization through up-regulation of MAPK-dependent alkaline phosphatase activity in osteoblasts," *In Vitro Cell Dev Biol Anim.* March–April 2009, 45(3-4):194–200.

21. K. Rajoria, S.K. Singh, R.S. Sharma, and S.N. Sharma, "Clinical study on Laksha Guggulu, Snehana, Swedana & traction in osteoarthritis (knee joint)," *Ayu.*, Jan. 2010 31(1):80–87.

22. K. Srisook, M. Palachot, N. Mongkol, E. Srisook, and S. Sarapusit, "Anti-inflammatory effect of ethyl acetate extract from Cissus quadrangularis Linn may be involved with induction of heme oxygenase-1 and suppression of NF-κB activation," *J. Ethnopharmacol.*, Feb. 2011, 16;133(3):1008–1814.

23. S. Hasani-Ranjbar, N. Nayebi, B. Larijani, and M. Abdollahi, "A systemic review of efficacy and safety of herbal medicines used in the treatment of obesity," *World Journal of Gastroenterology*, July 7, 2009, 15(25):3073–3085.

24. J.E. Oben, J.L. Ngondi, C.N. Momo, G.A. Aqbor, and C.S. Sobqui, "The use of Cissus quadragularis / Irvingia gabonensis combination in the management of weight loss: A double blind placebo-controlled trial," *Lipids Health Disease*, March 31, 2008, 7:12.

25. J.E. Oben, D.M. Enyegue, G.I. Fomekong, Y.B. Soukonkoua, and G.A. Aqbor, "The effect of Cissus quadrangularis and Cissus formulation on obesity and obesity induced oxidative stress," *Lipids Health Disease*, Feb. 4, 2007, 6:4.

26. M. Jainu, K. Vijai Mohan, and C.S. Shyamala Devi, "Gastroprotective effect of Cissus quadrangularis extract in rats with experimentally induced ulcer," *Indian J Med Res.*, June 2006, 123(6):799–806.

27. M. Jainu and K.V. Mohan, "Protective role of ascorbic acid isolated from Cissus quadrangularis on NSAID induced toxicity through immunomodulating response and growth factors expression," *Int. Immunopharmacol.*. Dec. 20, 2008, 8(13–14):1721–1727.

28. Jha, M.K., *The Folk Veterinary System of Bihar—A Research Survey* (Anand, Gujra: NDDB, 1992).

29. S.C. Kothari, P. Shivarudraiah, S.B. Venkataramaiah, K.P. Koppolu, S. Gavara, R. Jairam, S. Krishna, R.K. Chandrappa, and M.G. Soni, "Safety assessment of Cissus quadrangularis extract (CQR-300): Subchronic toxicity and mutagenicity studies," *Food Chem Toxicol.*, Dec. 2011, 49(12):3343–3357.

Commiphora mukul

Introduction

Commiphora mukul, also known as Guggul, is a small, spiny tree renowned for the medicinal properties of its sap, or gum. Also called Mukul myrrh, Guggul has been used in the Middle East, India, and China for thousands of years to treat conditions as diverse as infections, bronchial conditions, and digestive complaints. It is associated particularly with women's health and purification rituals. Commiphora mukul is referred to in ancient Hebrew, Greek, and Latin texts as bdellium.

Guggul grows in arid regions of North Africa and Central Asia. In India and Pakistan, the Guggul tree is cultivated commercially for its gum, which is used in incense and perfumes, as well as for a wide variety of medical conditions. Research has supported the use of Guggul gum in treating osteoarthritis. This substance also has been shown to have potential anti-cancer potential.

Guggulsterone, a compound isolated from Guggul gum, received regulatory approval in India in 1987 and is used to treat a range of conditions including obesity and lipid disorders. Clinical trials have demonstrated the compound's effectiveness in lowering blood cholesterol levels by inhibiting its production. Human studies also have indicated that Guggulsterone may assist obese patients in losing weight. Nutritional supplements containing extracts of Guggul gum have become popular in many Western countries.

Synonymous Names

English: Indian bdellium tree
Hindi: Guggul
Sanskrit: Guggulu

Habitat

Guggul is native to the arid, rocky regions of northern Africa and central Asia. In India, it is widespread and is found in Rajasthan, Gujarat, Maharashtra, Tamil Nadu, Karnataka, and Assam. The Guggul tree prefers arid and semi-arid climates and is tolerant of poor soil.

Botanical Characteristics

A small tree or shrub with thorny branches, Guggul grows to a maximum height of 4 meters and has thin, ash-colored, papery bark that is easily peeled away. Its leaves are simple or trifoliate, with ovate leaflets 1–5 cm long, 0.5–2.5 cm broad, and irregularly toothed. Some Guggul plants bear both bisexual and male flowers, and others bear only female blooms. The flowers are pink to red, with four small petals.

Guggul's gum resin is harvested in the winter via incisions made in its bark. The resin is pale yellow, brown, or dull green in color. It has a bitter, aromatic taste and a balsamic odor. Fumes from burning Guggul have been recommended to treat hay fever, nasal catarrh, laryngitis, bronchitis, and phthisis.

Chemical Composition

The following compounds have been isolated through chemical analysis of Guggul:[1,2,3,4]

- The lignans guggullignan-I and guggullignan-II
- Long-chain aliphatic tetrols: octadecan-1,2,3,4-tetrol, eicosan-1,2,3,4-tetrol and onadecan-1,2,3,4-tetrol.
- The terpenes Cembrene-A and mukulol and phenylpropanoids Cembrene-A and mukulol[5] were isolated from gum resin.
- An essential oil, prepared by the steam distillation of the gum resin, contains myrcene and eugenol.
- The following sterols also have been isolated: Z-guggulsterone, E-guggulsterone, guggulsterol I, II, and III, and β-sitosterol.

Pharmacological Activity

Anti-Inflammatory Activity

Guggul has been shown to have anti-inflammatory activity. At doses of 200 and 500 mg/kg, a petroleum ether extract of Guggul's gum resin significantly blocked carrageenan-induced rat paw edema.[6]

Guggulipid and nimesulide studied on lipopolysaccharides stimulated neuroinflammatory changes in the rat astrocytoma cell line. Rat astrocytoma cells were stimulated with lipopolysaccharides (10 microg/ml) alone and in combination with different concentrations of guggulipid or nimesulide for 24 hours of incubation. Both guggulipid and nimesulide significantly attenuated nitrite release, ROS generation, and also downregulated expressions of COX-2, glial fibrillary acidic protein (GFAP), and TNF-alpha. The anti-inflammatory effect of guggulipid was comparable to that of nimesulide, which suggests the potential use of guggulipid in treating inflammation of the nervous system.[7]

Inflammatory bowel diseases are chronic inflammatory and relapsing diseases of the gut that may manifest as Crohn's disease or ulcerative colitis. Crohn's disease and ulcerative colitis are immunologically different diseases characterized by exacerbated Th1 and Th2 response. T-cell resistance against apoptosis contributes to inappropriate T-cell accumulation and chronic mucosal inflammation. Guggulsterone was studied in two models of intestinal inflammation induced in mice by trinitro-benzene sulfonic acid and oxazolone. E-guggulsterone protected the mice against developing signs and symptoms of colon inflammation, whereas Z-guggulsterone did not show the protection, but it effectively regulates the function of effector T cells by modulating the cell signaling activation pathway caused by CD3/CD28. The net biological effects resulting from exposure to guggulsterone includes attenuation of generation of interleukin-2 and -4 and interferon-gamma, as well as T cell proliferation.[8]

Anti-Obesity Activity

To assess the effectiveness of Guggul in facilitating weight loss, 22 obese patients were studied in a clinical trial. All of the patients had hypercholesterolemia, hypertension, heart disease, and diabetes associated with their obesity. The study subjects were given oral Guggul supplements for 15 days to one month. At the end of the study period, all of the patients had experienced significant weight loss, as well as reductions in serum cholesterol and serum lipid phosphorus.[9,10]

Cholesterol-Lowering and Cardioprotective Activity

Guggul's cholesterol-lowering properties have been observed in several clinical trials.[11] During a clinical study, 35 patients received purified Guggul gum resin at doses of 4.5 grams daily for 16 weeks. The patients' serum triglyceride and cholesterol levels were measured at the end of the 4th, 8th, and 16th weeks of the study. All of the study participants experienced significant reductions in VDL and LDL cholesterol levels at all intervals. A gradual increase in HDL cholesterol was observed.[12]

In a randomized, double-blind study model, 31 patients with hypercholesterolemia were given Guggul supplements for a period of 24 weeks, along with a fruit and vegetable-enriched diet. These patients were compared with a control group of 30 patients who received a placebo. In the treated group, Guggul decreased total cholesterol levels by 11.7%. LDL cholesterol was reduced by 12.5%, triglycerides by 12%, and HDL cholesterol by 11%, whereas the control subjects showed no change. In addition, oxidative stress, as measured by lipid peroxide levels, declined 33.3% in the treated group, whereas no decrease was seen in the placebo group. After a rest period of 12 weeks, the patients treated with Guggul showed sustained reductions in blood lipoproteins, equivalent to the effects of modern drugs. The side-effects of Guggulipid were mild and included headache, mild nausea, eructation, and hiccups.[13]

In a clinical study, the effects of Guggal gum in patients with ischemic heart disease were studied. Guggul gum increased the fibrinolytic activity in these patients, with no effect on platelet aggregation. Increased clotting time with changes in the plasma fibrinogen level was also observed.[14]

Animal studies also have verified Guggulsterone's cardioprotective effects. The effects of Guggulsterone were studied on biogenic monoamine levels and dopamine activity in the brain and heart of rats, and indicated that Guggulsterone inhibited brain dopamine levels, with marked stimulation of the heart both in-vitro and in-vivo. Guggulsterone also was found to inhibit catecholamine levels, while increasing serotonin and histamine levels in the brain and decreasing the levels in the heart. These results suggest that Guggulsterone's anti-lipidemic activity may be the result of its alteration of biogenic amines and dopamine activity.[15] When Guggul gum resin was incorporated into the diet of Wistar rats, it lowered liver cholesterol and serum cholesterol, triglycerides and phospholipid levels. The petroleum ether and alcoholic extracts of the gum resin also lowered serum cholesterol in hypercholesterolemic chicks, rabbits, and domestic pigs.

In the same study, a pure steroid of Guggul and its alcoholic extract lowered serum cholesterol in triton-treated rats. The steroid fraction lowered LDL cholesterol by 65%, triglycerides by 39.4%, phospholipids and non-esterified fatty acids by 42.9%. This effectiveness was comparable to the drug Clofibrate. Guggul also lowered LDL cholesterol and VLDL cholesterol significantly.

Laboratory studies conducted on albino rats showed significant prevention of experimental atherosclerosis when ethyl acetate extracts of Guggal were given. The Guggal extract was found to increase plasma fibrinolytic activity. Deteriorative changes were also seen in serum cholesterol, triglycerides and in fibrinogen level.[16]

Research was conducted to determine the potential cardioprotective effects of Guggal when myocardial infarction was induced with isoproterenol in rats. Guggal's hydroalcoholic extract was found to significantly improve cardiac function and prevent myocardial ischemic impairment in the study animals. After treatment with Guggal, decreases were seen in heart rate and arterial pressure, and increases were observed in left ventricular and diastolic pressure. Myocardial contractility was altered as well.[17]

Treatment with Guggal extract also produced significant increases in lactate dehydrogenase levels and prevented the decline of protein content in the heart. Guggal preserved the structural integrity of the myocardium, reduced leakage of myocyte enzyme lactate dehydrogenase, enhanced modulation of cardiac function, and improved cardiac performance.

High-fat diet-induced diabetic rodent models resembling the type II diabetic condition in the human population were used to assess the anti-diabetic and hypolipidemic activity of guggulsterone. Four groups of rats were fed the high-fat diet for 16 weeks. Upon feeding the normal rats with the fat-rich diet, they showed increased serum glucose, cholesterol, and triglyceride levels, along with a significant increase in insulin resistance ($p<0.05$) in comparison to the control animals. Different biochemical parameters such as GTT, glycogen content, glucose homeostatic enzymes (e.g., glucose-6-phosphatase, hexokinase), insulin release in-vivo, and expression profiles of various genes involved in carbohydrate and lipid metabolism clearly demonstrated the hypoglycemic effect of this extract. Guggulsterone demonstrated a differential effect with a significantly improved peroxisome proliferator-activated receptor gamma (PPARgamma) expression and activity in-vivo and in-vitro conditions, respectively. PPAR gamma has diverse functions, the most notable of which is to regulate development of adipose tissue. It inhibited 3T3-L1 preadipocytes differentiation in-vitro. Guggulsterone has both hypoglycemic and hypolipidemic effects, which can help type II diabetes.[18]

Osteoarthritis Activity

Clinical investigations have been conducted to determine Guggul's effects on pain and stiffness in osteoarthritis patients. Older patients with osteoarthritis of the knee were given special attention to determine their tolerance of the herb. Thirty patients were studied, all of whom scored 2 or more on the Kellegran-Lawrence osteoarthritis scale in at least one knee. The patients were administered 500 mg of Guggul extract delivered three times a day with food for one month. After one month of supplementation with Guggul, all these patients showed significant improvement in pain, stiffness, and function. The WOMAC total score improved significantly ($P < 0.0001$), and the patients continued to improve after 2 months of treatment. No side-effects were reported during the study. Thus, Guggul appears to be a safe and effective supplement to reduce the symptoms of osteoarthritis.[19]

Anti-Cancer Activity

Effect of Guggulsterone was studied using PC-3, a human prostate cancer cell lines. Guggulsterone reduced number of proliferating PC-3 cells but had no effect on normal prostate epithelial cell lines. Effect of Guggulsterone on PC-3 was dose dependent. Guggulsterone induced apoptosis as characterized by the appearance of subdiploid cells and cytoplasmic histone-associated DNA fragmentation. Guggulsterone-induced apoptosis was associated with induction of Bcl-2 family members Bax and Bak. Guggulsterone treatment resulted in activation of caspase-9, caspase-8, and caspase-3, and guggulsterone-induced cell death was significantly attenuated in the presence of general caspase inhibitor, as well as specific inhibitors of caspase-9 and caspase-8.[20]

Guggulsterone induced apoptosis and cell cycle arrest, inhibited invasion in head and neck squamous cell carcinoma cell lines, and enhanced the efficacy of erlotinib, cetuximab, and cisplatin. Guggulsterone decreased the expression of both phosphotyrosine and the total signal transducer and activator of transcription (STAT)-3. Hypoxia-inducible factor (HIF)-1alpha also was decreased in response to guggulsterone treatment. In a xenograft model of head and neck squamous cell carcinoma, guggulsterone treatment resulted in increased apoptosis and decreased expression of STAT3, decreased rates of tumor growth, and enhancement of cetuximab activity.[21]

Guggulsterone can suppress tumor initiation, promotion, and metastasis. This steroid has been shown to bind to the farnesoid X receptor and modulate expression of proteins with antiapoptotic (IAP1, XIAP, Bfl-1/A1, Bcl-2, cFLIP, survivin), cell survival, cell proliferation (cyclin D1, c-Myc), angiogenic activity, and metastatic (MMP-9, COX-2, VEGF) activities in tumor cells. Guggulsterone mediates gene expression through regulation of various transcription factors, including NF-kappaB, STAT-3, and C/EBP alpha,This is fine and various steroid receptors such as androgen receptor and glucocorticoid receptors. Modulation of gene expression by guggulsterone leads to inhibition of cell proliferation, induction of apoptosis, suppression of invasion, and abrogation of angiogenesis.[22]

Bone resorption is commonly associated with aging and in cancers such as multiple myeloma and breast cancer. What induces bone resorption is not fully understood, but the role of osteoclasts is well established. Receptor activator of nuclear factor kappaB (NF-kappaB) ligand (RANKL), a member of the tumor necrosis factor, has been shown to be major mediator of bone resorption. This suggests that agents that can suppress RANKL signaling have the potential to inhibit bone resorption.

It was investigated whether guggulsterone could modulate RANKL (Receptor activator of nuclear factor kappa-B ligand) signaling and osteoclastogenesis induced by RANKL or tumor cells. Treatment of monocytes with guggulsterone suppressed RANKL and activated NF-kappaB activation. Suppression of NF-Kappa B correlated with inhibition of IkappaB alpha kinase, phosphorylation, and degradation of IkappaB alpha, an inhibitor of NF-kappaB. Guggulsterone also suppressed the differentiation of monocytes to osteoclasts in a dose-dependent and time-dependent manner. Finally, differentiation to osteoclasts induced by co-incubating Guggulsterone completely suppressed osteoclastogenesis in human breast tumor cells (MDA-MB-468) and human multiple myeloma (U266) cells.[23]

Anti-Diabetic Effects

Guggulsterone has been shown to exhibit protection for pancreatic beta cells. IL-1beta and IFN-gamma-induced beta-cell damage was investigated in RINm5F (RIN) rat insulinoma cells. Guggulsterone completely prevented cytokines-mediated cytotoxicity, as well as NO and PGE2 production, evidenced by reduced levels of the inducible form of NO synthase (iNOS) and cyclooxygenase-2 (COX-2) mRNA and protein expressions. Guggulsterone inhibited NF-kappaB activation. The cytoprotective effects of guggulsterone also were mediated through suppression of the JAK/STAT pathway. Cells treated with the cytokines downregulated the protein level of the suppressor of cytokine signaling 3 (SOCS-3); however, pre-treatment with guggulsterone reduced this decrease. Guggulsterone prevented cytokines-induced NO and PGE2 production, iNOS and COX-2 expressions, JAK/STAT activation, NF-kappaB activation, downregulation of SOCS-3, and impairment of glucose-stimulated insulin secretion in rat's islets cells. Collectively, this showed that guggulsterone may be used to preserve functional beta-cell mass.[24]

Ethnoveterinary Usage

Guggul gum resin is used in veterinary practice to treat rheumatism, cold, and cough.[25]

Dr. Sodhi's Experience

When considering treatment with Guggal, the following questions are relevant:

- Does the patient have dyslipidemia?
- Is the patient's HDL low?
- Is the lipoprotein a(Lpa) high?
- Is VLDL high?
- Is the LDL cholesterol particle size small?
- Is there an inflammatory disease of autoimmune origin?
- Is there a history of stroke, ischemic heart disease, or atherosclerosis?

Guggul is my favorite herb for treating dyslipidemias. Although it is not the best method for lowering overall cholesterol, it exerts specific action upon lipid metabolism that makes it unique in herbal medicine. First, it increases HDL, and no other herbs have been found to do this. In addition, Guggul decreases lipoprotein a (Lpa), an independent marker of cardiac risk. It also lowers VLDLs and increases cholesterol particle size in general.

In addition to its lipidemic effects, Guggul stimulates the thyroid and cleanses atherosclerotic plaque from the arteries. Because of this, it was used in traditional Ayurveda to treat stroke patients and in the treatment of atherosclerosis and ischemic heart disease.

Guggul also has anti-inflammatory action and is extremely useful in the treatment of arthritis, especially rheumatoid and psoriatic arthritis. It should be considered for any autoimmune inflammatory condition and has been used successfully in the treatment of inflammatory disorders. Guggul also has shown great results in cystic acne.

Because it is a resin, Guggul absorption is increased significantly if it is taken with an oil. Olive, hemp seed, coconut, and walnut oils, as well as ghee and fish oil, are all good transport vehicles. It also is well absorbed with pomegranate juice. Taking Guggul with food further enhances its activity.

Case Histories

Hyperlipidemia

The 45-year-old wife of an allopathic physician with high cholesterol came to our clinic for treatment. Her total cholesterol was 488, her HDL value was 29, and her triglycerides were were 622. We gave her the following herbal protocol:

For lipid support:

Commiphora mukul (Guggulu) extract, in combination with Triphala, a compound formula consisting of equal parts of Emblica officianalis (amalaki), Terminalia bellerica (bibhitaki), and Terminalia chebula (haritaki) extracts, with Vitamin B6 and folic acid, three times a day.

For digestive support:

Trifala, a compound formulation consisting of equal parts Emblica officinalis (Amalaki), Terminalia bellerica (Bibhitaki), and Terminalia chebula (Haritaki), three times a day.

A full-spectrum enzyme combination (amylase, amylase II, protease I, II, III, peptidase, lipase, cellulase, hemicellulase, lactase, maltase, invertase, and bromelain), to be taken with each meal, along with a probiotic of 100 billion organisms: three times a day.

For liver support:

Tinospora cardifolia (guduchi), Picrorrhiza kurnoa (kutki), and Boerhaavia diffusa (purnarnava) extracts, 50 mg of each herb in a proprietory blend of Phyllanthus amarus (bhumyamalaki), Swertia chirayita (kiraata), Calotropis gigantis (ark), Raphanus sativa (malaka), Berberis aristata (daaru Curcuma), Terminalia arjuna (arjun), Terminalia bellerica (bibhitaki), Terminalia chebula (haritaki), Emblica officinalis (amalaki), Solanum nigrum (kakmachi), and Andrographis paniculata One tablet three times a day.

For enhanced nutrient absorption:

500 mg of Piper longum (Pippli) extract One cap with meals

For inflammation and liver congestion:

500 mg Curcumin longum (Curcuma) extract, one cap three times a day, and 1000 mg high quality fish oil: one cap a day.

Diet and exercise recommendations were made according to the patient's Ayurvedic constitution, as well as her medical condition. She was expected to take curcumin and fish oil indefinitely, while the Guggulu formula was to be taken for only one year, after which diet and exercise were expected to be sufficient to control her cholesterol levels. After 3 months of treatment, the patient's total cholesterol had fallen to 167, her triglycerides were at 322, and her HDLs had risen to 46.

Stroke

A 76-year-old man, who had a stroke recently, came to our clinic in India. He was experiencing difficulty walking and was not responding well to physical therapy. We checked his copper, magnesium, and B12 levels and found all to be below normal. He was given B-complex injections with oral copper and magnesium supplementation. In addition, he received the Guggulu formula described in the case above, except at twice the dose, to be taken three times a day.

In addition, I prescribed the following heart protective formula, also to be taken three times a day:

Arjuna terminalia (Arjuna), Inula racemosa (pushkarmuul), coral powder, and CoQ10.

After the herbal therapy was begun, the patient's symptoms improved quickly, he began responding to physical therapy, and his speech became much better. Although total recovery of certain functions was not to be expected, the patient, as well as his family and his physical therapist, noticed significant changes and all were pleased with the outcome of the treatment.

Cystic Acne

A young girl came to our clinic with severe cystic acne and depression because of her appearance. Her face looked as though it had multiple bee stings. She had taken minocycline and erythromycin for the previous 3 years. When she took the antibiotics, her acne subsided, only to return 1½ months later. We gave her the following Guggul protocol:

Commiphora mukul (Guggulu) extract, in combination with Triphala, a compound formula consisting of equal parts of Emblica officianalis (amalaki), Terminalia bellerica (bibhitaki), and Terminalia chebula (haritaki) extracts, with Vitamin B6 and folic acid: three times a day.

For Skin Support:

Azadirachta indica (neem), in a proprietary blend of Emblica officinalis (amalaki), Terminalia chebula (haritaki), Terminalia bellerica (bibhitaki), Tinospora cordifolia (guduchi), and Rubia cordifolia (manjistha), One cap three times a day

For Inflammation:

500 mg Curcumin longum (Curcuma) extract 500 mg. One cap three times a day.

The patient's skin is now smooth and free from acne, with some dark pigmentation, which will take some time to go away. The patient reports that her confidence has returned and she is feeling much happier overall.

Chronic Inflammatory Diseases

I have treated several hundred patients with chronic inflammatory disease including osteoarthritis, rheumatoid arthritis, psoriatic arthritis, fibromyalgia, systemic lupus erythematous, polymyalgia, Crohn's disease, ulcerative colitis, bronchial asthma, and others with great success.

The patients were weaned off their medications between 3 and 9 months, and maintained solely on natural herbal treatment or with very low doses of immune-modulating drugs. I have been following some of the patients for 20 years with no signs of relapse. Here are my protocols:

Osteoarthritis, rheumatoid arthritis, psoriatic arthritis, polymyalgia, and fibromyalgia:

For inflammation modulation:

Commiphora mukul (Guggulu) extract, in combination with Triphala, a compound formula consisting of equal parts of Emblica officianalis (amalaki), Terminalia bellerica (bibhitaki), and Terminalia chebula (haritaki) extracts, with Vitamin B6, and folic acid two tablets three times a day.

Boswellia protocol: Boswellia serrata (Boswellia) extract, with Zingiber officinale and Withania somnifera (Ashwagandha) extracts, and Curcumin longum (Curcuma) extract, in a base of bromelain 1600 GDU glucosamine sulphate and chondroitin sulphate: two tablets three times per day.

Ashwagandha, 500 mg: two or three capsules three times per day

A medium-chain triglyceride bound to curcumunoids, a highly bio-available compound: one teaspoon twice a day dissolved in rice milk or coconut milk. This will yield 4 grams of curcumonoids per teaspoon.

Systemic lupus erythematous:

Add the following to to the above protocol:

Combination of extracts of Bacopa monnieri, Centella asiatica, Ginkgo biloba, Convolvulus pluricaulis (Shankhapushpi), and Withania Somnifera (Ashwagandha): three times a day.

Centella asiatica extract: 500 mg three times per day

Brahmi oil for local massage on the body

For Liver Support:

Tinospora cordifolia (guduchi), Picrorrhiza kurroa (kutki), and Boerhaavia diffusa (Punarnava) extracts , each herb in a proprietory blend of Phyllanthus amarus (bhumyamalaki), Swertia chirayita (kiraata), Calotropis gigantis (ark), Raphanus sativa (malaka), Berberis aristata (daaruCurcuma), Terminalia arjuna (arjun), Terminalia bellerica (bibhitaki), Terminalia chebula (haritaki), Emblica officinalis (amalaki), Solanum nigrum (kakmachi), and Andrographis paniculata (bhuunimb): one tablet three times per day.

For Digestive Support:

Triphala, a compound formulation consisting of standardized extracts of equal parts Emblica officinalis (Amalaki), Terminalia bellerica (Bibhitaki), and Terminalia chebula (Haritaki): 500 mg three times a day.

A full-spectrum enzyme combination (amylase, amylase II, protease I, II, III, peptidase, lipase, cellulase, hemicellulase, lactase, maltase, invertase, and bromelain): to be taken with each meal, along with a probiotic of 100 billion organisms: three times a day.

500 mg of Piper longum (Pippli) extract: three times per day with food

Crohn's Disease and Ulcerative Colitis

Commiphora mukul (Guggulu), in combination with Triphala, a compound formula consisting of equal parts of Emblica officinalis (amalaki), Terminalia bellerica (bibhitaki), and Terminalia chebula (haritaki) extracts, with Vitamin B6, and folic acid: two tablets three times a day.

Boswellia protocol: Boswellia serrata (Boswellia) extract, with Zingiber officinale and Withania somnifera (Ashwagandha) extracts, Curcumin longum (Curcuma) extract, in a base of bromelain glucosamine sulphate and chondroitin sulphate: two tablets three times per day.

500 mg Curcumin longum (Curcuma) extract

Asparagus racemosus (Shatavari) extract: 500 mg three times per day

Probiotic 100 billion three times per day 10–15 minutes before meals

Colostrum, 1 tablespoon three times per day; can be added to coconut milk, coconut yogurt, rice milk, hemp milk, or almond milk.

Bronchial Asthma

Boswellia protocol: Boswellia serrata (Boswellia) extract, Zingiber officinale, Withania somnifera (Ashwagandha) extracts, Curcumin longum (Curcuma) extract, in a base of bromelain 1600 GDU glucosamine sulphate and chondroitin sulphate: two tablets three times per day.

Commiphora mukul (Guggulu), in combination with Triphala, a compound formula consisting of equal parts of Emblica officinalis (amalaki), Terminalia bellerica (bibhitaki), and Terminalia chebula (haritaki) extracts, with Vitamin B6 and folic acid : two tablets three times a day.

Tylophora asthmatica (antraapaachak) extract, 150 mg in a blend with Piper longum,

Emblica officinalis, and Zingiber officinale extract: three times a day.

For immune support:

400 mg each Emblica officinalis (Amalaki), Ocimum sanctum (tulsi), Terminalia bellerica (bibhitaki/bahera), with Tinospora cordifolia (guduchi), and Glycyrrhiza glabra, Terminalia chebula (haritaki) and Adhatoda vasica (vasaka): three times a day.

Obesity

One or two capsules of the Guggul formulation may be taken once or twice a day, together with one or two cloves of fresh Allium sativum (lasuna), three times a day. The garlic can be chopped into small pieces and put into salads and other dishes. Fresh garlic is recommended for best results.

High Cholesterol

Commiphora mukul (Guggulu), in combination with Triphala, a compound formula consisting of equal parts of Emblica officinalis (amalaki), Terminalia bellerica (bibhitaki), and Terminalia chebula (haritaki) extracts, with Vitamin B6 and folic acid: two tablets three times a day.

If cholesterol is not sufficiently lowered using the Guggulu formulation, add the following supplements should be added:

500 mg niacin twice a day.

For Heart Support:

Arjuna terminalia (arjun), mg of Inula racemosa (pushkarmuul), coral powder, andCoQ10. one cap three times a day

If this still does not work, a very low dose of red rice yeast should be added. As cholesterol levels are lowered, statin dosages may be gradually lowered, under a doctor's supervision. This is especially true if LDLs drop below 70.

Hypothyroidism

The Guggul protocol is especially good if T3 is low. The formulation should be taken three times daily. The dose may be doubled if the initial response is not sufficient. In addition, the following herbal formulation should be given three times a day:

Combination of potassium iodide 7.5 mg, L-Tyrosine 100 mg and proprietary blend of Withania somnifera, Bacopa monnieri, Bauhinia tomentosa, Piper longum, Piper nigrum, Zingiber officinale, Crataeva nurvula, Cinnamomum zeylanicum, Cinnamomum tamala, Commiphora mukul, and Elettaria cardamomum: one capsule twice a day. There may be a slight rise in TSH in the beginning, but after 6 to 9 months, the TSH, free T3, and T4 will normalize. Many patients on levothyroxine sodium (Synthroid) or thyroid extract either reduced the dose to a minimal amount or got off completely.

Combination of Bacopa monniera (indriya brahmi) and Ginkgo biloba extracts, Centella asiatica (brahmi) extract, and Convolvulus pluricaulis (shankhapushpi) extract, Withania somnifera (Ashwagandha): 500 mg.one cap three times a day

Additional actions: Head, neck and metastatic cancers

A preparation of Laksha Guggul has shown great results in osteoporosis. Molecular biology concepts are now clearly indicating its usefulness in osteoporosis and metastatic cancer.

Safety Profile

Guggulipid does not appear to have any adverse effects when administered at a dose of 400 mg three times daily. It is contraindicated during pregnancy and internal inflammatory conditions, and it may cause gastrointestinal discomfort. In clinical studies, the crude resin revealed mild side-effects such as skin rashes, diarrhea, menorrhagia, and irregular menstruation.[26]

Guggul has a heating nature, so people with a pitta constitution have to be careful not to take too much, because they may become overheated. In rare conditions— for example, when the patient has a history of alcohol consumption—Guggal may cause a skin rash.

Dosage

Powdered gum resin: 0.4–1.5 g

Guggul extract 300 mg two to three times per day

Ayurvedic Properties

Rasa: Katu (pungent), tikta (bitter)
Guna: Laghu (light), ruksha (dry), tikshna (sharp), vishad (conspicuous), sukshma (minute), sugandhi (aromatic), snigdha-pichchhil (unctuous-sticky)
Veerya: Ushna (hot)
Vipaka: Katu (pungent)
Dosha: Pacifies tridosha

Notes

1. A. Fiatterjee and C.S. Pakrashi, *The Treatise of Indian Medicinal Plants*. New Delhi, India: PID, CSIR, 1994.

2. V.D. Patil, U.R. Nayak, and D. Sukh, "Chemistry of Ayurvedic crude drugs—III, guggulu (resin from Commiphora mukut)-3, long chain aliphatic tetrols, a new class of naturally occurring lipids," *Tetrahedron*, 1973, 29:1595.

3. V.D. Patil, U.R. Nayak, and D. Sukh, "Chemistry of Ayurvedic crude drugs—II, guggulu (resin from Commiphora mukul)~2 diterpenoid constituents," *Tetrahedron*, 1973, 29:341.

4. V.D. Patil, U.R. Nayak, and D. Sukh, "Chemistry of Ayurvedic crude drugs—1, guggulu (resin from Commiphora mukul) steroidal constituents," *Tetrahedron*, 1972, 28:2341.

5. A. Saukhla, P.N. Mathur, A.K. Saukhla, and P.K. Dashora, "Comparative efficiency of Shilajeet and gum guggal (Commiphora mukul) in preventing diet induced hypercholesterolemia in Wistar rats," *Indian Journal of Clinical Biochemistry*, 1992, 7(1):45.

6. J.N. Sharma M.N. Rajpal, T.S. Rao, and S.K. Gupta, "Some pharmacological investigations on the alcoholic extract of Triphala alone and in combination with petroleum ether extract of oleogum resin of Commiphora mukul," *Indian Drugs*, 1988, 25(6):220.

7. Author?, Niranjan R, Kamat P, Nath C, Shukla R "Evaluation of guggulipid and nimesulide on production of inflammatory mediators and GFAP expression in LPS stimulated rat astrocytoma, cell line (C6)," *J Ethnopharmacol.* , Feb. 17, 2010, 127(3):625–630.

8. A. Mencarelli, B. Renga, G. Palladino, E. Distrutti, and S. Fiorucci, "The plant sterol guggulsterone attenuates inflammation and immune dysfunction in murine models of inflammatory bowel disease," *Biochem Pharmacol.*, Nov. 1, 2009, 78(9):1214–1223.

9. G.V. Satyavati, "Effect of an indigenous drug on disorders of lipid metabolism with special reference to atherosclerosis and obesity (Medaroga)," MD thesis (Doctor of Ayurvedic Medicine), Banaras Hindu University, Varanasi, 1966.

10. K. Kuppurajan, S.S. Rajagopalan, Rao T. Koteswara, A.N. Vijayalakshmi, and C. Dwarkanath, "Effect of guggulu (Commiphora mukul-Engl) on serum lipids in obese subjects," *Journal of Research in Indian Medicine*, 1973, 8:4.

11. W.S. Sastry, "Experimental and clinical studies on the effect of oleogum resin of Commiphora mukul on thrombotic phenomenon associated with hyperlipaemia (Snehavyapat)." MD thesis (Doctor of Ayurvedic Medicine), Banaras Hindu University, Varanasi, 1967.

12. S.K. Verma and A. Bordia, "Effect of Commiphora mukul (gum guggul) in patients of hyperlipidemia with special reference to HDL-cholesterol," *Indian Journal of Medical Research*, 1988, 87:356.

13. R.B. Singh, M.A. Niaz, and S. Ghosh, "Hypolipidemic and anti-oxidant effects of Commiphora mukul as an adjunct to dietary therapy in patients with hypercholesterolemia," *Cardiovasc Drugs Ther.* Aug. 1994, 8(4):659–664.

14. H.A. Motani, "The effect of guggul (Commiphora mukul) on lipid profile and coagulation in ischaemic heart disease," PhD thesis, Nagpur University, 1981.

15. M. Srivastava and N.K. Kapoor, "Guggulsterol induced changes in the levels of biogenic monoamines and dopamine p-hydroxylase activity of rat tissue," *Journal of Bioscience*, 1986, 10:15.

16. See Saukka et al., Note 5.

17. S.K. Ojha, M. Nandave, S. Arora, R.D. Mehra, S. Joshi, R. Narang, and D.S. Arya, "Effect of Commiphora mukul extract on cardiac dysfunction and ventricular function in isoproterenol-induced myocardial infarction," *Indian J Exp Biol.*, Sept. 2008, 46(9):646–652.

18. B. Sharma, R. Salunke, S. Srivastava, C. Majumder, and P. Roy, "Effects of guggulsterone isolated from Commiphora mukul in high fat diet induced diabetic rats," *Food Chem Toxicol.*, Oct. 2009, 47(10):2631-9.

19. B.B. Singh, L.C. Mishra, S.P. Vinjamury, N. Aquilina, V.J. Singh, and N. Shepard, "The effectiveness of Commiphora mukul for osteoarthritis of the knee: an outcomes study," *Altern Ther Health Med.*, May–June, 2003, 9(3):74–79.

20. S.V. Singh, Y. Zeng, D. Xiao, V.G. Vogel, J.B. Nelson, R. Dhir, and Y.B. Tripathi, "Caspase-dependent apoptosis induction by guggulsterone, a constituent of Ayurvedic medicinal plant Commiphora mukul, in PC-3 human prostate cancer cells is mediated by Bax and Bak," *Mol Cancer Ther.*, Nov. 2005, 4(11):1747–1754.

21. R.R. Leeman-Neill, S.E. Wheeler, S.V. Singh, S.M. Thomas, R.R. Seethala, D.B. Neill, M.C. Panahandeh, E.R. Hahm, S.C. Joyce, M. Sen, Q. Cai, M.L. Freilino, C. Li, D.E. Johnson, and J.R. Grandis JR, "Guggulsterone enhances head and neck cancer therapies via inhibition of signal transducer and activator of transcription-3," *Carcinogenesis*, Nov. 2009, 30(11):1848-1856.

22. S. Shishodia, K.B. Harikumar, S. Dass, K.G. Ramawat, B.B. Aggarwal, "The guggul for chronic diseases: Ancient medicine, modern targets," *Anticancer Res.*, Nov–Dec 2008, 28(6A):3647–3664.

23. H. Ichikawa and B.B. Aggarwal, "Guggulsterone inhibits osteoclastogenesis induced by receptor activator of nuclear factor-kappaB ligand and by tumor cells by suppressing nuclear factor-kappaB activation," *Clin Cancer Res.*, Jan. 15, 2006, 12(2):662–668.

24. N. Lv, M.Y. Song, E.K. Kim, J.W. Park, K.B. Kwon, and B.H. Park, "Guggulsterone, a plant sterol, inhibits NF-kappaB activation and protects pancreatic beta cells from cytokine toxicity, *Mol Cell Endocrinol.*," July 16, 2008, 289(1–2):49–59.

25. M.K Jha, Folk *Veterinary Medicine of Bihar—A Research Project*. Anand, Gujrat: NDDB, 1992.

26. S.K. Bhargava, "Hypolipidemic activity of a steroid fraction of guggal resin (Commiphora mukul Hook. Ex Stocks) in monkeys (Presbytis entellus entellus Dufresne)," *Plantes Medicinales et Phytotherapie*, 1984, 18:68.

Additional Resources

S.N Vyas and C.P. Shukla, "A clinical study on the effect of Guggulu in rheumatoid arthritis," *Rheumatism*, 1987, 23(1):15. Let's leave it in further readings. We are not using any referencing in case studies

Number 9 did not appear as a superscript, so it either could be placed under a new Further Reading heading, or possibly it applies to the rheumatoid arthritis discussion on p. 16 – which could be added but would require numbering as #26.

V.K. Srivastava, S. Lata, R.S. Saxena, A. Kumar, and A.K. Saxena, "Beneficial effects of ethyl acetate extract of Commiphora mukul (guggulu) in experimental atherosclerosis." Proceedings of a Conference on Pharmacology and Herbal Drugs, New Delhi, India, March 15, 1991.

Number 11 did not appear as a superscript, so it either could be placed under a new Additional Resources heading, or possibly it applies to the atherosclerosis discussion on p. 16 – which could be added but would require additional numbering as #27 Same would be true for this

S. Panda and Kar A.1? Gugulu (commiphora mukul) induces triiodothyronine production: possible involvement of lipid peroxidation, *Life Sciences*, 65(12), PL137–PL141(1). Abstract, retrieved July 3, 2007. [No superscript 18 in text. Either place a superscript where appropriate and renumber subsequent notes OR place under Additional Resources heading] Additional references

D. Xiao and S.V. Singh, " z-Guggulsterone, a constituent of Ayurvedic medicinal plant Commiphora mukul, inhibits angiogenesis in vitro and in vivo," *Mol Cancer Ther.*, Jan. 2008,7(1):171-180. [Again, no superscript f 21 in text. What to do with this entry?] Additional references

Convolvulus pluricaulis

Introduction

Convolvulus pluricaulis, or Shankhapushpi, is a morning-glory-like creeping herb that grows throughout the plains of India. It has been used commonly in Ayurvedic medicine to treat nervous and brain disorders. Shankhpushpi is believed to calm the nerves by regulating the body's production of the stress hormones adrenaline and cortisol.

Shankhpushpi also is known widely as a memory improving drug and is used as a psycho-stimulant and tranquilizer. The ethanolic extract of the plant has been found to reduce total serum cholesterol, triglycerides, phospholipids, and non-esterified fatty-acids. The whole herb is used as a treatment for fever, insomnia, fatigue, and low energy level.

Shankhapushpi is an excellent treatment for bowel complaints, especially dysentery. This herb improves digestion and prevents water retention and constipation. Animal research investigating the effectiveness of Shankhapushpi in treating gastric ulcers revealed that it augments mucosal defensive factors in the digestive system.[1] Additional research showed that Shankhapushpi has significant anti-epileptic activity compared to a placebo.[2] Another study showed that Shankhapushpi may be helpful in improving symptoms of hyperthyroidism by reducing the activity of a key liver enzyme.[3]

Synonymous Names

Latin: Convolvulus pluricaulis
English: Bindweed
Hindi: Kaudiali, Shankhahuli
Sanskrit: Shankhapushpi, Vishnukranta

Habitat

Shankhapushpi grows in the plain areas of northern India.

Botanical Characteristics

Shankhapushpi is a low-growing creeping herb, with small, linear to oblong sessile leaves. Shankhapushpi's morning glory-like flowers appear from December to April. The axillary, pedicelled blossoms grow in groups of one to three. The axillary, pedicelled flowers have linear to lanceolate hair sepals. The shape of the blooms resembles a marine shell, or Shankh (conch); thus, the derivation of the plant's name, pushpa (meaning flower).

Chemical Composition

Chemical analysis of Shankhapushpi has revealed the presence of alkaloids, glycosides, coumarins, and flavonoids. An active alkaloid, termed Shankhapushpine has been identified as the plant's active principle. Beta sitosterol glycoside, Hydroxy cinnamic acid, and Octacosanol tetracosane, along with glucose and sucrose, also have been isolated from the plant. Additional alkaloids have been identified, including convolvine, convolamine, phyllabine, convolidine, confoline, convoline, subhirsine, convosine, convolvidine, and scopoline.[7]

Pharmacological Activity

Anti-Cholesteremic Activity

Shankhapushpi's ethanolic extract was shown to reduce total serum cholesterol, triglycerides, phosopholipids, and non-esterified fatty-acids when administered to hyperlipidemia rats for 30 days. At the same time, high-density lipoprotein was significantly raised in these animals.[4]

Anti-Depressant and Brain Tonic Activity

During the course of routine plasma drug level monitoring, an unexpected loss of seizure control and reduction in plasma phenytoin levels was noticed in two patients who also were taking Shankhapushpi. Therefore, a study was undertaken in rats to investigate any Shankhapushpi–phenytoin interaction from both pharmacokinetic (serum) levels and pharmacodynamic (electroshock seizure prevention) aspects.[2]

Single doses of Shankhapushpi did not have an effect on plasma phenytoin levels; however, phenytoin's anti-epileptic activity was decreased significantly. When multiple doses of the herb were given, Shankhapushpi not only reduced phenytoin's anti-epileptic activity but lowered plasma phenytoin levels as well. Shankhapushpi itself showed significant anti-epileptic activity compared to placebo.[2]

Shankhapushpi's ethanolic extract enhanced neuropeptide synthesis in the brain of laboratory animals. Increases were observed in brain protein, indicating increased memory and acquisition efficiency.[10]

An alcoholic extract of Shankhapushpi depressed myocardial activity in the brain of amphibians and mammals; however, the negative inotropic action was not sustained. The extract demonstrated spasmolytic activity on the smooth muscle of isolated rabbit ileum, rat uterus, and intact intestine of dog. The dog's tracheal muscle behaved differently and exhibited potentiation of the acetylcholine response.[3] Shankhpushpi also was shown to be a powerful tranquilizer in animal investigations.[6]

A study investigated the effects of petroleum ether, chloroform, and ethyl acetate fractions of shankhapushpi on depression in mice.[8] Petroleum ether, chloroform, and ethyl acetate fractions were administered orally for 10 successive days to separate groups of Swiss young male albino mice. Effects of the extracts on the mice's immobility periods were assessed in the forced swim and tail suspension tests. The added effects of reserpine, sulpiride, prazosin, and p-chlorophenylalanine were studied as well. The extracts' anti-depressant-like effect was compared with that of imipramine and fluoxetine when administered for 10 successive days.

Only the chloroform fraction in doses of 50 and 100 mg/kg significantly reduced the immobility time in both tests. This fraction did not significantly affect locomotor activity. Its efficacy was found to be comparable to that of imipramine and fluoxetine. The chloroform fraction reversed the reserpine induced extension of immobility period in both tests. Prazosin, sulpiride, and p-chlorophenylalanine significantly attenuated the chloroform fraction induced anti-depressant-like effect as observed in the tail suspension test. The chloroform fraction of the total ethanolic extract of Shankhapushpi elicited a significant anti-depressant-like effect in mice via its interactions with the adrenergic, dopaminergic, and serotonergic systems.

Immunomodulatory Activity

Shankhapushpi's immunomodulatory activity was studied in a rat model of arthritis. For the study, Freund's adjuvant was used to induce inflammation in the right hind paw of study animals and, subsequently, the crude extract of Shankhapushpi was administered intraperitoneally. Shankhapushpi's anti-inflammatory response was assessed by observing lymphocyte proliferation and the histopathological severity of synovial hyperplasia. These results indicated that treatment with Shankhapushpi significantly reduced both inflammation and edema. At the cellular level, immunosuppression occurred during the early phase of the disease. The animals treated with Shankhapushpi also showed mild synovial hyperplasia and infiltration of mononuclear cells. The induction of nitric oxide synthase was significantly decreased in the treated animals compared to the controls. These observations suggest that the herbal extract caused immunosuppression, indicating that it may provide a useful alternative treatment for arthritis.[9]

Anti-Ulcer Activity

A study was conducted to evaluate the anti-ulcerogenic effects of the juice of fresh whole Shankhpushpi plants. Various experimental models of gastric ulcer induction were used for the study, including ethanol, aspirin, 2-hour cold restraint stress, and 4-hour pyloric ligation in rats. Shankhapushpi juice was given to the animals twice daily for 5 days at doses of 375 and 750 mg/kg body weight. The herbal extract demonstrated an anti-ulcerogenic effect at both dosages in all the experimental gastric ulcer models used, with effectiveness comparable to the reference drug Sucralfate. Gastric juice secretion and mucosal levels were monitored to determine the possible mechanisms of action of this effect by studying both offensive and defensive mucosal factors. The anti-ulcerogenic effect of Shankhpushpi was found to result from augmentation of mucosal defensive factors such as mucin secretion, lifespan of mucosal cells, and glycoproteins, rather than offensive factors such as acid-pepsin.[1]

Shankhapushpi is unctuous, sticky and sweet after digestion and is cold in potency, alleviating Vatta (Air) and Pitta (Fire). It acts as a digestive tonic and a light sedative. Because of its cold potency, it is tonic to heart, helping blood coagulation and high blood pressure.

Dr. Sodhi's Experience

When considering herbal treatment with Shankhapushpi, the practitioner should consider the following:

- Is there any type of mental disturbance such as anxiety, depression, anger, psychosis, frustration or irritation?

Shankhapushpi is classified as a rasayana, one of a valuable class of herbs that have adaptogenic properties and enhance longevity. Like Centella asiatica (brahmi) and Bacopa monniera (indriya brahmi), Shankhapushpi is used to enhance mental and emotional health. It has a cooling, calming energy, and for this reason it is commonly used in India to treat hypertension.

Combined with brahmi, indriya brahmi, and almonds, Shankhapushpi is made into a chewable preparation thought to improve intelligence and memory in children. Like brahmi and indriya brahmi, Shankhapushpi is used to treat mental disturbances of all types, including anxiety, depression, psychosis, and excess anger. To ease frustration and calm excessive anger, a topical preparation of Shankhapushpi, Brahmi, Indriya brahmi, and milk is often used in traditional Ayurveda.

Safety Profile

No known safety concerns or interactions have been reported with recommended dosages of Shankhpushpi.

Although care must be taken when patients are on anti-seizure medication, anti-depressant and anti-anxiety medication.

Ayurvedic Properties

Rasa: Tikta
Guna: Snigdha; Pichchhila
Veerya: Sheeta
Vipaka: Madhura
Dosha: Pacifies Vata, Pitta and Kapha

Notes

1. K. Sairam, C.V. Rao, and R.K, Goel, "Effect of Convolvulus pluricaulis Chois on gastric ulceration and secretion in rats," *Indian Journal of Experimental Biology,* April 2001, 39(4):350–354.

2. U.P. Dandekar, R.S. Chandra, S.S. Dalvi, M.V Joshi, P.C. Gokhale, A.V. Sharma, P.U. Shah, and N.A Kshirsagar, "Analysis of a clinically important interaction between phenytoin and Shankhapushpi, an Ayurvedic preparation," *Journal of Ethnopharmacology*, **Jan. 1992, 35(3):285-288.**

3. Panda S, Kar A. Inhibition of T3 production in levothyroxine-treated female mice by the root extract of Convolvulus pluricaulis. Horm Metab Res. 2001 Jan;33(1):16-8.

4. F.S. Barar and V.N. Sharma, "Preliminary pharmacological studies on Convolvulus pluricaulis chois —an Indian indigenous herb," *Indian J Physiol Pharmacol.*, April 1965, 9(2):99-102.

5. B. Syed, M. Waseem Sharma, A.P. Singh, and M. Tiwari, "Neuroprotective role of Convolvulus pluricaulis on aluminium induced neurotoxicity in rat brain," *Journal of Ethnopharmacology,* July 2009, 124(3) 409–415.

6. N.H. Indurwade and K.R. Biyani, "Evaluation of comparative and combined depressive effect of Brahmi, Shankhpushpi and Jatamansi in mice," *Indian J Med Sci.*, Aug. 2000, 54(8):339–341.

7. G.K. Singh and A. Bhandari, *Text Book of Pharmacognosy* (1st ed.). (New Delhi: CBS Publishers, 2000), pp. 193–194.

8. D. Dhingra and R. Valecha, "Evaluation of the anti-depressant-like activity of Convolvulus pluricaulis choisy in the mouse forced swim and tail suspension tests," *International Medical Journal of Experimental and Clinical Research* (Med Sci Monit), July 2007, 13(7): BR155–61.

9. L. Ganju, D. Karan, S. Chanda, K.K. Srivastava, R.C. Sawhney, and W. Selvamurthy, "Immunomodulatory effects of agents of plant origin," *Biomed Pharmacother.*, Sept. 2003, 57(7):296–300.

10. S.N. Sinha, V.P. Dixit, A.V.S. Madnawat, and O.P. Sharma, "The possible potentiation of cognitive processing on administration of Convolvulus microphyllus in rats," *Indian Medicine,* 1989, 1(3):1–6.

11. V. Mudgal, "Studies on medicinal properties of Convolvulus pluricaulis and Boerhaavia diffusa," *Planta Med.*, Aug. 1975, 28(1):62–68.

12. R.H. Singh and A.K. Mehta, "Studies on the psychotropic effect of the Medhya Rasayana drug 'Shankapushpi' (Convolvulus pluricaulis), Part 1" (clinical studies), *Journal of Research in Indian Medicine, Yoga and Homeopathy*, 1977, 12(3):18.

Crataeva nurvala

Introduction

Crataeva nurvala, also known as Varuna, is a small tree that grows wild along riverbanks throughout India, where it also is widely cultivated. The stem and root bark are the parts of this plant that are most often used medicinally. Its Sanskrit name, Varuna, is taken from one of the oldest of the Vedic deities. The Latin name Crataeva derives from Crataevus, an ancient Greek botanist. The plant was well known to ancient Ayurvedic physicians, who used it as a blood purifier and to maintain homeostasis. It has been used in Ayurvedic tradition to treat a variety of disorders and is especially valued for its therapeutic effect on the urinary organs.

The triterpene Lupeol has been isolated from Varuna and is considered to be the active element responsible for the plant's extensive pharmacological value. Lupeol has been widely investigated in recent years for its potential anti-cancer effects. Lupeol also is used to treat hypercrystalluria, hyperoxaluria, and hypercalciuria.[1] The compound, too, is widely used to treat other urinary disorders such as urolithiasis, and it has been found to lower excess concentrations of oxalate, phosphorus, and magnesium in renal tissue.[2]

In addition to its usefulness in treating urinary disorders, Varuna is valued in Ayurvedic tradition as a laxative, antipyretic, antilithic, anti-helminthic, demulcent, stomachic, and alterative this is fine tonic for chest and blood diseases.[3] It is also useful as an anti-inflammatory drug and as a female contraceptive.

An herbal preparation combining Varuna with Eclipta, Picrorrhiza, and Achillea (yarrow) is used in Ayurvedic tradition as a specific therapy for hepatic inflammation, a disorder that can have secondary effects on urinary secretion. In this preparation, cassia seed, cichorium (chicory), and solanum—which are also useful for liver inflammation—are often added to treat fluid retention. In Ayurveda, Crataeva is valued as a bitter, antiperiodic, aperitif, astringent, demulcent, laxative, rubefacient, tonic, liver stimulant, and vesicant.

Synonymous Names

English: Three-leaved caper
Hindi: Barna, barun
Sanskrit: Varuna

Habitat

Varuna grows wild along riverbanks throughout India, where it is cultivated, too. It is distributed in sub-Himalayan tracts and is indigenous to Tamil Nadu, Kerala, and Karnataka.

Botanical Characteristics

Varuna is a deciduous tree that bears many branches. Its trifolate leaves are glabrous and consist of ovate leaflets. The large, greenish-white flowers grow in dense terminal clusters. The fruits are ovoid, with a tough rind and brown seeds embedded in a fleshy pulp. When mature, Varuna's bark is wrinkled and rough with visible lenticels. The tree's outer surface is gray to brown in color.

Chemical Composition

Chemical analysis of Varuna has revealed the following chemical constituents:[4]

Alkaloids:
  Cadabicine and cadabicine diacetate are present in the stem bark.

Tannins:
  The tannins (-) Epiafzelechin, (-) epiafzelechin-5-O-β-D glucoside, and catechin, also are present in the bark.

Triterpenes:
In addition to Lupeol, the triterpene diosgenin has been isolated from Varuna's stem, and β-sitosterol, and the acetates arunol, spinasterol acetate, taraxasterol, 3-pilupeol, and lupenone are present in the stem, root, and seeds.

Flavonoids:
  Varuna contains the flavonoids rutin, quercetin, and isoquercetin are also present.[5,6]

Pharmacological Activity

Anti-lithic activity

Varuna has been studied clinically to determine its anti-lithic effect in patients with calcium oxalate and calcium phosphate nephrolithiasis.[7] Treatment with Varuna provided symptomatic relief of pain and dysuria and the disappearance of urinary crystals in 65% to 70% of patients in the calcium oxalate group and 50% to 70% in the calcium phosphate group. Radiological reduction in size was observed as well.

Varuna's anti-lithic activity also was verified in animal studies. A study using rats measured the effect of the triterpene Lupeol on calcium oxalate stones. Ammonium oxalate was administered to adult male Wistar rats to induce a hyperoxaluric condition of increased oxalate excretion and elevation in urinary marker enzymes, indicating renal tissue damage. Lupeol, at a dose of 25 mg/kg, reduced the levels of urinary marker enzymes, suggesting a beneficial effect in reducing the deposition of stone-forming constituents in the kidney.[8,9]

In a prospective randomized, double-blind, placebo control trial, a total of 77 patients with calculi of more than 5 mm were included.[10] All patients were evaluated either by x-ray KUB or by USG KUB for 3 months. All of the patients were divided into two groups: Group A consisted of patients with calculi 5–10 mm (n = 31), and Group B had calculi > 10 mm (n = 30) with either active treatment or placebo in both groups. All of the patients were asked to keep a record of number of pain episodes, and the severity of pain was measured on a visual analogue scale (VAS). Group A showed a 33.04% reduction in the size of calculi in the active arm, while there was a 5.13% increase in the same group in the placebo arm ($p = 0.017$). In Group B, there was an 11.25% reduction in the active arm compared to a 1.41% reduction in the same group with the placebo. In the active arm there was statistically significant lower VAS compared to the placebo arm in the form of the highest VAS ($p = 0.008$), average VAS ($p = 0.001$), and VAS at the first episode of pain ($p < 0.0001$).

The authors' preliminary experience suggests that the Ayurvedic formulation "Varuna and banana stem" has promise for management of upper urinary-tract calculi, especially renal calculi. It helps to dissolve renal calculi and facilitate their passage. In addition, it helps to reduce pain from renal/

ureteric calculus disease. A larger phase III study with a longer follow-up is required.

In another experiment[11] the effects of Varuna were studied in rats predisposed to calcium oxalate stone formation. The control animals showed significant increases in the activity of the major oxalate synthesizing enzymes in the liver, in particular glycolate oxidase (GAO) and lactate dehydrogenase (LDH). A significant decrease in liver GAO activity was observed in the rats treated with the bark decoction. Marginal decreases in Na+, K+ -ATPase levels, and an increase in the activity of aspartate aminotransferase were produced when the decoction was fed to experimental rats along with a calculi-producing diet. Other enzyme levels were unaffected. The decrease in liver GAO activity seen during treatment with Varuna suggests that the herb may prove beneficial as a prophylactic in preventing oxalate stone recurrence. The bark decoction also lowered levels of small intestinal Na+, K+ -ATPases. Varuna's action on the small intestinal tract seems to be mediated through these substances, which in turn may affect the transport of metabolites.[12]

Anti-Inflammatory Activity

In an animal study, the anti-inflammatory effects of the triterpenes Lupeol and Lupeol linoleate, isolated from Varuna, were investigated in comparison with indomethacin, a commonly used non-steroidal anti-inflammatory drug.[13] In an adjuvant arthritis model of inflammation, Lupeol, lupeol linoleate, and indomethacin reduced paw swelling by 39%, 58%, and 35%, respectively. Unlike indomethacin, the triterpenes did not show antinociceptive, anti-pyretic, and ulcerogenic actions. These results suggest that the mechanism of action of triterpenes is different from the non-steroidal anti-inflammatory drug.

In an adjuvant-induced model of inflammation in rats, Lupeol, administered orally at a dose of 50 mg/kg for 8 days reduced the alterations in the enzyme levels in arthritic rats compared to normal rats.[14]

Anti-Cancer Activity

Pancreatic cancer is an extremely aggressive disease that is difficult to treat. Pancreatic cancer cells notoriously resist conventional cancer treatments including surgery, radiation, and chemotherapy. Research has targeted the role of RAS oncoprotein in inducing multiple signaling pathways, increasing pancreatic cancer cells' resistance to apoptosis. This research seeks to develop new chemotherapeutic agents that will target such multiple pathways and make pancreatic cancer cells more responsive to death signals.

The triterpene Lupeol, isolated from Varuna, has showed promise in the search for chemotherapeutic agents to effectively combat pancreatic cancer cells. In a study using human pancreatic adenocarcinoma cells, the effect of Lupeol on cell growth and the modulation of multiple RAS-induced signaling pathways was investigated.[15] The results of this research indicated that Lupeol caused a dose-dependent inhibition in pancreatic cancer cell growth, as assessed by MTT assay and apoptosis rates. Lupeol significantly reduced the expression of RAS oncoprotein, as well as inhibiting signaling pathways. These data suggest that Lupeol may act by targeting multiple signaling pathways, leading to increased apoptosis and inhibition in the growth of pancreatic cancer cells.

Cyclophosphamide (CP), an alkylating agent widely used in cancer chemotherapy, causes cardiac membrane damage. Lupeol, a pentacyclic triterpene isolated from Crataeva nurvala stem bark and its ester, lupeol linoleate, possess a wide range of medicinal properties. The effects of lupeol and its ester were evaluated in CP-induced alterations of cardiac electrolytes in rats.[16] Male albino rats of the Wistar strain were categorized into six groups. Group I served as the control. Rats in groups II, V, and VI were injected intraperitoneally with a single dose of CP (200 mg/kg body weight) dissolved in saline. The CP treated groups V and VI received lupeol and lupeol linoleate (50 mg/kg body weight), respectively, dissolved in olive oil for 10 days by oral gavage. At the end of the experimental period, urinary risk factors, activities of ATPases, and electrolytes were measured using standard procedures. The CP-administered rats showed a significant decrease ($P < 0.001$) in the activities of ATPases. This was associated with significant alterations ($P < 0.001$) of electrolytes in both serum and cardiac tissue. The levels of urea, uric acid, and creatinine also were significantly ($P < 0.001$) altered in the serum and urine. Lupeol and its ester reversed the above alterations induced by CP. These findings demonstrate that supplementation with lupeol and its ester could preserve membrane permeability, highlighting their protective effect against CP-induced cardiotoxicity.

Anti-oxidant Activity

Varuna is one of several Ayurvedic herbs that have shown anti-oxidant potency. Bark extracts from several medicinally active Ayurvedic plants, including Varuna, were investigated for their anti-oxidant potential.[17] Standardized aqueous alcoholic extracts taken from the selected barks were prepared and screened by multiple in-vitro assays. The extracts also were tested for their total phenolic and tannin content and correlated with anti-oxidant capacity. The results of this research showed that Varuna had the highest total concentrations of phenols and tannins. Lipid peroxidation and SOD mimetic activity also were found to be highest in Varuna, which in addition showed a comparatively high capacity to destroy nitrous oxide.

Further research showed that Lupeol, isolated from Varuna's stem bark, given in doses of 40 and 80 mg/kg body weight for 10 days, decreased the concentration of blood urea nitrogen, creatinine, and lipid peroxidation and increased glutathione and catalase activities in cisplatin-induced nephrotoxicity in rats. Lupeol's anti-oxidant properties also are indicated by increased glutathione and catalase activity.[18]

Ethnoveterinary Usage

The stem bark of Varuna is used in ethnoveterinary practice to treat renal lithiasis, swelling of the liver, and diarrhea.

Safety Profile

The leaves of Varuna are reported to cause reddening and possible blistering of the skin when applied topically. Decoctions of Varuna's root bark and stem bark appear to be well tolerated. The LD_{50} of a 50% ethanolic extract of stem bark was found to be >1000 mg/kg administered IP to adult rats.[19]

Dosage

Leaf paste: topical use
Decoction: 50 ml twice a day
Extract : 100 mg -200 mg two to three times per day

Ayurvedic Properties

Rasa: Tikta (bitter), kashaya (astringent)
Guna: Laghu (light), ruksha (dry)
Veerya: Ushna (hot)
Vipaka: Katu (pungent)
Dosha: Pacifies kapha and vata; promotes pitta

Notes

1. R. Anand, G.K., Patnaik, D.K.Kulshershta, and B.N. Dhawan, "24th Proceeding of Indian Pharmacol. Soc. Conference, Ahmedabad, Gujarat, India, 1994, A10.

2. K. Saleem, A. Kweon, and M. Afaq, "Lupeol, a fruit and vegetable based triterpene, induces apoptotic death of human pancreatic adenocarcinoma cells via inhibition of Ras signaling pathway," *Molecular Epidemiology and Cancer* :Oxford University Press. 2005).

3. C.H. Drury, In *The Useful Plants of India* (Dehradun: International Book Distributors, 1978), p. 353.

4. V.U Ahmed, K. Fizza, A.U.R. Amber AUR, and S.T. Arif7? "Cadabicine and cadabicine diacetate from *Crataeva nurvala* and *Cadabafarinosa*," *Journal of Natural Products*, 198R, 50(6):1186.

5. V. Sharma and M.A. Pandhya, "Screening of *Crataeva nurvala* for glucosinolate-glucocapparin," *Indian Drugs*, 1989, 26(10):572.

6. Y.S. Prabhakar and K.D. Suresh, "The varuna tree, *Crataeva nurvala*, a promising plant in the treatment of urinary stones—a review," *Fitoterapia*, 1990, 61(2):99.

7. S. Patankar, S. Dobhada, M. Bhansali, S. Khaaladkar, and J. Modi, "A prospective randomized controlled study to evaluate the efficacy and tolerability of Ayurvedic formulation 'Varuna and Banana stem' in the management of urinary stones," *Journal of Alternative Complementary Medicine*, Dec.. 2008 Dec;14(10):1287-90.

8. M.M. Malini, R. Bhaskar, and P. Varalakshm, "Effect of lupeol, a pentacyclic triterpene, on urinary enzymes in hyperoxaluric rats," *Japanese Journal of Medical Science and Biology*, 1995, 48(5–6):211.

9. P. Varalakshmi, Y. Shamila, and E. Latha, "Effect of *Crataeva nurvala* in experimental urolithiasis," *Journal of Ethnopharmacology*, 1990, 28(3):313.

10. See Note 9, Varalakshmi et al.

11. R. Bhaskar, N. Saravanan, and P. Varalakshmi, "Effect of *Crataeva nurvala* bark decoction on enzymatic changes in liver of normal and stone forming rats," *Indian Journal of Clinical Biochemistry*, 1995, 10(2):98.

12. P. Varalakshmi, E. Latha, Y. Shamila, and S. Jayanthi, "Effect of *Crataeva nurvala* on the biochemistry of the small intestinal tract of normal and stone forming rats," *Journal of Ethnopharmacology*, 1991, 31:67.

13. Geetha T, Varalakshmi P0 "Anti-inflammatory activity of lupeol and lupeol linoleate in rats," *J Ethnopharmacology*,.J Ethnopharmacol. 2001 Jun;76(1):77-80.

14. T. Geetha, P. Varalakshmi, and R.M. Latha, "Effects of triterpenes from *Crataeva nurvala* stembark on lipid peroxidation in adjuvant induced arthritis in rats," *Pharmacological Research*, 1998, 37(3):191.

15. See Note 2, Saleem et al.

16. P.T. Sudharsan, Y. Mythili, E. Selvakumar, and P. Varalakshmi, "Lupeol and its ester inhibit alteration of myocardial permeability in cyclophosphamide administered rats," *Mol Cell Biochem.*, Nov. 2006, 292(1–2):39–44.

17. A. Kumari and P. Kakkar, "Screening of anti-oxidant potential of selected barks of Indian medicinal plants by multiple in vitro assays," *Biomed Environ Sci.*, Feb. 2008, 21(1):24–29.

18. A Shirwaikar, M. Setty, and P. Bommu, "Effect of lupeol isolated from Crataeva nurvala Buch.-Ham. stem bark extract against free radical induced nephrotoxicity in rats," *Indian J Exp Biol.*, July 2004, 42(7):686–690.

19. D.S Bhakuni, M.L Dhar, M.M Dhar, B.N. Dhawan, B. Gupta, and R.C. Srimal, "Screening of Indian plants for biological activity," *Indian Journal of Experimental Biology*, 1971, 9:92.

Additonal Resources

R.G. Singh, D. Usha, and S. Kapoor, "Evaluation of antilithic properties of Varuna (*Crataeva nurvala*): An indigenous drug," *Journal of Research and Education in Indian Medicine*, 1991, 1092:35.

J. Buckingham (Ed.), In *Dictionary of Natural Products* (London: Chapman and Hall, 1994), p. 2570.

?Bharatiya Vidya Bhavan's Swami Prakashananda Ayurveda Research Centre. *Selected Medicinal Plants of Indi* (Mumbai: Chemexcil, 1992).

Indian Drug Manufacturers' Association. *Indian Herbal Pharmacopoeia, Vol 1*. Jammu: DMA/Regional Research Laboratory, 1998.

S.K Bhattacharjee, In *Handbook of Medicinal Plants* (Jaipur: Pointer Publishers, 1998), p. 228.

K.R. Kirtikar, B.D. Basu, Indian Medicinal Plants, Vol. I, Second ed., International Book Distributors, Dehradun, India, 1984, pp. 168-169

16

Curcuma Longa

Introduction

Curcuma longa, known in Sanskrit as Curcuma, is a perennial herb that is cultivated widely in tropical regions of India and Asia. Its rhizome is the source of the spice turmeric, which is used in cooking in many parts of the world, mainly as a principle seasoning and coloring in curried dishes. Curcumin, feruloyl methane, is the yellow pigment extracted from turmeric. Curcumin has become widely used as a food coloring and dietary additive. Extracts containing curcumin also have been used in medicine in India and Southeast Asia for generations, and according to tradition, they are useful in treating inflammation, skin wounds, hepatic and biliary disorders, cough, and coryza, as well as certain tumors.[1,2,3] Dietary intake of curcumin is especially high in these areas of Asia, where adults consume up to 200 mg of curcumin per day.[4]

The name "curcuma" is derived from the word "kurkum," the Arabic term for the plants of this genus. Among the several varieties of curcuma, Bengal turmeric is the best known. Because of its vivid yellow-orange pigment, turmeric often is used in dyeing fabrics. It is an important substance in the Hindu religion, a part of all religious occasions.

In Ayurvedic tradition, turmeric is a general tonic and blood purifier, an anti-inflammatory agent and analgesic in arthritis and rheumatism, and is used in treating the common cold. It has a particular role in diseases of the liver such as jaundice and as a cholagogue. It also has been used as an anodyne, antimalarial, antiepileptic, aperitif, carminative, diuretic, and vermifuge. Externally it can be applied to insect bites and wounds as an antiseptic.[5]

Synonymous Names

English: Turmeric
Hindi: Haldi
Sanskrit: Curcuma

Habitat

Curcuma is native to south Asia, especially India, but is cultivated in many other warm regions of the world as well. It is found in all states of India but particularly in Tamil Nadu, West Bengal, and Maharashtra.

Botanical Characteristics

Curcuma is a perennial, stemless herb that reaches up to 1.5 m in height. Its leaves are large, pale green, elongated, and tufted. The rhizome is short, branched, and bright yellow within. The pale yellow flowers blossom in dense, cylindrical inflorescences, from

10 to 15 cm long, which develop in the center of the leaves.

Chemical Composition

Phenylpropanoids:

Curcuma's main active principle, curcumin, is present in concentrations of 2% to 5% in the plant's rhizome. Curcumenone, curlone, bis-desmethoxycurcumin, bis-(para-hydroxycinnamoyl) methane, L-α-curcumene, cyclocurcumin, curcumenol, curdione, curzerenone, dehydroturmerone, dihydrocurcumin, eugenol, turmerin, turmerone, turmeronol, and others.[6,7]

Monoterpenes:

More than 20 components have been identified from Curcuma's leaf oil, of which the major monoterpenes are α-phellandrene, 1,8-cineole, p-cymene, and β-pinene. Others include α-terpinene, γ-terpinene and terpinolene.[8] Curcuma also contains the glycans Ukonans A, B, C and D,[9] as well as the sesquiterpenes zingiberene, bisabolol, germacrone, and sabinene. Additional chemical constituents include arabinose, ascorbic acid, ortho and p-coumaric acid, and phytosterols.[10,11]

Pharmacological Activity
Anti-inflammatory Activity

Curcumin, a component of Curcuma longa, conveys a variety of biological functions, including anti-inflammatory activity. In a cell culture system using the mouse macrophage cell line RAW264.7, monoacetylcurcumin, a synthetic analogue, strongly inhibited IkappaB phosphorylation, nuclear factor (NF)-kappaB activation, and tumor necrosis factor (TNF)-alpha production induced by lipopolysaccharide (LPS). In addition, oral administration of monoacetylcurcumin in mice led to greater suppression of TNF-alpha production after LPS stimulation than the administration of curcumin or tetrahydrocurcumin in-vivo. Monoacetylcurcumin also inhibited LPS-induced NF-kappaB activation in the liver. Collectively, monoacetylcurcumin is a potential chemopreventive agent for treating inflammatory responses more effectively than curcumin.[12]

In one study, several fractions of the herb's volatile oil acted as anti-inflammatory agents when tested against carrageenan-induced rat paw edema. The volatile oil at a dose of 1.6 ml/kg exhibited activity comparable to that of phenylbutazone.[13]

The same Curcuma activity was evaluated in human subjects in a clinical trial in which rheumatoid arthritis (RA) patients were given both curcumin and phenylbutazone. A significant improvement in symptoms was observed with the administration of curcumin, although phenylbutazone was found to be more potent overall, probably because it has analgesic action as well.[14]

In a postoperative inflammation model for evaluating anti-inflammatory activity, Curcuma was found to have greater activity than phenylbutazone or a placebo in a double-blind clinical trial.[15] The study was aimed at evaluating and comparing the effects of curcumin and the methylprednisolone sodium succinate (MPSS) functionally, biochemically, and pathologically after experimental spinal cord injury (SCI). Forty rats were randomly allocated into five groups: Group 1 was performed using only with laminectomy. Group 2 was introduced to 70-g closing force aneurysm clip injury. Group 3 was given 30 mg/kg MPSS intraperitoneally immediately after the trauma. Group 4 was given 200 mg/kg of curcumin immediately after the trauma. Group 5 was the vehicle, and immediately after the trauma, 1 mL of rice bran oil was injected. The animals were examined by inclined plane score and Basso-Beattie Bresnahan scale 24 hours after the trauma. At the end of the experiment, spinal cord tissue samples were harvested to analyze tissue concentrations of malondialdehyde (MDA) levels, glutathione peroxidase (GSH-Px), superoxide dismutase (SOD) activity, and catalase (CAT) activity and a pathological evaluation. The curcumin treatment improved the neurologic outcome, which was supported by a decreased level of tissue MDA and increased levels of tissue GSH-Px, SOD, and CAT activity.

Light microscopy results also showed preservation of tissue structure in the treatment group. This study indicated the neuroprotective effects of curcumin on an experimental model. By increasing tissue levels of GSH-Px, SOD, and CAT, curcumin seems to reduce the effects of injury to the spinal cord, which may be beneficial for neuronal survival.[16]

Most moderate-to-severe juvenile Crohn's disease patients are in a constant catabolic state resulting in poor weight gain and growth failure. Anti-inflammatory, immunomodulatory, and monoclonal antibody drugs, as well as growth hormone (GH), frequently fail to achieve sustained remission or to reverse growth failure. A test was conducted to see whether an exclusion diet with nutraceutical therapy could induce sustained clinical remission and weight gain, and if this would enhance the ability of GH to reverse growth failure.[17] The uncontrolled prospective case study was undertaken in six moderate-to- severe Crohn's disease patients, two of whom had completed growth. All were treated with nutraceuticals with adequate protein (>or= 3g/kg/d). Dairy products, certain grains, and carrageenan-containing foods were eliminated. Nutraceuticals, consisting of fish peptides, bovine colostrum, Boswellia serrata, curcumin, and a multivitamin were administered daily. Lactobacillus GG, a probiotic, was administered twice weekly. Recombinant human GH (rhGH) was administered daily. Within 2 months after starting this treatment, all six patients went into remission, with discontinuation of all pharmacological drugs.

Three patients have remained in sustained remission for 4 to 8 years; one patient with severe Crohn's had a recurrence of CD symptoms after being in complete remission for 18 months; one patient was in remission for 3 years but the symptoms recurred when she became less compliant to treatment; and one patient remained in remission after 6 months. With the addition of GH, the four growing patients had a good-to-excellent growth response. Treatment prolonged remission and restoration of normal weight in moderate-to severe juvenile Crohn's patients, providing conditions that enabled GH to stimulate growth. These findings justify larger controlled trials to evaluate the long-term benefits in Crohn's disease.

Sustained chronic inflammation in the prostate promotes prostate carcinogenesis. Because an elevated level of prostate-specific antigen (PSA) per se reflects the presence of inflammation in the prostate, intervention to improve the PSA value has potentially beneficial effects for preventing the development of prostate cancer. Isoflavones and curcumin have anti-inflammatory and anti-oxidant properties.[18] The biological effects of soy isoflavones and curcumin on LNCaP cells have been examined. Following that study, a clinical trial was conducted for men who received prostate biopsies but were not found to have prostate cancer, to evaluate the effects of soy isoflavones and curcumin on serum PSA levels. Expressions of androgen receptor and PSA were examined in LNCaP cells before and after treatment of isoflavones and/or curcumin. Eighty-five participants were randomized to take a supplement containing isoflavones and curcumin or placebo daily in the double-blind study. The subjects were subdivided by the cut-off of their baseline PSA value at 10 microg/ml. The values of PSA were evaluated before and 6 months after treatment. The production of PSA was decreased markedly by the combined treatment of isoflavones and curcumin in the prostate cancer cell line LNCaP. Expression of the androgen receptor also was suppressed by the treatment. In clinical trials, PSA levels decreased in the patient group with PSA > or = 10 treated with the supplement containing isoflavones and curcumin (P = 0.01). Curcumin presumably synergizes with isoflavones to suppress PSA production in prostate cells through the action of anti-androgen.

Ischemia-reperfusion of the rat pancreas induces acute pancreatitis with a systemic inflammatory response. Activated inflammatory cells are sequestered in the lung, to increase airway reactivity. A study characterized the effect of the anti-oxidant curcumin on airway hyper-reactivity induced by pancreatic ischemia-reperfusion. Ischemia of the pancreas was induced by clamping the gastroduodenal and the splenic artery for 2 hours followed by reperfusion for 6 hours. The pulmonary function test, were used to show the airway responses to a methacholine challenge. The blood concentration of oxygen radicals, nitric oxide, and tumor necrosis factor-alpha (TNF alpha) were measured after pancreatic ischemia-reperfusion. mRNA expressions of inducible nitric oxide synthase (iNOS) and TNFalpha in lung tissues were measured after pancreatic ischemia-reperfusion. Pre-treatment with curcumin (20 mg/ kg) was administered by intraperitoneal injection 2 hours before pancreatic ischemic-reperfusion (I/R). The protocol resulted in significant elevations of the blood concentrations of amylase, hydroxyl radical, nitric oxide, TNF alpha, and white cells among the I/R group. iNOS and TNFalpha mRNA expressions also increased significantly in lung tissues. Pulmonary function data showed that pancreatic I/R induced significant increases in responses to methacholine challenge.: Pre-treatment with curcumin significantly attenuated the inflammatory, oxidative, and nitrosative responses and lung tissue iNOS and TNF alpha expressions. Curcumin also attenuated airway reactivity to the methacholine challenge. I/R of the pancreas induced systemic inflammatory responses with respiratory burst, nitrosative stress, and hyperresponses in the airways. Curcumin, which has anti-oxidant and antiinflammatory effects, significantly attenuated the inflammatory responses and airway hyperreactivity induced by pancreatic I/R.[19]

The effectiveness of lung radiotherapy is limited by radiation tolerance of normal tissues and by the intrinsic radio sensitivity of lung cancer cells. The chemopreventive agent curcumin has known antioxidant and tumor cell radiosensitizing properties. An orthotopic model of lung cancer using intravenously injected Lewis lung carcinoma (LLC) cells was used. In-vitro, curcumin boosted anti-oxidant defenses by increasing heme oxygenase 1 (HO-1) levels in primary lung endothelial and fibroblast cells and blocked radiation-induced generation of reactive oxygen species (ROS). Dietary curcumin increased HO-1 in the lungs significantly as early as 1 week after feeding, coinciding with a steady-state level of curcumin in plasma. Although both 1% and 5% w/w dietary curcumin exerted physiological changes in lung tissues by significantly decreasing LPS-induced TNF-alpha production in lungs, only 5% dietary curcumin significantly improved the survival of mice after irradiation and decreased radiation-induced lung fibrosis. Importantly, dietary curcumin did not protect Lewis lung carcinoma metastases from radiation killing. Curcumin ameliorated radiation-induced pulmonary fibrosis and increases mouse survival while not impairing tumor cell killing by radiation.[20]

The bioflavonoids quercetin and curcumin has renal protective actions. To examine their effects on early graft function (EF), between September 2002 and August 2004, 43 dialysis dependent cadaveric kidney recipients were enrolled in a study using Oxy-Q, which contains 480 mg of curcumin and 20 mg of quercetin, started after surgery and taken for 1 month. They were randomized into three groups: control (placebo), low dose (one capsule) and high dose (two capsules). Delayed graft function (DGF) was defined as first week-dialysis need and slow function (SGF) as Cr >2.5 mg/dl by day 10. Category variables were compared by chi squared and continuous variables by Kruskal-Wallis. There were four withdrawals— one by patient choice and three for urine leak. The control group had 2 of 14 patients with DGF versus none in either treatment group. The incidence of EF was: control 43%, low-dose 71%, and high-dose 93% (P = 0.013). Serum creatinine was significantly lower at 2 days (control 7.6+/-2.1, low 5.4+/-0.6, high 3.96+/-.35 P = 0.0001) and 30 days (control 1.82+/-.16, low 1.65+/-.09, high 1.33 +/-.1, P=0.03). The incidence of acute rejection within 6 months was: control 14.3%, low-dose 14.3% and high-dose 0%. Tremor was detected in 13% of the high-dose patients versus 46% of the others. Urinary HO-1 was higher in the bioflavonoid groups. Bioflavonoid therapy improved early graft function. Acute rejection and neurotoxicity were lowest in the high-dose group. Curcumin and quercitin improve early outcomes in cadaveric renal transplantation, possibly through HO-1 induction.[22]

Anti-microbial Activity

Curcuma's essential oil has showed activity against Gram-negative bacteria and pathogenic fungi. The herb's alcoholic extract inhibited the growth of Gram-positive bacteria in several in vitro studies.[23]

Curcumin exerts its anti-inflammatory activity via inhibition of the nuclear factor kappaB. Oropharyngeal epithelia and residing bacteria closely interact in inflammation and infection. An in-vitro model investigated the effects of curcumin on bacterial survival, adherence to, and invasion of upper respiratory tract epithelia, and studied its antiinflammatory effect. It aimed to establish a model that could offer insights into the host–pathogen interaction in cancer therapy-induced mucositis.[24] Moraxella catarrhalis (Mcat) and the oropharyngeal epithelial cell line Detroit 562 were used. Time-kill curves assessed the inhibition of bacterial growth and adherence assays, and gentamicin protection assays determined the effect of curcumin-preincubated cells on bacterial adherence and invasion. Curcumin-mediated inhibition of pro-inflammatory activation by Mcat was determined via interleukin-8 concentrations in the supernatants. The synergistic role of secretory IgA (sIgA) on adherence was investigated. Curcumin was bactericidal at concentrations >50 microM. Preincubation of Detroit cells for 60 minutes demonstrated that concentrations >100 microM inhibited bacterial adherence. Together with sIgA, curcumin inhibited adherence at concentrations of >/=50 microM. Both 100 and 200 microM curcumin significantly inhibited Mcat cell invasion. Curcumin inhibited Mcat induced pro-inflammatory activation by strongly suppressing IL-8 release. At a concentration of 200 microM, 10 minutes of curcumin exposure inhibited IL-8 release significantly, and complete suppression required a pre-exposure time of >/=45 min. Curcumin, in clinically relevant concentrations for topical use, displayed strong anti-bacterial effect against a facultative upper respiratory tract pathogen by inhibiting bacterial growth, adherence, invasion, and pro-inflammatory activation of upper respiratory tract epithelial cells in-vitro.

Keeping these properties in mind, the antiinflammatory properties of curcumin were investigated in a mouse model of acute inflammation by introducing Klebsiella pneumoniae B5055 into BALB/c mice via the intranasal route.[25] Intranasal instillation of bacteria in this mouse model of acute pneumonia-induced inflammation resulted in a significant increase in neutrophil infiltration in the lungs along with increased production of various inflammatory mediators [i.e. malondialdehyde (MDA), myeloperoxidase (MPO), nitric oxide (NO), tumor necrosis factor (TNF)-alpha] in the lung tissue. The animals that received curcumin alone orally or in combination with augmentin, 15 days prior to bacterial instillation into the lungs via the intranasal route, showed a significant (P <0.05) decrease in neutrophil influx into the lungs and a significant ($P < 0.05$) decrease in the production of MDA, NO, MPO activity, and TNF-alpha levels. Augmentin treatment alone did not decrease the MDA, MPO, NO and TNF-alpha levels significantly ($P > 0.05$) compared to the control group. Curcumin can ameliorates lung inflammation induced by K. pneumoniae B5055 without significantly ($P < 0.05$) decreasing the bacterial load in the lung tissue, where as augmentin takes care of bacterial proliferation. Hence, curcumin can be used as an adjunct therapy along with antibiotics as an anti-inflammatory or an immunomodulatory agent in the case of acute lung infection.

Methicillin-resistant staphylococcus aureus (MRSA) has been emerging worldwide as one of the most significant hospital and community pathogens. Therefore, new agents are needed to treat MRSA associated infections. A study investigated the antimicrobial activity of ethyl acetate, methanol and water extracts of Curcuma longa against MRSA.[26] The ethyl acetate extract of C. longa demonstrated a higher anti-bacterial activity than the methanol extract or water extract. Because the ethyl acetate extract was more active than the other extracts, the study examined whether the ethyl acetate extract could restore the anti-bacterial activity of beta-lactams and alter the MRSA invasion of human mucosal fibroblasts (HMFs). In the checker board test, the ethyl acetate extract of C. longa markedly lowered the MICs of ampicillin and oxacillin against MRSA. In the bacterial invasion assay, MRSA intracellular invasion was decreased significantly in the presence of 0.125-2 mg/mL of Curcuma longa extract compared to the control group. These results suggest that the ethyl acetate extract of Curcuma longa may have anti-bacterial activity and the potential to restore the effectiveness of beta-lactams against MRSA, and inhibits the MRSA invasion of HMFs.

Anti-mutagenic Activity

Curcuma's extract and its isolated curcumin have been observed to have anti-mutagenic activity in a number of studies.[27] The isomer Curcumin III was shown to be active against dimethylbenzanthracene induced mutagenesis in Salmonella typhimurium TA 98.[28,29] Curcumin also showed a dose dependent inhibition of the in vitro mutagenicity of cayenne extract and capsaicin.[30,31]

Anti-Asthmatic Activity

Clinical studies have shown Curcuma's effectiveness in treating bronchial asthma.[32] Given at a dosage of 200 mg/kg for 7 days to rats, Curcuma's volatile oil exerted a protective effect on lung tissue.[32]

Anti-oxidant Activity

Extracts prepared from Curcuma's rhizome have demonstrated significant anti-oxidant properties. The plant's curcuminoid alkaloids are believed to be the source of this action.[33] Curcuma showed better anti-oxidant activity against air oxidation of linoleic acid than did dl-cc-tocopherol at the same concentration. A heat-stable protein isolated from Curcuma's aqueous extract also demonstrated significant anti-oxidant activity.[34]

In further research, three curcuminoids isolated from Curcuma—curcumin, demethoxy curcumin, and bis-desmethoxycurcumin—protected human and rat endothelial cells from oxidative stress from p-amyloid, as measured by a bromide reduction assay. Oxidative stress induced by p-amyloid is a well-established pathway of neuronal cell death in Alzheimer's disease.[35]

Hepatoprotective Activity

Curcumin extracted from Curcuma was tested for its hepatoprotective activity against CCl_4, aflatoxin Bl, paracetamol, iron, and cyclophosphamide induced liver damage in the livers of mice, rats, and ducklings.[36] Over a period of 10 days, curcumin prevented CCl_4-induced liver damage when given in combination with the herbs Phyllanthus niruri and Eclipta alba. Curcumin also reduced hepatic levels of lipids and serum bilirubin to near normal levels; however, increases in serum triglycerides, pre-β-lipoproteins, and cholesterol levels were noted with herbal treatment, as well as increased levels of glycogen.[37]

Chronic cholangiopathies have limited therapeutic options and represent an important indication for liver transplantation. Curcumin has pleiotropic actions and attenuates hepatic damage in animal models of chemically induced liver injury.

Potential anticholestatic, anti-inflammatory, and antifibrotic mechanisms of curcumin were explored in-vivo in Mdr2(-/-) mice as a murine model of chronic cholangiopathy, as well as in-vitro in a cholangiocyte cell line (HuCCT1) and portal myofibroblasts (MFBs) isolated from Mdr2(-/-) mice. Liver damage, cholestasis and fibrosis were reduced in Mdr2(-/-) mice after curcumin feeding.[38] Curcumin inhibited cholangiocyte proliferation and expression of activation marker vascular cell adhesion molecule-1 in Mdr2(-/-) mice. Curcumin- similar to PPARgamma synthetic agonist troglitazone directly inhibited TNF-alpha-induced inflammatory activation of cholangiocytes in-vitro, whereas these beneficial effects of curcumin were largely blocked by a PPAR-gamma synthetic antagonist. In addition, curcumin blocked proliferation and activation of portal MFBs by inhibiting ERK1/2 phosphorylation, thereby contributing to reduced fibrogenesis. These results show that curcumin may have multiple targets in liver, including activation of PPAR-gamma in cholangiocytes and inhibition of ERK1/2 signaling in MFBs, thus modulating several central cellular events in a mouse model of cholangiopathy. Targeting these pathways may be a promising therapeutic approach to cholangiopathies.

Anti-cancer Activity

Curcuma has been the subject of anti-cancer research. Several studies have investigated its impact on apoptosis, or programmed cell death. Various reports have suggested that the alkaloid curcumin inhibits apoptosis in human and rat T lymphocytes, whereas others have documented an induction of apoptosis in HL60 cancer cells, and in azoxymethane-induced colon tumors.

In one case report, life-threatening infantile hemangioendothelioma of the liver in a 6-month old infant was treated successfully with the dietary supplement curcumin, with a 6-year follow-up. Implications for pathogenesis based on sites of action of curcumin are considered.[40]

A phase 2 clinical trial was conducted at the M. D. Anderson cancer center. In the Phase II study of 25 patients, curcumin was given on its own without chemotherapy. The patients received 8 grams of curcumin by mouth every day for 2 months. Maintenance therapy was continued at the same dose and schedule until the disease progressed. Of the 25 patients, curcumin resulted in the following:

- Prolonged stable disease: Two patients temporarily experienced no significant tumor growth; one for 8 months and another for just over 2.5 years (an additional 12 months after the study was compiled for publication).

- Tumor regression: One patient experienced a decrease in tumor size of 73%, although the tumor grew back soon afterward. "Interestingly, at the time of progression, the lesions that had shrunk remained small, but other lesions grew larger," according to the study. "That suggests that a resistant clone of cancer cells emerged, which is a real problem in treating cancer," Kurzrock said.[41]

In addition, no side-effects were observed in the patients.

Curcumin activates diverse anti-cancer activities that lead to inhibition of cancer cell and tumor growth, induction of apoptosis, and antiangiogenic responses. This study observed that curcumin inhibits Panc28 and L3.6pL pancreatic cancer cell and tumor growth in nude mice bearing L3.6pL cells as xenografts.[42] In addition, curcumin decreased expression of p50 and p65 proteins and NF-kappaB dependent transactivation and also decreased Sp1, Sp3, and Sp4 transcription factors that were overexpressed in pancreatic cancer cells. Because both Sp-transcription factors and NF-kappaB regulate several common genes such as cyclin D1, survivin, and vascular endothelial growth factor that contribute to the cancer phenotype, interactions between Sp and NF-kappaB transcription factors also were investigated. Results of Sp1, Sp3, and Sp4 knock down by RNA interference demonstrate that both p50 and p65 are Sp-regulated genes and that inhibition of constitutive or tumor necrosis factor induced NF-kappaB by curcumin is dependent on downregulation of Sp1, Sp3, and Sp4 proteins by this compound. Curcumin also decreased mitochondrial membrane potential and induced reactive oxygen species in pancreatic cancer cells, and this pathway is required for downregulation of Sp proteins in these cells, demonstrating toxic effects to mitochondria of cancer cells, important for its anti-cancer activities.

In many of these investigations, curcumin has been given to study animals at high concentrations, exceeding the amounts that realistically could be consumed through diet alone. For this reason, further research has attempted to verify the chemopreventive effects of curcumin in amounts and under conditions that more closely resemble typical dietary consumption.

Despite the use of surgical resection and aggressive chemotherapy, nearly 50% of patients with colorectal carcinoma develop recurrent disease, highlighting the need for improved therapies.

Curcumin (diferuloylmethane) has shown to inhibit the growth of transformed cells and colon carcinogenesis at the initiation, promotion, and progression stages in carcinogen-induced rodent models. In a Phase I clinical trial, curcumin was given in combination with current chemotherapeutics such as 5-fluorouracil, oxaliplatin, and gemcitabine in treating gastrointestinal cancers, with particular reference to colorectal cancer. Curcumin in combination with chemotherapy is a superior strategy for treating gastrointestinal cancer.[43]

Curcumin (diferuloylmethane), which has no discernible toxicity, inhibits initiation, promotion, and progression of carcinogenesis. 5-Fluorouracil (5-FU) or 5-FU plus oxaliplatin (FOLFOX) remains the backbone of colorectal cancer chemotherapeutics but produces an incomplete response resulting in survival of cells (chemo-surviving cells) that may lead to the recurrence of cancer. A investigation was done to examine whether the addition of curcumin to FOLFOX is a superior therapeutic strategy for chemo-surviving cells.[44] A 48-hour treatment of colon cancer HCT-116 and HT-29 cells with FOLFOX resulted in 60%–to–70% survival, accompanied by a marked activation of insulin-like growth factor-1 receptor (IGF-1R) and a minor-to-moderate increase in epidermal growth factor receptor (EGFR), v-erb-b2 erythroblastic leukemia viral oncogene homolog 2 (HER-2), as well as v-akt murine thymoma viral oncogene homolog 1 (AKT), cyclooxygenase-2 (COX-2), and cyclinD1. Inclusion of curcumin to continued FOLFOX treatment for another 48 hours, however, greatly reduced the survival of these cells, accompanied by a concomitant reduction in activation of EGFR, HER-2, IGF-1R, and AKT, as well as expression of COX-2 and cyclin-D1. EGFR tyrosine kinase inhibitor gefitinib or attenuation of IGF-1R expression by the corresponding siRNA caused a 30%-to-60% growth inhibition of chemo-surviving HCT-116 cells. Curcumin alone, however, was found to be more effective than both gefitinib and IGF-1R si-RNA mediated growth inhibition of chemo-surviving HCT-116 cells. The data suggest that inclusion of curcumin in conventional chemotherapeutic regimens could be an effective strategy to prevent the emergence of chemoresistant colon cancer cells.

The value of a curcumin regimen in addition to conventional hormone refractory prostrate cancer treatment remains largely unknown. In combination with a taxane agent, curcumin may enhance cytotoxicity and retard prostrate cancer cell resistance to taxane.[45]

This study investigated the possible protective role of curcumin against renal damage caused by the administration of cyclosporine A (CsA) in adult male rats.[46] 27 adult male albino rats were divided into three equal groups. Group I (the control group) and Group II (the CsA-treated group) received a daily subcutaneous injection of CsA at a dose of 20 mg/kg b.w. Group III (the prophylactic group) received a daily dose of oral curcumin at 15 mg/kg b.w. simultaneously with CsA. After 21 days, all the animals were anaesthetized and the kidneys were rapidly removed and processed to prepare paraffin sections stained with H&E, PAS, and Masson's trichrome. In addition, the glutathione S-transferase (GST) enzyme was detected immunohistochemically. The optical density and the area (in %) of positive GST immunoreactions were measured in the cytoplasm of renal tubules and glomeruli and the data were analyzed statistically. Examination of sections from the CsA-treated group showed renal tubules with vacuolated cytoplasm, and others with darkly stained pyknotic nuclei. Apical brush borders of proximal tubules were undefined, and PAS-positive granules were noticed in their cytoplasm. The renal corpuscles contained shrunken glomeruli with widening of their Bowman's spaces. Inflammatory cellular infiltrate and an increase in the collagen fibers were observed between the renal tubules. In the prophylactic group, the structure of renal tubules and corpuscles was preserved except for a few tubular darkly stained pyknotic nuclei.

Numerous blood vessels, a few cellular infiltration, and thin collagen fibers were observed between the renal tubules. A statistical analysis of morphometric data showed a significant increase in the optical density of GST immunoreactivity in the cells of renal tubules and glomeruli of the CsA-treated group compared to the control or prophylactic groups. A significant decrease was observed in the area of GST immunoreactivity in sections from the prophylactic group compared to the control or CsA-treated groups. Curcumin protected cyclosporine-induced nephrotoxicity.

Neurological Activity

Overexpression and abnormal accumulation of aggregated alpha-synuclein (alphaS) have been linked to Parkinson's disease (PD) and other synucleinopathies. Although alphaS can misfold and adopt a variety of morphologies, studies implicate oligomeric forms as the most cytotoxic species. Genetic mutations and chronic exposure to neurotoxins both increase alphaS aggregation and intracellular reactive oxygen species (ROS), leading to mitochondrial dysfunction and oxidative damage in PD cell models. Curcumin can alleviate alphaS-induced toxicity, reduce ROS levels, and protect cells against apoptosis. It also shows that both intracellular overexpression of alphaS and extracellular addition of oligomeric alphaS increases ROS, which induces apoptosis, suggesting that aggregated alphaS may induce similar toxic effects whether generated intracellulary or extracellulary. Because curcumin can cross the blood-brain barrier it has potential therapeutic value for treating Parkinson's disease and other neurodegenerative disorders.[47]

Studies have shown that the c-Jun N-terminal kinase (JNK) signaling pathway is involved in dopaminergic neuronal degeneration, and direct blockade of JNK by specific inhibitors may prevent or effectively slow the progression of Parkinson's disease .

A study investigated whether curcumin protects against 1-methyl-4-phenyl-1,2,3,6-tetrahydropyridine- (MPTP) or 1-methyl-4-phenylpyridnium ion- (MPP(+)) induced dopaminergic neurotoxicity in C57BL/6N mice or SH-SY5Y cells by inhibiting JNK pathways both in-vivo and in-vitro. The curcumin treatment significantly improved behavioral deficits and enhanced the survival of tyrosine hydroxylase positive neurons in the substantia nigra (SN) in the MPTP-induced PD model mice. Curcumin treatment significantly inhibited MPTP/ MPP(+)-induced phosphorylation of JNK1/2 and c-Jun, and cleaved caspase-3. The study suggests that the neuroprotective effect of curcumin is not related simply to its anti-inflammatory and anti-oxidant properties but, rather, involves other mechanisms, particularly by targeting the JNK pathways.[48]

UCLA scientists and colleagues from U. C Riverside and the Human BioMolecular Research Institute have found that a form of vitamin D, together with curcumin, may stimulate the immune system to clear the brain of amyloid beta, which forms the plaques that are considered to be the hallmark of Alzheimer's disease. The early research findings, which appeared in the July 2009 issue of the *Journal of Alzheimer's Disease*, may lead to new approaches in preventing and treating Alzheimer's by utilizing the property of vitamin D3 both alone and together with natural or synthetic curcumin to boost the immune system in protecting the brain against amyloid beta.[49]

Anti-ulcer Activity

Curcuma's ethanolic extract was given to rats with ulceration induced by hypothermic restraint stress, pyloric ligation, indomethacin, and reserpine. The extract showed significant anti-ulcer action, thought to be a result of increasing gastric mucus and restoring non-protein sulfhydryl content in the stomach.[50]

Hypoglycemic Activity

A 50% ethanolic extract of Curcuma's rhizome lowered blood sugar levels.[51] In another study, when given together with Momordica charantia and Phyllanthus emblica (all in powder form), curcumin exhibited an even more pronounced anti-diabetic action.[52]

Immune Modulation and Immunostimulant Activity

Neutrophils (PMN) are the first cells recruited at the site of inflammation. They play a key role in the innate immune response by recognizing, ingesting, and eliminating pathogens and participate in the orientation of the adaptive immune responses in inflammatory bowel disease (IBD); however, transepithelial neutrophil migration leads to an impaired epithelial barrier function, perpetuation of inflammation, and tissue destruction via oxidative and proteolytic damage. Curcumin (diferulolylmethane) displays a protective role in mouse models of IBD and in human ulcerative colitis, a phenomenon consistently accompanied by reduced mucosal neutrophil infiltration.

The effect of curcumin on mouse and human neutrophil polarization and motility in-vitro and in-vivo was studied. Curcumin attenuated lipopolysaccharide (LPS)-stimulated expression and secretion of macrophage inflammatory protein (MIP)-2, interleukin (IL)-1beta, keratinocyte chemoattractant (KC), and MIP-1alpha in colonic epithelial cells (CECs) and in macrophages. Curcumin significantly inhibited PMN chemotaxis against MIP-2, KC, or against conditioned media from LPS-treated macrophages or CEC, as well as the IL-8-mediated chemotaxis of human neutrophils. Curcumin inhibited random neutrophil migration, suggesting a direct effect on neutrophil chemokinesis. Curcumin-mediated inhibition of PMN motility could be attributed to a downregulation of

PI3K activity, AKT phosphorylation, and F-actin polymerization at the leading edge.[53]

The inhibitory effect of curcumin on neutrophil motility was further demonstrated in-vivo in a model of aseptic peritonitis. The results indicate that curcumin interferes with colonic inflammation partly through inhibition of the chemokine expression and through direct inhibition of neutrophil chemotaxis and chemokinesis.[54]

Glycans isolated from a hot water extract of Curcuma exhibited reticuloendothelial system potentiating activity in a carbon clearance test.[55] Another immunostimulant polysaccharide, similar to bacterial lipopolysaccharide, has been isolated as well.[56]

To investigate the anti-angiogenic effect of topical curcumin on corneal neovascularization in a rabbit model one week after suturing, six eyes were treated with balanced salt solution (BSS) (Group A), and six eyes were treated with curcumin 40, 80, or 160 micromol/L (Groups B, C, and D, respectively), topically two times a day. After one week, light microscopy was used to analyze corneal neovascularization. The concentration of vascular endothelial growth factor (VEGF) mRNA in the corneal tissue was measured by reverse transcriptase-polymerase chain reaction (RT-PCR), and the activation of NF-kappaB was examined by immunofluorescent staining. Seven days after treatment, the sizes of the neovascularized areas were significantly reduced in Groups B (50.1% +/- 6.7%), C (43.2% +/- 8.1%), and D (29.5% +/- 7.8%) compared to Group A (69.5% +/- 1.5%) ($p < 0.05$). The corneal VEGF mRNA levels were significantly lower in Groups C and D than in Group A ($p < 0.05$). Immunofluorescent staining showed that phospho-NF-kappaB staining of the corneal tissue was weaker in Group C than it was in Groups A and B. Topical application of curcumin was useful in reducing experimental corneal neovascularization and can be used to inhibit angiogenesis in the cornea.[57]

Curcumin was administered orally to patients with chronic anterior uveitis (CAU) at a dose of 375 mg three times a day for 12 weeks. Of the 53 patients enrolled, 32 completed the 12-week study. They were divided into two groups: One group of 18 patients received curcumin alone, and the other group of 14 patients, who had a strong PPD (tuberculin) reaction, in addition received antitubercular treatment. The patients in both the groups started improving after 2 weeks of treatment. All of the patients who received curcumin alone improved, whereas the group receiving antitubercular therapy along with curcumin had a response rate of 86%. A follow-up of all the patients for the next 3 years indicated a recurrence rate of 55% in the first group and of 36% in the second group. Four of 18 (22%) patients in the first group and 3 of 14 patients (21%) in the second group lost their vision in the follow-up period because of various complications in the eyes (e.g. vitritis, macular edema, central venous block, cataract formation, glaucomatous optic nerve damage). None of the patients reported any side effects from curcumin. The efficacy of curcumin and recurrence following treatment are comparable to corticosteroid therapy, which presently is the only available standard treatment for this disease.[58]

A review studying effects of curcumin and autoimmune diseases concluded the following: The immune system has evolved to protect the host from microbial infection; nevertheless, a breakdown in the immune system often results in infection, cancer, and autoimmune diseases. Multiple sclerosis, rheumatoid arthritis, Type 1 diabetes, inflammatory bowel disease, myocarditis, thyroiditis, uveitis, systemic lupus erythromatosis, and myasthenia gravis are organ-specific autoimmune diseases that afflict more than 5% of the population worldwide. Although the etiology is not known and a cure is still wanting, the use of herbal and dietary supplements is on the rise in patients having autoimmune diseases, mainly because these treatments are effective, inexpensive, and relatively safe. Curcumin is a polyphenolic compound isolated from the rhizome of the plant Curcuma longa that traditionally has been used to treat pain and for wound-healing. Studies have shown that curcumin ameliorates multiple sclerosis, rheumatoid arthritis, psoriasis, and inflammatory bowel disease in human and animal models. Curcumin inhibits these autoimmune diseases by regulating inflammatory cytokines such as IL-1beta, IL-6, IL-12, TNF-alpha, and IFN-gamma and associated JAK-STAT, AP-1, and NF-kappaB signaling pathways in immune cells. Although the beneficial effects of nutraceuticals traditionally have been achieved through dietary consumption at low levels for long periods of time, the use of purified active compounds such as curcumin at higher doses for therapeutic purposes requires extreme caution. Precise understanding of effective doses and safe regimens and mechanisms of action is required for the use of curcumin in treating human autoimmune diseases.[59]

Hypocholesterolemic Activity

In a human clinical trial, an extract of Curcuma was given for a period of 12 weeks to patients with high cholesterol levels. The effect of the extract in lowering plasma cholesterol levels was almost equivalent to that of the drug clofibrate. Another study showed that Curcuma produced a reduction of cholesterol and triglycerides in nearly all of the cases. Patients in both of these studies also experienced an improvement in the symptoms of angina pectoris.[60]

Cardiac activity

To investigate the effects of curcumin on sarcoplasmic reticulum Ca^{2+}-ATPase in rabbits with heart failure, a rabbit heart failure model was developed with aortic regurgitation and abdominal aorta constriction, and 40 rabbits were divided randomly into four groups:

1. heart failure treated with curcumin;
2. heart failure treated with placebo;
3. healthy control treated with curcumin, and
4. healthy control treated with placebo.

All the rabbits were administrated with curcumin capsules or placebo capsules 100 mg x kg(-1) x d(-1), respectively. All of the groups were sacrificed after 8 weeks. The myocardial ultrastructural organization was detected by transmission electron microscope. RT-PCR and Western blot were used to measure the expression of sarcoplasmic reticulum Ca^{2+}-ATPase in mRNA and protein levels, respectively. A malachite green colorimetric assay was used to evaluate the activity of sarcoplasmic reticulum Ca^{2+}-ATPase. All of the detected parameters were similar between the control curcumin group and the control placebo group. Compared to the control groups (Groups 3 and 4), the heart-to-body weight ratio was increased significantly in the heart failure-curcumin group (Group 1) and the heart failure-placebo group (Group 2, all $P < 0.05$), but the ratio was significantly lower in heart failure curcumin group than in heart failure-placebo group ($P < 0.05$). The degree of heart failure was decreased by curcumin activity. Additionally, mRNA, and protein expression for sarcoplasmic reticulum Ca^{2+}-ATPase were significantly reduced in the heart failure-placebo group that could be significantly attenuated by curcumin (all $P < 0.05$). Curcumin could improve cardiac function via upregulating the expression of sarcoplasmic reticulum Ca^{2+}-ATPas in this model.[61]

Female Reproductive System Activity

Uterine leiomyomas are highly prevalent and symptomatic tumors of women in their reproductive years. The morbidity caused by these tumors is related directly to increasing size. Leiomyoma cells do not rapidly proliferate; instead, the tumors grow primarily because of excessive production of disorganized extracellular matrix (ECM). The aberrant ECM results from excessive production of collagen subtypes and proteoglycans increased profibrotic cytokines, including transforming growth factors beta1 and beta3, and decreased or disrupted matrix metalloproteinases. These alterations resulted in the development of an exceptionally stable ECM. As a result, therapeutic interventions must redirect leiomyoma cells toward extracellular matrix dissolution rather than solely inhibiting cell proliferation. Gonadotropin-releasing hormone analogues and selective progesterone receptor modulators with demonstrated clinical efficacy provide such a change in abnormal extracellular matrix formation by leiomyoma cells, inhibiting and reversing the fibrotic process. Novel therapies using pathways distinct from gonadal hormones, including antifibrotics, retinoic acid, peroxisome-proliferator-activated receptor gamma ligands, and curcumin, offer promise for a future with improved therapeutic options for women having uterine leiomyomas.[62]

Ethnoveterinary Usage

Curcuma has been used in ethnoveterinary usage for centuries to treat conditions such as abscesses, ulcers, ticks, castration wounds, bleeding, eye disorders, and fungal diseases. It also is used to treat diarrhea, rheumatism, and intestinal worms in poultry, and in ruminants for constipation, infection, and swollen teeth, sprains, coughs and colds, jaundice, and swinepox.

The rhizome of Curcuma also is used in veterinary practice to treat many digestive disorders, including E. coli bacillosis, glossitis, threadworm, and indigestion. Additional uses of the herb include treatment of irregular growth of teeth, holes in the hard palate, loss of appetite, and colic. It also has been used to relieve respiratory disorders, swelling of the throat, tonsillitis, asthma, pneumonia, and renal disorders such as polyuria.

Dr. Sodhi's Experience

Herbal treatment with Curcuma should be considered under the following conditions:

- Is inflammation present?
- Is cancer present?
- Is there liver or spleen congestion?
- Is there a need for an anti-oxidant?

Curcuma is one of Ayurveda's primary herbs for treating inflammation. This useful herb is believed to act by inhibiting many inflammatory pathways, including COX 1 and 2, by blocking leukotriences and antibody formation. Curcuma is the preferred herb for many inflammatory conditions, including osteoarthritis, rheumatoid arthritis, polymyalgia rheumatica, dermatitis, and other skin infections. It often is used successfully in combination with Azadirachta indica (Neem) to treat bacterial and fungal skin infections.

Because it stains skin and fabric, Curcuma often is prescribed for internal use, although it also is effective when applied topically for certain skin conditions. Like Emblica officinalis (amla), Withania somnifera (ashwagandha), and Bacopa monniera (indriya brahmi), Curcuma is a powerful anti-oxidant and is an effective adjunct to chemotherapy and radiation, for all types of cancer. The herb, too, relieves congestion of the liver and spleen.

Protocols

For inflammation and osteoporosis:

Curcuma at a dose of 500 mg is effective against inflammation and osteoporosis.

For dermatitis:

An external preparation made from 500 mg of Curcuma extract dissolved in 10 cc of DMSO, with 10 cc of water, may be applied directly to the skin to treat dermatitis. Curcuma also may be dissolved in ghee to make a paste that can be applied directly to the skin. Also useful is Azadirachta indica (Neem), 300 mg in a proprietary blend of Emblica officinalis (amalaki), Terminalia chebula (haritaki), Terminalia bellerica (bahera), Tinospora cordifolia (guduchi), and Rubia cordifolia (manjistha).

For eye conditions:

Uveitis: 500 mg Curcuma extract and given three times a day with coconut milk.

Viral conjunctivitis:

500 mg Curcuma extract dissolved in cold water may be combined with Santalum album (chandana), strained through cheesecloth and used as eye drops. This formulation is extremely cooling.

As an alternative, 500 mg Curcuma extract may be dissolved in one tablespoon of melted and filtered ghee, and applied as eye drops. The ghee should be appropriately cooled before placing it in the eyes.

For peptic ulcers:

500–1000 mg Curcuma extract, three times a day, provides relief for peptic ulcers.

For H. pylori:

Curcuma extract 500 mg three times per day.

A compound formulation of 600 mg Azadirachta indica (neem), Embelia ribes (vidang), Piper longum (Pippli), Aegle marmelos (bilva), Momordica charantia (karela), Berberis aristata (daaruhaldi), Holarrhena antidysenterica (kutaj), and Ocimum santum (tulsi) extracts an effective treatment for H. pylori. This protocol should be continued for at least two months

For constipation:

500 mg Curcuma extract three time a day helps to relieve constipation. If there is very little stool, or if stool is very dry, use Terminalia chebula (haritaki) 500 mg extract three times a day.

For burns, trauma, and surgical healing:

500–1000 mg Curcuma extract, three times a day, is an effective treatment for burns, trauma, and surgical healing. For external use, the following herbs should be combined with ghee along with Curcuma: Glycyrrhiza glabra (yastimadhu), and Centella asiatica (brahmi).

For ulcerative colitis and prostate cancer:

A retention enema composed of 1000 mg Curcuma extract, 500 mg Shatavari (for intestinal soothing), and 100 billion probiotic organisms dissolved in ghee should be given in cases of ulcerative colitis and prostate cancer. To administer the enema, a urethra catheter is placed on the syringe so it may be inserted deeply. Ghee may be used as a lubricant prior to insertion. The enema should be administered while the patient is lying on his or her back, and should be retained for 15–20 minutes.

To ensure proper absorption, Curcuma must be taken along with an appropriate transport medium such as an oil. If there is no evidence of kapha excess, such as mucus or congestion, coconut milk is a good vehicle. The herbal formulation Trikatu (Piper longum, Piper nigrum, and Zingiber officinalis) may be combined with this preparation. If evidence of excess kapha exists, fish oil or olive oil may be used. In addition, cayenne pepper, coconut curry, galangal, garlic, and basil all enhance absorption.

Safety Profile

Because it is widely used as a culinary spice, Curcuma is generally considered safe for oral use.[63] Large amounts, however, should not be given in cases of biliary obstruction, duodenal and gastric ulcers, and by pregnant women. Curcumin has been known to cause contact allergy; in one case, a positive patch test was observed at its most intense at 48 hours.[54]

Dosage

Infusion: 1–5 ml
Powder: 1–4 g
Curcumin: 250 mg to 500 mg, three times per day

Ayurvedic Properties

Rasa: Tikta (bitter), katu (pungent)
Guna: Laghu (light), ruksha (dry)
Veerya: Ushna (hot)
Vipaka: Katu (pungent)
Dosha: Balances tridosha

Notes

1. Ivan A. Ross, *Medicinal Herbs of the World, Vol. 1* (Totowa, New Jersey: Humana Press, 1999).
2. J.A Duke, *Handbook of Phytochemical Constituents of GRAS Herbs and Other Economic Plants* (Boca Raton, Louisiana: CRC Press, 1992).
3. S. Yano, M. Terai, K.I. Shimizu K.I., et al., Proceedings of the 2nd International Congress on Phytomedicine, Munich, Germany, Sept. 1996, pp. 11–14.
4. N. Mulky, A. J. Amonkar, and S.V. Bhide, "Antimutagenicity of curcumins and related compound: The structural requirement for the antimutagenicity of curcumins," *Indian Drugs*, 1987, 25(3):91.
5. See Note 1, Ross.
6. S. Toda, T. Miyase, H. Arichi, H. Tanizawa, and Y. Takino, "Natural anti-oxidants. III. Antioxidative components isolated from rhizome of Curcuma longa," *Chemical and Pharmaceutical Bulletin*, 1985, 33:1725.
7. See Note 3, Yano et al.
8. N.X. Dung, N.T.B. Tuyet, and P.A. Leclercq, "Constituents of the leaf oil of Curcuma domestica L. from Vietnam," *Journal of Essential Oil Research*, 1995, 7(6):701.
9. See Note 3, Yano et al.
10. See Note 3, Yano et al.
11. See Note 3, Yano et al.
12. M. Nishida, S. Nishiumi, Y. Mizushina, Y. Fujishima, K. Yamamoto, A. Masuda, S. Mizuno, T. Fujita, Y. Morita, H. Kutsumi, H. Yoshida, T. Azuma, and M. Yoshida M., "Monoacetylcurcumin strongly regulates inflammatory responses through inhibition of NF-kappaB activation," *Int J Mol Med.*, May 2010, 25(5):761–767.
13. H.P.T. Ammon and M.A. Wahl, "Pharmacology of Curcuma longa," *Planta Medica*, 1991, 57(1):1.
14. M.A., Lyengar, M.P. Rama Rao, S. Gurumadhva Rao, and M.S. Kamath, "Anti-inflammatory activity of volatile oil of Curcuma longa leaves," *Indian Drugs*, 1994, 31(11):S28.
15. R.C. Srimal and B.N. Dhawan, "Pharmacology of diferuloyl methane (curcumin), a non-steroidal anti-inflammatory agent," *Journal of Pharmacy and Pharmacology*, 1973, 25:447.

16. B. Cemil, K. Topuz, M.N. Demircan, G. Kurt, K. Tun, M. Kutlay, O. Ipcioglu, and Z. Kucukodaci, "Curcumin improves early functional results after experimental spinal cord injury," *Acta Neurochir (Wien)*, Sept. 2010, 152(9):1583–1590.

17. A.E. Slonim, M. Grovit, and L. Bulone, "Effect of exclusion diet with nutraceutical therapy in juvenile Crohn's disease," *J Am Coll Nutr,* June 2009, 28(3):277–285.

18. H. Ide, S. Tokiwa, K. Sakamaki, K. Nishio, S. Isotani, S. Muto, T. Hama, H. Masuda, and S. Horie. "Combined inhibitory effects of soy isoflavones and curcumin on the production of prostate-specific antigen," *Prostate*, July 1, 2010, 70(10):1127–1133.

19. K.H Chen, D. Chao, C.F. Liu, C.F. Chen, and D. Wang, "Curcumin attenuates airway hyperreactivity induced by ischemia-reperfusion of the pancreas in rats," *Transplant Proc.*, April 2010, 42(3):744–747.

20. ? Lee JC, Kinniry PA, Arguiri E, Serota M, Kanterakis S, Chatterjee S, Solomides CC, Javvadi P, Koumenis C, Cengel KA, Christofidou-Solomidou M. Dietary curcumin increases anti-oxidant defenses in lung, ameliorates radiation-induced pulmonary fibrosis, and improves survival in mice. Radiat Res. 2010 May;173(5):590-601.

21. D. Shoskes, C. Lapierre, M. Cruz-Correa, N. Muruve, F. Rosario, B. Fromkin, M. Braun, and J. Copley, "Beneficial effects of the bioflavonoids curcumin and quercetin on early function in cadaveric renal transplantation: a randomized placebo controlled trial," *Transplantation,* Dec 15, 2005, 80(11):1556–1559.

22. M.A. Lyengar, M. Rao, I. Rama, and M.S. Kamath, "Antimicrobial activity of the essential oil of Curcuma longa leaves," *Indian Drugs*, 1995, 32(6):249.

23. S. Lüer, R. Troller, M. Jetter, V. Spaniol, and C. Aebi, "Topical curcumin can inhibit deleterious effects of upper respiratory tract bacteria on human oropharyngeal cells in vitro: Potential role for patients with cancer therapy induced mucositis?" *Support Care Cancer*, 2011 Jun;19(6):799-80

24. S. Bansal and S. Chhibber S., "Curcumin alone and in combination with augmentin protects against pulmonary inflammation and acute lung injury generated during Klebsiella pneumoniae B5055-induced lung infection in BALB/c mice," *J Med Microbiol.,* April 2010, 59(Pt 4):429–437.

25. Kim KJ, Yu HH, Cha JD, Seo SJ, Choi NY, You YO. Anti-bacterial activity of Curcuma longa L. against methicillin-resistant Staphylococcus aureus. Phytother Res. 2005 Jul;19(7):599-604

26. See Note 13, Ammon & Wahl.

27. See Note 1, Ross.

28. See Note 13, Ammon & Wahl.

29. See Note 4, Miulky et al.

30. See Note 6, Toda et al.

31. N. Venkatesan and G. Chandrakasan, "Modulation of cyclophosphamide-induced early lung injury by curcumin, an anti-inflammatory anti-oxidant," *Molecular and Cellular Biochemistry*, 1995, 142:79.

32. See Note 1, Ross.

33. R. Selvam, L. Subramanian, R. Gayathri, and N. Angayarkanni, "The anti-oxidant activity of turmeric (Curcuma longa),"*Journal of Ethnopharmacology*,1995, 7(2):59.

34. A.S. Darvesh, R.T. Carroll, A. Bishayee, W. J. Geldenhuys, and C.J. Van der Schyf, "Oxidative stress and Alzheimer's disease: Dietary polyphenols as potential therapeutic agents," *Expert Rev Neurother.*, May 2010, 10(5):729–745.

35. R.C Srimal, "Turmeric: A brief review of medicinal properties," *Fitoterapia*, 1997, 68:483.

36. T. Chandra and J. Sadique, "A new recipe for liver injury," *Ancient Science of Life*, 1987, 7(2):99.

37. A. Baghdasaryan, T. Claudel, A. Kosters, J. Gumhold, D. Silbert, A. Thüringer, K. Leski, P. Fickert, S.J. Karpen, and M. Trauner, "Curcumin improves sclerosing cholangitis in Mdr2-/- mice by inhibition of cholangiocyte inflammatory response and portal myofibroblast proliferation," *Gut.*, April 2010, 59(4):521–530.

38. N. Venkatesan and G. Chandrakasan, "Modulation of cyclophosphamide-induced early lung injury by curcumin, an anti-inflammatory anti-oxidant," *Mol. Cell. Biochem.*, 1995, 142:79–87.

39. L.A. Hassell and le D. Roanh, "Potential response to curcumin in infantile hemangioendothelioma of the liver," *Pediatr Blood Cancer*, Aug. 2010, 55(2):377–379.

40. Dhillon N, Aggarwal BB, Newman RA, Wolff RA, Kunnumakkara AB, Abbruzzese JL, Ng CS, Badmaev V, Kurzrock R. Phase II trial of curcumin in patients with advanced pancreatic cancer. Clin Cancer Res. 2008 Jul 15;14(14):4491-9.

41. I, Jutooru, G. Chadalapaka, P. Lei, and S. Safe, "Inhibition of NFkappaB and pancreatic cancer cell and tumor growth by curcumin is dependent on specificity protein down-regulation," *J Biol Chem.*, Aug. 13, 2010, 285(33):25332–25344.

42. B.B. Patel and A.P. Majumdar, "Synergistic role of curcumin with current therapeutics in colorectal cancer: Mini review," *Nutr Cancer.*, Nov. 2009, 61(6):842–846.

43. B. B Patel, D. Gupta, A.A. Elliott, V. Sengupta, Y. Yu, and A.P. Majumdar, "Curcumin targets FOLFOX-surviving colon cancer cells via inhibition of EGFRs and IGF-1R," *Anticancer Res.*, Feb. 2010, 30(2):319–325.

44. A. Cabrespine-Faugeras, M. Bayet-Robert, J.O. Bay, P. Chollet, and C. Barthomeuf, "Possible benefits of curcumin regimen in combination with taxane chemotherapy for hormone-refractory prostate cancer treatment," *Nutr Cancer*, 2010, 62(2):148–153.

45. E.A. Abdel Fattah, H.E. Hashem, F.A. Ahmed, M.A. Ghallab, I. Varga, and W. Polak, "Prophylactic role of curcumin againset cyiclosporine-induced nephrotoxicity: Histological and immunohistological study," Gen Physiol Biophys, March 2010, 29(1):85–894.

46. M.S, Wang, S. Boddapati, S. Emadi, and M.R. Sierks, "Curcumin reduces alpha-synuclein induced cytotoxicity in Parkinson's disease cell model," *BMC Neurosci.*, April 30, 2010, 11:57.

47. S. Yu, W. Zheng, N. Xin, Z.H. Chi, N.Q. Wang,Y.lX. Nie, W.IY. Feng, and Z.YI. Wang, "Curcumin prevents dopaminergic neuronal death through inhibition of the c-Jun N-terminal kinase pathway," *Rejuvenation Res.*, Feb. 2010, 13(1):55–64.

48. Masoumi A, Goldenson B, Ghirmai S, Avagyan H, Zaghi J, Abel K, Zheng X, Espinosa-Jeffrey A, Mahanian M, Liu PT, Hewison M, Mizwickie M, Cashman J, Fiala M. 1alpha,25-dihydroxyvitamin D3 interacts with curcuminoids to stimulate amyloid-beta clearance by macrophages of Alzheimer's disease patients. J Alzheimers Dis. 2009;17(3):703-17

49. S. Rafatullah, M. Tariq, M.A. Al-Yahya, J.S. Mossa, and A.M. Ageel, "Evaluation of turmeric (Curcuma longa), for gastric and duodenal antiulcer activity in rats," *Journal of Ethnopharmacology*, 1990, 29(1):25.

50. R.Tank, N. Sharma N, Sharma I, Dixit VP 1990 Antidiabetic activity of Curcuma longa in alloxan induced diabetic rats. Indian Drugs 27(11):587

51. J. Sankaranarayanan and C.I. Jolly, "Phytochemical, anti-bacterial and pharmacological investigations on Momordica charantia Linn., Emblka offitinalis and Curcuma longa Linn.," *Indian Journal of Pharmaceutical Sciences*, 1993, 55(1):6.

52. Larmonier CB, Midura-Kiela MT, Ramalingam R, Laubitz D, Janikashvili N, Larmonier N, Ghishan FK, Kiela PR. Modulation of neutrophil motility by curcumin: Implications for inflammatory bowel disease. Inflamm Bowel Dis. 2010 Jul 13

53. Provide note

54. M. Tomoda, R. Gonda, N. Shimizu, M. Kimura, and M. Kanari, "A reticuloendothelial system activating glycan from the rhizomes of Curcuma longa," *Phytochemistry*, 1990, 29(4):1083.

55. H. Inagawa, T. Nishizawa, D. Tsukioka, et al., "Homeostasis as regulated by activated macrophage," *Chemical and Pharmaceutical Bulletin*, 1992, 40:994.

56. J.S. Kim, J.S. Choi, and S.K. Chung, "The effect of curcumin on corneal neovascularization in rabbit eyes," *Curr Eye Res.*, April 2010, 35(4)274–280.

57. B. Lal, A.K. Kapoor, O.P. Asthana, P.K. Agrawal, R. Prasad, P. Kumar, and R.C. Srimal, "Efficacy of curcumin in the management of chronic anterior uveitis," *Phytother Res.*, June 13, 1999, 3(4):218–322.

58. J.J. Bright, "Curcumin and autoimmune disease," *Adv Exp Med Biol.*, 2007, 595:425–451.

59. See Note 3, Srimal.

60. Y. Zhang, G.S. Lin, M.W. Bao, Y.Y. Wu, C. Wang, and B. Yang, "Effects of curcumin on sarcoplasmic reticulum Ca2+ATPase in rabbits with heart failure," Zhonghua Xin Xue Guan Bing Za Zhi????, April, 2010, 38(4):369–373.that's the name Please see this http://www.ncbi.nlm.nih.gov/pubmed/20654087

61. M. Malik, J. Norian, D. McCarthy-Keith, J. Britten, and W.H. Catherino, "Why leiomyomas are called fibroids: The central role of extracellular matrix in symptomatic women," *Semin Reprod Med.*, May 2010m, 28(3):169–179

62. A.V. Krishnaraju, D. Sundararaju, K. Senugupta, S. Venkateswarulu, and G. Trimurtulu , "Safety and toxicological evaluation of demethylated curcumonoids: A novel standardized curcumin product," *Toxicology Mechanisms and Methods*, Sept. 2009, 19(6–7):447–460.

63. C.L. Goh and S.K. Ng, "Allergic contact dermatitis to Curcuma longa (turmeric)," *Contact Dermatitis*, 1987, 17(3):186

ADDITIONAL RESOURCES

L.D. Kapoor, *Handbook of Ayurvedic Medicinal Plants*. Boca Raton, Louisiana, CRC Press, 1990.

Ministry of Health and Family Welfare. *The Indian Pharmacopoeia*. New Delhi, Government of India, 1966.

Ministry of Health and Family Welfare, *Ayurvedic Pharmacopoeia of India*. New Delhi, Government of India, 1989

A.K. Nadkarni, Indian Materia Medica. Bombay: Popular Prakashan PVT Ltd, 1976.

D.S. Kirn, S.Y Park, and J.K. Kirn, "Curcuminoids from Curcuma longa L. (Zingiberaceae) that protect PCI 2 rat pheochromocytoma and normal human umbilical vein endothelial cells from beta-amyloid (l->42) insult," *Neuroscience Letters*, 2001, 303(1):57.

R. Gonda, M. Tomoda, N. Shimizu, and M. Kanari, "Characterization of polysaccharides having activity on the reticuloendothelial system from the rhizome of Curcuma longa," *Chemical and Pharmaceutical Bulletin*, 1990, 38(2):482.

J. P. Jain, S.M.A. Naqvi, and K.D. Sharma, "A clinical trial of volatile oil of Curcuma longa Linn. (Curcuma) in cases of bronchial asthma (Tamaka Swasa)," *Journal of Research in Ayurveda and Siddha*, 1990, vol(number):pp. 11, 1(4), pg. 20--30

D.A. Liebermann, B. Gregory, and B. Hoffman, "AP-1 transcription factors in hematopoietic differentiation and apoptosis," *Int. J. Oncol.*, June 1998, 12:685–700.

O. S. Frankfurt and A. Krishan, "Identification of apoptotic cells by formamide-induced DNA denaturation in condensed chromatin,"*J. Histochem. Cytochem.*, 2001, 49:369–378.

C. B. Hendricks, E. K., Rowinsky, L. B., Grochow, R. C. Donehower, and S. H. Kaufmann, "Effect of P-glycoprotein expression on the accumulation and cytotoxicity of topotecan (SK&F 104864), a new camptothecin analogue," *Cancer Res.*, 1992, 52: 2268–2278.

W. Hiraoka, N. Vazquez, W. Nieves-Neira, S.J. Chanock, and Y. Pommier, "Role of oxygen radicals generated by NADPH oxidase in apoptosis induced in human leukemia cells," *J. Clin. Investig.*, 1998, 102:1961–1968.

S. Kharbanda, E. Rubin, H. Gunji, H. Hinz, B. Giovanella, P. Pantazis, and D. Kufe, "Camptothecin and its derivatives induce expression of the c-jun proto-oncogene in human myeloid leukemia cells," *Cancer Res.*, 1991, 51:6636–6642.

M. Sulkowska, S. Sulkowski, E. Skrzydlewska, and R. Farbiszewski, "Cyclophos-phamide-induced generation of reactive oxygen species. Comparison with morpho-logical changes in type II alveolar epithelial cells and lung capillaries," *Exp. Toxicol. Pathol.*, 1998, 50:209–220.

K Ikeda, K. Kajiwara, E. Tanabe, S. Tokumaru, E. Kishida, Y. Masuzawa, and S. Kojo, "Involvement of hydrogen peroxide and hydroxyl radical in chemically induced apoptosis of HL-60 cells," *Biochem. Pharmacol.*, 1999, 57:1361–1365.

C. Friesen, S. Fulda, and K.M. Debatin, "Induction of CD95 ligand and apoptosis by doxorubicin is modulated by the redox state in chemosensitive- and drug-resistant tumor cells," *Cell Death Differ.*, 1999, 6:471–480.

J. Dosch and B. Kaina, "Induction of c-fos, c-jun, junB, and junD mRNA and AP-1 by alkylating mutagens in cells deficient and proficient for the DNA repair protein O6-methylguanine-DNA methyltransferase and its relationship to cell death, mutation induction, and chromosomal instability, *Oncogene*, 1996, 13:1927–1935.

M. T. Osborn and T. C. Chambers, "Role of the stress-activated/c-Jun NH2-terminal protein kinase pathway in the cellular response to adriamycin and other chemotherapeutic drugs," *J. Biol. Chem.*, 1996, 271:30950–30955.

L. B. Grochow, "Covalent DNA-binding drugs," in M. C. Perry (Ed.), *The Chemotherapy Source Book, 2nd ed.* (Baltimore: Williams and Wilkins, 1997), pp. 293–316.

E. M. Creagh and T. G. Cotter, "Selective protection by hsp 70 against cytotoxic drug-, but not Fas-induced T-cell apoptosis," *Immunology*, 1999, 97:36–44,

Y. Y. Lo, J. M Wong, and T. F Cruz, "Reactive oxygen species mediate cytokine activation of c-Jun NH2-terminal kinases," *J. Biol. Chem.*, 1996, 271:15703–15707.

C. Tournier, G. Thomas, J. Pierre, C. Jacquemin, M. Pierre, and B. Saunier, "Mediation by arachidonic acid metabolites of the H2O2-induced stimulation of mitogen-activated protein kinases (extracellular signal-regulated kinase and c-Jun NH2-terminal kinase," *Eur. J. Biochem.*, 1997, 244:587–595,

J. T. Hancock, R. Desikan, and S. J. Neill, "Does the redox status of cytochrome C act as a fail-safe mechanism in the regulation of programmed cell death?" *Free Radic. Biol. Med.*, 2001, 31:697–703.

C. Tournier, P. Hess, D. D., Yang, J. Xu, T.K. Turner, A. Nimnual, D. Bar-Sagi, S. N. Jones, R. A. Flavell, and R. J. Davis, "Requirement of JNK for stress-induced activation of the cytochrome c-mediated death pathway," *Science*, (),2000, 288:870–874.

X. Wang, "The expanding role of mitochondria in apoptosis," *Genes Dev.*, 2001, 15:2922–2933.

H. S. Samaha, G.J. Kelloff, V. Steele, C.V. Rao, and B.S. Reddy, "Modulation of apoptosis by sulindac, curcumin, phenylethyl-3-methylcaffeate, and 6-phenylhexyl isothiocyanate: apoptotic index as a biomarker in colon cancer chemoprevention and promotion," *Cancer Res.*, 1997, 57:1301–1305.

M. C Jiang, H. F. Yang-Yen, J. J. Yen, and J.K. Lin, "Curcumin induces apoptosis in immortalized NIH 3T3 and malignant cancer cell lines," *Nutr. Cancer*, 1996, 26:111–120.

E. Jaruga, A. Bielak-Zmijewska, E. Sikora, J. Skierski, E. Radziszewska, K. Piwocka, and G. Bartosz, "Glutathione-independent mechanism of apoptosis inhibition by curcumin in rat thymocytes," *Biochem. Pharmacol.*, 1998, 56:961–965.

W. D. Jarvis, C. R. Johnson, F. A. Fornari, J. S., Park, P. Dent, and S. Grant, "Evidence that the apoptotic actions of etoposide are independent of c-Jun/activating protein-1-mediated transregulation," *J. Pharmacol. Exp. Ther.*, 1999, 290:1384–1392.

R. Clarke, F. Leonessa, N. Brunner, and E. W Thompson," "In vitro models of breast cancer," in J. R. Harris, M. E. Lippman, M. Morrow, and S. Hellman (Eds.), *Diseases of the Breast*, (Philadelphia: Lippincott-Raven Publishers, 1996), pp. 245–261.

S. Bhaumik, R. Anjum, N. Rangaraj, B.V. Pardhasaradhi, and A. Khar, "Curcumin mediated apoptosis in AK-5 tumor cells involves the production of reactive oxygen intermediates, " *FEBS Lett.*, 1999, 456:311–314.

Y. Huang, K.R. Johnson, J.S. Norris, and W. Fan, "Nuclear factor-B/IB signaling pathway may contribute to the mediation of paclitaxel-induced apoptosis in solid tumor cells," *Cancer Res.*, 2000, 60:4426–4432.

C. Ireson, S. Orr, D. J. Jones, R. Verschoyle, C.K. Lim, J. L. Luo, L. Howells, S. Plummer, R. Jukes, M. Williams, W.P. Steward, and A. Gescher, "Characterization of metabolites of the chemopreventive agent curcumin in human and rat hepatocytes and in the rat in vivo, and evaluation of their ability to inhibit phorbol ester-induced prostaglandin E2 production," *Cancer Res.*, 2001, 61:1058–1064.

J.C. Lee, P.A. Kinniry, E. Arguiri, M. Serota, S. Kanterakis, S. Chatterjee, C.C. Solomides, P. Javvadi, C. Koumenis, K.A. Cengel, and M. Christofidou-Solomidou, "Dietary curcumin increases anti-oxidant defenses in lung, ameliorates radiation-induced pulmonary fibrosis, and improves survival in mice," *Radiat Res.*, May 2010, 173(5):590-601.

M.L Dhar, M.M, Dhar, B.N. Dhawan, B.N. Mehrotral, and C. Ray C, "Screening of Indian plants for biological activity: Part I," *Indian Journal of Experimental Biology*, 1968, 6:232.

K. J Kim, H. H Yu, J.D. Cha, S.J. Seo, N.Y. Choi, and Y.O. You, "Anti-bacterial activity of Curcuma longa L. against methicillin-resistant Staphylococcus aureus, " *Phytother Res.*, July 2005, 19(7):599–604.

17

Cyperus rotundus

Introduction

Cyperus rotundus, or purple nutsedge, is a fast-growing plant considered mainly as a weed in many parts of the world but valued for its medicinal uses in others. In Ayurvedic tradition, the plant's tuberous roots and rhizomes are used to treat abdominal disorders, particularly peptic ulcers, diarrhea, and dyspepsia. Cyperus rotundas also is credited with antipyretic, carminative, demulcent, analgesic, emmenagogue, stomachic, diuretic properties, and finds uses in treating amenorrhea, dysmenorrhea, nasal congestion, impotence, and hypertension.

Known in Ayurvedic tradition as mustak, Cyperus rotundus is a perennial sedge grass that grows from a system of underground tubers. These tubers contain an essential oil that is diaphoretic and astringent. An ethanolic extract of the rhizome of Cyperus rotundus has been observed to have tranquilizing, hypotensive, and muscle-relaxant properties.

Topical preparations made from Cyperus are used to treat skin conditions, including scorpion bites, inflammation, wounds, sores, and edema. The plant is known to have anthelmintic, anti-bacterial, and fungicidal activities. Dried Cyperus tubers are used in perfumery and to make fragrant sticks called "agarbatties."

Synonymous Names

English: Nutgrass, sedge weed, nutsedge, chido
Hindi: Motha
Sanskrit: Mustak

Habitat

Mustak is a highly invasive weed found in most soils in sunny areas. It grows easily in sandy and loamy soils and is even found in tropical rainforests. It is found throughout most regions of the world, particularly in the Pacific Islands and India.

Botanical Characteristics

Mustak is notoriously fast-growing, filling the soil with its tangle of roots and rhizomes. The rhizomes are slender, scaly, and bulbous at the base, growing singly from tubers that are black outside and reddish inside, and have a characteristic odor. Aerial parts of the plant grow up to 25 cm tall as a sedge grass. The narrow, dark-green leaves are grooved on the upper surfaces. The reddish-purple flowers appear as small spikelets, growing in clusters at the ends of the plant's solitary stems. The plant's triangular nut is yellow when young and turns black as it ripens.

Chemical Composition

Steam distillation of mustak tubers and rhizomes has yielded an essential oil consisting mainly of sesquiterpene hydrocarbons, epoxides, and ketones, along with monoterpene and aliphatic alcohols.[1] These alcohols have been identified as isocyperol, cyperone rotundines A-C, cyperene, cyperol, cyperlolonecyperotundone, rotundene, (β-selinene, patchoulenone, isopatchoula-3,5-diene, caryophyllene-6,7 oxide, caryophyllene-α-oxide, caryophylla-6-one, caryophyllene and 10,12-peroxycalamenene, 4,7-dimethyl-1-tetralone. The essential oil also contains the monoterpenes cineole, limonene, and camphene. The triterpenes β-Sitosterol and oleanolic acid also have been isolated from mustak.[1]

Pharmacological Activity

Anti-diabetic activity

Animal investigations have verified traditional claims of mustak in the treatment of diabetes. In one such experiment, alloxan-induced diabetic rats were given mustak extracts at a dosage of 500 mg/kg over a period of 7 days. Results of this research showed a significant reduction in blood glucose levels in the study animals.[3]

Anti-inflammatory activity

Various extracts of mustak exerted significant anti-inflammatory activity against carageenan-induced edema in albino rats. The anti-inflammatory properties of the petroleum ether, chloroform, and methanolic extracts of mustak were all found to exceed that of hydrocortisone.[4]

Anti-pyretic activity

An alcoholic extract of mustak tubers demonstrated potency comparable to sodium salicylate in suppressing yeast-induced pyrexia. Researchers believe this activity to be the result of the anti-inflammatory properties of the compound. Mustak's anti-pyretic capacity appears to be independent of the pituitary adrenal system.[5]

Anti-emetic activity

The ethanolic extract of Mustak's rhizome demonstrated anti-emetic activity in dogs. The extract was shown to antagonize apomorphine-induced vomiting.[6]

Anti-malarial activity

Endoperoxide sesquiterpene, isolated from mustak tubers, was shown in laboratory research to have anti-malarial properties.[7]

Anti-obesity activity

A clinical study was conducted to assess the capacity of mustak to aid in weight control. Thirty obese subjects were given a powdered supplement prepared from mustak tubers over a period of 90 days. All of the study subjects experienced weight loss. Decreases in serum cholesterol and triglycerides were observed as well.[8] Results of animal studies on mustak's anti-obesity activity have affirmed these claims. When obese Zucker rats were given an extract made from mustak's tubers at two different dosages over a period of 60 days, a significant reduction in weight gain was observed. This effect was independent of food consumption and did not induce toxicity.[9] The extract was able to stimulate lipolysis, suggesting that mustak activates beta-adrenoreceptors.

Anti-oxidant activity

The anti-oxidant activity of mustak's hydroalcoholic extract was evaluated using various experimental models, including the phosphomolybdenum method, total anti-oxidant activity in linoleic acid emulsion systems, 1,1-diphenyl-2-picrylhydrazyl, superoxide, hydroxyl radicals, and nitric oxide scavenging. In addition, the reducing potential of mustak extract, as well as Fe(2+)-ascorbate-induced lipid peroxidation, was studied in rat liver homogenate. These anti-oxidant activities were compared to standard anti-oxidants such as butylated hydroxytoluene, tocopherol, L-ascorbic acid, and catechin. Total phenolic and flavonoid content of CRE also was determined by a colorimetric method. The extract exhibited high reduction capability and powerful free radical scavenging, especially against DPPH and superoxide anions, and with a moderate effect on nitric oxide. The extract also inhibited lipid peroxidation in rat liver homogenate induced by Fe(2+)/ascorbate, and prevented deoxyribose degradation in both non-site-specific and site-specific assays. This indicates that the extract stimulated hydroxyl radical scavenging and metal chelating activity. These results support the anti-oxidative potency of mustak, which may account for many of the medical claims attributed to this plant.[10]

Anti-cancer activity

Apoptosis, or programmed cell death, a highly organized physiological response mechanism to eliminate injured or abnormal cells, is implicated in multistage carcinogenesis. Mustak extracts have been observed to suppress the growth and proliferation of cancerous cells derived from murine lymphoblastic leukemia. The morphological features of treated cells and their characteristic DNA fragmentation revealed that the cytotoxicity exerted by mustak extract was a result of the induction of apoptosis.[11]

Cytoprotective activity

A decoction of mustak rhizome was evaluated to determine whether it may be effective against ethanol-induced gastric damage. The extract exhibited anti-ulcer activity in a dose-dependent manner. This protective action appears to be the result of inhibition of gastric motility and endogenous prostaglandins.[12]

Anti-bacterial activity

Anti-bacterial activity of different extracts was evaluated against five bacterial reference strains. A marked inhibitory effect was observed against Salmonella enteritidis, Staphylococcus aureus, and Enterococcus faecalis with total oligomers of flavonoids and ethyl acetate extracts of mustak.[13]

In further studies, mustak's essential oil totally inhibited the growth of Staphylococcus aureus. Of the fractions, cyperone was completely inert and the hydrocarbon fractions cyperene I and II were more potent than the oil and cyperol.[14] Other forms of the extract were found to be active against various bacterial strains.[14]

Neurological activity

Ethanol extract of Cyperus rotundus (EECR) was tested for possible pharmacological effects on experimental animals. Extract of Cyperous significantly potentiated the sleeping time of mice induced by standard hypnotics, viz. phenobarbitone sodium, diazepam, and meprobamate, in a dose-dependent manner. Extract of Cyperus showed significant analgesic properties, as evidenced by the significant reduction in number of writhes and stretches induced in mice by 1.2% acetic acid solution. It also potentiated analgesia induced by morphine and pethidine in mice. Pre-treatment with extract of Cyperus caused significant protection against strychnine and leptazol-induced convulsions. The behavioral studies on mice indicate CNS-depressant activity of the ethanol extract of C. rotundus.[15]

Cyperus rotundus, is a well-known functional food and traditional herbal medicine in Korea. It has been reported to have anti-oxidant and free radical scavenging activities playing a major role in protection of neurodegenerative disorders such as Parkinson's disease. In a study, the neuroprotective effects of a water extract of Cyperus rotundus against 6-hydroxydopamine (6-OHDA)-induced neuronal damage were evaluated in an experimental model of Parkinson's disease. In PC12 cells, Cyperus extract showed a significant protective effect on cell viability at 50 and 100 microg/mL. Cyperus extract inhibited generation of reactive oxygen species and nitric oxide, reduction of mitochondrial membrane potential, and caspase-3 activity, which were induced by 6-OHDA. Cyperus extract also showed a significant protective effect against damage to dopaminergic neurons in a primary mesencephalic culture.[16]

Anti-diarrheal activity

Various alcohol extracts of mustak's rhizome, given orally at doses of 250 and 500 mg/kg, showed significant anti-diarrheal activity in castor oil-induced diarrhea in mice. Among the fractions, the petroleum ether fraction and residual methanol fraction were found to provide the best diarrhea control, the latter being more active than the control. The ethyl acetate fraction did not show any anti-diarrheal activity.[17]

Ethnoveterinary Usage

Mustak tubers are used in traditional veterinary practice to treat wounds, tuberculosis, pneumonia, scabies, and pox, and to help heal cracked tail.[18]

Dosage

Powder: 1–3 g
Decoction: 56–112 ml

Ayurvedic Properties

Rasa: Tikta (bitter), kashaya (astringent)
Guna: Laghu (light), ruksha (dry)
Veerya: Shita (cold)
Vipaka: Katu (pungent)
Dosha: Pacifies kapha and pitta

Notes

1. V.H. Kapadia, V.G. Naik, M. S Wadia, and S. Sukhdev, "fSesquiterpenes from essential oils from Cyperus rotundus," *Tetrahedron*, 19671. 4661–4667 [**I added a hyphen between 4661. Verify or reinstate.**] **there are no issure it only goes with page numbers**

2. S.J. Jeong, T. Miyamoto, M. Inagaki, Y.C, Kirn, and R. Higuchi, "Rotundines A-C, three novel sesquiterpene alkaloids from Cyperus rotundus," *Journal of Natural Products*, 2000, 63(5): 673.

3. N.A Raut and N.J. Gaikwad, "Antidiabetic activity of hydro-ethanolic extract of Cyperus rotundus in alloxan induced diabetes in rats," *Fitoterapia,* Dec. 2006, 77(7–8):585–588.

4. M.B. Gupta, T.K. Palit, N. Singh, K.P. Bhargava. Pharmacological studies to isolate the active constituents from Cyperus rotundus possessing anti-inflammatory, anti-pyretic and analgesic activities Indian Journal of Medical Research, 59 (1971), pp. 76–8

5. M. B Gupta, R. Nath, N. Srivastava, K. Shanker, K. Kishor, and K.P. Bhargava, "Anti-inflammatory and antipyretic activities of (5-sitosterol)" *Planta Medica*, 1980, 39:157.

6. N. Singh, V.K. Kulshreshtha, M.B. Gupta, and K.P. Bhargava, "A pharmacological study of Cyperus rotundus," *Indian Journal of Medical Research*, 1970, 58(1):103.

7. C. Thebtaranonth, Y. Thebtaranonth, S. Wanauppathamkul, and Y. Yuthavong, "Antimalarial sesquiterpenes from tubers of Cyperus rotundus: structure of 10,12-peroxycalamenene, a sesquiterpene endoperoxide," *Phytochemistry*, 1995, 40(1):125.

8. C. R. Karnick, "Clinical evaluation of Cyperus rotundus Linn (Motha) on obesity: A randomised double blind placebo controlled trial on Indian patients," *Indian Medicine*, 1992, 4(2):7.

9. B. Lemaure, A. Touché, I. Zbinden, J. Moulin, D. Courtois, K. Macé, and C. Darimont, "Administration of Cyperus rotundus tubers extract prevents weight gain in obese Zucker rats," *Phytother Res.*, Aug. 2007, 21(8):724–730.

10. R.Yazdanparast and A. Ardestani, "In vitro antioxidant and free radical scavenging activity of Cyperus rotundus," *J Med Food*, Dec. 2007, 10(4):667–674.

11. S. Kilani, M. Ben Sghaier, I. Limem, J. Bouhlel, J. Boubaker, W. Bhouri, I. Skandrani, A. Neffatti, R. Ben Ammar, M.G. Dijoux-Franca, K. Ghedira, and L. Chekir-Ghedira, "In-vitro evaluation of anti-bacterial, anti-oxidant, cytotoxic and apoptic activities of the tubers infusion and extracts of Cyperus rotundas," *Bioresource Techology*, Dec, 2008, 99(18):9004–9008.

12. M. Zhu, H. H Luk, H. S, Fung, and C.T. Luk, "Cytoprotective effects of Cyperus rotundus against ethanol induced gastric ulceration in rats," *Phytotherapy Research*, 1997, 11:392.

13. S. Radomir, D. Sukh, and M. Sirsi, "Chemistry and anti-bacterial activity of nut grass," *Current Science*, 1956, 4:118.

14. **[first initial]** Ivan A. Ross, "Cyperus rotundus," in *Medicinal Plants of the World (Vol 1)* (Totowa, NJ: Humana Press, 1999).

15. D. Pal, S. Dutta, and A. Sarkar, "Evaluation of CNS activities of ethanol extract of roots and rhizomes of Cyperus rotundus in mice," *Acta Pol Pharm.*, Sept-Oct 2009, 66(5):535–541.

16. C. H Lee, D.S. Hwang, H.G. Kim, H. Oh, H. Park, J.H. Cho, J.M. Lee, J.B. Jang, K.S. Lee, and M.S. Oh, "Protective effect of Cyperi rhizoma against 6-hydroxydopamine-induced neuronal damage," *J Med Food.*, June 2010, 13(3):564–571.

17. S. J Uddin, K. Mondal, J.A. Shilpi, and M.T. Rahman,5"Antidiarrhoeal activity of Cyperus rotundus," *Fitoterapia*, Feb. 2006, 77(2):134–136. **[Check the dates. Something is wrong here]**

18. M.K. Jha, *Folk Veterinary Medicine of Bihar—A Research Project* (Anand, Gujrat: NDDB, 1992).

Additional Reading

P.S, Kalsi, A.Sharma, A. Singh, I.P. Singh, and B.R. Chhabra, "Biogenetically important sesquiterpenes from Cyperus rotundus," *Fitoterapia*, 1995, 66(1):94. This number had no corresponding superscript.

M. Alain, B. Frederic, and D. Marc, "Cosmetic or pharmaceutical composition containing a Cyperus extract for pigmentation of the skin or hair," *International Patent Application*, 1992, 92(20):322.

M. Indira, M. Sirsi, S. Radomir, and S. Dev, "Occurrence of estrogenic substances in plants I. Estrogenic activity of Cyperus rotundus," *Indian Journal of Science Research*, 1956, 15:202.

Council for Scientific and Industrial Research, *The Wealth of India* (New Delhi: PID, CSIR, 1985).

18

DIDYMOCARPUS PEDICELLATA

INTRODUCTION

Didymocarpus pedicellata is a valuable, although somewhat lesser known, medicinal plant called Shilpushpa in Sanskrit, Didymocarpus has been shown to be effective as a diuretic and to promote a healthy urinary tract. Together with several other Ayurvedic herbs, Didymocarpus is an ingredient in the popular herbal remedy for kidney diseases.[1] Didymocarpus is mentioned in the ancient Sanskrit texts, as well as in early Arabian and Persian manuscripts. Traditionally, Didymocarpus was used to treat various renal diseases, especially kidney stones.[2] This action is believed to be the result of its regulatory action on calcium absorption. The herb also is especially valuable in these conditions because it helps to prevent new calculi from mineralizing in the kidneys.

SYNONYMOUS NAMES

English: Stone flower
Hindi: Charlea, patharphori
Sanskrit: Shilapushpa, shantapushpi, pasanbheda

HABITAT

Didymocarpus pedicellata is native to the tropical regions of Asia. It grows in the subtropical western Himalayas, reaching altitudes from 2,500 feet up to 5,500 feet.

BOTANICAL CHARACTERISTICS

A small herb with a reduced stem, Didymocarpus bears two or three pairs of opposite, roundly ovate, glabrous, gland-punctated, highly folded leaves 3-to-6 inches in diameter. The dried leaves have a characteristic spicy odor and appear to be dusted with a reddish color.

CHEMICAL COMPOSITION

A chemical investigation of Didymocarpus pedicellata revealed the presence of the novel compounds.[3,4,5,6,7,8,9,10,11,12,13] Chalcones: Pashanone, 8-hydroxy-5, 6, 7-trimethoxy-flavanone, 2'-hydroxy-4', 5', 6'-trimethoxychalcone, Polyterpenes: Didymocarpol and didymacarpenol, Flavonoids: Didmyocarpin, isodidmyocarpin, pedicin, isopedicin, pedicellin,

Pediflavone, 5, 6, 7, 8-tetramethoxy flavanone Dicarboxylic acid: Pedicellic acid. The main constituent of Didymocarpus' essential oil is didymocarpene.

Pharmacological activity

Anti-oxidant activity

An ethanolic extract of the aerial parts of Didymocarpus pedicellata demonstrated significant anti-oxidant and protective activity against ferric nitriloacetate induced renal oxidative stress, nephrotoxicity, and tumor promotion response. The extract also significantly protected against ferric nitriloacetate mediated damage to lipids and DNA in a dose-dependent manner. The nephroprotective activity of the plant is attributed to polyphenolic compounds. These results further confirm and support the ancient use of Didymocarpus in the treatment of kidney diseases.[14]

Renal activity

Didymocarpus pedicellata is widely used in traditional Indian medicines against renal afflictions. A study revealed the significant anti-oxidant effects of an ethanolic extract of the aerial parts of Didymocarpus against ferric nitrilotriacetate-mediated renal oxidative stress, nephrotoxicity, and tumor promotion response.[8] The extract also was shown to have a protective effect. Didymocarpus extract was found to possess a high content of total polyphenolics, to exhibit potent reducing power, and to significantly scavenge free radicals including several reactive oxygen species and reactive nitrogen species. The extract also significantly and dose-dependently protected against Fe-NTA plus H_2O_2-mediated damage to lipids and DNA.

The protective efficacy of the extract also was tested in-vivo against Fe-NTA mediated nephrotoxicity and tumor promotion response. Administration of Fe-NTA to Swiss albino mice depleted renal glutathione content and activities of anti-oxidant and phase II metabolizing enzymes, with concomitant induction of oxidative damage. Fe-NTA also incited hyperproliferation response-elevating ornithine decarboxylase activity and [3H]-thymidine incorporation into DNA. An elevation in serum creatinine and blood urea nitrogen, and histopathological changes also were evident, suggesting that Fe-NTA afflicts damage to the kidneys. Pre-treatment of mice with Didymocarpus extract for 7 days not only restored anti-oxidants to near-normal values but also significantly protected against renal oxidative stress and damage, restoring normal renal architecture and levels of renal damage markers. The results of this study indicate that Didymocarpus pedicellata possesses potent anti-oxidant and free radical scavenging activities and precludes oxidative damage and hyperproliferation in renal tissues.

Oncology support

A polyherbal formulation in ayurvedic medicine which has Didymocarpus as its main ingredient has shown to ameliorate renal toxicity induced by cisplatin in rats. The rats pretreated with with polyherbal formula (1000 mg/kg i.p.) had significantly lower blood urea nitrogen (BUN) and serum creatinine (33.8 and 0.92 mg/dl, respectively) compared to cisplatin alone (51.5 and 1.41 mg/dl, respectively). The control animals had 17.1 and 0.63 mg/dl, respectively. The with polyherbal formula treated animals lost 5.63 g body weight compared to 12.5 g for cisplatin alone treated animals on day 5. Renal functions like urine to serum creatinine ratio and creatinine clearance showed significant improvement when with polyherbal formula was given 1 h before cisplatin.[15]

Antimicrobial activity

The essential oil of Didymocarpus pedicellata has antimicrobial activity.[17]

Safety Profile

No safety contraindications are known for Didymocarpus pedicellata.

Notes

1. S.C. Agarwal, A. Bhaskar, and T.R. Sheshadri, "Constituents of the roots of Didymocarpus pedicellata: Isolation and structure of pashanone, a new chalcone," *Indian J Chem.*, 1972, 12:2–5.

2. C.P Bahl and T.R. Seshadri (Eds.), "Pashanbhedi: drugs for urinary calculus," K.N. Udupa, 1978, 77–98.

3. P.C. Bose and N. Chauadhary, "Didmyocarpin, a new flavanone from Didymocarpus pedicellata," Phytochem., 1978, 17:587–588.

4. P.C. Bose and N. Chauadhary, "Isodidmyocarpin, a new chalcone from Didymocarpus pedicellata," *J Indian Chem.*, 1978, 25:1198–1200.

5. S.K Garg, S.R. Gupta, and N.D. Sharma, "Synthesis of 7-hydroxy-5, 6, 8-trimethoxyflavone: Revision of structure of didmyocarpin," *Indian J Chem.*, 1979, 17B:394–295.

6. P.K. Guha and A. Bhattacharya, "5, 8-dihgydroxyflavone from the immature leaves of Didymocarpus pedicellata," *Phytochem.*, 1992, 31(5):1833–1834.

7. S.L Kapoor and L.D. Kapoor, "On the botany and distribution of 'pashanbheda,'" *Sachitra Ayurved*, 1976, 28(12), 769–791.

8. G. Kaur, et al.. "Protective effect of Didymocarpus pedicellata on ferric nitriloacetate induced renal oxidative stress and hyperproliferative response," *Chem Biol Interact*, 2007, 165(1):33–34. 2007.

9. M. McGuffinet et al., Eds., "Herbs of commerce," 2nd ed. (Herbs Commerce ed2)

10. [Complete city: publisher, year for this entry – or delete, if not cited]

11. K.V. Rao, et al., "Isolation and constitution of pedicellic acid a new dicarboxylic acid from the leaves of Didymocarpus pedicellata," *Tetrahedron*, 1966, 22(4):1495–1498.

12. J.S. Rathore, S.K. Garg, and S.R. Gupta, "A chalcone and flavanones from Didymocarpus pedicellata," *Phytochem.*, 1981, 20:1755–1756.

13. J.S. Rathoreet, et al., "New phenolic compounds of Didymocarpus pedicellata," *Phytochem.*, 1981, 43:86–88.

14. C.S. Shah, N. Shah, and K.D. Mody, "Pharmacognostic study of pashanbhed: I-III: Bergenia ciliata and Didymocarpus pedicellata," *Quarterly Journal of Crude Drug Research*, 1972, 12(1):182–193.

15. V. Sharma and S. Siddiqui, "The constituents of Didymocarpus pedicellata. Part II. Comparative studies in the constitution of pedicin, isopedicin and pedicellin," *J Indian Chem Soc.*,1939, 16:1–8.

16. S. Siddiqui, "The constituents of Didymocarpus pedicellata. Part I. Isolation of a new series of colouring matter," *J Indian Chem Soc.*, 1937, 12:703–708.

17. A. Singh and A.S. Sandhu, *A Dictionary of Medicinal Plants*. New Delhi. Sundeep Publishers, 2005.

18. P Singh, G.K. Sinha, and R. C. Pathak, "Antimicrobial activity of some essential oils," *JRIM*, [Write out] 1978, 13(4):111–114.

Additional Resources

Mahadev Rao, M.N.A Rao "Protective effects of cytone, a polyherbal ayurvedic preparation, on cisplatin-induced renal toxicity in rats," Journal of Ethnopharmacology, Aug 1998, 62(1): pp 1–6.

S.L Kapoor and L.D. Kapoor, "On the botany and distribution of 'pashanbheda,'" *Sachitra Ayurved*, 1976, 28(12), 769–791.

S.C. Agarwal, A. Bhaskar, and T.R. Sheshadri, "Constituents of the roots of Didymocarpus pedicellata: Isolation and structure of pashanone, a new chalcone," *Indian J Chem.*, 1972, 12:2–5.

P.C. Bose and N. Chauadhary, "Didmyocarpin, a new flavanone from Didymocarpus pedicellata," Phytochem., 1978, 17:587–588.

P.C. Bose and N. Chauadhary, "Isodidmyocarpin, a new chalcone from Didymocarpus pedicellata," *J Indian Chem.*, 1978, 25:1198–1200.

S.K Garg, S.R. Gupta, and N.D. Sharma, "Synthesis of 7-hydroxy-5, 6, 8-trimethoxyflavone: Revision of structure of didmyocarpin," *Indian J Chem.*, 1979, 17B:394–295.

P.K. Guha and A. Bhattacharya, "5, 8-dihydroxyflavone from the immature leaves of Didymocarpus pedicellata," *Phytochem.*, 1992, 31(5):1833–1834.

K.V. Rao, et al., "Isolation and constitution of pedicellic acid a new dicarboxylic acid from the leaves of Didymocarpus pedicellata," Tetrahedron, 1966, 22(4):1495–1498.

J.S. Rathore, S.K. Garg, and S.R. Gupta, "A chalcone and flavanones from Didymocarpus pedicellata," Phytochem., 1981, 20:1755–1756.

J.S. Rathoreet, et al., "New phenolic compounds of Didymocarpus pedicellata," Phytochem., 1981, 43:86–88.

C.S. Shah, N. Shah, and K.D. Mody, " Pharmacognostic study of pashanbhed: I-III: Bergenia ciliata and Didymocarpus pedicellata," Quarterly Journal of Crude Drug Research, 1972, 12(1):182–193.

V. Sharma and S. Siddiqui, "The constituents of Didymocarpus pedicellata. Part II. Comparative studies in the constitution of pedicin, isopedicin and pedicellin," J Indian Chem Soc.,1939, 16:1–8.

S. Siddiqui, "The constituents of Didymocarpus pedicellata. Part I. Isolation of a new series of colouring matter," J Indian Chem Soc., 1937, 12:703–708.

G. Kaur, et al.. "Protective effect of Didymocarpus pedicellata on ferric nitriloacetate induced renal oxidative stress and hyperproliferative response," Chem Biol Interact, 2007, 165(1):33–34. 2007.

See note 1

P Singh, G.K. Sinha, and R. C. Pathak, "Antimicrobial activity of some essential oils," *JRIM,* [Write out] This is fine 1978, 13(4):111–114.

19

Dioscorea bulbifera

Introduction

Dioscorea bulbifera, or "air potato," is a species in the yam family that, like others in this family, bears multiple underground tubers, which are used as food and also have a variety of medicinal uses. Known by its Sanskrit name, Varahi, the air potato is a perennial vine with broad leaves and two types of storage organs. As the plant grows, bulbs form in the leaf axils of the twining stems, and tubers resembling small, oblong potatoes grow underground. The air potato is cultivated as a food crop in West Africa.

The air potato has been used as a folk remedy to treat conjunctivitis, diarrhea, and dysentery, among other ailments. It is important to note that uncultivated forms of Dioscorea bulbifera, such as those found growing wild in Florida, can be poisonous. These Dioscorea bulbifera contain the steroid diosgenin, which is a principal material used in the manufacture of a number of synthetic steroidal hormones, such as those used in hormonal treatments.

The plant is native to Africa and Asia. In some areas it is considered to be an invasive species because of its quick-growing, large-leafed vine that spreads tenaciously and shades any plants growing beneath it. The bulb on the vines sprout and become new vines, twisting around each other to form a thick mat. If the plant is cut to the ground, the tubers can survive for extended periods and send up new shoots later.

In both traditional Chinese medicine and Ayurvedic medicine, Dioscorea has a history of therapeutic use. Its use as a folk remedy dates back to around 500–600 AD. There are a number of different indications for use of the dried tuber, decoctions, and tinctures, including its use in uterine bleeding, vomiting of blood, sore throat, gastric cancer, carcinoma of the rectum, goiter, hemoptysis, epistaxis, and pharyngitis. Dioscorea is used topically for sores and for snake and dog bites.

The dried bulbs have been used topically to treat sores and internally to treat syphilis.

Synonymous Names

English: Air potato, air yam, bitter yam
Sanskrit: Varahi
Marathi: Dukkar Kand
Chinese: Huang Yao Zi
Japanese: Oyakushi

Habitat

Dioscorea bulbifera is widely distributed around the world in tropical and subtropical regions of all continents. In the Himalayas, the plant is found at altitudes of up to 6000 feet.

Botanical Characteristics

The air potato is dormant in winter, when the stems die back to their underground tubers. The vine's round stems grow rapidly from the tubers and can reach 65.6 feet (20 meters) in height. The stems are herbaceous, and the plant's large cordate heart-shaped leaves are up to 20 cm long.

The flowers of Dioscorea bulbifera are small and greenish in color and hang in clusters up to 10 cm long. The plant bears aerial bulbs that may be attached to the stems where the leaves meet the stem. These bulbs are gray and irregular in shape. The air potato's tubers grow underground and are larger than the bulbs. They are yellowish-brown on the outside and have a yellowish-white flesh inside. The tubers often are described as having a bitter taste, which is removed by boiling.

Chemical Composition

Chemical analysis of Dioscorea bulbifera has revealed the presence of the following active constituents[1,2]:

Sapponins: dioscorecin, dioscoretoxin and tannin.

Alkaloids: dihydrodioscorine

Sapogenins: diosgenin

Pharmacological Activity

Anti-cancer activity

An in-vivo investigation was conducted with mice to assess the anti-cancer activities of Dioscorea bulbifera. The herb was extracted sequentially with petroleum ether, ethanol, and water. The inhibitory effects on the formation of ascites volume and HepA cell viability in ascites were found in those extracted fractions except the water fraction; the petroleum ether fraction was the strongest. The life span of mice bearing HepA ascites was prolonged after exposure to a petroleum ether fraction and was shortened significantly after exposure to the water fraction. Abnormal microstructure on HepA cells surface was found, and the extract was postulated to have an effect against the viability of HepA. This theory was confirmed with the regeneration of HepA cells from ascites in mice exposed to petroleum ether fraction. Anti-cancer active compounds are extracted mainly by petroleum ether from hydrophobic constituents of Dioscorea bulbifera. The anti-cancer effects were related to direct toxicity on the tumor cell.[3] Additional research showed that the Diosbulbins A and B inhibited tumor growth in mice inoculated with Sarcoma 180, Hep-A, and U14 cells.

Herbal mixture containing Dioscorea as one of its ingredient showed to decrease the development of oral cancer induced by 4-nitroquinoline-1-oxide in mice. The herbal formulation contained Sophora tonkinensis, Polygonum bistorta, Prunella vulgaris, Sonchus arvensis L., Dictamnus dasycarpus, and Dioscorea bulbifera.[4]

Various fractions of the 75% ethanol extract of Dioscorea showed weak cytotoxic activity against neoplastic transformation assay of mouse epidermal JB6 cell lines.[5] The most cytotoxic constituent was kaempferol-3,5-dimethylether.

Anti-hypercholesterolemic activity

Diosgenin given to mice and rats was reported to be anti-hypercholesterolemic and led to an increase of biliary cholesterol concentrations in a rat studies.[6]

Hypoglycemic activity

Preliminary studies on Dioscorea had showed it to be a very potent Amylase and Glucosidase Inhibitor. Glucosidase inhibitor and α-amylase inhibitors are class of compounds that help in managing post prandial hyperglycemia. The preparation of Dioscorea with Gnidia glauca showed to considerable inhibit action of amylase and glucosidase.[7]

Diosgenin produced hypoglycemic effects in STZ-diabetic rats. Oral diosgenin attenuated the acute cholestatic effects of estradiol derivatives in the rat study.[8]

Estrogenic activity

In a randomized blind, placebo controlled trial was done to evaluate effect of Dioscorea on fifty menopausal women. Patients were administered 12mg/sachet extracts of Dioscorea. At 6 months and at the end of treatment, those women who received Diascorea showed general improvement in almost all the clinical symptoms investigated. A significant reduction was noted in the total Greene scores in the Dioscorea group assessed at the end of 12 month's treatment ($p<0.01$). This phenomenon was more significant for the psychological parameters of anxiety than for other parameters. Apparent improvements were noted in the parameters 'feeling tense or nervous' ($p=0.007$), 'insomnia' ($p=0.004$), 'excitable' ($p=0.047$) and 'musculoskeletal pain' ($p=0.019$) among those receiving Dioscorea. Diascorea consumption also resulted in positive effects on blood hormone profiles.[9]

Twenty-four apparently healthy postmenopausal women were recruited to replace their staple food (rice for the most part) with 390 g of yam (Dioscorea alata) in 2 of 3 meals per day for 30 days and 22 completed the study. Fasting blood and first morning urine samples were collected before and after yam intervention for the analyses of blood lipids, sex hormones, urinary estrogen metabolites and oxidant stress biomarker. The design was a one arm, pre-post study. A similar study of postmenopausal women (n = 19) fed 240 g of sweet potato for 41 days was included as a control study. Serum levels of estrone, estradiol and SHBG were analyzed for this control group. After yam ingestion, there were significant increases in serum concentrations of estrone (26%), sex hormone binding globulin (SHBG) (9.5%), and near significant increase in estradiol (27%). No significant changes were observed in serum concentrations of dehydroepiandrosterone sulfate, androstenedione, testosterone, follicular stimulating hormone, and luteinizing hormone. Free androgen index estimated from the ratio of serum concentrations of total testosterone to SHBG decreased. Urinary concentrations of the genotoxic metabolite of estrogen, 16alpha-hydroxyestrone decreased significantly by 37%. Plasma cholesterol concentration decreased significantly by 5.9%. Lag time of low-density lipoprotein oxidation prolonged significantly by 5.8% and urinary isoprostane levels decreased significantly by 42%. Elevated levels of isoprostanes are suspected of contributing to increased risk of heart attack in patients taking Cox-2 inhibitors. Isoprostanes and their metabolites have also been shown to be elevated in the urine of cigarette smokers, and have been suggested as biomarkers of oxidative stress in smokers. For the control subjects fed with sweet potato, all three hormone parameters measured were not changed after intervention.[10]

Ovariectomized (OVX) rat model of postmenopausal osteoporosis was used to examine the effect of the oral administration of different dosages of Dioscorea, red mold Dioscorea (RMD), and soy isoflavones on bone mineral density (BMD). Three months after osteoporosis had been induced and 4 weeks after feeding had begun, the tibia and femur BMD of OVX rats administered RMD showed significant increases compared with that of all other groups of OVX rats. Closer examination using microcomputed tomography also revealed that the RMD-administered rats had denser trabecular bone volume and a higher trabecular number compared to all other rat groups. Reconstructed 3D imaging indicated increases in cancellous bone mineral content, cancellous bone mineral density, and cortical bone mineral content of the proximal tibia in OVX rats. These findings indicate that administration of red mold Dioscorea and phytoestrogen diosgenin could prevent bone loss induced by estrogen deficiency.[11]

Neurological activity

A study evaluated the effects of the methanol extract of the bulbs of Dioscorea bulbifera in inflammatory and neuropathic models of pain and further investigated its possible mechanism of action.[12] The effects of Dioscorea bulbifera administered orally at the doses of 250 and 500mg/kg were tested in mechanical hypernociception induced by intraplantar (i.pl.) injection of complete Freund's adjuvant (CFA), lipopolysaccharides (LPS), or prostaglandin-E(2) (PGE(2)), as well as in partial ligation sciatic nerve (PLSN), nociception induced by capsaicin and thermal hyperalgesia induced by i.pl. injection of CFA. The therapeutic effects of Dioscorea bulbifera on PGE(2)-induced hyperalgesia were evaluated in the absence and in the presence of l-NAME, an inhibitor of nitric oxide synthase (NOS) and glibenclamide, an inhibitor of ATP-sensitive potassium channels. The extract showed significant antinociceptive effects in persistent pain induced by CFA and on neuropathic pain induced by PLSN. The effects of Dioscorea bulbifera persisted for 5 days after two administrations in CFA-induced hypernociception. Dioscorea bulbifera significantly inhibited acute LPS-induced pain but failed to reduce thermal hypernociception and capsaicin-induced spontaneous nociception. The antinociceptive effects of this plant extract in the PGE(2) model was antagonized by either l-NAME or glibenclamide. This demonstrates the antinociceptive activities of Dioscorea bulbifera both in inflammatory and neuropathic models of pain, and these effects may result, at least partially, from its ability to activate the NO-cGMP-ATP-sensitive potassium channels pathway.

Antimicrobial activity

Bioassay-guided fractionation of an aqueous methanolic extract of Dioscorea bulbifera was performed using organic solvents. A novel plasmid curing compound was identified as 8-epidiosbulbin E acetate (EEA) (norditerpene) on the basis of modern spectroscopic analysis and X-ray crystallography. EEA exhibited broad-spectrum plasmid-curing activity against multidrug-resistant (MDR) bacteria, including vancomycin-resistant enterococci. EEA cured antibiotic resistance plasmids (R-plasmids) from clinical isolates of Enterococcus faecalis, Escherichia coli, Shigella sonnei, and Pseudomonas aeruginosa with 12-48% curing efficiency. The reference plasmids of Bacillus subtilis (pUB110), E. coli (RP4), P. aeruginosa (RIP64), and Salmonella typhi (R136) were cured with efficiencies ranging from 16% to 64%. EEA-mediated R-plasmid curing decreased the minimal inhibitory concentration of antibiotics against MDR bacteria, thus making antibiotic treatment more effective. The antibiotic resistance pattern revealed that the compound was effective in reversing bacterial resistance to various antibiotics.[13]

Safety Profile

The single-dose toxicity findings for dihydrodioscorine and diosgenin have been reported. In mice, the IP LD50 for dihydrodioscorine was 65 mg/kg with some animals (presumably those given the higher doses) showing clonic and tonic convulsions, followed by death. After cases of human poisoning indicating the substance is also convulsant after an oral overdose, dihydrodioscorine was isolated from a related yam species, but no data exist for the acute human toxicity from an oral route.[14] Other experimental data suggest that some ingredients in Dioscorea can cause hepatotoxicity via liver oxidative stress.[15]

Notes

1. Wang G, Lin B, Liu J, Wang G, Wang F, Liu J. Chemical constituents from tubers of Dioscorea bulbifera. Zhongguo Zhong Yao Za Zhi. 2009 Jul;34(13):1679-82.

2. Liu H, Chou GX, Wu T, Guo YL, Wang SC, Wang CH, Wang ZT. Steroidal sapogenins and glycosides from the rhizomes of Dioscorea bulbifera. J Nat Prod. 2009 Nov;72(11):1964-8.

3. Z. L. Yu, X.R. Liu, M. McCulloch, and J. Gao, "Anticancer effects of various fractions extracted from Dioscorea bulbifera on mice bearing HepA," Zhongguo Zhong Yao Za Zhi, June, 2001, 29(6):563–567.

4. Wang Y, Yao R, Gao S, Wen W, Du Y, Szabo E, Hu M, Lubet RA, You M. Chemopreventive effect of a mixture of Chinese Herbs (antitumor B) on chemically induced oral carcinogenesis. Mol Carcinog. 2011 Nov 15. They can find this reference even with no page numbers as it is ahead online print. No changes needed.

5. H. Gao, M. Kuroyanagi, L.Wu, N. Kawahara, T. Yasuno, and Y. Nakamura, "Antitumor-promoting constituents from Dioscorea bulbifera L. in JB6 mouse epidermal cells," Biological and Pharmaceutical Bulletin, 2002, 25(9):1241–1243.

6. A. Thewles, R.A. Parslow, and R. Coleman, "Effect of diosgenin on biliary cholesterol transport in the rat," Biochem J, 1993, 291:793–798.

7. Ghosh S, Ahire M, Patil S, Jabgunde A, Bhat Dusane M, Joshi BN, Pardesi K, Jachak S, Dhavale DD, Chopade BA. Antidiabetic Activity of Gnidia glauca and Dioscorea bulbifera: Potent Amylase and Glucosidase Inhibitors. Evid Based Complement Alternat Med. 2012 same here it is advanced online print

8. Ahmed Z, Chishti MZ, Johri RK, Bhagat A, Gupta KK, Ram G. Antihyperglycemic and antidyslipidemic activity of aqueous extract of D. bulbifera tubers. Diabetologia Croatica. 2009;38(3):63–72.

9. Hsu CC, Kuo HC, Chang SY, Wu TC, Huang KE. The assessment of efficacy of Diascorea alata for menopausal symptom treatment in Taiwanese women. Climacteric. 2011 Feb;14(1):132-9.

10. Wu WH, Liu LY, Chung CJ, Jou HJ, Wang TA. Estrogenic effect of yam ingestion in healthy postmenopausal women. J Am Coll Nutr. 2005 Aug;24(4):235-43.

11. Chiang SS, Chang SP, Pan TM. Osteoprotective effect of Monascus-fermented dioscorea in ovariectomized rat model of postmenopausal osteoporosis. J Agric Food Chem. 2011 Sep 14;59(17):9150-7.

12. T.B. Nguelefack, R.C. Dutra, A.F. Paszcuk, E.L. Andrade, L.A. Tapondjou, and J.B. Calixto, "Antinociceptive activities of the methanol extract of the bulbs of Dioscorea bulbifera L. var sativa in mice is dependent of NO-cGMP-ATP-sensitive-K(+) channel activation," J Ethnopharmacol,, Apr 21, 2010, 128(3):567–574.

13. V. Shriram, S. Jahagirdar, C. Latha, V. Kumar, V. Puranik, S. Rojatkar, P.K. Dhakephalkar, and M.G. Shitole, "A potential plasmid-curing agent, 8-epidiosbulbin E acetate, from Dioscorea bulbifera L. against multidrug-resistant bacteria," Int J Antimicrob Agents, Nov. 2008, 32(5):405–410.

14. Su L, Zhu JH, Cheng LB. Experimental pathological study of subacute intoxication by Dioscorea bulbifera L. Fa Yi Xue Za Zhi. 2003;19(2):81-3.

15. J.Wang, L Ji, H. Liu, and Z. Wang Z., "Study of the hepatotoxicity induced by Dioscorea bulbifera L. rhizome in mice," Biosci Trends. April 2010, 4(2):79-85.

20

Eclipta Alba

Introduction

Eclipta alba, known in Sanskrit as Bhringaraj, is an herbaceous plant belonging to the daisy family that grows as a weed throughout many areas of the world, including India, China, Thailand, and Brazil. In Ayurvedic tradition, the leaf extract of Eclipta alba is considered to be a powerful liver tonic and rejuvenative, or rasayana herb. A black dye obtained from the plant is often used for dyeing hair and tattooing.

Known as one of the "Ten Auspicious Flowers" of Ayurveda, Eclipta alba has been used for thousands of years to enhance the appearance of the skin and hair. Preparations from the plant are used externally to treat athlete foot, eczema, and dermatitis, and are applied to the scalp to reduce hair loss. The leaves are used in the treatment of scorpion stings, and as an anti-venom against snakebite.

Eclipta alba is considered to be a rasayana in Ayurveda because of its rejuvenative properties. Research also has indicated its profound antihepatotoxic activity. Cardio-depressant activity has been observed when Eclipta alba is used for hepatic congestion. Symptomatic relief for epigastric pain, nausea, and vomiting in ulcer patients have been observed as well.

In traditional Chinese medicine, Eclipta alba is used as a cooling and restorative herb supporting the mind, nerves, liver, and eyes. Chinese practitioners use the herb to treat bleeding, hepatitis, diphtheria, and diarrhea. In India, the expressed leaf juice of Eclipta alba, applied along with honey, is a popular remedy for catarrh in infants. A preparation obtained from the leaf juice, combined with sesame or coconut oil, is used to make the hair black and luxuriant. The leaf juice also may be rubbed on the gums to relieve toothache. The roots are considered to be emetic and purgative.

Synonymous Names

English: Trailing eclipta, false daisy
Hindi: Bhangra, babri
Sanskrit: Bhringaraj, tekarajah

Habitat

Eclipta alba is a common weed that grows in moist areas, usually in waste places. The plant grows natively throughout India, China, Thailand, Brazil, and other areas of the world, up to an altitude of 2000 meters.

Botanical Characteristics

Bhringaraj is a prostrate, creeping herb that thrives in moist soil. It is a much-branched plant with a short, brown stem that usually does not grow more than 3 inches above the ground. The lance-shaped leaves are opposite and pubescent on both upper and lower surfaces, reaching 10 cm in length. The herb's composite flowers are white with compressed rays, 6-to-8 millimeters in diameter. The flowers grow on short, solitary stalks.

Chemical Composition

Eclipta alba contains mainly coumestans such as wedelolactone (I) and demethylwedelolactone (II), polypeptides, polyacetylenes, thiophene-derivatives, steroids, triterpenes, and flavonoids. Ecliptal, a terthienyl aldehyde, has been isolated from the whole plant and L-terthienyl methanol and wedelic acid from leaves and stem, and the sesquiterpene lactone columbin.[1,2]

Triterpene glycosides and saponins :
Six new oleanane glycosides, the eclalbasaponins I-VI, as well as β-amyrin and other sterols have been isolated from the aerial parts.[3,4]

Flavonoids and isoflavonoids:
Apigenin, luteolin and their glucosides have been isolated from the leaves and stem; and the isoflavonoids wedelolactone, desmethylwedelolactone and its 7-0-glucoside from the whole plant.[5]

Pharmacological Activity

Hepatoprotective Activity

An extract of Eclipta alba was studied under laboratory conditions to ascertain its action against hepatotoxicity in rats. The study results showed that the extract provided protection by regulating the levels of hepatic drug-metabolizing enzymes.[6]

Eclipta alba exhibited similar activity when administered in combination with the herbs Phyllanthus niruri and curcumin. High levels of hepatic lipids and serum bilirubin were decreased and normalized. The herbal preparation also increased the levels of serum triglyceride, pre-β-lipoproteins, and cholesterol, and decreased levels of glycogen were elevated.[7]

An ethanolic extract of the fresh Eclipta alba showed significant hepatoprotective activity in CCl_4-induced liver damage in rats and mice in a dose-dependent manner, with no signs of toxicity observed up to levels of 2.0 g/kg given either orally or intraperitoneally.[8]

In another animal study, significant hepatoprotective action was observed at 100 mg/kg body weight.[9] A freeze-dried aqueous extract of Eclipta alba was studied for its hepatoprotective effects in acute hepatitis that was induced in mice by a single dose of CCl_4 or acetaminophen (paracetamol), and in rats by β-D-galactosamine. The extract also showed significant inhibition of acute elevation of serum transaminases induced by CCl_4 in mice and by β-D-galactosamine in rats; however, no significant improvement was observed in acetaminophen induced liver damage.[10]

Hypotensive Activity

The combined effect of dried Eclipta alba leaf powder (3 g/day) in encapsulated form was studied in a blood pressure, diuresis, and lipid profile of 60 mildly hypertensive male subjects ages 40 to 55 years. The subjects were divided into two groups— a control (placebo) and the Eclipta group—and were given six capsules (500 mg each) per day in three equal doses for 60 days. Clinical parameters, viz., blood pressure, urine volume, electrolytes (Na and K) in serum and urine, lipid profile, and plasma lipid peroxides, were analyzed before and after the feeding trials. The findings revealed that the Eclipta supplemented group had a marked reduction in mean arterial pressure (by 15%), total cholesterol (17%), low-density lipoprotein fraction (24%), triglycerides (14%), very-low-density lipoprotein fraction (14%), and plasma lipid peroxides (18%). The results also revealed a remarkable increase in urine volume (34%), urine sodium (24%), serum vitamin C (17%), and serum tocopherols (23%) of the Eclipta group. Eclipta alba showed diuretic, hypotensive, and hypocholesterolemic effects and helped to alleviate oxidative stress-induced complications in hypertensives.[11]

A mixture of polypeptides from Eclipta alba exhibited hypotensive activity in dogs, and columbin isolated from the ethanolic extract of the whole plant showed remarkable antihypertensive action on anesthetized rats.[12]

Antimicrobial activity

The anti-malarial activity of an extract of Eclipta alba leaves was evaluated against the Plasmodium' berghei ANKA strain in mice. A standard inoculum of 1 x 10(6) infected erythrocytes was used. The methanolic leaf extract (250–750 mg/kg) produced a dose-dependent chemosupression or schizontocidal effect during early and established infection and high mean survival time values particularly in the group that was administered 750 mg/kg/day of extract. The plant extract also exhibited repository activity.[13]

Central Nervous System Activity

An animal study was conducted to assess the ability of an aqueous extract of Eclipta alba to ease aggressive behavior. Foot shock induced aggression and water competition tests were used as models for screening for anti-aggressive activity. The results showed that Eclipta alba significantly minimized dominance, which is correlated with the level of aggression. A dosage of 200mg/kg of the extract was particularly effective in the water competition test. A tangible change in behavioral submission was observed with 100 and 200mg/kg of Eclipta alba in the foot shock induced test.[14]

In another experiment in similar path Eclipta was studied for its effect during the postpartum aggressive behavior. Prolonged aggression during the postpartum period could affect maternal care. Eclipta alba is traditionally known to induce neuropsychiatric alterations, however its ability to circumvent maternal aggression has not been elucidated. A study was aimed to investigate the ability of the aqueous extract of Eclipta alba to suppress maternal aggression. In the single dose study, 100, 200 and 500 mg/kg body weight of the aqueous extract of Eclipta alba was administered to parturient females 30 minutes prior to maternal aggression testing against intruder males. In the multiple dose study, 100, 200 and 500 mg/kg of the extract were administered for 15 and 30 days and maternal aggression was quantified. Administration of the extract for 15 and 30 days in dose schedules of 200 and 500 mg/kg body weight significantly suppressed antagonistic encounters by the dams and therefore had beneficial anti-aggressive activity.[15]

Short-term and long-term memory loss may result from deteriorating cerebral mechanisms with varied causes which could have a tremendous impact on the quality of life. Eclipta alba has shown memory-enhancing qualities. The shade-dried leaves of Eclipta alba were extracted with distilled water. The suspension of Eclipta alba containing 100 and 200 mg/kg was administered to rats to evaluate transfer latency on an elevated plus maze. Transfer latency was a measure of acquisition and retrieval learning. The rats were placed at the center of an open-field apparatus to assess spatial habitual learning. They were observed for 20 minutes for rearing and time spent during rearing using varied doses for 30 minutes, 24 hours, 96 hours, and 144 hours. The results revealed significant improvement of retrieval memory.[16]

Anti-inflammatory activity

An extract of Eclipta alba, tested in both acute and chronic anti-inflammatory models, significantly inhibited chronic inflammation.[17] In the search for potent and selective 5-lipoxygenase-inhibitors, extracts of medicinal plants were screened for their potency in inhibiting the formation of inflammatory acting products of arachidonic acid metabolism using a porcine-leukocytes test system. The wedelolactone isolated from Eclipta alba has been found to be a potent and selective 5-lipoxygenase-inhibitor with an IC (50) of 2,5 microMol. As found by chemoluminescence, wedelolactone inhibits 5-lipoxygenase by an oxygen radical scavenger mechanism.[18]

Immunomodulation Activity

An attempt has been made to assess the immunomodulatory activity of methanol extracts of the whole plant of Eclipta alba (1.6% wedelolactone) and Centella asiatica (0.18% of asiaticoside) at five dose levels (dose-response relationship) ranging from 100 to 500 mg/kg body wt. using carbon clearance, antibody titer, and cyclophosphamide immunosuppression parameters. In the case of Eclipta alba, the phagocytic index and antibody titer increased significantly and the F ratios of the phagocytic index and white blood cell (WBC) count also were significant. Regression analysis showed linearity in patterns of the dose response relationship, greatest in the case of the phagocytic index, moderate in the WBC count, and lowest in the antibody titer. Centella asiatica, increases in the phagocytic index and total WBC count were observed, and the F ratio of the phagocytic index also was significant. Regressed values revealed maximum linearity in the case of the phagocytic index, moderate linearity in the total WBC count, and lowest linearity in the antibody response.[19]

Anti-nociceptive Activity

Various analgesics are used to treat acute and chronic pain in different disease states. New options for narcotic or non-narcotic analgesics that do not cause respiratory depression and addiction are needed.

Research was undertaken to determine the analgesic activity of the total ethanol extract of Eclipta alba and its isolated alkaloids using standard experimental models such as the tail clip method, the tail flick method, and the acetic acid induced writhing response. Results from this study showed that both the ethanol extract and the total alkaloids of Eclipta alba produced good analgesic activity in all the different models of analgesia used. The total alkaloidal fraction was the most efficacious in all the models tested.[20]

In a further study using mice, a hydroalcoholic extract of the herb inhibited acetic acid-induced writhing by 35% to 55%. At the same dose, the effect ranged from 41% to 77% using the formalin test in mice. The herbal extract preferentially inhibited the second phase of the response.[21]

Hair Growth

Alopecia is a dermatological disorder with psychosocial implications for patients with hair loss. Eclipta alba is a well-known Ayurvedic herb with claims of hair growth promotion. In the reported work, attempts were undertaken to evaluate petroleum ether and ethanol extract of Eclipta alba for their effects on promoting hair growth in albino rats. The extracts were incorporated into oleaginous cream (water in oil cream base) and applied topically on the shaved denuded skin of albino rats. The times (in days) required for hair growth initiation as well as completion of hair growth cycle were recorded. A minoxidil 2% solution, applied topically, served as the positive control for comparison. After treatment with the hair growth initiation, the time was significantly reduced by half, compared to the control animals.

The time required for complete hair growth also was significantly reduced. The quantitative analysis of hair growth after treatment with petroleum ether extract (5%) exhibited a greater number of hair follicles in the anagenic phase (69 +/- 4), higher than the control (47 +/- 13). Results of treatment with 2% and 5% petroleum ether extracts were better than the positive control minoxidil 2% treatment.[22]

Similar results were found in another study of which Eclipta alba was part of the polyherbal formulation for Alopecia.[23] In the study, the hair growth initiation time was markedly reduced to one third after treatment with the prepared formulation compared to the control animals. The time required for complete hair growth also was reduced by 32%. Quantitative analysis of the hair growth cycle after treatment with formulations and minoxidil (2%) exhibited a greater number of hair follicles in the anagenic phase compared to the control. Minoxidil was used as the control in the study.

Ethnoveterinary Usage

The leaves, herb, and root of Eclipta alba are used in veterinary practice to treat wounds, blisters, broken horns, cracked tail, scratching, scabies, abscess in the ear, hemorrhagic septicemia, mastitis, rabies, jackal bites, glossitis, oral lesions, jaundice, leeches in the nostril, pneumonia, swelling of the throat and nasal mucus membranes, epistaxis, and tetanus.[24]

Dr. Sodhi's Experience

Many studies have shown Bhringaraj to be hepatoprotective. Some practitioners believe that simply drinking smoothies made with the herb may reverse the effects of all forms of hepatitis. Bhringaraj is a potent remedy for all kinds of liver congestion, whether from heavy metals, environmental toxins, or drug toxicity. It also is effective against digestive disorders involving the liver, such as cirrhosis and fatty liver degeneration. Bhringaraj also is widely believed to stimulate hair growth.

Case History

A physician from Colorado came to our clinic reporting extreme fatigue. When we tested her liver enzymes, we found that they were elevated into the 80s. Her TSH level, too, was elevated at 7.4, indicating hypothyroidism. Upon further testing, we determined that she had been exposed to hepatitis B. We put her on the herbal following protocol:

For hepatitis B:
  Bhringaraj, 500 mg extract three times a day

For thyroid support:
  Commiphora mukul (Guggul), 300 mg extract with 80 mg of triphala, consisting of equal parts Emblica officinalis (amalaki), Terminalia bellerica (bibhitaki), Terminalia chebula (haritaki), with 20 mg vitamin B6 and 400 mcg of folate, three times a day.

For liver support:
  250 mg Phyllanthus amarus extract, three times a day.

After 1½ months of treatment, the patient's liver enzymes were back to normal, and her TSH had dropped to 4.9. Three months later, she had developed antibodies to hepatitis B, indicating that she was no longer a carrier. Her thyroid levels also were within a normal range.

Safety Profile

The maximum tolerated dose of the 50% ethanolic extract of the whole Eclipta alba plant was found to be 1000 mg/kg body weight when given intraperitoneally to adult albino mice.[11]

Dosage

Infusion: 4–12 ml
Powder: 3-6 g
Extract: 100 mg to 200 mg, three times per day

Ayurvedic Properties

Rasa: Katu (pungent), tikta (bitter)
Guna: Laghu (light), ruksha (dry)
Veerya: Ushna (hot)
Vipaka: Katu (pungent)
Dosha: Balances kapha and vata

Notes

1. L.K Leal, A.A Ferreira, G.A. Bezerra, F.J. Matos, and G.S.Viana, "Antinociceptive, anti-inflammatory and bronchodilator activities of Brazilian medicinal plants containing coumarins: A comparative study," *Journal of Ethnopharmacology*, 2000, 70(2):151.

2. H. Wagner, B. Geyer, Y. Kiso, H. Hikino, and G.S. Rao, "Coumestans as main active principles of the liver drugs Eclipta alga and Wedelia calendulaceae," *Planta Medica*, 1986, 5:370–373.

3. S. Yahara, N. Ding, and T. Nohara, "Oleanane glycosides from Edipta alba," *Chemical and Pharmaceutical Bulletin*, 1994, 42(6):1336.

4. R.K. Upadhyay, M.B. Pandey, R.N. Jha, and V.B. Pandey, "Eclalbatin, a triterpine saponins from Eclipta alba," *J Asian Nat Prod Res*, 2001, 3:213–217.

5. See Note l, Leal et al.

6. A. K. Saxena, B. Singh, and K.K. Anand, "Hepatoprotective effects ofaEclipta alba on subcellular levels in rats," *Journal of Ethnopharmacology*, 1993, 40(3):155.

7. T. Chandra and J. Sadique, "A new recipe for liver injury," *Ancient Science of Life*, 1987, 7(2):99.

8. B. Singh, A.K. Saxena, B.K. Chandan, S.G. Agarwal, M.S. Bhatia, and K.K. Anand, "Hepatoprotective effect of ethanolic extract of Edipta alba on experimental liver damage in rats and mice," *Phytotherapy Research*, 1993, 7(2):154.

9. T.S. Murthy, B.G. Rao, T. Satyanarayana, and R.V.K. Rao, "Hepatoprotective activity of Edipta alba," *Journal of Research and Education in Indian Medicine*, 1993, 12(2):41.

10. S-C Lin, C-J Yao, C-C Lin, and Y-H Lin, "Hepatoprotective activity of Taiwan folk medicine: Edipta prostrata Linn, against various hepatotoxins induced acute hepatotoxicity," *Phytotherapy Research*, 1996 10:483.

11. V. Rangineni, D. Sharada, and S. Saxena, "Diuretic, hypotensive, and hypocholesterolemic effects of Eclipta alba in mild hypertensive subjects: A pilot study," *J Med Food.*, March 2007 10(1):143–148.

12. M.D. Rashid, V. Karim, M. Ahmed, and A.R. Choudhuiy, "Antihypertensive activity of Eclipta alba," International Seminar on Traditional Medicine, Calcutta, India, November 7–9, 1992.

13. S. Bapna, S. Adsule, S. Shirshat Mahendra, S. Jadhav, L.S. Patil, and R.A. Deshmukh, "Anti-malarial activity of Eclipta alba against Plasmodium berghei infection in mice," *J Commun Dis.*, June 2007, 39(2):91–94.

14. O.J. Lobo, D. Banji, A.R. Annamalai, and R. Manavalan R., "Evaluation of antiaggressive activity of Eclipta alba in experimental animals," *Pak J Pharm Sci.*, April 2008, 21(2):195–199.

15. D. Banji, O.J. Banji, A.R. Annamalai, and M. Shanthmurthy, "Impact of the aqueous extract of Eclipta alba on maternal aggression in rats," *Pak J Pharm Sci.*, April 2010, 23(2):138–142.

16. O. Banji, D. Banji, A.R. Annamalai, and R. Manavalan, "Investigation on the effect of eclipta alba on animal models of learning and memory," *Indian J Physiol Pharmacol.*, July-Sept. 2007, 51(3):274–278.

17. K.R.K. Reddy, S.S. Tehara, P.V. Goud, and M.M. Alikhan, "Comparison of the anti-inflammatory activity of Edipta alba (Bhangra) and Solanum nigrum (Mako Khushk) in rats," *Journal of Research and Education in Indian Medicine*, 1990, 9(4):43.

18. See Note 2, Wagner et al. –Verify, as SS & Note 16 is about liver, not anti-inflammatory I am not sure what the question was. Note 2 is about drugs which are predominately liver remedies but also have anti-inflammatory actions

19. M.G. Jayathirtha and S.H. Mishra, "Preliminary immunomodulatory activities of methanol extracts of Eclipta alba and Centella asiatica," *Phytomedicine*, 2004, 11(4):361–365.

20. M. Sawant, J. C. Isaac, and S. Narayanan, "Analgesic studies on total alkaloids and alcohol extracts of Eclipta alba (Linn.) Hassk.," *Phytother Res.*, Feb. 2004, 18(2):111–113.

21. See Note 1, Leal et al.

22. Roy RK, Thakur M, Dixit VK. Hair growth promoting activity of Eclipta alba in male albino rats. Arch Dermatol Res. 2008 Aug;300(7):357-64.

23. R.K. Roy, M. Thakur, and V.K. Dixit, "Development and evaluation of polyherbal formulation for hair growth-promoting activity," *J Cosmet Dermatol.*, June 2007, 6(2):108–112.

24. M.K. Jha, *Folk Veterinary Medicine of Bihar —A Research Project* (Anand, Gujrat: NDDB, 1992).

Additional Resource

M. L Dhar, M.M, Dhar, B.N Dhawan, B.N. Mehrotra, and C. Ray, "Screening of Indian plants for biological activity: Part I," *Indian Journal of Experimental Biology*, 1968 6:232.

R.N Chopra, S.L.Nayar, and I.C. Chopra, *Glossary of Indian Medicinal Plants* (New Delhi., India: C.S.I.R., 1955).

J.H Everitt, R.L. Lonard, and C.R. Little, *Weeds in South Texas and Northern Mexico*. (Lubbock: Texas Tech University Press, 2007).

K. R Kritikar and B.D. Basu, *Chronica Botanica Indian Medicinal plants* (New Delhi, India: Publisher, 1975). I don't have details on this.

H. S Puri, *Rasayana: Ayurvedic Herbs for Longevity and Rejuvenation* (London: Taylor & Francis, 2003), pp. 80–85.

B. Singh, A.K. Saxena, B.K. Chandan, S.G. Agarwal, and K.K.Anand, "In vivo hepatoprotective activity of active fraction from ethanolic extract of Eclipta alba leaves," *Indian J Physiol Pharmacol.*, Oct. 2001, 45(4):435–441.

Council of Scientific and Industrial Research, *The Wealth of India* (New Delhi, India: PID, CSIR, 1985).

L.D. Kapoor, *Handbook of Ayurvedic Medicinal Plants* (Boca Raton, Louisiana: CRC Press, 1990).

A.K. Nadkarni, *Indian Materia Medica* (Bombay, India: Popular Prakashan PVT Ltd, 1976).

G.S. Pandey, G.S. (Ed.), *Bhavprakash Nighantu* (Gokul Bhawan,Varanasi: Chaukhambha Bharati Academy, 1998).This is what it is referenced as

T.V. Sairam,. *Home Remedies, Vol II* (New Delhi, India: Penguin, 1999).r?*The wealth of India* (New Delhi: PID, CSIR, date) I really have no details on this. Please see this http://www.niscair.res.in/activitiesandservices/products/woi1.htm

Embelia ribes

Introduction

Embelia ribes, or vidanga, is an important Ayurvedic herb, used as a primary ingredient in many herbal formulations. Records of the use of Embelia ribes are found in ancient Ayurvedic and Unani texts. An important antihelmintic, vidanga traditionally has been used to purge the body of parasites and intestinal bacteria, including E. coli. This herb has the ability to expel tapeworms and detoxify the blood and the liver. Embelia ribes also possesses decongestant, carminative, antihelmintic, anti-bacterial, diuretic, stimulant, alterative, and antiinflammatory properties. Modern medical research has investigated Embelia ribes' potential use as a contraceptive agent.

Traditional practitioners use a powder made from embelia's berries to treat worm infestations, particularly ringworm. The plant's pulp has purgative properties, and its cooling juice has both laxative and diuretic effects. Embelia also is valued for its astringent and nervine properties. A preparation made from the plant's leaves eases sore throat and heals mouth ulcers. The root is effective in treating digestive complaints such as dyspepsia, constipation, colic, flatulence, and hemorrhoids.

Synonymous Names

English: Embelia
Hindi: Vayvidanga
Sanskrit: Vidanga

Habitat

Embelia is native to the Himalayas, Singapore, Sri Lanka, and India, growing primarily in hilly regions of India and southeast Asia, and is found in hilly regions of the central and lower Himalayas as far as Sri Lanka and Singapore.

Botanical Characteristics

Embelia ribes is a large, climbing shrub, with simple, alternate leaves, which are narrowly elliptical to lanceolate in shape. The leaves are coriaceous and about 14 cm long and 4 cm wide, glossy green on the upper surface and more silvery on the lower surface, with scattered, tiny, sunken glands.

The flowers are small, white or greenish, in terminal or axillary panicles; the calyx is five-lobed, corolla puberulous, with five stamens. The fruits are globose berries, up to 4 millimeters in diameter, dull red or brownish-black when dried, with a wrinkled or warty surface. The berries' thin pericarp encloses a single red seed, enveloped in a delicate membrane.

The berries have a faint spicy odor and a pungent and astringent taste.

Chemical Composition

Quinones:
The fruit contains embelin (embelic acid), which is considered to be the major active principle, and vilangin.[1]

Fatty acids:
The seed oil contains palmitic, oleic, and linoleic acids.[2]

Alkaloid:
The fruit contains christembine.[3]

Pharmacological Activity

Contraceptive activity

The active agent embelin, isolated from Embelia ribes, has shown promising contraceptive properties in fertility research.[4] In a study using dogs, a dose of 80 mg/kg embelin was given orally for 100 days. At the close of the study, epididymis were found to be devoid of spermatozoa. Histological, blood chemistry, and tissue biochemistry examinations showed that embelin had caused complete inhibition of spermatogenesis. Blood serum parameters revealed normal liver and kidney functions. When administration of embelin was discontinued, complete recovery of spermatogenesis occurred after 250 days, suggesting that the substance could be an effective, reversible, male contraceptive.[5]

In additional research, powdered Embelia berries were given to male bonnet monkeys by mouth for 3 months at a dose of 100 mg/day. Ingestion of the berries adversely affected the quantity and quality of semen and caused a reduction in circulating testosterone levels. Testicular biopsies revealed normal spermatogenesis, but a reduction in testosterone levels may be responsible for reduced secretory activity of the accessory glands, resulting in a decrease in volume of the semen.[6]

The effect of embelin as an oral contraceptive was demonstrated in pregnant rats. Biochemical changes in the uterus and uterine fluid were observed when 10 mg/kg was administered orally from days 1 to 5 of pregnancy. Decreased glycogen content of the uterus, lactic acid in uterine fluid, and increased alanine aminotransferase activity were observed, suggesting an anti-implantation effect by decreasing the energy available to the blastocyst for survival.[7]

When 20 mg/kg of herbal extract was given to male albino rats for 15 or 30 days, embelin caused an inhibition of epididymis motile sperm count and fertility parameters such as pregnancy attainment and litter size. These changes were reversible. The addition of embelin to epididymis sperm suspensions caused a dose- and duration-dependent inhibition of spermatozoal motility, and increased the activity of the enzymes of carbohydrate metabolism. Light and SEM microscopy revealed that both in-vivo and in-vitro treatment caused profound morphological changes in spermatozoa, such as decapitation of the spermatozoal head, discontinuity of the outer membranous sheath in the mid-piece and the tail region, and alteration in the shape of cytoplasmic droplets in the tail.[8]

Embelin also significantly reduced the sperm count and motility and the weight of the testes in rats[9] and has been shown to alter rat testicular histology and glycogen levels, gametogenic counts, and accessory sex gland fructose levels at doses of 0.3, 0.4 and 0.5 mg/kg when administered subcutaneous for 35 days. In female rats, embelin demonstrated 57.9% and 55.5% anti-fertility activity at doses of 100 and 50 mg/kg, respectively.[10]

Anti-tumor activity

Embelia ribes has demonstrated cytotoxicity against fibrosarcoma cells. A fibrosarcoma cell line was exposed to increasing concentrations of embelin in an in-vitro study, followed by inoculation with (3H)-thymidine. The results showed a dose-dependent decrease in labeled thymidine uptake, lipid peroxide and glutathione levels.[11] Embelin was shown to decrease tumor size and prevent an increase in serum enzymes activity in rats with experimental fibrosarcoma, indicating that it interfered with carbohydrate and amino acid metabolism in tumor bearing animals.[12]

Antihelmintic activity

Both the alcoholic and aqueous extracts of Embelia berries were tested on 40 children infested with ascarides. The alcoholic extract cured 80% of cases, and the aqueous extract cured 55%, expelling the worms and rendering the stool free from ova. No toxicity was observed during and after the treatment.[13]

Anti-diabetic activity

Forty days of oral administration of aqueous Embelia ribes extract to streptozotocin-induced diabetic rats produced significant decreases in heart rate, systolic blood pressure, blood glucose, blood glycosylated hemoglobin, serum lactate dehydrogenase, and creatine kinase, and an increase in blood glutathione levels, compared to pathogenic diabetic rats.

Further, the extract significantly decreased levels of pancreatic lipid peroxides and increased levels of pancreatic superoxide dismutase, catalase, and glutathione. The results also suggest that aqueous Embelia ribes extract has a significant blood glucose and blood pressure-lowering potential. Further, it enhances the endogenous anti-oxidant defense against free radicals produced under hyperglycemic conditions, and thus seemingly protects the pancreatic beta-cells against loss in streptozotocin-induced diabetic rats.[14]

A study was designed to examine the anti-oxidant defense by ethanolic extract of Embelia ribes on streptozotocin-(40 mg/kg, intravenously, single injection)-induced diabetes in Wistar rats.[15] Forty days of oral feeding of the extract (100 mg/kg and 200 mg/kg) to diabetic rats resulted in a significant (P < .01) decrease in blood glucose, blood glycosylated hemoglobin, serum lactate dehydrogenase, creatine kinase, and an increase in blood glutathione levels compared to pathogenic diabetic rats. Further, the extract significantly (P < .01) decreased the pancreatic thiobarbituric acid-reactive substances (TBARS) levels and significantly (P < .01) increased the superoxide dismutase, catalase, and glutathione levels, compared to the above levels in the pancreatic tissue of pathogenic diabetic rats. The islets were shrunken in the diabetic rats in comparison to the normal rats. The drug-treated diabetic rats had an expansion of islets. Results of test drug were comparable to gliclazide (25 mg/kg, daily), a standard antihyperglycemic agent. The study concludes that Embelia ribes enhances the anti-oxidant defense against reactive oxygen species produced under hyperglycemic condition and this protects beta-cells against loss and exhibits an anti-diabetic property.

The lipid-lowering and anti-oxidant potential of an ethanolic extract of Embeila was investigated in streptozotocin-induced diabetes in rats.[16] Twenty days of orally feeding the extract to diabetic rats resulted in a significant decrease in blood glucose, serum total cholesterol, and triglycerides, along with an increase in HDL-cholesterol levels compared to the levels of pathogenic diabetic rats. Further, the extract lowered the liver and pancreas thiobarbituric acid-reactive substances values when compared to similar values of the liver and pancreas of pathogenic diabetic rats. The results were comparable to those of gliclazide, a standard antihyperglycemic agent.

Cardioprotective activity

The cardioprotective effect of aqueous extract of Embelia fruit was evaluated in animals with acute myocardial infarction, induced by isoproterenol. Pre-treatment with Embelia for a 40-day period before induction of myocardial infarction significantly decreased the heart rate and systolic blood pressure, increased levels of serum lactate dehydrogenase, serum creatine kinase, and myocardial lipid peroxides, and significantly increased the myocardial endogenous anti-oxidants levels (glutathione, superoxide dismutase, and catalase).

Results of biochemical observations in serum and heart tissues were supplemented by histopathological examination of rat's heart sections to confirm the myocardial injury. The results were comparable to that of a gliclazide-treated group. These results provide evidence that pre-treatment with aqueous Embelia extract ameliorated myocardial injury, enhanced the anti-oxidant defense against isoproterenol-induced myocardial infarction in rats, and exhibited cardioprotective property.[17]

Anti-microbial activity

Embelin was demonstrated to have anti-bacterial activity against the following Staphylococcus strains: Staphylococcus aureus, albus, and citreus.[18]

Analgesic activity

Potassium embelate has been shown to have an analgesic value.[19] Laboratory research with mice and rats showed the substance to be a centrally acting analgesic. This activity may involve mixed binding sites in the brain. Embelin's analgesic activity was comparable to that of morphine, although it was not antagonized by naloxone, which indicates that it may involve a central site of action different from opiates.[20]

Anti-oxidant activity

Anti-oxidants have been the focus of studies for developing neuroprotective agents to be used in the therapy for stroke, which is an acute and progressive neurodegenerative disorder and is the second leading cause of death throughout the world. Many herbal anti-oxidants have been developed in in-vitro and in-vivo experiments, and some of these have been tested in clinical studies for stroke.

Embelia ribes has been reported to have neuroprotective effect of ethanolic extract of Embelia fruits on middle cerebral artery occlusion induced focal cerebral ischemia in rats. Male Wistar albino rats were fed an ethanolic Embelia extract for 30 days. After the 30 days, all of the animals were anesthetized with chloral hydrate. The right middle cerebral artery was occluded with a 4-0 suture for 2 hours. Then the suture was removed to allow reperfusion injury. Ischemia, followed by reperfusion in the ischemic-group rats, significantly reduced the grip strength activity and non-enzymatic and enzymatic anti-oxidant levels in the hippocampus and frontal cortex compared to the sham-operated rats.[21] Serum lactate dehydrogenase and thiobarbituric acid reactive substance levels in the hippocampus and frontal cortex were increased significantly in the ischemic group compared to the sham-operated rats. Pre-treatment with ethanolic Embelia extracts significantly increased the grip strength activity, and GSH, GPx, GR, and GST levels in the hippocampus and frontal cortex, with a significant decrease in LDH levels in serum and TBARS levels in hippocampus and frontal cortex compared to the middle cerebral artery occlusion group rats. These results suggest that chronic treatment with ethanolic Embelia extract enhances the anti-oxidant defense against middle cerebral artery occlusion induced focal cerebral ischemia in rats and exhibits neuroprotective activity.

A study aimed to find out the protective effect of ethanolic extract of Embelia ribes fruits on homocysteine, lactate dehydrogenase (LDH), and lipid profile in serum, lipid peroxidation (LPO), and non-enzymatic anti-oxidant glutathione (GSH) levels in brain homogenates and histopathological examination of brain tissue in methionine (1 g/kg body weight, orally for 30 days) induced hyperhomocysteinemic rats.[22] A significant increase in homocysteine, LDH, total cholesterol, triglycerides, low density lipoprotein (LDL-C), and very low density lipoprotein (VLDL-C) levels was observed in serum. Other salient features observed in the methionine-treated pathogenic control rats were increased LPO levels in brain homogenates with reduced serum high density lipoprotein (HDL-C) levels and decreased GSH content. Administration of ethanolic Embelia ribes extract (100 mg/kg body weight, orally) for 30 days to methionine-induced hyperhomocysteinemic rats produced a significant decrease in the levels of homocysteine, LDH, total cholesterol, triglycerides, and LDL-C, VLDL-C in serum and LPO levels in brain homogenates, with a significant increase in serum HDL-C levels and GSH content in brain homogenates, when compared with pathogenic control rats. Biochemical observations were further substantiated with a histological examination of the brain. Degenerative changes of neuronal cells in methionine-treated rats were minimized to near normal morphology by administration of ethanolic Embelia ribes extract, as evidenced by histopathological examination.

Anti-plaque activity

Fruit extracts of Embelia ribes prevented the adherence of viable cells of Staphylococcus mutans to smooth surfaces, and also had anti-enzymatic action against glucosyltransferase. The principle constituent in this activity was found to be embelin, which inhibited the bacterial growth at a concentration of 62.5 Ug/ml and glucan synthesis at an IC_{50} of 125 ug/ml.[23] Staphylococcus mutans has been implicated in pathogenesis of periodontal disease. Embelia ribes has shown in-vitro to prevent adhesion of staphylococcus mutans, there by preventing plaque formation which eventually can lead to severe periodontal disease.

Chemoprotective activity

The effects of embelin (50 mg/kg/day), a benzoquinone derivative of Embelia ribes, and the effects of curcumin (100 mg/kg/day)—the active principle of Curcuma longa, against N-nitrosodiethylamine (DENA)-initiated and phenobarbital (PB)-promoted hepatocarcinogenesis—were studied in Wistar rats. This prevented the induction of hepatic hyperplastic nodules, body weight loss, increase in the levels of hepatic diagnostic markers, and hypoproteinemia induced by DENA/PB treatment.[24]

Insecticidal activity

Embelin was evaluated for its potential to control Tribolium castaneum, a common pest that destroys wheat crops. Embelin caused adult mortality in this species, which lasted even after 8 months of wheat storage. The pest's reproduction rate also declined significantly.[25]

Also, embelin has been shown to protect wheat against several other insect species, including Sitophilus oryzae, Rhyzopertha dominica, and Ephestia cautella. Embelin increased mortality and decreased reproduction rates in Sitophilus oryzae and Rhyzopertha dominica, and significantly reduced the adult emergence of Ephestia cautella.[26]

Ethnoveterinary Usage

Embelia fruits are used to treat bloating in ruminants.[27]

Dr. Sodhi's Experience

Vidanga is highly useful as an antiparasitic and antihelmintic. It quickly and effectively expels many intestinal parasites, including roundworms, tapeworms, and pinworms. Its action against worms is so rapid that dead parasites are visible in the stool almost immediately after the herb is ingested.

Case History

A 5-year-old boy came to my clinic in India reporting constant vomiting that had lasted 5 days. His parents had taken him to several doctors, and he had been given various antiemetics, which had not been able to cure vomiting. After only a few hours with one of these treatments, the child's vomiting had started again.

When I examined the boy's throat, I noticed something that looked like a worm at the back. I used a forceps to remove it and found that it was a roundworm almost 9 inches long. Somehow it had become lodged in the boy's esophagus and was causing the incessant vomiting. Even though he had complained about feeling irritation in his throat, no one had realized that this was the source of the vomiting.

I gave the boy ½ teaspoon of Embelia powder immediately, and instructed the parents to examine the boy's stool the next day. They reported that he had voided bunches of roundworms resembling balls of hair.

At the Ayurvedic and Naturopathic Clinic, we routinely treat roundworm infections with a combination formula containing Embelia ribes (vidanga), along with Azadirachta indica (neem), Piper longum (Pippli), Aegle marmelos (bilva), Momordica charantia (karela), Berberis aristata (daaruhaldi), Holarrhena antidysenterica (kutaj), and Ocimum sanctum (tulsi).

Herbal Protocol

For roundworm:

> First, the patient should drink a sweetened solution made from sweet juices and/or honey to attract the worm. Then, 15 to 20 minutes later, the patient should take 1000 mg of the following herbal formula: Azadirachta indica (neem), Embelia ribes (vidanga), Piper longum (Pippli), Aegle marmelos (bilva), Momordica charantia (karela), Berberis aristata (daaruhaldi), Holarrhena antidysenterica (kutaj), and Ocimum sanctum (tulsi). This formulation should be continued three times a day for 7 days. After one week, the formulation may be reduced to 500 mg for one month. During this time, the pre-dose of sweetened solution is not necessary.

Safety Profile

Embelia generally is regarded as safe for short-term use at its recommended doses. Because of its contraceptive properties, using Embelia for several months can eventually cause infertility. Its safety with pregnant or nursing women and those with severe liver or kidney diseases is not known. The 50% alcoholic extract of the seed showed an LD_{50} value of 750 mg/kg body weight when administered IP in mice.[28]

Dosage

Powder: 6–12 g (adult), 2–3 grams (children)
Decoction: 14-28 ml

Ayurvedic Properties

Guna: Laghu (light), ruksha (dry), tikshna (sharp)
Rasa: Katu (pungent)
Veerya: Ushna (lukewarm)
Vipaka: Katu (pungent)
Dosha: Balances kapha and vata

Notes

1. T.V. Rao and W. Padmanabha, "Some natural and synthetic methyl-enebisbenzoquinones," *Bulletin of the National Institute of Science of India*, 1965, 28:14.

2. R. Ahmad, I. Ahmad, A. Mannan, F. Ahmad, and S.M. Osman, "Studies on minor seed oils XI," *Fette Seifen Arzneimittel*, 1986, 88(4):147.

3. See Notes 1 and 2.

4. T. Namba, M. Tsunezuka, DMRB Dissanayake, et al., "Studies on dental caries prevention by traditional medicines (Part VII): Screening of Ayurvedic medicines for anti-plaque action," *Shoyakugaku Zasshi*, 1985, 39(2):146.

5. V.P. Dixit and S.K. Bhargava, "Reversible contraception-like activity of embelin in male dogs *(Canis indicus* Linn)," *Andrologia*, 1983, 15(5):486.

6. T.V. Purandare, S.D. Kholkute, and A. Gurjar, et al., "Semen analysis and hormonal levels in bonnet macaques administered *Embelia ribes* berries, an indigenous plant having contraceptive activity," *Indian Journal of Experimental Biology*, 1979, 17(9):935.

7. C. Seshadri, D. Suganthan, G. Santhakumari, and G.Y.N. Lyer, "Biochemical changes in the uterus and uterine fluid of mated rats treated with embelin—a nonsteroidal oral contraceptive," *Indian Journal of Experimental Biology*, 1978, 16(11): 1187.

8. S. Gupta, S.N, Sanyal, and U. Kanwar, "Antispermatogenic effect of embelin, a plant benzoquinone, on male albino rats *in vivo* and *in vitro*," *Contraception*, 1989, 39(3):307.

9. S.D Seth, N. Johri, and K.R. Sundaram, "Antispermatogenic effect of embelin from *Embelia ribes*," *Indian Journal of Pharmacology*, 1982, 14(2):207.

10. M. Krishnaswamy and K.K. Purushothaman, "Antifertility properties *of Embelia ribes* (embelin)," *Indian Journal of Experimental Biology*, 1980, 18(11):1359.

11. M. Chitra, E. Sukumar, and C.S. Shyamala, "[3H]-Thymidine uptake and lipid peroxidation by tumor cells on embelin treatment: An *in vitro* study," Oncology, 1995, 52(1):66.

12. M. Chitra, E. Sukumar, V. Suja, and C.S. Shyamala Devi , "Effect of embelin on enzyme profile in experimental fibrosarcoma," *Indian Journal of Medical and Scientific Research*, 1994, 22(12):877.

13. L.V. Guru and D.N. Mishra, "Effect of the alcoholic and aqueous extractives *of Embelia ribes* (Burm.) in patients infested by ascarides," *Journal of Research in Indian Medicine*, 1966, 1:47.

14. U. Bhandari and M.N. Ansari, "Antihyperglycemic activity of aqueous extract of Embelia ribes Burm in streptozotocin-induced diabetic rats," *Indian J Exp Biol.*, Aug. 2008, 46(8):607–613.

15. U. Bhandari, N. Jain, and K.K. Pillai, "Further studies on anti-oxidant potential and protection of pancreatic beta-cells by Embelia ribes in experimental diabetes," *Exp Diabetes Res.*, 2007, 2007volume?:Article: 15803. THERE is no page number for this this is fine and can be searched very easily using the article ID

16. Bhandari U, Kanojia R, Pillai KK. Effect of ethanolic extract of Embelia ribes on dyslipidemia in diabetic rats. Int J Exp Diabetes Res. 2002 Jul-Sep;3(3):159-62.

17. U. Bhandari, M.N. Ansari, and F. Islam, "Cardioprotective effect of aqueous extract of Embelia ribes Burm fruits against isoproterenol-induced myocardial infarction in albino rats," *Indian J Exp Biol.*, Jan. 2008, 46(1):35-40.

18. R.H Gopal and K.K.,"Purushothaman, Effect of new plant isolates and extracts on bacteria," *Bulletin of Medical Ethnobotany Research*, 1986, 7(l–2):78.

19. U. Zutshi, R.K. John, and C.K. Atal, "Possible interaction of potassium embelate, a putative analgesic agent, with opiate receptors," *Indian Journal of Experimental Biology*, 1989, 7(7):656.

20. C.K. Atal, M.A. Siddiqui, U. Zutshi, et al., "A non-narcotic, orally effective, centrally acting analgesic from an Ayurvedic drug," *Journal of Ethnopharmacology*, 1984, 11(3):309.

21. M. Nazam Ansari, U. Bhandari, F. Islam, and C.D. Tripathi CD, "Evaluation of anti-oxidant and neuroprotective effect of ethanolic extract of Embelia ribes Burm in focal cerebral ischemia/reperfusion-induced oxidative stress in rats," *Fundam Clin Pharmacol.*, June 2008, 22(3):305–314.

22. M.N. Ansari and U. Bhandari, "Protective effect of Embelia ribes Burm on methionine-induced hyperhomocysteinemia and oxidative stress in rat brain," *Indian J Exp Biol.*, July 2008, 46(7):521–527.

23. Chitra M, Devi CS, Sukumar E. Anti-bacterial activity of embelin. Fitoterapia. 2003 Jun;74(4):401-3.

24. M. Sreepriya and G. Bali, "Chemopreventive effects of embelin and curcumin against N-nitrosodiethylamine/phenobarbital-induced hepatocarcinogenesis in Wistar rats," *Fitoterapia*. Sept. 2005, 76(6):549–555.

25. H. Chander and S.M. Ahmed, "Efficacy of natural embelin against the red flour *beetle, Tribolium castaneum* Herbst," *Insect Science and its Application*, 1985, 6(2):217.

26. H. Chander and S.M. Ahmed, "Comparative evaluation of fungicidal quinones and natural embelin against some insect pests of storage," *Journal of Stored Products Research*, 1989, 25(2):87.

27. International Institute of Rural Reconstruction Ethnoveterinary Medicine in Asia, "An information kit on traditional animal health care practices" (Silang, Philippines: IIRR, 1994).

28. B.N. Dhawan, M.P. Dubey, B.N. Mehrotra, R.R. Rastogi, and J.S.Tandon, "Screening of Indian medicinal plants for biological activity: Part-IX," *Indian Journal of Experimental Biology*, 1980, 18:594.

22

Glycyrrhiza glabra

Introduction

Glycyrrhiza glabra, commonly known as licorice, has been used for centuries in the traditional and folk medicines of Asia and Europe to treat ailments ranging from the common cold to liver disease. Historical mention of licorice as a curative plant dates back thousands of years. Hippocrates first recorded the use of licorice as early as 300 B.C. The first century Roman naturalist Pliny noted that licorice is native to Sicily. Theophrastus mentioned the sweet flavor of licorice root and cited it as useful for treating asthma, dry cough, and all diseases of the lungs. Though not native to Germany, licorice was well-known there by the eleventh century and was extensively grown in Bavaria by the end of the sixteenth century. Cultivation of licorice was recorded in Spain during the thirteenth century.

Licorice stick is the sweet, distinctively-flavored root of the plant. The sweetest sections are found in the horizontal stems (or stolons) that grow off of the vertical taproot and may extend as far as 8 meters) from the main root. Cut into small sections, these underground stems are widely available in the herb market. Licorice root often is made into candy because of its distinctive taste and intense sweetness.

In Ayurvedic tradition, licorice is considered to be a rasayana. It is an important ingredient in many herbal preparations, and is used especially for bronchial conditions. Western herbalists use licorice to treat ulcers, as an anti-inflammatory, and as an expectorant, and in Chinese herbal medicine, licorice is valued as a rejuvenative and an aphrodisiac.

Because of its expectorant properties, powdered licorice has been used for centuries to treat cough and bronchial conditions. Modern cough syrups often contain licorice extract. Licorice also is contained in tooth powders and for freshening the breath. Because of its significant anti-ulcer properties, licorice is included in conventional and naturopathic preparations to treat mouth ulcers as well as peptic ulcers.

In Ayurveda, licorice is described as a tonic, laxative, demulcent, and emollient. It finds particular use in cough, catarrh, bronchitis, fever, gastritis, gastric and duodenal ulcers, and skin diseases and as a general tonic. A tincture made from licorice root may be applied externally to cuts and wounds, and in the treatment of hyperdipsia, genitourinary diseases, and as a corticosteroid replacement agent.

Synonymous Names

English: Licorice
Hindi: Mulethi
Sanskrit: Yashtimadhu, madhuka

The name Glycyrrhiza was given to this plant in the first century. It is derived from the Greek words "glukos," meaning "sweet," and "rhiza," meaning "root." Theophrastus referred to it as "Radix Dulcis," from the Latin equivalent.

Habitat

Glycyrrhiza glabra is indigenous to the Mediterranean region and the Middle East, and varieties of the genus grow in many other temperate and subtropical regions of the world. The plant is cultivated in Greece, Russia, Turkey, China, and parts of Europe. It is commercially available in many forms virtually everywhere. The licorice plant grows best in deep, fertile, well-drained soils with full sun, and is harvested in the autumn two to three years after planting.

Botanical Characteristics

Licorice is a hardy, perennial shrub, which typically reaches a height of 3 to 7 feet. Its leaves are compound and alternate, having four-to-seven pairs of oblong, elliptical, or lanceolate leaflets. The lavender-to-violet flowers are narrow and grow in axillary spikes. The calyx is short, campanulate, with lanceolate tips and glandular hairs. The fruit is a compressed legume or pod, up to 1.5cm long, erect, glabrous, somewhat reticulately pitted, and usually contains three-to-five brown, reniform seeds.

The licorice taproot is approximately 4-5 feet long and subdivides into three-to-five subsidiary roots from which the horizontal woody stolons arise. These may reach 8 meters, and when dried and cut, together with the root, constitute commercial licorice. The taproot may be found peeled or unpeeled. The pieces of root break with a fibrous fracture, revealing the yellowish interior with a characteristic odor and sweet taste.

Chemical Composition

Triterpene saponins:
  A unique saponin, Glycyrrhizin (glycyrrhizic acid), and its aglycone, glycyrrhetmic acid, are the chemicals responsible for the sweet taste of licorice. Other derivatives and glycosides are present such as glycyrrhizol, glabrins A and B, glycyrrhetol, glabrolide, isoglabrolide and others.[1]

Flavonoids and isoflavonoids:
  During drying and storage, liquiritin undergoes partial conversion to isoliquiritin and the aglycones, liquiritigenin and isoliquirkigenin, isolicoflavonol, licoagrodione, glucoliquiritin apioside, prenyllicoflavone A, shinflavone, shinpterocarpin, 1-methoxyphyaseollin and rhamnoliquirilin.[2]

  A variety of isoflavones also have been isolated from the licorice plant, including formononetin, glabrene, neoliquiritin, hispaglabridin A and B, glabridin, glabrol, 3-hydroxyglarol. glycyrrhisflavone, 4-O-methylglabridin, 3'-hydroxy-4'-O-methylglabridin, and many 2-methyl isoflavones.

Coumarins and coumestan derivatives:
  Herniarin, C-liqucoumarin, 6-acetyl-5,hydroxy-4-methylcoumarin, glycycoumarin and licopyanocoumarin have been identified.

Phytosterols:
  Stigmasterol, onocerin, p-sitosterol and beta-amyrin.

Volatile oils:
  Licorice contains a trace amount (0.5%) of volatile oil containing anethole, estragole, eugenol, and hexanoic acid as the main constituents.

Pharmacological Activity

Anti-ulcerogenic activity

Licorice has demonstrated anti-ulcerogenic properties. Research has shown the plant to be as effective as the drugs cimetidine and pirenzapine in its healing properties for peptic ulcers. One study showed that an Ayurvedic preparation containing licorice increased p-glucuronidase activity in the Brunner's glands, making it effective against duodenal ulcers.[3,4,5]

Health-care practitioners in Europe and Japan often prescribe a synthetic form of licorice to treat stomach ulcers. Although this drug is not available in the United States, many health-care providers use deglycyrrhizinated licorice (DGL) to treat gastric ulcers. DGL is a licorice supplement in which the component glycyrrhizin is removed. Glycyrrhizin has been reported to cause increases in blood pressure.

Animal studies and early trials in humans support the value of licorice to treat stomach ulcers. One animal study found that aspirin coated with licorice reduced the number of ulcers in rats by 50%. (High doses of aspirin often cause ulcers in rats).[6] Earlier studies in humans have found that preparations containing glycyrrhizin may be as effective as leading anti-ulcer medications in relieving the pain associated with stomach ulcers. The substance also may prevent the ulcers from recurring. In one study, licorice root fluid extract was used to treat 100 patients with stomach ulcers (of which 86 had not improved after using conventional medication) for 6 weeks. Of these patients, 90% improved, and the ulcers totally disappeared in 22 of them.[7]

Licorice has been widely used in European herbal medicine as a treatment for gastric ulcers. Modern use began in 1946, when the Dutch physician F. E. Revers demonstrated that licorice was the active ingredient in a domestic medicine used in the Netherlands. When the substance was studied for this use, good results were obtained in treating stomach ulcers in 32 patients.[8]

In the 1950s, research indicated that licorice derived compounds can raise the concentration of prostaglandins in the digestive system that promote mucous secretion from the stomach, and also produce new cells in the stomach lining. It also was shown that licorice prolongs the lifespan of surface cells in the stomach and has an antipepsin effect. These combined effects lead to the healing of ulcers.[9]

A study from Germany had shown that Glycyrrhiza significantly inhibited the adhesion of Helicobacter pylori to human stomach tissue. According to the study, this effect was related to the polysaccharides isolated from the extract, with one purified acidic fraction as the main active polymer. In addition, raw polysaccharides from Glycyrrhiza were shown to have strong anti-adhesive effects against Porphyromonas gingivalis.[10] A review of the literature suggests that Glycyrrhiza also has moderate cytotoxic effect on H.pylori.[11,12]

Lipids, heart, and anti-obesity activity

Emerging studies are beginning to suggest that licorice may play a role in the treatment of heart disease by reducing LDL cholesterol levels. In one study, people with high cholesterol experienced a significant reduction in total cholesterol, LDL cholesterol, and triglyceride levels after taking licorice root extracts for one month. The extract also reduced systolic blood pressure. Unfortunately, however, these decreases in cholesterol levels were followed by a "rebound effect" when therapy with the licorice was discontinued. When these subjects stopped taking the licorice, cholesterol levels reverted to the previous elevated condition.[13]

Another study concluded that glycyrrhizic acids could counteract the development of visceral obesity and improve dyslipidemia via selective induction of tissue lipoprotein lipase LPL expression and a positive shift in serum lipid parameters, respectively, and retard the development of insulin resistance associated with tissue steatosis[14]

A study in humans showed that a preparation of licorice may reduce body fat. Fifteen normal weight subjects consumed licorice for 2 months (3.5 grams a day). Body fat mass was measured before and after treatment. The licorice was able to reduce body fat mass and to suppress the hormone aldosterone.[15] Another study found that a topical preparation of glycyrrhetinic acid resulted in reduction in the thickness of fat on the thighs of the human subjects.[16]

Acyl-coenzyme A, diacylglycerol acyltransferase (DGAT) catalyzes triglyceride synthesis in the glycerol phosphate pathway. It has a relationship with the excess supply and accumulation of triglycerides. Therefore, DGAT inhibitors may offer potential therapy for obesity and type 2 diabetes.

Five flavonoids were isolated from the ethanol extracts of licorice roots, using an in-vitro DGAT inhibitory assay. One isoprenyl flavonoid showed the most potential inhibition of DGAT of the five flavonoids (1-5). On the basis of spectral evidences, the compound was identified as glabrol (5). Compound 5 glabrol inhibited rat liver microsomal DGAT activity with an IC50 value of 8.0 microM, but the IC50 value for four flavonoids (1–4) was more than 100 microM. In addition, glabrol showed a noncompetitive type of inhibition against DGAT. These data suggest that potential therapy for the treatment in obesity and type 2 diabetes patients by licorice roots might be related to its DGAT inhibitory effect.[17]

Hepatoprotective activity

An alcoholic extract of licorice increased the cumulative biliary and urinary excretion of acetaminophen without affecting the thioether or sulphate conjugates. It also increased glucuronidation in rats, suggesting that it may influence the detoxification of xenobiotics.[18]

Liver fibrosis has been characterized as chronic inflammatory processes involving multiple molecular pathogenetic pathways. A therapeutic study investigated whether a combination regimen of Salvia miltiorrhiza (S), Ligusticum chuanxiong (L), and Glycyrrhiza glabra (G) exerted in-vivo antifibrotic effects on rats with hepatic fibrosis.[19] Fibrosis was induced in rats by dimethylnitrosamine (DMN) administration for 4 weeks. The fibrotic rats were randomly assigned to one of the three groups: control, combination of Salvia, Ligusticum and Glycyrrhiza (SLG) (50 mg/kg), or silymarin (50 mg/kg), and each received gavage twice daily for 3 weeks starting one week after DMN injection. The results showed that fibrosis scores of livers from DMN-treated rats with SLG (1.13 +/- 0.13) were significantly reduced in comparison to the DMN-treated rats receiving vehicle (1.63 +/- 0.18). Moreover, the hepatic collagen content of DMN rats was significantly reduced by either SLG or silymarin treatment. The double immunohistochemical staining results also showed that alpha-SMA positive cells with NF kappa B nuclear translocation were decreased in the fibrotic livers after SLG and silymarin treatments. The mRNA expression levels of TGF-beta1, alpha-SMA, collagen1 alpha 2, iNOS, and ICAM-1 genes were attenuated by SLG and silymarin treatment. The results showed that SLG exerted antifibrotic effects in the rats with DMN-induced hepatic fibrosis.

A systematic review reported significant improvements in virological and/or biochemical response in trials of vitamin E, thymic extract, zinc, traditional Chinese medicine, Glycyrrhiza glabra, and oxymatrine.[20]

Anti-oxidant activity

Traditionally, licorice has been used in the prevention of liver diseases.[21] An increase was seen in the lag phase of oxidation of ascorbate free radicals in the liver and myocardia of experimental animals when licorice was administered. The anti-oxidant activity of the root powder was comparable to that of beta-carotene and caused markedly decreased lipid peroxides in the liver.[22]

Isoflavonoids extracted from licorice examined the protective ability in liver mitochondria against oxidative stresses. This effect was determined to be caused by inhibition of mitochondrial lipid peroxidation-related respiratory electron transport.[23]

Low-density lipoprotein (LDL) oxidation is a prominent risk factor of early arteriosclerosis. The isoflavonoid glabridin and its derivatives were shown to contribute to the anti-oxidant activity induced by heavy metal ions and macrophages against low density lipoprotein oxidation.[24] The isoflavonoids also showed a potent scavenging effect on the DPPH radical and were able to chelate heavy metals.

Glabridin also inhibited the susceptibility of LDL to oxidation in an atherosclerotic apolipoprotein E deficient and in-vitro human LDL oxidation model and prevented the consumption of beta-carotene and lycopene.[25]

Further experiments with glabridin and accompanying isoflavans suggested that glabridin is a potent isoflavones of cholesterol linoleate hydroperoxide formation.[26]

In an ex-vivo study, LDL isolated from the plasma of 10 normolipidemic subjects who were orally supplemented for 2 weeks with 100 mg licorice/d was more resistant to oxidation than was LDL isolated before licorice supplementation. Dietary supplementation of each E-zero mouse with licorice (200 micrograms/d) or pure glabridin (20 micrograms/d) for 6 weeks resulted in a substantial reduction in the susceptibility of their LDL to oxidation along with a reduction in the atherosclerotic lesion area. These results could be related to the absorption and binding of glabridin to the LDL particle and subsequent protection of the LDL from oxidation by multiple modes as shown in humans and in E-zero mice.[27]

DHC-1, an herbal formulation derived from the popular plants Bacopa monniera, Emblica officinalis, Glycyrrhiza glabra, Mangifera indica, and Syzygium aromaticum was studied for its anti-oxidant activity. The protective effect of DHC-1 in isoproterenol-induced myocardial infarction and cisplatin-induced renal damage was studied. A significant reduction in the serum markers of heart and kidney damage and the extent of lipid peroxidation with a concomitant increase in the enzymatic (SOD and CAT) and non-enzymatic anti-oxidants (reduced glutathione) were observed in the DHC-1 pre-treated animals compared to the isoproterenol or cisplatin alone-treated animals.[28]

Some studies had different view, though. Antinephritis activity of glabridin, a pyranoisoflavan isolated from Glycyrrhiza glabra, was evaluated after its oral administration to mice with glomerular disease (Masugi-nephritis) by measuring the urinary protein excretion, total cholesterol, serum creatinine, and blood urea nitrogen levels. Administration of glabridin for 10 days (30 mg kg(-1) day(-1)) reduced the amount of urinary protein excretion from the control level (100+/-23 mg/day) to a significantly lower level (47+/-4 mg/day). ESR spectroscopy demonstrated that glabridin neither produced radical nor affected the radical intensity of, sodium ascorbate, suggesting the lack of correlation between the antinephritis activity and radical scavenging activity.[29]

Anti-cancer activity

Licorice potentiated the antitumor and antimetastatic activity of cyclophosphamide when tested in metastasising Lewis lung carcinoma.[30] Extracts have been assayed for cytotoxicity in-vitro using the Yoshida ascites sarcoma. The petroleum ether extract exhibited a more potent activity than other solvent extracts.[31]

Licorice has been shown to be a protective against skin tumorigenesis caused by DMBA (7,12-dimethyl-benz [a] anthracene) initiation and 12-O-tetradecanoylphorbol-13-acetate promotion. The latency period of tumor onset was increased and the number of tumors decreased, possibly because the carcinogen metabolism was inhibited after DNA adduct formation.[32]

Licochalcone-A, a substance in licorice root, has been discovered to kill cancer cells in the laboratory. Laboratory cultures of cancer cells from human leukemia, breast, and prostate cancers were killed when the licorice extract was added.[33]

Anti-mutagenic activity

The anti-mutagenic activity of Glycyrrhiza glabra root and its isolated constituents was assessed for its effectiveness against ethyl methanesulphonate, N-methyl-N'-nitro-N-nitrosoguanidine, and ribose-lysine Maillard models of mutagenesis, using a salmonella microsome reversion assay. Glycyrrhiza extract showed marked antimutagenicity against the ethyl methanesulphonate and 18-p glycyrrhetinic acid, and demonstrated a significant desmutagenic activity against a ribose-lysine mutagen browning mixture.[34]

Anti-microbial activity

Licorice extracts contain flavonoids, which showed significant antimycotic activity when evaluated using strains of Candida albicans isolated from clinical samples of acute vaginitis.[35] The flavonoid constituents isolated from licorice root cultures also exhibited antimicrobial activity when tested by the disc diffusion method.[36] Hispaglabridin A and B, glabridin, glabrol, 3-hydroxyglabrol, and 4'-O-methylglabridin also have demonstrated significant anti-microbial activity.[37]

A double-blind, placebo-controlled, randomized pilot clinical trial of ImmunoGuard—a standardized combination of Andrographis, Eleutherococcus, Schizandra, and Glycyrrhiza—was conducted in patients with Familial Mediterranean Fever (FMF). The study was conducted in 24 (3-to-15 years of age of both genders) patients with FMF. Of these, 14 were treated with ImmunoGuard and 10 received the series B product (placebo). The study medication was taken three times, four tablets daily, for 1 month. The primary outcome measures in the physician's evaluation were related to duration, frequency, and severity of attacks in the FMF patients (attacks characteristics score). Each patient's self-evaluation was based mainly on symptoms—abdominal, chest pains, temperature, arthritis, myalgia and erysipelas-like erythema. All three features (duration, frequency, severity of attacks) showed significant improvement in the ImmunoGuard group compared to the placebo. In both the clinical and the self evaluations, the severity of attacks was found to show the most significant improvement in the ImmunoGuard group. Both the clinical and the laboratory results of the phase II (pilot) clinical study suggest that ImmunoGuard is a safe and efficacious herbal drug for the management of patients with FMF.[38]

Anti-viral activity

Glycyrrhizin demonstrated anti-viral activity against Japanese encephalitis virus and inhibited plaque formation at a concentration of 500 ug.[39] It also was shown to inhibit viral growth and deactivate viral particles.[40]

Further research suggests that licorice may play a role in the treatment of human immunodeficiency virus (HIV). A preliminary study conducted with three HIV patients suggested that intravenous glycyrrhizin may prevent replication of HIV.[41]

Historical sources for the use of Glycyrrhiza species include ancient manuscripts from China,

India, and Greece. They all mention its use to alleviate symptoms of viral respiratory tract infections and hepatitis.

Randomized controlled trials confirmed that the Glycyrrhiza glabra-derived compound glycyrrhizin and its derivatives alleviated hepatocellular damage in chronic hepatitis B and C. In hepatitis C virus-induced cirrhosis, the risk of hepatocellular carcinoma was reduced. Animal studies demonstrated a reduction of mortality and viral activity in herpes simplex virus encephalitis and influenza A virus pneumonia. In-vitro studies revealed anti-viral activity against HIV-1, SARS related coronavirus, respiratory syncytial virus, arboviruses, vaccinia virus, and vesicular stomatitis virus. Mechanisms for anti-viral activity of Glycyrrhiza spp. include reduced transport to the membrane and sialylation of hepatitis B virus surface antigen, reduction of membrane fluidity leading to inhibition of fusion of the viral membrane of HIV-1 with the cell, induction of interferon gamma in T-cells, inhibition of phosphorylating enzymes in vesicular stomatitis virus infection, and reduction of viral latency.[42]

Several investigations were undertaken to identify the definite root by which glycyrrhizin protects cells from infection with influenza A virus (IAV). The researchers found that glycyrrhizin treatment leads to a clear reduction in the number of IAV-infected human lung cells, as well as a reduction in the CCID50 titer by 90%. The anti-viral effect, however, was limited to one or two virus replication cycles. Analysis of different glycyrrhizin treatment protocols suggested that the anti-viral effect of glycyrrhizin was limited to an early step in the virus replication cycle.

A direct inhibitory action of glycyrrhizin on IAV particles could be excluded, and did not interact with the virus receptor binding either. The anti-viral effect of glycyrrhizin was abolished by treatment 1 hour after virus infection, whereas pre-treatment and treatment during and after virus adsorption led to a reduction in the cytopathic effect, reduced viral RNA within the cells and in the cell supernatants, and reduced viral hemagglutination titers. Detailed virus uptake analyses unambiguously demonstrated reduced virus uptake in various glycyrrhizin-treated cells. Glycyrrhizin showed anti-viral activity by an interaction with the cell membrane, which most likely results in reduced endocytotic activity and hence reduced virus uptake.[43]

Immune modulation

The increasing use of medicinal herbs by the general public has piqued the need for scientific-based research to determine the action of herbs administered orally in human subjects. The ability of three herbs—Echinacea purpurea, Astragalus membranaceus, and Glycyrrhiza glabra—to activate immune cells in human subjects was assessed in this pilot study. The effect of these herbs when ingested for 7 days was measured both when administered singly and in combination, using flow cytometry. The primary cell activation marker measured was CD69. The results demonstrate that Echinacea, Astragalus, and Glycyrrhiza herbal tinctures stimulated immune cells, as quantified by CD69 expression on CD4 and CD8 T cells. This activation took place within 24 hours after ingestion, and continued for at least 7 days. These three herbs also had an additive effect on CD69 expression when used in combination.[44]

Anti-inflammatory activity

Glycyrrhizin, a major active constituent of licorice root (Glycyrrhiza glabra), has a free radical scavenging property, and its effects were evaluated on an animal model of spinal cord injury induced by the application of vascular clips (force of 24 g) to the dura via a T5-T8 laminectomy. Spinal cord injury in mice resulted in severe trauma characterized by edema, tissue damage, and apoptosis (measured by terminal deoxynucleotidyltransferase-mediated dUTP-biotin end labeling staining, Bax, and Bcl-2 expression). Immunohistochemical examination demonstrated a marked increase in immunoreactivity for nitrotyrosine, iNOS, and poly adenosine diphosphate-ribose in the spinal cord tissue. These inflammatory events were associated with the activation of nuclear factor-kappaB. In contrast, the degree of (1) spinal cord inflammation and tissue injury (histological score), (2) nitrotyrosine and poly(adenosine diphosphate [ADP] ribose) formation, (3) iNOS expression, (4) nuclear factor kappaB activation, and (5) apoptosis (terminal deoxynucleotidyltransferase-mediated dUTP-biotin end labeling, Bax, and Bcl-2) was markedly reduced in spinal cord tissue obtained from mice treated with glycyrrhizin extract (10 mg/kg, i.p., 30 min before and 1 and 6 h after SCI).[45]

In a separate set of experiments, the researchers clearly demonstrated that glycyrrhizin extract treatment significantly ameliorated the recovery of limb function (evaluated by motor recovery score). Taken together, the results clearly demonstrate that treatment with glycyrrhizin extract reduces the development of inflammation and tissue injury events associated with spinal cord trauma.[46]

The saponin Glycyrrhizin was shown to inhibit thrombin-induced platelet aggregation, which indicates anti-inflammatory activity. Glycyrrhizin also prolonged plasma re-calcification and extended fibrogen clotting times. Glyderinine, a derivative of glycyrrhizic acid, reduced inflammation via the adrenal cortex and suppressed vascular permeability and antipyretic activity without causing ulceration.[47]

Oral administration of Licorice extract reduced clinical arthritis score, paw swelling, and histopathological changes in a murine CIA. Licorice extract decreased the levels of pro-inflammatory cytokines in serum and matrix metalloproteinase-3 expression in the joints. Cell proliferation and cytokine secretion in response to type II collagen or lipopolysaccharide stimulation were suppressed in spleen cells from Licorice extract-treated CIA mice and prevented oxidative damages in liver and kidney tissues of CIA mice.[48]

Hormonal activity

Studies have shown that glycyrrhizin stimulates the excretion of hormones by the adrenal cortex. Some researchers have suggested it as a possible drug to prolong the action of cortisone. Glycyrrhizin has a chemical structure similar to corticosteroids released by the adrenals, and further studies have suggested that it might one day prove useful in improving the function of hormone drugs, or be used as an aid in reducing withdrawal symptoms from dependency on some corticosteroid hormones. Glycyrrhizin also has shown estrogenic activity in laboratory animals.[49]

Abnormal levels of androgens cause many diseases such as benign prostatic hyperplasia, and hormone-dependent cancers. Although the reduction in serum testosterone (T) by Glycyrrhiza glabra has been reported, its effects on seminal vesicle (SV) and prostate tissues have never been reported.

A study was carried out to investigate different aspects of anti-androgenic properties of this plant. Immature male rats were divided into five groups (n = 7): castrated rats without any treatment received only vehicle; castrated rats plus T replacement; and three castrated groups with T replacement plus various doses of Licorice extract (75, 150 and 300 mg/kg). All of the injections were carried out once daily in a subcutaneous manner for 7 days. On the eighth day, blood samples were collected for total T measurement. Ventral prostate (VP), seminal vesicle (SV), and levator ani muscle were dissected and weighed. Slides prepared from the prostate were assessed histologically. The variation in the relative and absolute volume of the prostate tissue compartments was determined. Those receiving the doses of 150 and 300 mg/kg showed a significant reduction (p < 0.05) in prostate weight, total T, and VP epithelium/stroma ratio (V/V). These results in SV and levator ani were shown in response to 300 mg/kg of extract. Increasing in T metabolism, down regulation of androgen receptors, or activation of estrogen receptors could be the mechanisms involved. This study showed that alcoholic extract of Glycyrrhiza glabra has anti-androgenic properties.[50]

Bleeding and clotting time

Ankaferd contains a mixture of Thymus vulgaris, Glycyrrhiza glabra, Vitis vinifera, Alpinia officinarum, and Urtica dioica. Ankaferd Blood Stopper (ABS) has been approved in the management of bleeding. A study was aimed to evaluate the in-vivo hemostatic effect of ABS in rats pre-treated with warfarin. Wistar rats (210–270 g) were treated either with warfarin (2 mg/kg) or vehicle (0.9% NaCl) orally before bilateral hind-leg amputation. ABS was administered topically to one of the amputated legs. The duration of bleeding and the amount of bleeding were measured to evaluate the hemostatic effect of ABS. Topical ABS administration to the amputated leg shortened the duration of bleeding markedly in both untreated and warfarin-treated rats by 31.9% [1.42 min (95% CI: 0.35-2.49)] and 43.5% [5.12 min (95% CI: 2.16-8.07)] respectively. The amount of bleeding in the ABS-administered amputated leg showed a decrease by 53.8% in the warfarin-treated group. It was concluded that ABS has in-vivo hemostatic actions that may provide therapeutic potential for the management of patients with deficient primary hemostasis in clinical medicine.[51]

Similar results were obtained in using ABS for bleeding management after dental surgery. Authors of this study concluded that ABS has demonstrated potential for being an effective hemostatic agent for treating excessive bleeding following dental surgery in four patients with hemorrhagic diathesis.[52]

Glycyrrhizin, an anti-inflammatory compound isolated from licorice (Glycyrrhiza glabra), previously was identified as a thrombin inhibitor.[53] The in-vivo effects of Glycyrrhizin were reported on two experimental models of induced thrombosis in rats. Intravenous administration of Glycyrrhizin caused a dose-dependent reduction in thrombus size on a venous thrombosis model combining stasis and hypercoagulability. It was observed that Glycyrrhizin (GL) at doses of 180 mg/kg body weight produced a 93% decrease on thrombus weight. This effect showed that a time-dependent pattern was significantly reduced when the thrombogenic stimulus was applied 60 minutes after drug administration. GL also was able to prevent thrombosis using an arteriovenous shunt model. GL doses of 180 and 360 mg/kg decreased the thrombus weight by 35% and 90%, respectively. Accordingly, the APTT ex-vivo was enhanced 1.5-fold and 4.3-fold at GL doses of 180 and 360 mg/kg, respectively. In addition, GL doses above 90 mg/kg caused a significant hemorrhagic effect. In contrast to heparin, GL did not potentiate the inhibitory activity of antithrombin III or heparin cofactor II toward thrombin.

Altogether, the data indicate that GL is an effective thrombin inhibitor in-vivo. This may account for its other known pharmacological properties.[54]

Neurological activity

Stroke is a life-threatening disease characterized by rapidly developing clinical signs of focal or global disturbance of cerebral function from cerebral ischemia. A number of flavonoids have been shown to attenuate the cerebral injuries in stroked animal models. Glabridin, a major flavonoid of Glycyrrhiza glabra possesses multiple pharmacological activities.

A study aimed to investigate whether glabridin modulated the cerebral injuries induced by middle cerebral artery occlusion (MCAO) in rats and staurosporine-induced damage in cultured rat cortical neurons and the possible mechanisms involved. The study showed that glabridin at 25mg/kg by intraperitoneal injection, but not at 5mg/kg, significantly decreased the focal infarct volume, cerebral histological damage, and apoptosis in MCAO rats compared to the sham-operated rats.[55] Glabridin significantly attenuated the level of brain malonyldialdehyde (MDA) in the MCAO rats, while it elevated the level of two endogenous anti-oxidants in the brain involved—superoxide dismutase (SOD) and reduced glutathione (GSH). Co-treatment with glabridin significantly inhibited the staurosporine induced cytotoxicity and apoptosis of cultured rat cortical neurons in a concentration-dependent manner. Consistently, glabridin significantly reduced the DNA laddering caused by staurosporine in a concentration-dependent manner. Glabridin also suppressed the elevated Bax protein and caspase-3 proenzyme and decreased bcl-2 induced by staurosporine in cultured rat cortical neurons, facilitating cell survival. Glabridin also inhibited superoxide production in cultured cortical neurons exposed to staurosporine.

These findings indicated that glabridin had a neuroprotective effect via modulation of multiple pathways associated with apoptosis. Further studies are warranted to investigate the biochemical mechanisms for the protective effect of glabridin on neurons and the evidence for clinical use of licorice in the management of cerebral ischemia. A similar study was done using isoliquiritigenin (ISL), a flavonoid constituent in the root of Glycyrrhiza glabra.[56]

A study was undertaken to investigate the effects of aqueous extract of Glycyrrhiza glabra on depression in mice using the forced swim test (FST) and the tail suspension test (TST).[57] The extract of Glycyrrhiza glabra (75, 150, and 300 mg/kg) was administered orally for 7 successive days in separate groups of Swiss young male albino mice. The dose of 150 mg/kg of the extract significantly reduced the immobility times of mice in both FST and TST, without any significant effect on locomotor activity of the mice. The efficacy of extract was found to be comparable to that of imipramine (15 mg/kg i.p.) and fluoxetine (20 mg/kg i.p.). Licorice extract reversed the reserpine induced extension of immobility period of mice in FST and TST. Sulpiride (50 mg/kg i.p.; a selective D2 receptor antagonist) and prazosin (62.5 microg/kg i.p.; an alpha1-adrenoceptor antagonist) significantly attenuated the extract-induced anti-depressant-like effect in TST. Conversely, p-chlorophenylalanine (100 mg/kg i.p.; an inhibitor of serotonin synthesis) did not reverse anti-depressant-like effect of licorice extract. This suggests that the anti-depressant-like effect of licorice extract seems to be mediated by an increase of brain norepinephrine and dopamine, but not by an increase of serotonin. The monoamine oxidase-inhibiting effect of licorice may be contributing favorably to the anti-depressant-like activity.

Anti-allergic activity

Licorice frequently is used in traditional medicine to treat inflammatory and allergic diseases. In a study, the main components (glycyrrhizin, 18beta-glycyrrhetinic acid, isoliquiritin, and liquiritigenin) were isolated from licorice, and their anti-allergic effects, such as anti-scratching behavior and IgE production-inhibitory activity, were evaluated both in-vitro and in-vivo.[58] Liquiritigenin and 18beta-glycyrrhetinic acid most potently inhibited the degranulation of RBL-2H3 cells induced by IgE with the antigen (DNP-HSA) and rat peritoneal mast cells induced by compound 48/80. Liquiritigenin and 18betaglycyrrhetinic acid potently inhibited the passive cutaneous anaphylactic reaction, as well as the scratching behavior in mice induced by compound 48/80. These components inhibited the production of IgE in ovalbumin-induced asthma mice. This suggests that the anti-allergic effects of licorice are attributable mainly to glycyrrhizin,

18beta-glycyrrhetinic acid, and liquiritigenin, which can relieve IgE-induced allergic diseases such as dermatitis and asthma.

Asthma would benefit from a better therapeutic molecule, preferably of natural origin, that has negligible or no adverse effects. In view of this, researchers evaluated Glycyrrhizin, a major constituent of the plant Glycyrrhiza glabra, for its efficacy on asthmatic features in a mouse model of asthma.[59] The BALB/c mice were sensitized and challenged with ovalbumin (OVA) to develop asthmatic features such as airway hyperresponsiveness: allergen-induced airway constriction and airway hyperreactivity (AHR) to methacholine (MCh), and pulmonary inflammation. The mice were treated orally with glycyrrhizin (2.5, 5, 10 and 20 mg/kg) during or after OVA-sensitization and OVA-challenge to evaluate its protective or reversal effect, respectively, on the above asthmatic features. The status of airway hyperresponsiveness was measured by monitoring specific airway conductance (SGaw) using a noninvasive method, and the pulmonary inflammation was assessed by haematoxylin and eosin staining of lung sections. Several other parameters associated with asthma such as interleukin (IL)-4, IL-5 interferon-gamma (IFN-gamma), OVA-specific IgE, total IgG(2a), and cortisol were measured by ELISA. Glycyrrhizin (5 mg/kg) markedly inhibited OVA-induced immediate airway constriction, AHR to MCh ($p<0.01$), lung inflammation, and infiltration of eosinophils in the peribronchial and perivascular areas. It prevented the reduction of IFN-gamma ($p<0.02$), and decreased IL-4 ($p<0.05$), IL-5 ($p<0.05$) and eosinophils ($p<0.0002$) in the BAL fluid. Also, it reduced OVA-specific IgE levels ($p<0.01$) and prevented the reduction of total IgG(2a) ($p<0.01$) in serum. Researchers also have showed that it has no effect on serum cortisol levels.

Glycyrrhiza glabra has been used in herbal medicine to treat skin eruptions, including dermatitis, eczema, pruritus, and cysts. The effect of licorice extract as a topical preparation was evaluated on atopic dermatitis.[60] The plant was collected and extracted by percolation with a suitable solvent. The extract was standardized, based on Glycyrrhizinic acid, using a titrimetry method. Different topical gels were formulated using different co-solvents. After standardizing of topical preparations, the best formulations (1% and 2%) were studied in a double-blind clinical trial in comparison to the base gel on atopic dermatitis over 2 weeks (30 patients in each group). Propylene glycol was the best co-solvent for the extract and Carbopol 940 as gelling agent showed the best results in final formulations. The quantity of glycyrrhizinic acid was determined to be 20.3% in the extract and 19.6% in the topical preparation. The 2% licorice topical gel was more effective than the 1% in reducing the scores for erythema, edema, and itching over two weeks ($p<0.05$). The results showed that licorice extract could be considered as an effective agent for treating atopic dermatitis.

Ethnoveterinary Usage

In India, Glycyrrhiza glabra has been used extensively from ancient times for treating various ailments of domestic animals, with purposes similar to those in humans. For example, it is used for coughs and colds, as an expectorant, and as a wound-healing agent in ruminants.[61]

Safety Profile

Licorice is considered to be safe within the designated therapeutic dosage. Excessive consumption may lead to hypertension and the potentiation of diuretic and corticosteroid activity. Its use in cardiovascular and renal patients is contraindicated as it may lead to a disturbance of electrolytic balance and increased sensitivity to cardiac glycosides as a result of excess excretion of potassium. Its use during breastfeeding also is not recommended.[62]

Studies have demonstrated that licorice flavonoid oil (LFO) is safe when administered once daily up to 1200 mg/day. This is the first report on the safety of licorice flavonoids in an oil preparation.[63]

Dosage

Dried root: 1 – 5 g as an infusion or decoction, three times daily

Licorice 1:5 tincture: 2 – 5 mL, three times daily

Standardized extract: 250 – 500 mg, three times daily, standardized to contain 20% glycyrrhizinic acid

DGL extract: 0.4 – 1.6 g, three times daily, for peptic ulcer

DGL extract 4:1: chew 300 – 400 mg, three times daily 20 minutes before meals, for peptic ulcer

Ayurvedic Properties

Rasa: Madhur (sweet)
Guna: Guru (heavy), snigdha (unctuous)
Veerya: Shita (cold)
Vipaka: Madhur (sweet)
Dosha: Pacifies vata and pitta

Notes

1. Ivan A., Ross, *Medicinal Plants of the World* (Vol. 2). Totowa, New Jersey: Humana Press, 2001.

2. I. Kitagawa, W.Z. Chen, K. Hori, et al., "Chemical studies of Chinese licorice-roots. I. Elucidation of five new flavonoid constituents from the roots of Glycyrrhiza glabra L. collected in Xinjiang," *Chemical and Pharmaceutical Bulletin*, 1994, 42(S):1056.

3. A.G Morgan, W.A. F McAdam, and C. Pacsoo, "Comparison between cimetidine and Caved-S in the treatment of gastric ulceration, and subsequent maintenance therapy, *Gut*, 1982, 23:545.

4. P.G. Bianchi, M. Petrillo, and M. Lazzaroni, "Comparison of pirenzepine and carbenoxolone in the treatment of chronic gastric ulcer: A double-blind endoscopic trial," *Hepatogastroenterology*, 1985, 32:293.

5. T.S. Nadar and M. M. Pillai, "Effect of Ayurvedic medicines on beta-glucuronidase activity of Brunner's glands during recovery from cysteamine induced duodenal ulcers in rats," *Indian Journal of Experimental Biology*, 1989, 27(11):959.

6. Dehpour AR, Zolfaghari ME, Samadian T, Vahedi Y. The protective effect of liquorice components and their derivatives against gastric ulcer induced by aspirin in rats. J Pharm Pharmacol. 1994 Feb;46(2):148-9

7. Add Note 7

8. M. Blumenthal (Ed.) and S. Klein (Trans), "German Bundesgesuntheitsamt (BGA) Commission E, *Therapeutic Monographs on Medicinal Products for Human Use* (English translation). Austin, Texas: American Botanical Council, YEAR).

9. Baker ME. Licorice and enzymes other than 11 beta-hydroxysteroid dehydrogenase: an evolutionary perspective. Steroids. 1994 Feb;59(2):136-41

10. N. Wittschiera, G. Fallerb, and A. Hensela, "Aqueous extracts and polysaccharides from Liquorice roots (*Glycyrrhiza glabra* L.) inhibit adhesion of *Helicobacter pylori* to human gastric mucosa," *Journal of Ethnopharmacology*, Sept 7, 2009, 125(2):218–223.

11. T. Fukai, A. Marumo, K. Kaitou, T. Kanda, S. Terada, and T. Nomura, "Anti-helicobacter pylori flavonoids from licorice extract," *Life Science*, Aug. 2002, 71(12),1449–1463–1463.

12. R. Krausse, J. Bielenberg, W. Blaschek, and U. Ullmann, "In vitro anti-Helicobacter pylori activity of extractum liquiritiae, glycyrrhizin and its metabolites," *Journal of Antimicrobial Chemotherapy*, 2004, 54: 243–246.

13. J.A. Duke,. *CRC Handbook of Medicinal Herbs* (Boca Raton, Florida: CRC Press, 1985).

14. W.Y. Lim, Y.Y. Chia, S.Y, Liong, S. H. Ton, A.A. Kadir, and S.N. Husain, "Lipoprotein lipase expression, serum lipids and tissue lipid deposition in orally administered glycyrrhizic acid treated rats," *Lipids Health Disease,* July 29, 2009, 8:31.

15. Armanini D, De Palo CB, Mattarello MJ, Spinella P, Zaccaria M, Ermolao A, Palermo M, Fiore C, Sartorato P, Francini-Pesenti F, Karbowiak I. Effect of licorice on the reduction of body fat mass in healthy subjects. J Endocrinol Invest. 2003 Jul;26(7):646-50

16. V. E. Tyler, *Herbs of Choice—The Therapeutic Use of Phytomedicinals* (Binghamton, NY: Pharmaceutical Products Press, 1994)

17. J.H. Choi, J.N. Choi, S.Y. Lee, S.J. Lee, K. Kim, and Y.K. Kim, "Inhibitory activity of diacylglycerol acyltransferase by glabrol isolated from the roots of licorice," *Arch Pharm Res.*, Feb. 2010, 33(2):237–242.

18. A. Moon and S.H. Kim, "Effect of Glycyrrhiza glabra roots and glycyrrhizin on the glucuronidation in rats," *Planta Medica*, 1997, 63(2):115

19. Y.L. Lin, Y.C. Hsu, Y.T. Chiu, and Y.T. Huang, "Antifibrotic effects of a herbal combination regimen on hepatic fibrotic rats," *Phytother Res.*, Jan. 2008, 22(1):69–76.

20. J. T Coon and E. Ernst, "Complementary and alternative therapies in the treatment of chronic hepatitis C: A systematic review," *J Hepatol.*, March 2004, 40(3):491–500.

21. S. Luper, "A review of plants used in the treatment of liver disease: Part two," *Alternative Medicine Review*, 1999, 4(3):178.

22. G. G. Konovalova, A.K. Tikhaze, and V.Z. Lankin, "Anti-oxidant activity of parapharmaceuticals containing natural inhibitors of the free radical process," *Bulletin of Experimental Biology and Medicine*, 2000, 130(7):658.

23. H. Haraguchi, N. Yosida, H. Ishikawa, Y. Tamura, K. Mizutani, and T. Kinoshita, "Protection of mitochondria! functions against oxidative stresses by isoflavans from Glycyrrhiza glabra," *Journal of Pharmacy and Pharmacology*, 2000, 52(2):219.

24. P.A. Belinky, M. Aviram, B. Fuhrman, M. Rosenblat, and J. Vaya, "The antioxidative effects of the isoflavan glabridin on endogenous constituents of LDL during its oxidation," *Atherosclerosis*, 1998, 137(1):49.

25. P.A. Belinky, M. Aviram, S. Mahmood, and J. Vaya, "Structural aspects of the inhibitory effect of glabridin on LDL oxidation," *Free Radical Biology and Medicine*, 1998, 24(9):1419.

26. J. Vaya, P.A. Belinky, and M. Aviram, "Anti-oxidant constituents from licorice roots: Isolation, structure elucidation and antioxidative capacity toward LDL oxidation," *Free Radical Biology and Medicine*, 1997, 23(2):302.

27. B. Fuhrman, S. Buch, J. Vaya, P.A. Belinky, R. Coleman, T. Hayek, and M.Aviram, "Licorice extract and its major polyphenol glabridin protect low-density lipoprotein against lipid peroxidation: in vitro and ex vivo studies in humans and in atherosclerotic apolipoprotein E-deficient mice," *Am J Clin Nutr,* 1997, 66:267–275.

28. P.A. Bafna, and R. Balaraman, "Anti-oxidant activity of DHC-1, an herbal formulation, in experimentally-induced cardiac and renal damage," *Phytother Res.*, March 2005, 19(3):216–221.

29. T. Fukai, K. Satoh, T. Nomura, and H. Sakagami, "Preliminary evaluation of antinephritis and radical scavenging activities of glabridin from Glycyrrhiza glabra," *Fitoterapia*, Dec. 2003, 74(7–8):624–629.

30. T.G. Razina, E.P. Zueva, E.N.Amosova, and S.G. Krylova, "Medicinal plant preparations used as adjuvant therapeutics in experimental oncology," *Eksperimental'naia i Klinickaia Farmakologia*, 2000, 63(5):59.

31. A. Trovalo, M.T. Monforte, A. Rossitto, and A.M. Foresticri, "In vitrv cytotoxic effect of some medicinal plants containing flavonoids," *Bolletino Chimieo Farmaceutico*, 1996, 135(4):263.

32. R.Agarwal, Z.Y. Wang, and H. Mukhtar, "Inhibition of mouse skin tumor-initiating activity of DMBA by chronic oral feeding of glycyrrhizin in drinking water," *Nutrition and Cancer*, 1991, 15(3–4):187.

33. Rafi MM, Rosen RT, Vassil A, Ho CT, Zhang H, Ghai G, Lambert G, DiPaola RS. Modulation of bcl-2 and cytotoxicity by licochalcone-A, a novel estrogenic flavonoid. Anticancer Res. 2000 Jul-Aug;20(4):2653-8

34. F. Zani, M.T. Cuzzoni, M. Daglia, S. Bcnvenuti, G. Vampa, and A.P. Maz, "Inhibition of mutagenicity in Salmonella lyphirnurium by Glycyrrhiza glabra extract, glycyrrhizin acid, 18 alpha- and 18 beta-glycyrrhinic acids," *Planta Medica*, 1993, 59(61):502.

35. A. Trovato, M.T. Monforte, A.M. Forestieri, and F. Pizzimenti, "In vitro anti-mycotic activity of some medicinal plants containing flavonoids," *Bolletino Chimico Farmaceutico*, 2000, 139(5):225.

36. W. Li, Y. Asada, and T. Yoshikawa, "Antimicrobial flavonoids from Glycyrrhiza glabra hairy root cultures," *Planta Medica*, 1998, 64(8):746.

37. L.A. Mitscher, Y.H. Park, D. Clark, and J.L. Beal, "Antimicrobial agents from higher plants. Antimicrobial isoflavonoids and related substances from Glycyrrhiza glabra L. var. typica," *Journal of Natural Products*, 1980, 43(2):259.

38. G. Amaryan, V. Astvatsatryan, E. Gabrielyan, A. Panossian, V. Panosyan, and G. Wikman, "Double-blind, placebo-controlled, randomized, pilot clinical trial of ImmunoGuard—a standardized fixed combination of Andrographis paniculata Nees, with Eleutherococcus senticosus Maxim, Schizandra chinensis Bail, and Glycyrrhiza glabra L. extracts in patients with Familial Mediterranean Fever, *Phytomedicine*, May 2003; 10(4):271–285.

39. L. Badam, "In vitro anti-viral activity of indigenous glycyrrhizin, licorice and glycyrrhizic acid (Sigma) on Japanese encephalitis virus," *Journal of Communicable Diseases*, 1997, 29(2):91.

40. R. Pompei, O. Flore, M.A. Marccialis, A. Pani, and B. Loddo, "Glycyrrhizic acid inhibits virus growth and inactivates virus particles," *Nature*, 1979, 281(5733):689.

41. Hattori T, et al. Preliminary evidence for inhibitory effect of glycyrrhizin on HIV replication in patients with aids. Anti-viral Res. 1989;II:255-262

42. C. Fiore, M. Eisenhut, R. Krausse, E. Ragazzi, D. Pellati, D. Armanini, and J. Bielenberg, "Anti-viral effects of Glycyrrhiza species," *Phytother Res.*, Feb. 2008, 22(2):141–148.

43. A. Wolkerstorfer, H. Kurz, N. Bachhofner, and O.H. Szolar, Glycyrrhizin inhibits influenza A virus uptake into the cell," *Anti-viral Res.*, Aug. 2009, 83(2):171–178.

44. J. Brush, E. Mendenhall, A. Guggenheim, T. Chan, E. Connelly, A. Soumyanath, R. Buresh, R. Barrett, and H. Zwickey, "The effect of Echinacea purpurea, Astragalus membranaceus and Glycyrrhiza glabra on CD69 expression and immune cell activation in humans," Phytother Res., Aug. 2006, 20(8):687–695.

45. Genovese T, Menegazzi M, Mazzon E, Crisafulli C, Di Paola R, Dal Bosco M, Zou Z, Suzuki H, Cuzzocrea S. Glycyrrhizin reduces secondary inflammatory process after spinal cord compression injury in mice. Shock. 2009 Apr;31(4):367-75.

46. T. Genovese, M. Menegazzi, E. Mazzon, C. Crisafulli, R. Di Paola, M. Dal Bosco, Z. Zou, H. Suzuki, and S. Cuzzocrea, "Glycyrrhizin reduces secondary inflammatory process after spinal cord compression injury in mice," *Shock*, April 2009, 31(4):367–375.

47. M.M. Azimov, L.I.B. Zakirov, and S.D. Radzhapova, "Pharmacological study of the anti-inflammatory agent glyderinine," *Farcnakologika Toksikologica*, 1983, 51(4):90.

48. K.R. Kim, C.K. Jeong, K.K. Park, J.H. Choi, J.H. Park, S.S. Lim, and W.Y. Chung, "Anti-inflammatory effects of licorice and roasted licorice extracts on TPA-induced acute inflammation and collagen-induced arthritis in mice," *J Biomed Biotechnol.*, 2010: Article ID: 709378. OK? This is how this journal references.

49. Baschetti R. Chronic fatigue syndrome and liquorice. N Z Med J. 1995 Apr 26;108(998):156-77.

50. F. Zamansoltani, M. Nassiri-Asl, M.R. Sarookhani, H. Jahani-Hashemi, and A.A. Zangiv, "Antiandrogenic activities of Glycyrrhiza glabra in male rats," *Int J Androl.*, Aug. 2009, 32(4):417–422.

51. H.S. Cipil, A. Kosar, A. Kaya, B. Uz, I.C. Haznedaroglu, H. Goker, O. Ozdemir, M. Koroglu, S. Kirazli, and H.C. Firat, "In vivo hemostatic effect of the medicinal plant extract Ankaferd Blood Stopper in rats pretreated with warfarin," *Clin Appl Thromb Hemost.*, May–June 2009,15(3):270–276.

52. T. Baykul, E.G. Alanoglu, and G. Kocer, "Use of Ankaferd Blood Stopper as a hemostatic agent: A clinical experience," *J Contemp Dent Pract.*, Jan. 1, 2010, 11(1):E088-94.

53. M. Francischetii, R.Q. Moniiro, J.A. Giiimaraes, and B. Francischetli, "Identification of glycyrrhizin as a thrombin inhibitor," *Biochemistry and Biophysics Research Communications*, 1997, 235(1):259-263.

54. W. Mendes-Silva, M. Assafim, B. Ruta, R.Q. Monteiro, J.A. Guimarães, and R.B. Zingali, "Antithrombotic effect of Glycyrrhizin, a plant-derived thrombin inhibitor," *Thromb Res.* 2003,112(1–2):93–98.

55. X.Q Yu, C.C. Xue, A.W. Zhou, C.G. Li, Y.M. Du, J. Liang, and S.F. Zhou, "In vitro and in vivo neuroprotective effect and mechanisms of glabridin, a major active isoflavan from Glycyrrhiza glabra (licorice)," *Life Sci.*, Jan. 2, 2008, 82 (1–2):68–78.

56. C. Zhan and J. Yang, "Protective effects of isoliquiritigenin in transient middle cerebral artery occlusion-induced focal cerebral ischemia in rats," *Pharmacol Res.*, March 2006, 53(3):303–309.

57. D. Dhingra and A. Sharma, "Anti-depressant-like activity of Glycyrrhiza glabra L. in mouse models of immobility tests," *Prog Neuropsychopharmacol Biol Psychiatry*, May 2006, 30(3):449–454.

58. Y.W. Shin, E.A. Bae, B. Lee, S.H. Lee, J.A. Kim, Y.S. Kim, and D.H. Kim, "In vitro and in vivo antiallergic effects of Glycyrrhiza glabra and its components," *Planta Med.*, March 2007, 73(3):257–261.

59. A. Ram, U. Mabalirajan, M. Das, I. Bhattacharya, A.K. Dinda, S.V. Gangal, and B. Ghosh, "Glycyrrhizin alleviates experimental allergic asthma in mice," *Int Immunopharmacol.*, Sept. 2006, 6(9):1468–1477.

60. M. Saeedi, K. Morteza-Semnani, and M.R. Ghoreishi, "The treatment of atopic dermatitis with licorice gel," *J Dermatolog Treat.*, Sept. 2003, 14(3):153–157.

61. E. Mathias, D.V. Rangnekar, and C.M. McCorkle, "Ethnoveterinary medicine, alternative for livestock development." Proceedings of an International Conference, BAIF Development Research Foundation, Pune, India, 1988.

62. Hausen BM, In De Smet PAGM, Keller K, Hansel R, et al eds: Adverse effects of herbal drugs. Vol 1, Berlin, 1992, Springer Verlag, pp 227-236

63. F. Aoki, K. Nakagawa, M. Kitano, H. Ikematsu, K. Nakamura, S. Yokota, Y. Tominaga, N. Arai, and T. Mae, "Clinical safety of licorice flavonoid oil (LFO) and pharmacokinetics of glabridin in healthy humans," *J Am Coll Nutr.*, June 2007, 26(3):209–218.

Gymnema sylvestre

Introduction

Called Gurmar or Merasingi in Hindi, Meshasringi (or "ram's horn") in Sanskrit, and "Periploca of the Woods" in English, Gymnema sylvestre is a woody, climbing plant that grows in the tropical forests of central and southern India. It has been recognized for centuries as a highly effective anti-diabetic medicinal herb.

In Ayurvedic tradition, Gymnema sylvestre has been used for stomach upsets and as a diuretic. Ancient texts as long ago as the first century A.D. noted that Gymnema successfully "destroyed" excess sugars in the body, a condition now recognized as diabetes. In India, Gymnema has been used to treat diabetes for more than 2,000 years.

Gymnema, in the form of a tea, now is also used for controlling obesity. The active compounds of the plant have been isolated and identified as gymnemic acids. The leaves of gymnema, when chewed, interfere with the ability to taste sweetness; hence the herb's name Gurmar, which means "sugar destroyer."

Gymnema is a stomachic, diuretic, refrigerant, astringent, and tonic. In animal and human studies, it has been found to increase urine output and reduce hyperglycemia. Historically, Gymnema's primary medicinal use was for adult-onset diabetes, a condition for which it continues to be recommended today in India. The leaves also were used to alleviate stomach ailments, constipation, water retention, and liver disease.

Human and animal studies have confirmed that Gymnema has pronounced effects on blood sugar levels among diabetics. Within the past two decades, researchers have demonstrated that gymnema extracts may play a role in the treatment of Type I diabetics, who typically need daily injections of insulin to control the disease. Extracts of gymnema given to patients with Type I diabetes undergoing insulin therapy have reduced insulin requirements and fasting blood sugar levels, and improved blood sugar control.[1] Taken orally, gymnema lowers diabetics' blood glucose levels and improves blood fat and cholesterol profiles.[2,3]

Synonymous Names

English: Periploca of the Woods
Hindi: Gurmar, Merasingi, Gurmarbooti
Sanskrit: Meshashringi, Madhunashini
Marathi: Kavali, Kalikardori, Vakundi
Gujrathi: Dhuleti, Mardashingi
Telugu: Podapatri
Tamil: Adigam, Cherukurinja
Kannada: Sannagerasehambu

Habitat

Gymnema sylvestre is native to the tropical forests of southern and central India, Deccan peninsula, Assam, and some parts of Africa. It also is found in the Western Ghats in South India, and to the west of those mountains in the area around the coastal city of Goa.

Botanical Characteristics

Gymnema sylvestre is a large, more or less pubescent woody climber. Its leaves are opposite, usually elliptic or ovate, 1.25 to 2 inches long, and 0.5 to 1.25 inches wide. The leaves are base-acute to acuminate, glabrous above, and sparsely or densely tomentose beneath.

Gymnema's small, yellow flowers appear in axillary and lateral umbellate cymes with long pedicels. The long, fusiform follicles are terete and lanceolate, up to 3 inches in length. The calyx-lobes are long, ovate, obtuse, and pubescent; the corolla is pale yellow, and campanulate, valvate; and the corona is single, with five fleshy scales.

Chemical Composition

The major bioactive constituents of Gymnema sylvestris are a group of oleanan-type triterpenoid saponins known as gymnemic acids. The latter contain several acylated derivatives of deacylgymnemic acid.[4] The individual gymnemic acids (saponins) include gymnemic acids I-VII, gymnemosides A-F, and gymnemasaponins.[5,6]

The leaves of Gymnema sylvestre contain triterpene saponins belonging to the oleanane and dammarene classes. Oleanane saponins are gymnemic acids and gymnema saponins, and dammarene saponins are gymnemasides.[7,8,9,10]

Other plant constituents are flavones, anthraquinones, hentri-acontane, pentatriacontane, α and β-chlorophylls, phytin, resins, d-quercitol, tartaric acid, formic acid, butyric acid, lupeol, β-amyrin-related glycosides, and stigmasterol. The plant extract also tests positive for alkaloids. The leaves of this species yield acidic glycosides and anthroquinones and their derivatives.[11]

Pharmacological Activity

Anti-diabetic activity

The hypoglycemic action of Gymnema sylvestre leaves was first documented in the late 1920s. The plant's hypoglycemic action is gradual in nature, differing from the rapid effect of many prescription hypoglycemic drugs. Gymnema leaves raise insulin levels by causing regeneration of beta-cells in the pancreas, which secrete insulin.[12]

Research has shown that gymnema improves the uptake of glucose into cells by increasing the activity of glucose-metabolizing enzymes, and preventing adrenaline from stimulating the liver to produce glucose. The net effect is that blood sugar levels are reduced.[13]

Another anti-diabetic effect of gymnema is that it negates the taste of sugar, which has the effect of suppressing and neutralizing the craving for sweets.[14] Gymnemic acid found in the leaf extracts inhibits hyperglycemia and also acts as a cardiovascular stimulant.

Gymnema has been the subject of considerable research since the 1930s, which revealed its effectiveness in treating both Type I and Type II diabetes. Gymnema has been successful in controlling blood sugar levels without causing hypoglycemia—an effect seen with the use of insulin and oral hypoglycemic sulphonylurea compounds. Gymnema extract provides a simple and effective method to help maintain healthy glucose levels. Gymnema contains Gymnemic acid, quercitol, lupeol, ß-amyrin and stigmasterol, all of which have glucose-lowering properties.[15]

Researchers at India's University of Madras in the early 1990s found that high doses of Gymnema extract actually may help to repair or regenerate pancreas beta cells, which play a crucial role in the production and secretion of insulin.[16] Few other substances, synthetic or natural, offer such promise for reversing beta-cell damage and at least partially reducing diabetic's need for insulin and other drugs. Studies, however, indicate that animals that do not have diabetes do not produce more insulin after consuming gymnema.[17]

In a clinical trial, the hypoglycemic activity of Gymnema sylvestre was evaluated in 10 normal and 6 diabetic patients. The patients were subjected to glucose tolerance tests, and venous blood samples were collected at 30-minute intervals up to 2 hours. An aqueous decoction of the leaves was given at a dosage of 2 grams three times daily for 10 days in healthy volunteers. The diabetic patients with mild-to-moderate hyperglycemia were given this dosage for 15 days. Administration of the extract brought about a significant reduction in the fasting blood sugar levels in both the normal and the diabetic patients, suggesting definite hypoglycemic activity.[18] The hypoglycemic effect of Gymnema sylvestre was studied in 16 normal subjects and in 43 mild diabetic patients. All of the subjects were administered leaf powder 10 grams a day for 7 days. The results indicate that Gymnema sylvestre leaf powder has a hypoglycemic effect comparable to tolbutamide. Serum triacylglycerol, free fatty acids, and cholesterol levels in the normal subjects were unaffected, whereas in diabetic patients these were decreased significantly. Ascorbic acid and iron levels were elevated significantly in both groups. Excretion of creatine decreased in diabetic patients and remained unaffected in the normal volunteers.[19] Extracts of gymnema given to patients with Type II diabetes on insulin therapy led to reduced insulin requirements and fasting blood sugar levels and improved blood sugar control in clinical studies.[20]

In one study of Type II diabetics, gymnema extract, given along with oral hypoglycemic drugs, was shown to improve blood sugar control and either led to discontinuation of the medicine or a significantly reduced dosage. Gymnema extract given to healthy volunteers did not produce any blood sugar-lowering, or hypoglycemic, effects.[21]

The effectiveness of an extract from the leaves of Gymnema sylvestre in controlling hyperglycemia was investigated in 22 Type II diabetic patients taking conventional oral anti-hyperglycemic agents.[22] The extract, at a dose of 400 mg/day was administered for 18–20 months as a supplement to conventional oral drugs. During supplementation, the patients showed significant reductions in blood glucose, glycosylated hemoglobin and glycosylated plasma proteins. All of the patients treated with gymnema extract were able to maintain lower blood sugar levels with lower dosages of conventional anti-diabetic drugs. Five of the 22 patients were able to discontinue their conventional drugs completely and to maintain their blood glucose homeostasis with gymnema extract alone. These results suggest strongly that pancreatic beta-cells may be regenerated or repaired in Type II diabetic patients with gymnema supplementation. This is supported by raised insulin levels in the serum of patients after supplementation.

In another study, a water-soluble extract of the leaves of Gymnema sylvestre, was administered to 27 patients with insulin-dependent diabetes mellitus taking insulin therapy. After treatment with the extract, the patients' insulin requirements were reduced, along with fasting blood glucose, glycosylated hemoglobin, and glycosylated plasma protein levels. Serum lipids returned to near normal levels with gymnema therapy, but levels of glycosylated hemoglobin and glycosylated plasma protein remained higher than the controls. The patients on insulin therapy alone showed no significant reduction in serum lipids, HbA1c or glycosylated plasma proteins, when tested 10–12 months after the study's conclusion. Gymnema therapy seems to enhance endogenous insulin, possibly by regeneration or revitalization of the residual beta-cells in insulin-dependent diabetes mellitus.[23]

Extracts containing gymnemic acids from the leaves of Gymnema sylvestre has shown to block glucose transport in high K(+)-induced contraction in guinea pig ileal longitudinal muscles, inverted intestine of guinea-pig and rat.[24]

In another study, researchers investigated the hypoglycemic and anti-hyperglycemic potential of five extracts (water, ethanol, methanol, hexane, and chloroform) of four plants (i.e., seeds of Eugenia jambolana, fruits of Momordica charantia, leaves of Gymnema sylvestre, and seeds of Trigonella foenum-graecum alone and/or in combination with glimepiride in rats.[25] Ethanol extract of Eugenia jambolana, water extract of Momordica charantia, ethanol extract of Gymnema sylvestre, and water extract of Trigonella foenum graecum exhibited the highest hypoglycemic and anti-hyperglycemic activity in rats among all the extracts, and the hexane extracts exhibited the least activities. Most of the active extracts were studied further to dose-dependent (200, 100, and 50 mg/kg body weight (bw)) hypoglycemic and antihyperglycemic effects alone and in combination with glimepiride (20, 10, and 5 mg/kg bw). The combination of the most active extracts (200 mg/kg bw) and lower dose of glimepiride (5 mg/kg bw) showed safer and potent hypoglycemic as well as antihyperglycemic activities without creating severe hypoglycemia in normal rats. Higher doses (200 mg/kg bw of most active extracts, and 10 and 20 mg/kg bw of glimepiride) generated lethal hypoglycemia in normal rats. From this study, it may be concluded that the ethanol extract of Eugenia jambolana, water extract of Momordica charantia, ethanol extract of Gymnema sylvestre, and water extract of Trigonella foenum graecum seeds have higher hypoglycemic and anti-hyperglycemic potential and may be used as complementary medicine to treat the diabetic population by significantly reducing the dose of standard drugs.

Hypolipidemic activity

Gymnema leaves also are noted for lowering serum cholesterol and triglycerides. Gymnema leaf extract at a dosage of 25% 100 mg/kg administered orally to experimentally induced hyperlipidemic rats for 2 weeks reduced the elevated serum triglyceride, total cholesterol, very low density lipoprotein, and low density lipoprotein-cholesterol in a dose-dependent manner. The ability of the extract at 100 mg/kg to lower triglycerides and total cholesterol in serum and its anti-atherosclerotic potential was similar to that of the standard lipid-lowering agent clofibrate.[26] Researchers at Georgetown University compared the effects of chromium, vanadium, and gymnema in experimental rats experiencing sugar-induced hypertension. Unlike the trace minerals, the herb reduced blood cholesterol but did not reduce the high blood pressure caused by dietary sugar.[27]

Anti-obesity activity

The efficacy of optimal doses of highly bioavailable (-)-hydroxycitric acid alone and in combination with niacin-bound chromium and a standardized Gymnema sylvestre extract on weight loss in moderately obese subjects was evaluated by monitoring changes in body weight, body mass index (BMI), appetite, lipid profiles, serum leptin, and excretion of urinary fat metabolites. Hydroxycitric acid was shown to reduce appetite, inhibit fat synthesis, and decrease body weight without stimulating the central nervous system. Niacin-bound chromium demonstrated an ability to maintain healthy insulin levels, and gymnema extract was shown to regulate weight loss and blood sugar levels.[28]

A randomized, double-blind, placebo-controlled human study was conducted for 8 weeks with 60 moderately obese subjects ages 21 to 50.[29] The subjects were randomly divided into three groups. Group A was administered hydroxycitric acid; Group B was administered a combination of hydroxycitric acid, niacin-bound chromium, and gymnema extract; and Group C was given a placebo daily in three equally divided doses 30 to 60 minutes before meals. All of the subjects received a diet of 2000 calories per day and participated in supervised walking. At the end of 8 weeks, body weight and BMI had decreased by 5% to 6% in Groups A and B. Food intake, total cholesterol, low-density lipoproteins, triglycerides, and serum leptin levels were reduced significantly in both groups, and high-density lipoprotein levels and excretion of urinary fat metabolites increased in both groups. A marginal or non-significant effect was observed in all parameters in Group C. This study demonstrates that optimal doses of hydroxycitric acid and, to a greater degree, the combination of hydroxycitric acid, niacin-bound chromium, and Gymnema sylvestre extract can serve as an effective and safe weight-loss formula that can facilitate a reduction in excess body weight and BMI while promoting healthy blood lipid levels.

Dr. Sodhi's Experience

When considering treatment with Gymnema, the practitioner should consider the following:

- Is any dysglycemia present?
- Is there a need/desire to lose weight?
- Is there a desire to build muscle?

Gymnema is well known both in Ayurveda and Western herbal medicine for its superior ability to modulate sugar metabolism. In Hindi, the plant is called Gurmar which means, literally, "destroyer of sugar." This term applies to both external and internal uses of the plant. Indian chefs know that if excess sugar is added to a dish accidentally, a good dose of Gymnema will destroy the excess sweetness.

Gymnema is effective in treating both Type I and Type II diabetes and may be used to treat other disorders involving the need for improved glycogenesis. It also is useful for weight loss and for body-building, as increased glycogen leads inevitably to more muscle mass and less fat.

Case Histories

A medical doctor called our clinic seeking advice concerning his 7-year-old son, who had been diagnosed with diabetes and was taking insulin. The doctor said that reversing the boy's diabetes might be impossible but that he would seek a way to decrease the amount of insulin the boy required. After checking the boy's C-peptide levels to assess beta cell activity, we prescribed the following protocol:

To be taken once a day: Gymnema sylvestre (shardunika) extract, 300 mg, in combination with 200 mg betaine HCl, chromium nicotinate 105 mcg, biotin 2150 mcg, Pterocarpus marsupium (vijjayasaar) and Ocimum sanctuam (tulsi) extracts, 100 mg each, and Momordica charantia and Azadirachtia indica (neem) extracts, 50 mg each.

We also prescribed the following dietary supplements: fish oil 1000 mg, three times per day, and vitamin B3 (niacin) 300 mg. And we recommended dietary changes including eating protein and carbohydrates in equal amounts by weight, along with one piece of fresh fruit and two bowls of vegetables per day.

In just a few days the patient was able to receive a 50% reduction in his insulin dose. One week later, he needed only 25% of his original insulin dose. He has continued with the herbal protocol and is able to keep his insulin level at 25%. He is growing and developing well on the lower dose of insulin.

Another patient, an attorney, came into our clinic with glucose levels at 300 even though he was taking both Glucophage and Glucotrol. His blood pressure had been rising, and he had been put on a beta-blocker and an ACE-inhibitor. Because the beta-blocker inhibits all beta cells, the patient's blood sugar was continuing to increase. He was also under considerable stress, as he was working at two jobs. Blood work showed that the patient's HbA1c was 11.6, and his total cholesterol was 319 with an HDL of 26. His triglycerides were 625.

We prescribed the following herbal protocol, in addition to the same dietary guidelines as described in the previous case, and a regular exercise program:

For sugar metabolism:

To be taken one three times per day: Gymnema sylvestre (shardunika) extract, 300 mg, in combination with 200 mg betaine HCl, chromium nicotinate 105 mcg, biotin 2150 mcg, Pterocarpus marsupium (vijjayasaar) and Ocimum sanctuam (tulsi) extracts, 100 mg each, and Momordica charantia and Azadirachta indica (neem) extracts, 50 mg each.

For minerals and immune support:

Shilajit, 250 mg three times a day.

For lipid metabolism:

Three times a day: Commiphora mukul (guggulu), 300 mg extract, in combination with 80 mg of triphala, a compound formula consisting of equal parts of Emblica officinalis (amalaki), Terminalia bellerica (bibhitaki), Terminalia chebula (haritaki) extract.

For stress and improved overall metabolism:

Withania somnifera (ashwagandha) 500 mg three times a day and B-complex one cap twice a day. After one month of this therapy, this patient was able to stop taking the beta-blocker. In one month, his blood sugar had stabilized at 120–150. Because his blood pressure was dropping, we decided not to give him any additional therapy. We put him on the following formula so that he could get off of the Ace inhibitor:

For blood pressure:

To be taken once a day, in the evening: 100 mg each Convolvulus pluricaulis (shankhapushpi) and Tribulus terrestris (gokshura), with 50 mg Rauwolfia serpentina (sarpagandha) and 25 mg Rosa vinca.

We instructed the patient to check his blood pressure twice a day. Within a few days, his blood pressure had stabilized at 110/60, and he reported feeling light-headed, so we reduced the ACE-inhibitor by half. After another week, the patient's blood pressure had stabilized at 110/70 and he was feeling better, so we eliminated the rest of the ACE-inhibitor. After 3 months, his HbA1c was 6.1, blood pressure was 110/70, blood sugar was 120, total cholesterol was 178, HDL 46, and triglycerides were within the normal ranges, at 150.

Safety Profile

No side-effects have been reported from using gymnema. Its safety in pregnant and nursing women has not been established.

Diabetic patients using gymnema may require dosage adjustments in other anti-diabetic drugs. Some of Gymnema's effects may be enhanced by anti-depressant medications, fenfluramine, salicylates (including aspirin), and tetracyclines. Its actions may be decreased by the use of oral contraceptives, epinephrine, phenothiazines, and thyroid hormones.

Dosage

The typical dosage is 150 mg, three times a day. A 250-mg supplement dose, twice daily, represents the extract when the gymnemic acids have been standardized at 25%. The 75-mg extract, taken twice daily, provides 75% gymnemic acids.

Ayurvedic Properties

Rasa: Kashaya and Tikta
Guna: Laghu and Rukhsha
Vipak: Katu
Virya: Ushna

Notes

1. E. R. Shanmugasundaram, G. Rajeswari, K. Baskaran, B.R. Rajesh Kumarm, K. Radha Shanmugasundaram, and B. Kizar Ahmath, "Use of Gymnema sylvestre leaf extract in the control of blood glucose in insulin-dependent diabetes mellitus," *J Ethnopharmacol.*, Oct. 1990, 30(3):281–294.

2. A. Qayum, et al., "Pharmacological screening of medicinal plants," Journal *of the Pakistan Medical Association*, April 1982, pp. 103–105.

3. S.P. Wahi and K.X. Chukenar, "Pharmcological studies of gymnema sylvestre R.," *Br. Journal Sci. Res.* (Banaras Hindu University, Varanasi, India), 1964, 15, 205–210.

4. K. Baskaran, B. Kizar Ahamath, K. Radha Shanmugasundaram, and E.R. Shanmugasundaram, "Antidiabetic effect of a leaf extract from *Gymnema sylvestre* in non-insulin-dependent diabetes mellitus patients," *J Ethnopharmacol*, Oct.1990, 30(3):295–300.

5. G.P. Dateo and L. Long, "Gymnemic acid, the antisaccharine principle of Gymnema sylvestre. Studies on isolation and heterogenesity of gymnemic acid A1," *J. Agric. Food Chem.*, 1973, 21:899–903.

6. H.M. Liu, F. Kiuchi, and Y. Tsuda, "Isolation and structure elucidation of Gymnemic acids, antisweet principles of Gymnema sylvestre," *Chem. Pharm. Bull.*, 1992, 40:1366–1375.

7. J.E. Sinsheimer and P.E. Manni, "Constituents from Gymnema sylvestre leaves," *J. Pharm. Sci.*, 1965, 54:1541–1544.

8. J.E. Sinsheimer and G. Subbarao, "Constituents from Gymnema sylvestre leaves VIII: Isolation, chemistry and derivatives of gymnemagenin and gymnestrogenin," *J. Pharm. Sci.*, 1971, 60:190–193.

9. J.E. Sinsheimer, R.G. Subba, and H.M. McIlhenny8, "Constituents from Gyimnema syilvestre leaves V: Isolation and preliminary characterization of Gymnemic acids," J. Pharm. Sci., 1970, 59:622–628.

10. Yoshikawa, M. Nakagawa, R.Yamamoto, S. Arihara, and K. Matsuura, K., "Antisweet natural products V structures of gymnemic acids VIII-XII from Gymnema sylvestre R.," *Br. Chem. Pharm. Bull.*, 1992, 40:1779–1782.

11. See Note 6.

12. K. Shimizu, M. Ozeki, K. Tanaka, K. Itoh, S. Nakajyo, N. Urakawa, and M. Atsuchi, "Suppression of glucose absorption by extracts from the leaves of *Gymnema inodorum*, **Jpn J Pharmacol. 2001 Jun;86(2):223-9.**

13. K. Yoshikawa, M. Nakagawa, R. Yamamoto, S. Arihara, and K. Matsuura, K., "Antisweet natural products V structures of Gymnemic acids VIII-XII from Giymnema sylvestre R.," *Br. Chem. Pharm. Bull.*, 1992, 40:1779–1782.

14. N. Shigemura, K. Nakao, T. Yasuo, Y. Murata, K. Yasumatsu, A. Nakashima, H. Katsukawa, N. Sako, and Y. Ninomiya, "Gurmarin sensitivity of sweet taste responses is associated with co-expression patterns of T1r2, T1r3, and gustducin," *Biochem Biophys Res Commun.*, March 7, 2008, 367(2):356–363.

15. S.K. Agarwal, S.S. Singh, S. Verma, V. Lakshmi, and A. Sharma, "Chemistry and medicinal uses of Gymnema sylvestre (gur-mar) leaves: A review," *Indian Drugs*, 2000, 37:354–360.

16. See Note 1

17. Khare AK, Tondon RN, Tewari JP. Hypoglycaemic activity of an indigenous drug (Gymnema sylvestre, 'Gurmar') in normal and diabetic persons. Indian J Physiol Pharmacol. 1983 Jul-Sep;27(3):257-8.

18. Shanmugasundaram KR, Panneerselvam C, Samudram P, Shanmugasundaram ER. The insulinotropic activity of Gymnema sylvestre, R. Br. An Indian medical herb used in controlling diabetes mellitus. Pharmacol Res Commun. 1981 May;13(5):475-86.

19. Balasubramaniam k., Vasanthy A. Studies on the effect of Gymnema sylvestre on diabetics. J. Natn. Sci. Coun. Sri Lanka 1992; 20(1): 81-89

20. See Note 1.

21. A.K. Khare, R.N.Tondon, and J.P.Tewari, "Hypoglycemic activity of an indigenous drug Gymnema sylvestre in normal and diabetic persons," *Ind. J. Physiol. Pharmacol*, 1983, 27:257–261.

22. See Note 4.

23. M. Yadav, A. Lavania, R. Tomar, G.B. Prasad, S. Jain, and H. Yadav, "Complementary and comparative study on hypoglycemic and antihyperglycemic activity of various extracts of Eugenia jambolana seed, Momordica charantia fruits, Gymnema sylvestre, and Trigonella foenum graecum seeds in rats," *Appl Biochem Biotechnol..* April 2010, 160(8):2388–2400.

24. K. Shimizu, et al., "Suppression of glucose absorption by some fractions extracted from Gymnema sylvestre leaves," *J Vet Med Sci,* 1997, *59*(4):245–251.

25. See Note 23.

26. Dogar IA, Ali M, Yaqub M. Effect of Grewia asiatica, Gossypium herbacium and Gymnema sylvestre on blood glucose, cholesterol and triglycerides levels in normoglycaemic and alloxan diabetic rabbits. J Pak Med Assoc. 1988 Nov;38(11):289-95.

27. Preuss HG, Jarrell ST, Scheckenbach R, Lieberman S, Anderson RA. Comparative effects of chromium, vanadium and gymnema sylvestre on sugar-induced blood pressure elevations in SHR. J Am Coll Nutr. 1998 Apr;17(2):116-23.

28. H.G Preuss, R.I, Garis, J.D. Bramble, M. Bagchi, D. Bagchi, C.V. Rao, and S. Satyanarayana, "Efficacy of a novel calcium/potassium salts of (-)hydroxycitric acid in weight control," *International Journal of Clinical Pharmacology Research*, 2005, 25(3):133–144.

29. H.G. Preuss, D. Bagchi, M. Bagchi, C.V. Rao, D.K. Dey, and S. Satyanarayana, "Effects of natural extracts of (-)hydroxycitric acid (HCA-SX) and a combination of HCA-SX plus niacin-bound chromium and Gymnema extract on weight loss," *Diabetes Obesity Metabolism*, May 2004, 6(3) 171–180.

24

Inula Racemosa

Introduction

Inula Racemosa, an Ayurvedic herb that grows in high mountain areas, is highly valued for its cardioprotective properties. Its roots are treasured in Ayurveda for their expectorant action in cough, breathlessness, and chest pain. Inula, known in Sanskrit as Pushkaramoola, has been used traditionally in India to support a healthy cardiovascular system. Research indicates that this herb contributes to maintaining healthy cholesterol and triglyceride levels, thereby helping patients take control of their cardiac health.[1]

A member of the Asteraceae family, Inula grows in the temperate and alpine western Himalayas, and it is common in Kashmir. The roots are widely used locally in indigenous medicine as an expectorant and in veterinary medicine as a tonic.

A study published in the *Journal of Ethnopharmacology* suggests that Pushkaramoola is a natural beta-blocker, which could explain its cardioprotective capacity.[2] In Ayurvedic practice, it is used mainly as an expectorant and a bronchodilator. It has been used to treat tuberculosis and topically to treat skin diseases. With larger doses, it produces a laxative effect.

Inula exhibits anti-peroxidative and hypoglycemic properties. Its extracts are thought to regulate diabetes mellitus, and it possesses anti-allergic properties. Inula has been shown to lower the stress hormone cortisol, which in turn leads to lower blood sugar levels.

Synonymous Names

Sanskrit: Pushkaramoola, Pushkarmool

Habitat

Inula grows in the high mountain areas of India and neighboring countries.

Botanical Characteristics

Inula is a perennial plant that reaches about 6.6 feet (2 meters) in height. It flowers from July to August, bearing large, yellow flowers that have both male and female organs.

Chemical Composition

At least four sesquiterpene lactones have been isolated from Inula.[3] Along with other ingredients, these account for the healing medicinal properties of this herb. Other chemicals present include: alantolactone, isoalantolactone, dihydroalantolactone, dihydroisoalantolactone, beta sitosterol, daucosterol, and inunolide.[4]

Pharmacological Activity
Cardioprotective activity

Inula racemosa has demonstrated potential cardioprotective benefits. In human trials, a preparation containing Inula racemosa was shown to be superior to nitroglycerin in reducing the chest pain and dyspnea associated with angina.[5]

In one study, equal proportions of extracts of Terminalia arjuna, Inula racemosa, and latex of Commiphora mukul, in three different doses, was administered orally to experimental rats daily 6 days a week for 60-days.[6] Thereafter, the rats were subjected to isoproterenol (ISO)-induced (85 mg/kg, s.c. for 2 days) myocardial necrosis. Gross and microscopic examinations (histopathology) were done, along with estimations of myocardial tissue high-energy phosphate stores and lactate content. The gross examination showed significant cardioprotection in the treated animals. Upon microscopic examination, no statistically significant reduction in myocardial damage from taking 350 and 450 mg/kg of herbal combination was observed, although loss of myocardial high energy phosphate stores and accumulation of lactate were significantly prevented. The results of this study suggest the potential usefulness of herbal combination in preventing ischemic heart disease.

The petroleum ether extract of roots lowered plasma insulin and glucose levels within 75 minutes after oral administration to albino rats, and it significantly counteracted adrenaline-induced hyperglycemia in rats. The extract further showed negative inotropic and negative chronotropic effects on the frog heart. All these findings indicate that one of the constituents of Inula racemosa may have adrenergic beta-blocking activity.[7]

Inula was studied using a 1:1 mixture of Guggul (Commiphora mukul). The trial was conducted with 200 patients with ischemic heart disease. Approximately 80% had experienced dyspnea, and all 200 subjects had chest pain with positive indications of myocardial ischemia. At the end of the 6-month study period, 26% of the subjects had a complete restoration of normal ECG. Another 59% of the subjects showed improvement in ECG; 25% had no chest pain; and the patients experiencing dyspnea fell from 80% at the beginning of the study to 32%.[8] In another trial, the efficacy of Inula was compared to nitroglycerin in preventing anginal symptoms. Nine subjects with ischemic heart disease participated in the study. All of the patients experienced chest pain and tested positive for myocardial ischemia by their ECG ST-segment depression on exertion. The Inula group received 3 grams of root powder 90 minutes prior to testing, and the controls were given nitroglycerin. All nine subjects showed improvement in ST-segment depression on the ECG. Improvement, however, was greater for those who were given Inula.[9] In further research, myocardial infarction was induced experimentally in rats by injection of isoprenaline. Circulating GOT, LDH, CPK, cAMP, Cortisol, pyruvate, lactate glucose, and cardiac cAMP adenyl cyclase levels were increased gradually, and serum and cardiac cAMP-PDE levels were decreased gradually from 1 hour to 120 hours after the first injection of isoprenaline. In the rats pre-treated with beta-blocker or Pushkarmool, these changes were less when compared to untreated rats. Similar results were observed in the infarcted rats post-treated with Pushkaramoola. The pre-treatment with Pushkarmool was found to be more effective than post-treatment, suggesting both preventive and curative functions of the drug in myocardial infarction.[10] An animal study also showed that Inula can have an anti-atherosclerosis and anti-obesity effect. Compared to the positive control, alcoholic extract of Inula decreased total cholesterol, triglycerides, low-density lipoprotein cholesterol, and the atherogenic index, and increased high-density lipoprotein cholesterol. It scavenged thiobarbituric acid reactive substances and increased reduced glutathione in the liver, and it enhanced superoxide dismutase and glutathione peroxidase in the heart. Aortic lesion area and percent bodyweight increase was least in the Inula extract-treated group. Coronary artery changes resulting from the high-fat diet were reversed by the extracts.[11]

Anti-diabetic activity

The efficacy of Inula racemosa root extract was studied to determine the amelioration of corticosteroid-induced hyperglycemia in mice. Thyroid hormone levels were estimated by radio-immuno-assay to ascertain whether the effects are mediated through thyroid hormones. Administration of the corticosteroid (dexamethasone) increased the serum glucose concentration and decreased serum concentrations of the thyroid hormones thyroxine and triiodothyronine. Administration of the plant extract decreased the serum glucose concentration in dexamethasone-induced hyperglycemic animals. These effects were comparable to the standard corticosteroid-inhibiting drug ketoconazole. No marked changes in thyroid hormone concentrations were observed by administration of the plant extract in the dexamethasone-treated animals, so it may not prove to be effective in thyroid hormone mediated Type II diabetes but, rather, for steroid induced diabetes.[12]

Alcoholic extract of the root of Inula racemosa was found to lower blood glucose and enhance liver glycogen without increasing plasma insulin in rats. Also, there was no observed increase in degranulation of the beta cells of the pancreas. No effect on the activity of the adrenal glands was noticed; however, the thyroid gland showed activation in the later stage (delayed response). The hypoglycemic response of Inula racemosa seems to be a result not of enhanced secretion/synthesis of insulin but, rather, at the peripheral level by potentiating insulin sensitivity.[13]

Anti-asthmatic activity

The effect of Inula extract was studied in animal tissues. The extract showed potent, anti-inflammatory, antipyretic, and antispasmodic effect against bronchial spasms induced by histamine, 5-hydroxytryptamine, and the various plant pollens Zea mays and Acacia arabica.[14]

Anti-microbial activity

The essential oil of Inula racemosa was tested for anti-bacterial and anti-fungal activity. It was shown to be moderately effective against Staph aureus, Pseudomonas aeruginosa, and Bacillussubtillis, and mildly effective against E. coli and Bacillus anthracis.[15] Isoalantolactone, a major sesquiterpene lactone of Inula racemosa, was found to be active against the human pathogenic fungi Aspergillus flavus, Aspergillus niger, Geotrichum candidum, Candida tropicalis, and Candida albicans at concentrations of 50, 50, 25, 25, and 25 micrograms/ml, respectively.

Anti-allergy activity

An alcoholic extract of root of Inula racemosa was studied for its anti-allergic effect in experimental models of type I hypersensitivity—specifically, egg albumin-induced passive cutaneous anaphylaxis and mast cell degranulation in albino rats.[16] The alcoholic extract was prepared using the process of continuous heat extraction. The protective value of different doses of Inula extract against egg albumin-induced passive cutaneous anaphylaxis was evaluated by intraperitoneal or oral administration of the extract for 7 days or once only. Mast cell degranulation studies were conducted using a compound 48/80 as the degranulation agent with the same dosage schedule. Inula racemosa showed significant protection against egg albumin-induced passive cutaneous anaphylaxis via both methods of administration. Protection against the compound 48/80 induced mast cell degranulation by alcoholic extract of Inula racemosa (single dose) was similar to that of disodium cromoglycate. The 7-day drug treatment schedule showed greater protection than disodium cromoglycate intraperitoneally. The results suggest that Inula racemosa possesses significant anti-allergic properties in rats.

Anti-cancer activity

In this study, 95% ethanolic extract of Inula roots and its fractions (n-hexane, chloroform, n-butanol, and aqueous) were evaluated for in-vitro cytotoxicity against cancer cell lines of colon, ovary, prostate, lung, CNS, and leukemia.[19] The n-hexane fraction containing alantolactone and isoalantolactone as its major constituents was studied further for its mode of action in HL-60 cells. The lowest IC(50) value of n-hexane fraction was 10.25 mug/ml for Colo-205, a colon cancer cell line, whereas 17.86 mug/ml was the highest IC(50) value observed against the CNS cancer cell line SF-295. Further studies on HL-60 cells treated with n-hexane fraction at 10, 25, and 50 mug/ml for 6 hours revealed that it induces apoptosis through intrinsic as well as extrinsic pathways by generating reactive oxygen species (ROS) intermediates. The mitochondrial dysfunction prompted the release of cytochrome c, translocation of pro-apoptotic protein (Bax), activation of caspase cascade, resulting in the cleavage of some specific substrates for caspase-3 such as poly (ADP-ribose) polymerase (PARP), which eventually leads to apoptosis.

Inflammatory modulation

Eupatolide, a sesquiterpene lactone from Inula britannica, as an inhibitor of cyclooxygenase-2 (COX-2) and inducible nitric oxide synthase (iNOS) expression was investigated.[10] Eupatolide inhibited the production of nitric oxide (NO) and prostaglandin E(2) (PGE(2)) as well as iNOS and COX-2 protein expression in lipopolysaccharide (LPS)-stimulated RAW264.7 cells. Eupatolide dose-dependently decreased the mRNA levels and the promoter activities of COX-2 and iNOS in LPS-stimulated RAW264.7 cells. Eupatolide significantly suppressed the LPS-induced expression of nuclear factor-kappa B (NF-kappaB) and activator protein-1 (AP-1) reporter genes. Pre-treatment of eupatolide inhibited LPS-induced phosphorylation and degradation of I kappaB alpha, and phosphorylation of RelA/p65 on Ser-536, as well as the activation of mitogen-activated protein kinases (MAPKs) and Akt in LPS-stimulated RAW264.7 cells. Eupatolide induced proteasomal degradation of tumor necrosis factor receptor-associated factor-6 (TRAF6), and subsequently inhibited LPS-induced TRAF6 polyubiquitination. Eupatolide blocked LPS-induced COX-2 and iNOS expression at the transcriptional level through inhibiting the signaling pathways such as NF-kappaB and MAPKs via proteasomal degradation of TRAF6. Taken together, eupatolide may be a novel anti-inflammatory agent that induces proteasomal degradation of TRAF6, and a valuable compound for modulating inflammatory conditions.

Ayurvedic Properties

Rasa: Tikta (Bitter); Katu (Pungent)
Guna:Laghu (Light)
Veerya: Ushna (Warm)
Vipaka: Katu(Pungent)
Tridosha (three bio humors): Pacifies Vata and Kapha bio humors and is useful in

management of diseases with Kapha/ Vata origin or both.

Kasa-shwashara: Useful in cough and respiratory discomfort

Hikka nigrahana: Alleviates hiccough

Parshwa shoola hara: Helps with pain in thorax region

Shophaghna: Useful in all edematous conditions

Pandunashanam: Useful in anemia and its complications

Ardit vinashanam: Useful in conditions involving nervous system, especially facial paralysis

Hrich chhulaghna: Alleviates pain in the heart region

Notes

1. A.L. Miller, "Botanical influences on cardiovascular disease," *Alternative Med Rev.*, Dec. 1998, 3(6):422–431.
2. Y.B. Tripathi, P. Tripathi, and B.N. Upadhyay, "Assessment of the adrenergic beta-blocking activity of Inula racemosa," *J Ethnopharmacol.*, May–June, 1988, 23(1):3–9.
3. Y. Huo, H.M. Shi, M.Y Wang, and X.B. Li, "Chemical constituents and pharmacological properties of radix Inulae," *Pharmazie*, Oct. 2008, 63(10):699–703.
4. W. Ketai, L. Huitao, Z. Yunkun, C. Xingguo, H. Zhide, S. Yucheng, and M. Xiao, "Separation and determination of alantolactone and isoalantolactone in traditional Chinese herbs by capillary electrophoresis," *Talanta*, Sept. 5, 2000, 52(6):1001–1005.
5. R.P. Singh, R. Singh, P. Ram, and P.G.Batliwala, "Use of Pushkar-Guggul, an indigenous antiischemic combination, in the management of ischemic heart disease," *Int J Pharmacog*, 1993, 31:147–160.
6. See Note 1.
7. S.D. Seth, M. Maulik, C.K. Katiyar, and S.K. Maulik, "Role of Lipistat in protection against isoproterenol induced myocardial necrosis in rats: A biochemical and histopathological study," *Indian J Physiol Pharmacol.*, Jan. 1998, 42(1):101–106.
8. See Note 5
9. S.N. Tripathi, B.N. Upadhyaya, and V.K. Gupta, "Beneficial effect of Inula racemosa (pushkarmoola) in angina pectoris: A preliminary report," *Indian J Physiol Pharmacol.*, Jan.–March, 1984, 28(1):73–75.
10. V. Patel, N. Banu, J.K. Ojha, et al., "Effect of indigenous drug (Pushkarmula) on experimentally induced myocardial infarction in rats," *Act Nerv Super*, 1982, 3:387–394.
11. K. Mangathayaru, S. Kuruvilla, K. Balakrishna, and J. Venkhateshm, "Modulatory effects of Inula racemosa Hook. F. on experimental atherosclerosis in guinea-pigs," *Journal of Pharmacy and Pharmacology*, Aug. 2009, 61(8):1111–1118.
12. S. Gholap and A. Kar, "Effects of Inula racemosa root and Gymnema sylvestre leaf extracts in the regulation of corticosteroid induced diabetes mellitus: Involvement of thyroid hormones," *Pharmazie*, June 2003, 58(6):413–415.

13. Tripathi Y.B. and P. Chaturvedi, "Assessment of endocrine response of Inula racemosa in relation to glucose homeostasis in rats," *Indian J Exp Biol.*, Sept. 1995, 33(9):686–689.

14. N. Singh, R. Nath, M. L. Gupta, and R. P. Kohli. An Experimental Evaluation of Anti-Asthmatic Potentialitis of Inula racemosa (Puskar Mul). Pharmaceutical Biology, 1980, Vol. 18, No. 2 : Pages 89-9

15. R.X Tan, H.Q. Tang, J. Hu, and B. Shuai, "Lignans and sesquiterpene lactones from Artemisia sieversiana and Inula racemosa," *Phytochemistry*, Sept. 1998, 49(1):157–161.

16. S. Srivastava, P.P. Gupta, R. Prasad, K.S. Dixit, G. Palit, B. Ali, G. Misra, and R.C. Saxena, "Evaluation of antiallergic activity (type I hypersensitivity) of Inula racemosa in rats," *Indian J Physiol Pharmacol.*, April 1999, 43(2):235–241.

17. H.C. Pal, I. Sehar, S. Bhushan, B.D. Gupta, and A.K. Saxena, "Activation of caspases and poly (ADP-ribose) polymerase cleavage to induce apoptosis in leukemia HL-60 cells by Inula racemosa," *Toxicol In Vitro*, June 17, 2010.

18. J. Lee, N. Tae, J.J. Lee, T. Kim, and J.H. Lee, "Eupatolide inhibits lipopolysaccharide-induced COX-2 and iNOS expression in RAW264.7 cells by inducing proteasomal degradation of TRAF6," *Eur J Pharmacol.*, June 25, 2010, 636 (1–3):173–180.

Momordica charantia

Introduction

Momordica charantia, or bitter melon, is a common food in Indian cuisine and also is used as a medicine to treat a wide array of conditions in the tropical regions in which it grows. The leaves and fruit of Momordica are part of the folk medicine traditions of China, India, Africa, and the West Indies since ancient times.

The Latin name Momordica, meaning "to bite," refers to the jagged edges of the bitter melon leaves, which appear as if they have been bitten. All parts of the plant, including the fruit, taste extremely bitter. Bitter melon is used to make teas, to ferment local beers, and to season soups. The plant grows natively in many tropical regions of the world, including East Africa, Asia, the Caribbean, and South America.

An unusual-looking fruit, bitter melon resembles a cucumber covered with hard bumps. Its firm fruit covers bright red seeds, which are inedible. When steeped in salt water, the fruit loses its bitter taste. The fruit also may be pickled and used as a relish.

Bitter melon is highly recommended for treating diabetes, both as part of the general diet and in the form of an extract or as a herbal tea made from the leaf. It also is commonly used in treating asthma, gastrointestinal problems, and hypertension. Bitter melon is used topically for sores, wounds, rashes, eczema, leprosy and other infections, and internally for worms and parasites, inflammation, and colic.

Synonymous Names

Botanical name: Momordica charantia
English: Bitter melon, bitter gourd
Sanskrit: Karavella, angarvell
Hindi: Karela
Common names: Bitter Gourd, Balsam Pear

Habitat

Bitter melon grows commonly throughout India, and is a vegetable crop all over the tropics, including parts of East Africa, Asia, the Caribbean, and South America.

Botanical Characteristics

The bitter melon plant is an annual creeping plant with branched stems that are twining and slender. The leaf blades are 5 to 12 centimeters in diameter, reniform or suborbicular, prominently nerved, and 5 to 7 lobed with irregular margins.

Bitter melon's tendrils are simple, slender, and pubescent. The flowers are monocious, and yellow in color. The male flowers are solitary, and the female flowers are bracteate at the base with a fusiform and muricate ovary. Bitter melon's fruits are muricate or tuberculate, oblong, and 2.5 to 7 centimeters long with tapering ends, green or yellowish in color with numerous soft triangular spikes on the surface. The seeds are 1.3 centimeters long, compressed, with a sculptured surface.

CHEMICAL COMPOSITION

Active Constituents

The fruit of bitter melon has been shown to lower blood sugar and provide other benefits for diabetes patients. The chemical component believed to provide this action is a mixture of the steroidal saponin known as charantin, insulin-like peptides, and alkaloids. It still is unclear which of these is most effective or if all three work together.

In preliminary studies, two proteins, alpha- and beta-momorcharin, have been shown to inhibit the AIDS virus, but this research has been demonstrated only in test tubes and not in humans. Another unidentified constituent in bitter melon inhibits the enzyme guanylate cyclase, which is associated with psoriasis.

Terpenoids

A series of cucurbitane-type triterpene glycosides called goyaglycosides a-h have been isolated along with the momordicosides A-L. Oleanane-type triterpene saponins, termed goyasaponins I, II and III, were also identified in the herb. The pyrimidine arabinopyranosides charine, vicine and others, along with the triterpenes momordicin, momordicinin and cucurbitanes I, II and III, have also been reported.[1, 2, 4]

Proteins

Alpha, beta, and gama Momorcharins, with N-glycosidase activity, and momordins a and b, were identified along with ribosome-inactivating proteins (RIPs) and lectins.[4,5]

Sterols and fatty acids

Palmitic and oleic acids are the major components of Momordica. Its minor constituents include stearic, lauric, linoleic, arachidic, myristic and capric acids. Conjugated octadecatrienoic acids form 63%–68% of the oil content, together with beta-sitosterol, campesterol, daucosterol, stigmasterol, and momordenol (3-beta-hydroxystigmasta-5,14-dien-16-one). The 4-monomethylsterols obtusifoliol, cycloeucalenol, 4-alpha methylzymosterol, lophenol, the desmethylsterols spinasterol (chondrillasterol), and others also have been identified.[6, 7]

Volatile constituents

Valeric acid, aldehydes (mainly pentanal, 2-hexenal, 2-heptenal and nonadienal), amyl formate, amylvalerate, 2-butylfuran and 2-hexanone, p-cymene, menthol, nerolidol, pentadecanol, hexadecanol, myrtenol, 3-hexenol, benzyl alcohol, l-penten-3-ol, cis-2-penten-1-ol, trans-2-hexenal, cis-sabinol and others have been identified.[8]

PHARMACOLOGICAL ACTIVITY

Hypoglycemic activity

Various studies have demonstrated the blood sugar lowering effect of Momordica's bitter fruit. Bitter melon has been demonstrated to enhance the cell's uptake of glucose, to promote insulin release, and to potentiate the effect of insulin.

Extracts of Momordica charantia also have been shown to rapidly decrease and normalize blood sugar levels in alloxan- or streptozotocin-induced diabetes mellitus. A water-soluble peptide fraction of

Momordica was found to be effective in normalizing blood sugar levels through oral administration.[9]

Different fractions of the fruits and seeds exhibited antilipolytic activity resembling insulin by inhibiting hormone-induced lipolysis.[10] Two of the active compounds were identified as peptides with similar amino acid compositions.[11] The effect of the insulin-like peptide on the lipid profile is not clear because it had no action on steroidogenesis, but other studies demonstrated antilipolytic activity.[12] Extracts of the fruit reversed some of the complications of diabetes in the liver and kidneys in experimental diabetes, with effective glucose control,[13] and reversed the effect of chronic diabetes on the modulation of both P450-dependent monooxygenase activities and GSH-dependent oxidative stress.[14]

Few other clinical trials were done to demonstrate the hypoglycemic activity of Momordica. In one clinical trial nine patients with confirmed type 1 diabetes were given a subcutaneous injection of Momordica extract containing crystalline p-insulin (p-insulin is an insulin-like compound found in Momordica). The results showed that p-insulin significantly decreased blood sugar compared to the controls. The authors of this study concluded that it acted like a long-acting insulin as its action started 30 to 60 minutes after administration and peaking effect ranging from 4 to 12 hours.[15] In another clinical trial of type 2 diabetes, 18 subjects were given 100 milliliters of Momordica juice prior to a glucose load. Of the 18 patients, 13 had better control of glucose tolerance.[16] In an uncontrolled trial of diabetic patients, one group received fractions of Momordica, one group received fruit powder, and another received an aqueous extract of Momordica. Those in the fruit group experienced an average 25% drop in blood sugar, and those receiving the aqueous extract experienced a 54% drop. Glycosylated hemoglobin examined in seven subjects decreased by an average of 17% after a 3-week trial. In the same clinical trial, the hypoglycemic effects were accompanied by significant adaptogenic properties, indicated by a delay in the appearance of cataracts and other secondary complications of diabetes.[17] In a study comparing the effects of Momordica and Rosiglitazone (Avandia) in managing type 2 diabetes showed that Momordica was more effective, and its complications much better than Rosiglitazone. The study evaluated the effect of Momordica and Rosiglitazone on serum levels of sialic acid changes. The Momordica group showed no changes, but the Rosiglitazone group had an increase in sialic acid, which is implicated as an acute phase marker for changes in microvasculature in diabetic patients.[18]

Cholesterol-reducing activity

Bitter melon fruit and seeds have been shown to reduce total cholesterol. In one study, elevated cholesterol and triglyceride levels in diabetic rats were returned to normal after 10 weeks of treatment.[19]

Anti-cancer activity

Several studies have demonstrated the anti-tumor activity of the entire bitter melon plant. In one study, a water extract blocked the growth of rat prostate carcinoma.[20] A subsequent study reported that a hot water extract of the entire bitter melon plant inhibited the development of mammary tumors in mice.[21] Numerous in-vitro studies have also demonstrated the anti-cancerous and anti-leukemic activity of bitter melon against numerous cell lines, including liver cancer, human leukemia, melanoma, and solid sarcomas.

An aqueous extract of bitter melon killed human leukemia lymphocytes in a dose-dependent manner, while not affecting the viability of normal human lymphocytes. A partially purified factor showed an inhibitory action on both viral and host cell RNA and on protein synthesis. This factor was found to be a single component with a molecular weight of 40 000 daltons.[22] The crude extract acted rapidly on human lymphocytes and leukemic lymphocytic cells[23] and was reported to inhibit guanylate cyclase activity, preventing the growth of concanavalin A-stimulated rat splenic lymphocytes.[24] An injection of the extract resulted in cytotoxicity against YAC-1 targets in a short-term assay and implicated a non-adherent cell population, which was capable of killing NK-sensitive cell lines.[25] In experimental studies the ribosome-inactivating protein momordin was found to be specifically cytotoxic to the Thy 1.1-expressing mouse lymphoma cell line AKR-A in vitro.[26] A glycoprotein derived from bitter melon seeds inhibited protein synthesis by nitrogen stimulated normal and leukemic lymphocytes, with a subsequent decrease in DNA formation and cell viability, which was more potent than hemagglutinin, possibly resulting from a greater penetration of lymphocytes by the lectin.[27]

Application of Momordica proteins to MDA-MB-231 breast cancer cells resulted in inhibition of cell proliferation, as well as the inhibition of expression of the HER2 gene in-vitro, suggesting a potential therapeutic use against carcinoma of the breast.[28] Momordin 1 and momordin 2 from bitter melon seeds inhibited protein synthesis in rabbit reticulocyte lysate, and showed potent cytotoxic activity against target Molt-4 cells, making them useful in allogeneic bone marrow transplantation.[29] Momordin 2, conjugated to the H65 monoclonal antibody, recognized the human T lymphocyte CD5 surface antigen using a heterobifunctional cross-linking reagent, 2-iminothiolane.

The resulting immunotoxins had no effect on human hematopoietic cells but suppressed tumor growth.

Alpha-Momorcharin inhibited the incorporation of [3H]leucine and [3H]uridine into P388 (mouse monocyte-macrophage), J774 (Balb/c macrophage), JAR (human placental choriocarcinoma), and sarcoma SI 80 cell lines. The most potent inhibitory effect was exerted on the P388 cell line, with the enhancement of the tumoricidal effect on mouse mastocytomal (P815) cells.[30] Tumor cell lines from renal, non-small cell lung and breast responded better to the proteins isolated from the plant.[31]

A comparative study evaluating the inhibitory potential of Momordica peel, pulp, seed, and whole fruit extract on mouse skin papillomagenesis indicated that the peel was the most effective. Topical application also produced a significant elevation of sulfhydryl (-SH), cytosolic glutathione S-transferase (GST), and microsomal cytochrome b5.[32]

An anti-CD5 monoclonal antibody (mAb), linked to momordin (a type-1 ribosome-inactivating protein), was studied for in-vitro cytotoxicity, measured as the inhibition of protein and/or DNA synthesis using isolated human peripheral blood mononuclear cells (PBMC) and neoplastic T lymphocytes.

The potency of the immunotoxin on PBMC was high, and it was very efficient in the inhibition of the proliferative response in a mixed lymphocyte reaction, suggesting a possible use of anti-CD5-momordin conjugate in the treatment of some leukemias and lymphomas.[33] A clinical trial was conducted in Thailand to evaluate the effect of Momordica on level and function of natural killer cells in cervical cancer with radiotherapy.[34] There was a decrease in total white blood cell count including lymphocytes and natural killer (NK) cells. NK cells, one type of lymphocytes, play a role to eliminate cancer cells by an antibody-dependent cell mediated cytotoxicity (ADCC) mechanism. Previous studies have shown that P-glycoprotein (170 kDa, transmembrane protein) may be a transporter for cytokine releasing in ADCC mechanism. This study proposed to explore the role of bitter melon intake in cervical cancer patients undergoing normal treatment (radiotherapy). The subjects were divided into three groups: (1) normal control (women 35-55 years, n = 35), (2) patient control (n = 30), and (3) patient treatment (n = 30) groups. The patient control and patient treatment groups were cervical cancer patients (stage II or III) treated with radiotherapy (without or with bitter melon ingestion). Blood samples of the patient control and patient treatment groups were analyzed for NK cells percentage and P-glycoprotein level. The authors hoped that bitter melon could stimulate the increase in NK cells percentage and P-glycoprotein level on the membrane in blood samples from cervical cancer patients who ingested bitter melon. The results showed an increased percentage of NK cells in patient control and patient treatment groups. The increase in each group was significant ($p < 0.05$) when compared to the percentage of NK cells from the second and third blood sampling times (after radiation with or without bitter melon intake for 45 and 90 days) with the first blood sampling time (before treatment). The results also showed a significant decrease in P-glycoprotein level ($p < 0.05$) in second and third blood sampling times when compared to the first blood sampling time of the patient treatment group. There was no significant difference in the P-glycoprotein (P-gp) level from the first, second, and third blood sampling times in the patient control group. Bitter melon ingestion did not affect the NK cell level but did affect the decrease of P-gp level on NK cell membrane.

Anti-fertility activity

The momorcharins are effective in inducing early and mid-term abortions but have teratogenic effects.[35] The intraperitoneal administration to mice of momorcharin on days 4 and 6 of pregnancy led to an inhibition of pregnancy with the disturbance of peri-implantation development. The termination of early pregnancy in the mouse may have resulted from an inhibitory effect of the abortifacient protein on the differentiating endometrium.[36]

Alpha and beta-momorcharin both inhibit embryonic implantation, probably by inhibiting cell free protein synthesis.[37]

Anti-genotoxic activity

Momordica charantia decreased the genotoxic activity of methylnitrosamine, methanesulphonate, and tetracycline, as shown by the decrease in chromosome breakage.[38]

Anti-helmintic activity

Momordica was more effective than piperazine in the treatment of Ascaridia galli.[39]

Anti-microbial activity

Leaf extracts of bitter melon have demonstrated broad-spectrum anti-microbial activity. Various extracts of the leaves have demonstrated in-vitro anti-bacterial effectiveness against E. coli, Staphylococcus, Pseudomonas, Salmonella, Streptobacillus, and Streptococcus. An extract of the entire bitter melon plant was shown to have antiprotozoal activity against Entamoeba histolytica. The fruit and fruit juice have demonstrated the same type of anti-bacterial properties and in another study, a fruit extract demonstrated activity against the stomach ulcer-causing bacteria Helicobacter pylori.

Bitter melon has also been shown to have antibacterial effects in several standard test systems.[40] Extracts of the dried powder alone and in combination with the fruits of Emblica officinalis and rhizomes of Curcuma longa showed anti-bacterial activity.[41]

Anti-viral activity

Bitter melon, like several of its isolated plant chemicals, has been documented with respect to in-vitro anti-viral activity against numerous viruses, including Epstein-Barr, herpes, and HIV viruses. In-vivo study, a leaf extract increased resistance to viral infections and had an immunostimulant effect in humans and animals, increasing interferon production and natural killer cell activity.

The proteins MAP30 and GAP3Q, isolated from Momordica, are active against the infection and replication of Herpes simplex virus, comparable in effect to acyclovir.[42] MAP30 inactivated viral DNA and specific cleavage of 28 S RNA, which may regulate HIV replication in conjunction with steroidal and non-steroidal inhibitors of prostaglandin synthesis. Use of the plant protein, in combination with dexamethasone and indomethacin, therefore was suggested for anti-HIV therapy.[43]

The inhibition of HIV 1 integrase suggests that impediment of viral DNA integration may play a key role in the anti-HIV activity and the effect on cell-free HIV 1 infection. Replication was proportionate to the dose.[44,45]

Hepatoprotective activity

Feeding bitter melon to diabetic rats brought levels of aminopyrene N-demethylase close to that of control animals, while ethoxycoumarin-O-deethylase was further reduced to 60% of the control value, with the normalization of cytosolic glutathione.[46] These results indicate in-vitro metabolic activation of aflatoxin Bl and benzo(a)pyrene and demonstrates that the fruits contain monofunctional phase II enzyme inducers and compounds capable of repressing some monooxygenases, especially those involved in the metabolic activation of chemical carcinogens. This shows potential as a chemopreventive agent.[47]

ETHNOVETERINARY USAGE

Bitter melon is used widely in veterinary medicine for tetanus, eye disorders, abdominal pain, liver fluke, and constipation. It is given to animals to promote digestion and urination. In cattle, it is used to expel the placenta and stop lactation after the death of a calf.[48]

DR. SODHI'S EXPERIENCE

When considering herbal therapy with Momordica, the practitioner should consider the following:

- Is dysglycemia present?
- Are parasites present, or likely to be present?
- Is there a viral infection, or increased viral load?
- Is there a need/desire to lose weight?
- Is HER-2+ breast cancer present?
- Is Leukemia or Lymphoma present?

Because Momordica has an insulin-like structure and helps to lower blood sugar, it is highly useful in treating all types of diabetes. It lowers blood sugar and increases glycogen storage, which enhances weight loss. For controlling blood sugar, its effect is enhanced if taken in combination with Pterocarpus marsupin (vijjayasaar), Ocimum sanctum (tulsi) and Azadirachtia indica (neem). These herbs work synergistically to normalize blood sugar metabolism.

Momordica also is good for treating intestinal parasites, especially pinworms. Many of my patients in India thought that I could read their minds because when they came to me to tell me that their stool was filled with white bugs with little black heads, I would say to them, "Oh, you must have eaten some Momordica recently," which, of course, they admitted that they had with great amazement.

Also, Momordica is a phenomenal anti-viral herb, in part because it is a protease inhibitor. I use it to treat hepatitis B and C, as well as HIV patients. We have lowered hepatitis C viral load successfully without using ribavirin and interferon. This is demonstrated in the case history below.

Case Histories

A patient who was infected with hepatitis C came to my clinic seeking an alternative to conventional medical treatment. We found his viral load to be 22 million. We started him on the following herbal protocol, to be taken three times a day:

> Tinospora cardifolia (guduchi), Picrorrhiza kurnoa (kutki), and Boerhaavia diffusa (purnarnava) extracts, 50 mg of each herb in a proprietory blend of Phyllanthus amarus (bhumyamalaki), Swertia chirayita (kiraata), Calotropis gigantis (ark), Raphanus sativa (malaka), Berberis aristata (daaru Curcuma), Terminalia arjuna (arjun), Terminalia bellerica (bibhitaki), Terminalia chebula (haritaki), Emblica officinalis (amalaki), Solanum nigrum (kakmachi), Andrographis paniculata (bhuunimb).

> Phyllanthus amarus, 250 mg extract, Momordica extract, 500 mg and Azadirachta indica (neem) extract 300 mg, in a proprietary blend of Emblica officinalis (amalaki), Terminalia chebula (haritaki), Terminalia bellerica (bahera), Tinospora cordifolia (guduchi), and Rubia cordifolia (manjistha).

After 6 weeks the patient's viral load had dropped to 3 million, and in 3 months the level was only 120,000. He has been able to control the disease, keeping his levels between 100,000 and 500,000 as long as he continues with the protocol.

We use this protocol whenever we have hepatitis C patients. Although we are unable to achieve a 100% negative viral load unless we add the ribavirin and interferon protocol, everyone who has done this protocol in conjunction with ribavirin and interferon have achieved a negative 100% viral load by the end of treatment. It should be noted that this is not true for hepatitis C patients who use only ribavirin and interferon therapy; the success rate for achieving a 100% negative viral load with this protocol alone is only 25%–30%.

Protocols

For diabetes mellitus:

> For both insulin-dependent and independent diabetes: 250 mg extract one to three times a day, either alone or in combination with the following formulation:

> Gymnema sylvestre (shardunika) extract, 300 mg, in combination with 200 mg betaine HCl, Chromium nicotinate 105 mcg, biotin 2150 mcg, Pterocarpus marsupium (vijjayasaar) and Ocimum sanctum (tulsi) extracts, 100 mg each, and Momordica charantia and Azadirachta indica (neem) extracts, 50 mg each three times per day

This treatment must be accompanied by appropriate diet and lifestyle changes.

Adding Neem extract further enhances anti-diabetic properties.

Safety Profile

Because it is used so widely as a food, bitter melon is considered to be reasonably safe, although the cytotoxic and other effects indicate that caution is required. Pregnant women should avoid the fruit. Side-effects of excessive doses of bitter melon are stomach pain and diarrhea. Excessive intake of Momordica also may induce emesis, although some of the toxic proteins may be degraded during cooking.

Momordin 1 was shown to have an LD_{50} value of 8.8 mg/kg in mice.[49] The insulin-like polypeptide did not have any cross-reaction with bovine insulin. When used as an anti-obesity agent, no side effects were observed.[50]

Patients being treated for hypoglycemia should avoid bitter melon. Diabetic patients taking hypoglycemic drugs (such as chlorpropamide, glyburide, or phenformin) or insulin should use bitter melon only under medical supervision, as it may potentiate the effectiveness of the drugs and lead to severe hypoglycemia. Combining standard drugs with bitter melon may reduce blood sugar to dangerously low levels, so it should be taken only under the strict guidance of a physician.

Dosage

Expressed juice of the whole plant or fruit: 10–30 ml.

For those with a taste or tolerance for bitter flavor, a small melon can be eaten as food, or up to 50 ml of fresh juice can be drunk per day. Those who do not care for the bitter taste of Momordica may find success using bitter melon tinctures, of which 5 ml is generally taken two or three times per day.

Extract: 10:1 100 mg to 250 mg one to three times per day

Ayurvedic Properties

Rasa: Tikta (bitter), katu (pungent)
Guna: Ruksha (dry), laghu (light)
Veerya: Ushna (hot)
Vipaka: Katu (pungent)
Dosha: Pacifies pitta and kapha

Notes

1. Ivan Ross, *Medicinal Plants of the World, Vol. 1* (Totowa, New Jersey: Humana Press, 1999). Any more current revisions? NO this is what is been referred

2. S. Begum, M. Ahmed, B.S. Siddiqui, A. Khan, Z.S. Saify, and M. Arif, "Triterpenes, a sterol and a monocyclic alcohol from Momordica charantia," *Phytochemistry,* 1997, 44(7):1313.

3. B. Hayat, F. Jabeen, C.S Hayat, and M. Akhtar, "Comparative prophylactic effects of salinomycin and some indigenous preparations against Coccidiosis in broiler chicks," *Pakistan Veterinary Journal,* 1996, 16(4):164.

4. Z. Pu, B. Lu, W. Liu, and S. Jin, "Characterization of the enzymic mechanism of gamma-momorcharin. a novel ri bosom e-in activating protein with lower molecular weight of 11,500 purified from the seeds of bitter gourd (Momordica charanlia)," *Biochemistry and Biophysics Research Communications,* 1996, 229(1|:287.

5. Z. Feng, W.W. Li, H.W. Yeung, et al., "Crystals of alpha-momorcharin, A new ribosome-inactivating protein," *Journal of Molecular Biology,* 1990, 214(3):625.

6. R. Armougom, I. Grondin, and J. Smadja, "Composition of fatty acids in lipid extracts of seeds of tropical Cucurbitaccae," *Lipides,* 1998, 5(4):323.

7. M.K. Chang, E.J. Conkerton, D.C. Chapital, P.J. Wan, O.P. Vandhwa, and J.M. Spiers, "Chinese melon (Momordica charanria L.) seed: Composition and potential use," *Journal of the American Oil Chemistry Society,* 1996, 73(2):263.

8. R.G. Binder, R.A. Hath, and T.R. Mon, "Volatile components of bitter melon," *Journal of Agricultural and Food Chemistry,* 1989, 37(2):418.

9. T.B. Ng, W.W. Li, and H.W.Yeung, "Effects of ginsenosides, lectins and Momordica charantia insulin-like peptide on corticosterone production by isolated rat adrenal cells," *Journal of Ethnopharmacology,* 1987, 21(1):21.

10. C.M Wong, T.B Ng, and H.W.Yeung, "Screening of Trichosanthes kirilowii, Momordica charantia and Cucurbita maxima (family Cucurbitaceae) for compounds with antilipolytic activity," *Journal of Ethnopharmacology,* 1985, 13(3):313.

11. T.B Ng, C.M. Wong, W.W Li, and H.W. Yeung, Peptides with antilipolytic and lipogenic activities from seeds of the bitter gourd Momordica charantia (family Cucurbitaceae). General Pharmacology, 1987, 18(3):275.

12. T.B Ng, C.M. Wong, W.W. Li, and H.W Yeung, "Insulin-like molecules in Momordica charantia seeds," *Journal of Ethnopharmacology*, 1986, 15(1):107.

13. N.Z. Baquer, D. Gupta, and J. Raju, "Regulation of metabolic pathways in liver and kidney during experimental diabetes: effects of antidiabetic compounds," *Indian Journal of Clinical Biochemistry*, 1998, 13(2):63.

14. H. Raza, I. Ahmed, A. John, and A.K. Sharma, "Modulation of xenobiotic metabolism and oxidative stress in chronic streptozotocin-induced diabetic rats fed with Momordica charantia fruit extract," *Journal of Biochemical and Molecular Toxicology*, 2000, 14(3):131.

15. V.S Baldwa, C.M. Bhandari, A. Pangaria, and R.K. Goyal, "Clinical trial in patients with diabetes mellitus of an insulin like compound obtained from plant source," *Upsala Journal of Medical Science*, 1977, 82:39–41.

16. J. Welihinda, E.H. Karunanayake, M.H. Sheriff, K.S. Jayasinghe, "Effect of Momordica charantia on the glucose tolerance in maturity onset diabetes," *Journal of Ethnopharmacology* 1986,17:277–282.

17. Y. Srivastava, H. Venkatakrishna-Bhatt, Y. Verma, K. Venkaiah, and B.H. Raval, "Antidiabetic and adaptogenic properties of Momordica charantia extract: An experimental and clinical evaluation," *Phytotherapy Research*, 1993, 7(4):285.

18. Inayat-ur-Rahman, S.A Malik, M. Bashir, R. Khan, and M. Iqbal M., "Serum sialic acid changes in non-insulin-dependant diabetes mellitus (NIDDM) patients following bitter melon (Momordica charantia) and rosiglitazone (Avandia) treatment," *Phytomedicine*, May 2009,16(5):401–405.

19. Ahmed I, Lakhani MS, Gillett M, John A, Raza H. Hypotriglyceridemic and hypocholesterolemic effects of anti-diabetic Momordica charantia (karela) fruit extract in streptozotocin-induced diabetic rats. Diabetes Res Clin Pract. 2001 Mar;51(3):155-61.

20. Pitchakarn P, Suzuki S, Ogawa K, Pompimon W, Takahashi S, Asamoto M, Limtrakul P, Shirai T. Kuguacin J, a triterpeniod from Momordica charantia leaf, modulates the progression of androgen-independent human prostate cancer cell line, PC3. Food Chem Toxicol. 2012 Mar;50(3-4):840-7.

21. Fang EF, Zhang CZ, Fong WP, Ng TB. RNase MC2: a new Momordica charantia ribonuclease that induces apoptosis in breast cancer cells associated with activation of MAPKs and induction of caspase pathways. Apoptosis. 2012 Apr;17(4):377-87.

22. D.J. Takemoto, C. Jilka, S. Rockenbach, and J.V. Hughes, "Purification and characterisation of a cytostatic factor with anti-viral activity from the bitter melon," *Preparative Biochemistry*, 1983, 13(5):391.

23. D.J. Takemoto, C. Dunford, and M.M. McMurray, "The cytotoxic and cytostatic effects of the bitter melon (Momordica charantia) on human lymphocytes," *Toxicon*, 1982, 20(3):593.

24. D.J. Takemoto, R. Kresie, and D. Vaughn, "Partial purification and characterization of a guatiylate cyclasic inhibitor with cytotoxic properties from the bitter melon (Memordica charantia)," *Biochemistry and Biophysics Research Communications*, 1980, 94(1):332.

25. J.E. Cunnick, K. Sakamoto, S.K Chapes, G.W. Fortner, and D.J. Takemoio, "Induction of tumor cytotoxic immune cells using a protein from the bitter melon t/Aomordica charantia)," *Cellular Immunology*, 1990, 126(2):278.

26. F. Stirpe, E.J Wawrzynczak, A.N.F. Brown, et al., "Selective cytotoxic activity of immunotoxins composed of a monoclonal anti-Thy 1.1 antibody and the ribosome-in activatitig proteins bryodin and momordin," *British Journal of Cancer*, 1988, 58(5):S58.

27. M.O. Fatope, Y. Takeda, H. Yamashita, H. Okabe, and T. Yamauchi, "New cucurbitane triterpenoids from Momordica charantia," *Journal of Natural Products*, 1990, 53(6):149.

28. S. Lee-Huang, P.L. Huang, Y.Sun, et al., "Inhibition of MDA-MB-231 human breast tumor xenografts and HER2 expression by anti-tumor agents GAP31 and MAP30," *Anticancer Research*, 2000, 20(2A):653.

29. R. Wang, X. Chen, Y. Li, and P. Shen, "Immunotoxins composed of monoclonal antihuman T lymphocyte antibody and single chain ribosome-inactivating proteins: antitumor effects in vitro and in vivo," *Zhongguo Mianyixue Zazhi*, 1992, 8(6):356.

30. T.B. Ng, W.K. Liu, S.F. Sze, and H.W. Yeung, "Action of a-momorcharin, a ribosome inactivating protein, on cultured tumor cell lines," *General Pharmacology*, 25(1):75.

31. S.M Rybak, J.J. Lin, D.L.Newton, et al., "In vitro antitumor activity of the plant ribosome inactivating proteins MAP 30 and GAP 31," *International Journal of Oncology*, 1994, 5(5): 1171.

32. A. Singh, S.P. Singh, and R. Bamezai, "Momordica charantia (Bitter Gourd) peel, pulp, seed and whole fruit extract inhibits mouse skin papillomagenesis," *Toxicology Letters*, 1998, 94(1):37.

33. G. Porro, A. Bolognesi, P. Caretto, et al., "In vitro and in vivo properties of an anti-CD5-momordin immunotoxin on normal and neoplastic T lymphocytes," *Cancer Immunology and Immunotherapy*, 1993, 36(5):346.

34. S. Pongnikorn, D. Fongmoon, W. Kasinrerk, and P.N. Limtrakul, "Effect of bitter melon (Momordica charantia Linn) on level and function of natural killer cells in cervical cancer patients with radiotherapy," *J Med Assoc Thai.*, Jan. 2003, 86(1):61–68.

35. W.Y. Chan, P.P.L Tarn, H.L, Choi, T.B. Ng, and H.W. Yeung, "Effects of momorcharins on the mouse embryo at the early organogenesis stage," *Contraception*, 1986, 34(5):537.

36. W.Y. Chan, P.P.L. Tarn, K.G. So, and H.W. Yeung, "The inhibitory effects of B-momorcharin on endometrial cells in the mouse," *Contraception*, 1985, 31(1):83.

37. T.B. Ng, P.P.L Tarn, W.K. Hon, H.L. Choi, and H.W. Yeung, "Effects of momorcharins on ovarian response to gonadotropin-induced superovulation in mice," *International Journal of Fertility*, 1988, 33(2):123.

38. J.G Balboa and C.Y. Lim-Sylianco, "Antigenotoxic effects of drug preparations Akapulko and Ampalaya," *Philippine Journal of Science*, 1992, 121(4):399.

39. J. Lal, S. Chandra, V. Raviprakash, and M. Sabir, "In vitro anthelmintic action of some indigenous medicinal plants on Ascaridia galli worms," *Indian Journal of Physiology and Pharmacology*, 1976, 20(2):64.

40. See Note 1, Ross.

41. J. Sankaranarayanan and C.I. Jolly, "Phytochemical, anti-bacterial, and pharmacological investigations on Momordica charantia Linn., Emblica offidnalis Gaertn. and Curcuma longa Linn," *Indian Journal of Pharmaceutical Science*, 1993, 55(1):6.

42. A.S. Bourinbaiar and S. Lee-Huang, "The activity of plant-derived antiretroviral proteins MAP30 and GAP31 against herpes simplex virus infection in vitro," *Biochemistry and Biophysics Research Communications*, 1996, 219(3):923.

43. A.S Bourinbaiar and S. Lee-Huang, "Potentiation of anti-HIV activity of the anti-inflammatory drugs dexamethasone and indomethacin by MAP30, the anti-viral agent from bitter melon," *Biochemistry and Biophysics Research Communications*, 1995, 208(2):779.

44. S. Lee-Huang, P.L. Huang, A.S. Bourinbaiar, H.C. Chen, and H.F. Kung, "Inhibition of the integrase of human immunodeficiency virus (HIV) type 1 by anti-HIV plant proteins MAP30 and GAPS 1," *Proceedings of the National Academy of Science of the USA*, 1995, 92(19):8818.

45. S. Lee-Huang, P.L. Huang, P.L. Nara, et al., "MAP 30: a new inhibitor of HIV-1 infection and replication," *FEES Letters*, 1990, 272(1–2):12.

46. H. Raza, I. Amed, M.S. Lakhani, A.K. Sharma, D. Pallot, and W. Montague, "Effect of bitter melon (Momordica charantia) fruit juice on the hepatic cytochrome P-450-dependent monooxygenases and glutathione S-transferases in streptozotocin-induced diabetic rats," *Biochemistry and Pharmacology*, 1996, 52(10):1639.

47. W.R. Kusamran, A. Ratanavila, and A. Tepsuwan, "Effects of neem flowers, Thai and Chinese bitter gourd fruits and sweet basil leaves on hepatic monooxygenases and glutathione S-transferase activities, and in vitro metabolic activation of chemical carcinogens in rats," *Food Chemistry and Toxicology*, 1998, 36(6):475.

48. M.K. Jha, *Folk veterinary medicine of Bihar—a research project* (Anand, Gujrat: NDDB, 1992).

49. M.L Dhar, M.M. Dhar, B.N. Dhawan, B.N. Mehrotra, and C. Ray, "Screening of Indian plants for biological activity-I," *Indian Journal of Experimental Biology*, 1968, 6:232.

50. J. Yamahara, "D-Xylose and pharmaceutical natural products as anti-obesity agents," 1998. Japanese patent application JP 97-108130 19970409.

26

Mucuna pruriens

Introduction

Also known as velvet bean or cowhage, Mucuna pruriens is one of the most popular Ayurvedic herbs. Because it contains the chemical L-dopa, a precursor to the neurotransmitter dopamine, Mucuna has been used for generations in India to treat Parkinson's disease. In Ayurvedic tradition, Velvet bean is considered a diuretic, nerve tonic, and aphrodisiac. It also is used in India for conditions as diverse as worms, dysentery, diarrhea, snakebite, cough, tuberculosis, impotence, rheumatic disorders, muscular pain, sterility, gout, diabetes, and cancer.

In Central America, the seeds of velvet bean are roasted and ground to make a coffee substitute. For this reason, the plant is known by the common name nescafé in these regions, as well as in Brazil, Also in Brazil, the seed is used internally to treat Parkinson's disease, edema, impotence, intestinal gas, and worms. Velvet bean is used in many cultures as a nerve tonic for nervous system disorders.

The L-dopa in velvet bean converts into dopamine, an important brain chemical involved in mood, sexuality, and movement. For this reason, velvet bean now is being considered as an alternative to the pharmaceutical medication Levodopa in treating Parkinson's disease. Early studies have shown its capacity to slow the progression of Parkinson's symptoms such as tremors, rigidity, slurring, drooling, and balance, and to have none of the side-effects of the current pharmaceutical L-dopa.

Synonymous Names

Latin: Mucuna pruriens, Mucuna prurita
English: Cow-itch plant, velvet bean, cowhage
Hindi: Kaunch, kevanch
Sanskrit: Kapikachhu, atmagupta

Habitat

The velvet bean plant is indigenous to Africa, India, and the Caribbean.

Botanical Characteristics

Velvet bean is an annual climbing vine that usually grows to about 15 meters tall. When the plant is young, it is covered almost completely with fuzzy hairs, but when mature, most of the hairs disappear. The plant's leaves are tripinnate, ovate, reverse ovate, rhombus-shaped or widely ovate. The sides of the leaves are often heavily grooved, and the tips are pointed. The stems of the leaflets are 2 to 3 millimeters long. Additional adjacent leaves are present and are about 5 mm long.

Velvet bean bears white, lavender, or purple flowers. Its seed pods are about 10 cm long and are covered in loose orange hairs that cause a severe itch if they come in contact with skin. The chemical compounds responsible for the itch are a protein, mucunain, and serotonin. The seeds are shiny and black or brown.

Mucuna's flower heads are axially arrayed panicles. They are 15 to 32 centimeters long with two or three, or even many flowers. The accompanying leaves are about 12.5 millimeters long, and the flower stand axes are from 2.5 to 5 millimeters. The bell is 7.5 to 9 millimeters long and silky. The sepals are longer or of the same length as the shuttles. The crown is purplish or white.

Chemical Composition

The seeds of velvet bean are high in protein, carbohydrates, lipids, fiber, and minerals. They also are rich in novel alkaloids, saponins, and sterols. The seeds of all Mucuna species contain a high concentration of L-dopa; the velvet bean seeds contain 7% to 10% L-dopa. Concentrations of serotonin also have been found in the pod, leaf, and fruit. The stinging hairs of the seed pods contain the phytochemical mucunain, which is responsible for causing skin irritation and itch.

The main plant chemicals found in velvet bean include the following: alkaloids, alkylamines, arachidic acid, behenic acid, betacarboline, beta-sitosterol, bufotenine, cystine, dopamine, fatty acids, flavones, galactose d, gallic acid, genistein, glutamic acid, glutathione, glycine, histidine, hydroxygenistein, 5-hydroxytryptamine, isoleucine, l-dopa, linoleic acid, linolenic acid, lysine, mannose d, methionine, 6-methoxyharman, mucunadine, mucunain, mucunine, myristic acid, niacin, nicotine, oleic acid, palmitic acid, palmitoleic acid, phenylalanine, prurienidine, prurienine, riboflavin, saponins, serine, serotonin, stearic acid, stizolamine, threonine, trypsin, tryptamine, tyrosine, valine, and vernolic acid.[1]

Pharmacological Activity

Anti-Parkinsonian activity

Because of the high concentration of L-dopa in velvet bean seeds, it has been studied intensively for its potential use in treating Parkinson's disease, a common age-related neurodegenerative disorder that affects more than four million people worldwide. Parkinson's disease is associated with progressive degeneration of dopaminergic neurons in specific areas of the brain. Dopamine does not cross the blood-brain barrier and, therefore, cannot be used directly as a treatment. L-dopa, however, does gain access to the brain, where it is converted to dopamine.

The clinical effects of Mucuna were compared to standard doses of L-dopa in Parkinson's patients.[2,3] For the study, eight Parkinson's disease patients were treated with a short duration L-dopa response and completed a randomized, controlled, double blind crossover trial. Compared to the standard treatment, the Mucuna preparation led to a considerably faster onset of the effects. The average onset was approximately 22% faster with a dose of 30 grams of Mucuna than the standard drug treatment. No significant differences in dyskinesia or tolerability occurred.[4]

The rapid onset of action and longer on-time without a concomitant increase in dyskinesias on Mucuna seed powder formulation suggest that this natural source of L-dopa might have advantages over conventional L-dopa preparations in the long-term management of Parkinson's disease.

Parkinson's disease has a low prevalence in India except in its small Parsi (Persian) community. Although early onset Parkinson's and familial cases have been described from India, no genetic mutations have been identified as yet. Parkinson's disease has been known in India since ancient days, and the powder of Mucuna seeds has been used traditionally as its treatment.[12]

In a clinical prospective study, the efficacy of a traditional Ayurvedic treatment including Mucuna was studied in 18 clinically diagnosed Parkinson's disease patients. Thirteen of the patients underwent both cleansing (28 days) and palliative therapy (56 days), and five patients underwent palliative therapy alone (84 days). Only the former group showed significant improvement in activities of daily living and on motor examination. Symptomatically, they exhibited better response in tremor, bradykinesia, stiffness, and cramps compared to the latter group. Excessive salivation worsened in both groups. Analyses of powdered samples in milk, as administered in patients, revealed about 200 mg of L-dopa per dose.

This study establishes the necessity of cleansing therapy when using Ayurvedic medication prior to palliative therapy. It also reveals contribution of L-dopa in the recovery as observed in Parkinson's disease following Ayurvedic medication.[6]

In a rat model of Parkinson's disease, Mucuna was shown to possess significantly higher anti-Parkinson activity than Levodopa.[7] The study evaluated the neurorestorative effect of Mucuna pruriens cotyledon powder on the nigrostriatal tract of 6-OHDA lesioned rats. Mucuna pruriens powder significantly increased the brain mitochondrial complex-I activity but did not affect the total monoamine oxidase activity in-vitro.

Unlike synthetic Levodopa treatment, Mucuna powder treatment significantly restored the endogenous Levodopa, dopamine, norepinephrine, and serotonin content in the substantia nigra. Nicotine adenine dinucleotide (NADH) and coenzyme Q-10, which are known to have a therapeutic benefit in Parkinson's disease, were present in the Mucuna pruriens powder.

Neurorestorative benefit by Mucuna pruriens powder on the degenerating dopaminergic neurons in the substantia nigra may be attributable to increased complex-I activity and the presence of NADH and coenzyme Q-10.[8]

The chemical constituent HP-200, which contains Mucuna pruriens, has been shown to be effective in treating Parkinson's disease. Mucuna pruriens also has been shown to be more effective than synthetic Levodopa in an animal model of Parkinson's disease. A study was conducted to assess the long-term effect of Mucuna pruriens in HP-200 on monoaminergic neurotransmitters and its metabolite in various regions of the rat brain.[9]

The Mucuna constituent HP-200 was fed to rats for 52 weeks, after which a significant effect on dopamine content in the cortex was observed. No significant effect on Levodopa, norepinephrine or dopamine, serotonin, and their metabolites was found. The failure of Mucuna pruriens endocarp to significantly affect dopamine metabolism in the striatonigral tract, along with its ability to improve Parkinsonian symptoms in the 6-hydorxydopamine animal model and humans, may suggest that its anti-Parkinson effect may be attributable to components other than Levodopa or that it has an Levodopa enhancing effect.[10]

Other anti-dyskinesia activity

Neuroleptic-induced tardive dyskinesia (TD) is a motor disorder of the orofacial region resulting from chronic neuroleptic treatment. The agents improving dopaminergic transmission improve TD. Mucuna pruriens seed contains Levodopa and amino acids. The effect of methanolic extract of M. pruriens seeds was studied on haloperidol-induced TD, along with the changes in lipid peroxidation, reduced glutathione, superoxide dismutase (SOD), and catalase levels. The effect of Mucuna also was evaluated in terms of the generation of hydroxyl and 1,1-diphenyl,2-picrylhydrazyl (DPPH) radical. Mucuna (100 and 200 mg kg(-1)) inhibited haloperidol-induced vacuous chewing movements, orofacial bursts, biochemical changes and also inhibited hydroxyl radical generation and DPPH.[11]

Anti-venom activity

Extracts of Mucuna pruriens seeds have been shown to protect mice against Echis carinatus venom by an immunological mechanism. A study demonstrated that the Mucuna immunogen generating the antibody that cross-reacts with the venom proteins is a multiform glycoprotein whose immunogenic properties reside mainly in its glycan-chains.[12]

The anti-venom property of a water extract of Mucuna seeds was assessed in-vivo in mice. The serum of mice treated with the extract was tested for its immunological properties. Two proteins of Echis carinatus venom were detected. Through enzymatic in-gel digestion and electrospray ionization-mass spectrometry analysis of immunoreactive venom proteins, phospholipase A(2) the most toxic enzyme of snake venom, was identified. These results demonstrate that the observed anti-venom activity has an immune mechanism. Antibodies of mice treated with non-lethal doses of venom reacted against some proteins of Mucuna pruriens extract. Proteins of Echis carinatus venom and the Mucuna extract have at least one epitope in common, as confirmed by the immunodiffusion assay.[13]

The effect of a lethal Echis carinatus venom on serum enzyme levels and blood plasma coagulation was studied in rats pre-treated with Mucuna pruriens seed aqueous extract 24 hours and 3 weeks before venom injection. Rats injected with the venom alone were used as controls. Results of this study indicate that the increased enzymes lactate dehydrogenase, glutamic pyruvic transaminase, creatinine kinase, and changed coagulation parameters from the venom effect were inhibited by Mucuna seed extract in the pre-treated rats. Rats pre-treated with a single dose of extract maintained the normal enzyme levels and showed an anticoagulant effect, as evidenced by the high PTT level, which also was observed in the venom-treated animals; however, the extract seemed to significantly inhibit the lethal venom-induced myotoxic, cytotoxic, and coagulation activities in the experimental animals.[14]

In rats, Mucuna pre-treatment conferred effective protection against the lethality of Naja sputatrix venom and provided moderate protection against the Calloselasma rhodostoma venom. Indirect ELISA and immunoblotting studies revealed extensive cross-reactions between anti-Mucuna pruriens extract (MPE) IgG and venoms from many different genera of poisonous snakes. This suggests the involvement of immunological neutralization in the protective effect of Mucuna pruriens pre-treatment against snake venom poisoning. In-vitro neutralization experiments showed that the anti-MPE antibodies effectively neutralized the lethality of Asiatic cobra (Naja) venoms but were not effective against the other venoms tested.[15]

Anti-diabetic activity

Several in-vivo studies have been conducted on the blood-sugar-lowering effect of velvet bean. These studies all validate the traditional use of the plant for diabetes. An ethanol-water extract of the root, fruit, and seed decreased the blood sugar levels in rats by more than 30%. At 200 mg, an ethanol extract produced a 40% fall in blood glucose within one month, and a 51% reduction at 4 months.[16]

Mucuna was assessed for its effectiveness in preventing murine alloxan diabetic cataract. Rats received a lyophilized aqueous extract of Mucuna every day for 4 months. Serum glucose concentration was assessed, and cataracts were examined with both the naked eye and through a slit lamp. Of the eight animals in the diabetic control group, four developed a cortical cataract by day 90 and the remaining four developed it by day 100. None of the animals treated with the herbal extract had developed cataracts at the end of a 120- day period.[17]

Mucuna pruriens was assessed for its anti-hyperglycemic effect on varying degrees of hyperglycemia and diabetic complications. An alcohol extract of the herb was evaluated in a pilot study, a long term study in alloxanized rats, and streptozotocin induced mice. In the pilot study, the maximum antihyperglycemic effect occurred with an alcohol extract of Mucuna at week 6 at a dose of 200 mg/kg/day. In the chronic alloxanized rats, the selected dose of Mucuna led to a significant fall of in plasma glucose levels.[18]

A study was undertaken to investigate the effects of daily oral feeding of Mucuna pruriens and other Ayurvedic herbs for 40 days on blood glucose concentrations and kidney functions in streptozotocin (STZ)-diabetic rats. Plasma glucose levels, body weight, urine volume, and urinary albumin levels were monitored on every 10th day over a 40-day period, and plasma creatinine levels were assessed at the beginning and end of the experiment. Renal hypertrophy was assessed as the ratio between kidney weight and total body weight.

The plasma glucose concentrations in STZ-diabetic mice were reduced by the administration of extracts of several of the herbs, including Mucuna. After 10 days of STZ administration, urinary albumin levels were more than six times higher in the diabetic controls compared to the normal controls. Treatment with Mucuna and several other herbal extracts significantly prevented the rise in urinary albumin levels from day 0 to day 40 in comparison to the diabetic controls. Renal hypertrophy was significantly higher in the diabetic controls as compared to the non-diabetic controls.[19]

Sexual dysfunction is one of the major secondary complications in diabetic individuals. The objective of this study was to analyze the efficacy of Mucuna pruriens on male sexual behavior and sperm parameters in long-term hyperglycemic male rats.[20] The male albino rats were divided as: group I control; group II diabetes induced (streptozotocin [STZ] 60 mg/kg of body weight (b.w.) in 0.1 M citrate buffer); group III diabetic rats administered with 200 mg/kg b.w. of ethanolic extract of M. pruriens seed; group IV diabetic rats administered with 5 mg/kg b.w. of sildenafil citrate (SC); group V administered with 200 mg/kg b.w. of extract, and group VI administered with 5 mg/kg b.w. of SC. M. pruriens and SC were administered in single oral dosage per day for 60 days.

The mating behavior, libido, and test of potency, along with epididymal sperms, were studied. The study showed significant reduction in sexual behavior and sperm parameters in group II. Daily sperm production and levels of follicular stimulating hormone, luteinizing hormone, and testosterone were reduced significantly in group II, whereas the animals with diabetes administered with seed extract of Mucuna pruriens (group III) showed significant improvement in sexual behavior, libido, and potency, sperm parameters, daily sperm production, and hormonal levels compared to group II.

This work reveals the potential efficacy of ethanolic seed extract of M. pruriens to improve male sexual behavior with androgenic and anti-diabetic effects in the STZ-induced diabetic male rats. This study supports the use of Mucuna pruriens in the Ayurvedic medicine as a sexual invigorator in the diabetic condition and encourages performing a similar study in men.

Anti-oxidant activity

In-vitro and in-vivo studies were carried out with an alcohol extract of the seeds of Mucuna pruriens to investigate its anti-oxidant properties. In-vitro studies were carried out in rat liver homogenate to investigate the chemical interaction of various phytochemicals with different species of free radicals. The effect also was checked for iron-induced lipid peroxidation, oxidation of GSH content, and its interaction with hydroxyl and superoxide radicals. The rate of aerial oxidation of GSH content was unchanged, but it significantly inhibited $FeSO_4$ induced lipid peroxidation. It also inhibited the specific chemical reactions induced by superoxides and hydroxyl radicals. These species were removed through direct chemical interaction. [21, 22]

An in-vivo study on albino rats for 30 days showed no toxic effect up to an oral dose of 600 mg/kg body weight. There was no change in the level of TBA-reactive substances, reduced glutathione content, or SOD activity in the liver. The activity of serum GOT, GPT, and alkaline phosphatase also was unchanged. Mucuna pruriens has an anti-lipid peroxidation property that is mediated through the removal of superoxides and hydroxyl radicals.[23]

Male fertility

In a study to evaluate mechanism of action of Mucuna, seventy five healthy fertile men (control) were paired against seventy five infertile men. Full spectrum of diagnostic tests were done before and after the study. Estimation was done by RIA of hormonal parameters in blood plasma, namely Testosterone (T), luteinizing hormone (LH), Follicle stimulating hormone (FSH), and Prolactin (PRL). Before and after treatment, serum testosterone, LH, FSH, PRL, dopamine, adrenaline, and noradrenaline in seminal and blood plasma were measured. A decreased sperm count and motility were seen in the infertile subjects. Serum T and LH levels, as well as seminal plasma and blood levels of dopamine, adrenaline, and noradrenaline also were decreased in all groups of infertile men. This was accompanied by significantly increased serum FSH and PRL levels in the oligozoospermic subjects. Treatment with Mucuna pruriens significantly improved T, LH, dopamine, adrenaline, and noradrenaline levels in the infertile men, and reduced the levels of FSH and PRL. Sperm count and motility were recovered significantly in the infertile men after treatment. Mucuna pruriens regulated steroidogenesis and improved semen quality in infertile men.[24]

Another investigation was undertaken to assess the role of Mucuna pruriens in infertile men under psychological stress.[25] The study consisted of 60 subjects who were undergoing infertility screening and were found to be suffering from psychological stress, assessed on the basis of a questionnaire and elevated serum cortisol levels. The controls consisted of 60 age-matched healthy men having normal semen parameters and who previously had initiated at least one pregnancy. The infertile subjects were administered Mucuna pruriens seed powder (5 g day(-1)) orally. For carrying out morphological and biochemical analysis, semen samples were collected twice, first before starting treatment and then after 3 months of treatment. The results demonstrated a decreased sperm count and motility in the subjects who were under psychological stress. Serum cortisol and seminal plasma lipid peroxide levels were found to be elevated along with decreased seminal plasma glutathione (GSH), ascorbic acid contents, reduced superoxide dismutase (SOD) and catalase activity. Treatment with Mucuna pruriens significantly reduced psychological stress and seminal plasma lipid peroxide levels, along with an improved sperm count and motility. The treatment also restored the levels of SOD, catalase, GSH, and ascorbic acid in the seminal plasma of infertile men. Mucuna pruriens not only reactivates the anti-oxidant defense system of infertile men but also helps in the management of stress and improves semen quality. In animal studies the protective efficacy of Mucuna pruriens on reactive oxygen species (ROS)-induced pathophysiological alterations in structural and functional integrity of epididymal sperm in aged Wister albino rat was analysed.[26] The animals were grouped as groups I, II, III and IV—i.e. young (control), aged, aged treated with ethanolic extract

(200 mg/kg b.w.) of Mucuna Pruriens. After 60 days of the experimental period the animals were sacrificed and the epididymal sperm were collected and subjected to count, viability, motility, morphology, and morphometric analysis. Enzymatic and non-enzymatic anti-oxidants, ROS, lipid peroxidation (LPO), DNA damage, chromosomal integrity, and mitochondrial membrane potential were estimated. The results obtained from the aged animals showed significant reduction in sperm count, viability and motility, increased morphological damage, and an increase in the number of sperm with cytoplasmic remnant. These alterations were reversed significantly in the Mucuna pruriens-treated group.

A significant increase in LPO and H_2O_2 production and a significant decline in the levels of the enzymatic and non-enzymatic anti-oxidants were observed in the aged animals. Supplementation of Mucuna pruriens significantly reduced ROS and LPO production and significantly increased both enzymatic and non-enzymatic anti-oxidant levels. Significant DNA damage, loss of chromosomal integrity, and an increase in mitochondrial membrane permeability was seen in the aged rat sperm. This was significantly reduced in group III which were treated with Mucuna pruriens. Collectively, sperm damage from aging was reduced significantly by quenching ROS and improving the anti-oxidant defense system and mitochondrial function.[27]

Dr. Sodhi's Experience

When considering herbal treatment with Mucuna, the practitioner should consider the following:

- Has Parkinson's disease been diagnosed?
- Does the individual need more dopamine?
- Is sperm quality is a issue?

Mucuna is specific for Parkinson's disease, as well as for any disorder caused by insufficient levels of the neurotransmitter dopamine. Mucuna (Kapikachu) contains a natural form of dopamine, but its effectiveness against Parkinson's disease is not limited to this quality. Research has shown that when the natural dopamine is chemically removed, Kapikachu is still effective to some extent in treating Parkinson's disease. This indicates that the herb possesses additional active anti-Parkinsonian properties.

For centuries in India, Kapikachu has been used in conjunction with the herb Panchakarma to treat Parkinson's disease. Empirical evidence gathered over this time strongly suggests that this treatment halts the progress of the disease by helping to regenerate the nervous system and arresting damage caused by free radicals.

The Panchakarma (Ayurvedic detoxification) is believed to act by a process of systemic detoxification that significantly reduces the overall toxic burden on the body, thus returning it to normal physiology. In addition to providing natural dopamine, Kapikachu is also cholinesterase inhibitor.

Mucuna (Kapikachu) also is useful as a therapy for infertility, increasing sperm motility and sperm count. The herb enhances the sexual experience for both men and women, making it more satisfying while also increasing seminal and vaginal fluids.

Case Histories

For Parkinson's disease:

Whenever I am asked how we treat Parkinson's disease in Ayurveda, one patient in particular often comes to mind. This patient was a man in his 80s who had the disease. He was a Boeing engineer and thought that Ayurveda was nothing more than "hocus pocus." His wife first came to our clinic seeking medicine for him. When I told her that the Ayurvedic treatment of Parkinson's did not just involve taking a single herb or herbal formulation, she replied, "He won't come in to see you. Isn't there just one thing you could give me for him?" I gave her the following formulation and told her to have him take one three times a day in the beginning, but that we might have to increase the dose later:

> Mucuna pruriens (kapikachu) extract, 250 mg, in a proprietary blend of Centella asiatica (brahmi), Valeriana waliichii (tagara), and Ashwagandha.

At first, the patient refused to take this medication, but his wife kept the bottle on hand, ready in the event that he might change his mind. Some time later, they went to Hawaii for a vacation and, as always, she took the formula with her, tucked away in her luggage on this occasion. When they got to Hawaii, her husband realized that he had forgotten his prescription medications of L-dopa. His wife said, "Well, maybe this will work better. Why don't you try it?"

Because a few days were needed to have the L-dopa prescription mailed, even by express mail, he relented and took our formulation. After just one day, he noticed that he felt better and didn't have the usual side-effect of a dry mouth, which L-dopa caused. He didn't mention this to his wife, and she didn't ask, but he did take the herbs again. A couple of days later, his wife asked him how he was doing and commented that he seemed to be shaking less. He replied, "Oh, I'm taking Dr. Sodhi's formula, and I'm feeling fine."

The patient has continued taking the herbal formula for 4 or 5 years, and the disease has not progressed further. His hair is even growing back. But he has not come into the clinic for clinical evaluation, or for panchakarma (Ayurvedic detoxification) treatment.

For infertility:

A young Asian man with a low sperm count and decreased sperm motility came to my clinic after having seen many doctors for a skin rash. We discovered that he had an undiagnosed intolerance for gluten. His skin rash disappeared completely as soon as he stopped ingesting gluten. We also found that he had low testosterone levels, so we gave him the following herbal protocol:

> For sperm health: Mucuna pruriens (kapikachu) extract 250 mg in a proprietary blend of Centella asiatica (brahmi), Valeriana waliichii (tagara), and Ashwagandha, taken three times a day.

> For low testosterone: Withania somnifera (ashwagandha) 175 mg extract, Tribulus terristris (gokhru) 50 mg extract, Shilajiit (Black asphaltum) 25 mg, 25 mg extract, in a proprietary blend of Crocus sativus (kumkuma), Emblica officinalis (amalaki), Piper longum (Pippli), Glycyrrhiza glabra (yastimadhu), Bacopa monniera (indriya brahmi), Sida cordifolia (bala), Mucuna pruriens (kapikachu), Spilanthes acmella (akarkara).

After 4 months, the patient's sperm motility and count had increased to within a normal range, and his testosterone was increased to normal levels.

For impotence:

A 70-year-old man came to our clinic reporting that he gets erections without any ejaculate, which has made his erections quite painful. "The well is dried up," he said. We gave him the following herbal formulations, to be taken three times daily:

> Mucuna pruriens (kapikachu) extract, 250 mg, in a proprietary blend of Centella asiatica (brahmi), Valeriana waliichii (tagara), and Ashwagandha.

Four weeks later, the patient called to say that "The well is no longer dry, and things are going well."

Herbal Protocol

When replacing L-dopa with Mucuna (kapikachu), it is better to begin taking the herb first, preferably as part of a formulation such as that described in the first case above, and then to taper off the L-dopa gradually.

Safety Profile

Mucuna seed may cause birth defects, and has uterine stimulant activity. It should not be used during pregnancy. Velvet bean has shown to lower blood sugar. Those with hypoglycemia or diabetes should use velvet bean only under the supervision of a qualified healthcare practitioner. Velvet bean is contraindicated in combination with MAO. inhibitors. It also has androgenic activity, increasing testosterone levels. Individuals with excessive androgen syndromes should avoid using velvet bean.

Velvet bean inhibits prolactin. If you have a medical condition resulting in inadequate levels of prolactin in the body, do not use Velvet bean except under the direction of a healthcare practitioner.

Some studies showed adverse effect, either from allergic reactions or from contaminates found in the preparations.[28, 29, 30]

Notes

1. L. Misra and H. Wagner, 2004 Alkaloidal constituents of Mucuna pruriens seeds," *Phytochemistry*. Sept. 2004, 65(18):2565–2567.

2. B.V. Manyam, M. Dhanasekaran, and M, Hare, "Neuroprotective effects of the antiparkinson drug Mucuna pruriens," *Phytother Res.*, Sept. 2004, 18(9):706–712.

3. S. Kasture, S. Pontis, A. Pinna, N. Schintu, L. Spina, R. Longoni, N. Simola, and M. Ballero, "Assessment of symptomatic and neuroprotective efficacy of mucuna pruriens seed extract in rodent model of Parkinson's disease," *Neurotox Res.*, Feb. 2009, 15(2):111–122. Feb. 20, 2009.

4. R. Katzenschlager, A. Evans, A. Manson, P.N. Patsalos, N. Ratnaraj, H. Watt, and [initial?]Timmermann, "Mucuna pruriens in Parkinson's disease: A double blind clinical and pharmacological study," *J Neurol Neurosurg Psychiatry*, Dec. 2004, 75(12):1672–1677.

5. B. Singhal, J. Lalkaka, and C. Sankhla, "Epidemiology and treatment of Parkinson's disease in India," *Parkinsonism Relat Disord.*, Aug. 2003, 9 Suppl 2:S105–1059.

6. N. Nagashayana, P. Sankarankutty, M.R. Nampoothiri, P.K. Mohan, and K.P. Mohanakumar, "Association of L-DOPA with recovery following Ayurveda medication in Parkinson's disease," *J Neurol Sci.*, June 15, 2000, 176(2):124–127.

7. See Note 2

8. See Note 2

9. B.V. Manyam, M. Dhanasekaran, and T.A. Hare, "Effect of antiparkinson drug HP-200 (Mucuna pruriens) on the central monoaminergic neurotransmitters," *Phytother Res.*, Feb. 2004, 18(2):97–101.

10. See Note 9.

11. A. A., M.A.S. and S.B. , """ , July, –

12. R. Guerranti, J.C. Aguiyi, I.G. Ogueli, G. Onorati, S. Neri, F. Rosati, F. Del Buono, R. Lampariello, R. Pagani, and E. Marinello, "Protection of Mucuna pruriens seeds against Echis carinatus venom is exerted through a multiform glycoprotein whose oligosaccharide chains are functional in this role," *Biochem Biophys Res Commun.*, Oct. 15, 2004, 323(2):484–490.

13. R. Guerranti, J.C. Aguiyi, S. Neri, R. Leoncini, R. Pagani, and E Marinello, "Proteins from Mucuna pruriens and enzymes from Echis carinatus venom: Characterization and cross-reactions," *J Biol Chem.*, May 10, 2002, 277(19):17072–17078. Epub Feb. 26, 2002.

14. J.C. Aguiyi, R. Guerranti, R. Pagani, and E. Marinello, "Blood chemistry of rats pretreated with Mucuna pruriens seed aqueous extract MP101UJ after Echis carinatus venom challenge," *Phytother Res.*, Dec. 2001, 15(8):712–714.

15. N.H. Tan, S.Y. Fung, S.M. Sim, E. Marinello, R. Guerranti, and J.C. Aguiyi, "The protective effect of Mucuna pruriens seeds against snake venom poisoning," *J Ethnopharmacol.* June 22, 2009, 123(2):356–358. Epub March 26, 2009.

16. J.K. Grover, S.S. Rathi, and V. Vats, "Amelioration of experimental diabetic neuropathy and gastropathy in rats following oral administration of plant (Eugenia jambolana, Mucuna pruriens and Tinospora cordifolia) extracts," *Indian J Exp Biol.*, March 2002, 40(3):273–276.

17. S. S. Rathi, J.K. Grover, V. Vikrant, and N.R. Biswas, "Prevention of experimental diabetic cataract by Indian Ayurvedic plant extracts," *Phytother Res.*, Dec. 2002, 16(8):774–777.

18. S. S, Rathi, J.K. Grover, and V. Vats, "The effect of Momordica charantia and Mucuna pruriens in experimental diabetes and their effect on key metabolic enzymes involved in carbohydrate metabolism," *Phytother Res.*, May 2002, 16(3):236–243.

19. J. K Grover, V. Vats, S. S, Rathi, and R. Dawar, "Traditional Indian anti-diabetic plants attenuate progression of renal damage in streptozotocin induced diabetic mice," *J Ethnopharmacol*, Aug. 2001, 76(3):233–238.

20. S. Suresh and S. Prakash, "Effect of Mucuna pruriens (Linn.) on sexual behavior and sperm parameters in streptozotocin- induced diabetic male rat," *J Sex Med.*, April 26, 2010.

21. Y.B. Tripathi and A.K. Upadhyay, "Effect of the alcohol extract of the seeds of Mucuna pruriens on free radicals and oxidative stress in albino rats," *Phytother Res.*, Sept. 2002, 16(6):534–538.

22. M. Dhanasekaran, B. Tharakan, and B.V. Manyam, "Antiparkinson drug—Mucuna pruriens shows antioxidant and metal chelating activity," *Phytother Res.*, Jan. 2008, 22(1):6–11.

23. See Note 21.

24. K.K. Shukla, A.A. Mahdi, M.K. Ahmad, S.N., Rajender, and, S.P. Jaiswar, "Mucuna pruriens improves male fertility by its action on the hypothalamus-pituitary-gonadal axis," *Fertil Steril.*, Oct.28, 2008.

25. K.K. Shukla, A.A. Mahdi, M.K. Ahmad, S.P. Jaiswar, S.N. Shankwar, and S.C. Tiwari, "Mucuna pruriens reduces stress and improves the quality of semen in infertile men," *Evid Based Complement Alternat Med*, Dec. 18, 2007.

26. See Note 27

27. S. Suresh, E. Prithiviraj, and S. Prakash, "Effect of Mucuna pruriens on oxidative stress mediated damage in aged rat sperm," *Int J Androl.*, Jan. 8, 2009.

28. M.E Infante, A.M. Perez, M.R. Simao, F. Manda, E.F. Baquete, A.M. Fernandes, and J.L. Cliff, "Outbreak of acute toxic psychosis attributed to Mucuna pruriens," *Lancet,* Nov. 3, 1990, 336(8723):1129.

29. A.K Roy and H.K. Chourasia, "Effect of temperature on aflatoxin production in Mucuna pruriens seeds," *Appl Environ Microbiol.*, Feb.1989, 55(2):531–532.

30. Author, "Leads from the MMWR. Mucuna pruriens-associated pruritus—New Jersey,"*JAMA*, Jan. 17, 1986, 255(3):313.

Nigella sativa

Introduction

Nigella sativa, known in English as black cumin, is an annual flowering plant native to southwest Asia. An important part of herbal traditions in Asia, the Middle East, and Africa, it is known for its anti-hypertensive, carminative, and anthelminthic properties. Nigella seeds have a pungent bitter taste.

Nigella has been used for medicinal purposes for centuries, both as an herb and as an expressed oil. It is useful in promoting and maintaining respiratory health, liver and kidney function, and intestinal health, as well as to support the circulatory and immune systems, and as a general tonic for well-being.

In the Middle East and Southeast Asia, black cumin seeds are used to treat asthma, bronchitis, rheumatism, and related inflammatory diseases, to increase lactation, to promote digestion, and to fight parasitic infections. Nigella oil is also used to treat skin conditions such as eczema and boils, and to treat the symptoms of the common cold.

An active chemical, nigellone, has been isolated from Nigella and is believed to be responsible for the herb's effectiveness in treating respiratory disorders. An anti-tumor sterol, beta sitosterol, has also been isolated from Nigella, which may explain its effectiveness in treating abscesses and tumors of the abdomen, eyes, and liver.

Synonymous Names

English: Small fennel, black cumin
Hindi: Kalunji
Sanskrit: Kalajaji
Gujarati: Kalunji

Habitat

Nigella is a native of southern Europe. It is found growing in all parts of India, especially in the eastern region. It is cultivated commercially in Punjab, Himachal Pradesh, Bihar, and Assam.

Botanical Characteristics

Nigella grows to an average height of 20 to 30 centimeters tall. It has finely divided, linear (but not thread-like) leaves. The flowers are delicate, usually pale blue and white, with 5 to 10 petals per blossom. The fruit is a large, inflated capsule composed of 3 to 7 united follicles, each containing numerous seeds, which often are used as a spice.

Chemical Composition

Nigella seeds contain a brown-colored volatile oil at concentrations of 0.5% to 1.6% and red-colored stable oil at approximately 31%. In addition, Nigella contains albumin, sugar, carbonic acid, saponin, melanthin, Arabic acid, the bitter compound nigellin, resins, tannins, and ash. Also present are the volatile oils carvone, D-lymonine, and cymine. Its active agent nigellone is helpful in supporting the respiratory tract.

Pharmacological Activity

Anti-cestodal activity

The anti-cestodal effect of Nigella seeds was studied in children infected with various parasitic worms. A single oral administration of 40 mg/kg of Nigella seeds and an equivalent amount of its ethanolic extract was effective in reducing the egg count in the feces, with an effect comparable to that of niclosamide. The crude extracts did not produce any adverse side-effects.[1]

The anti-schistosomicidal properties of aqueous extract of Nigella seeds against Schistosoma mansoni miracidia, Schistosoma cercariae, and the adult worms in-vitro. Nigella showed strong biocidal effects against all stages of the parasite and inhibited egg-laying of adult female wors.[4]

Anti-inflammatory activity

Studies have been carried out that have substantiated the anti-inflammatory effects of Nigella. One study was conducted to explore the anti-inflammatory effects of the active principle thymoquinone on arthritis in rat models. The results of this study confirmed the function of thymoquinone in suppressing adjuvant-induced arthritis in rats.[3]

The effect of thymoquinone on the in-vivo production of prostaglandins and lung inflammation was studied in a mouse model of allergic airway inflammation. Mice sensitized and challenged through the airways with ovalbumin exhibited a significant increase in prostaglandin production in the airways. Intraperitoneal injection of thymoquinone derived from Nigella seeds for five days before airway inflammation demonstrated a significant decrease in all of the inflammatory factors measured. These findings suggest that Nigella has an anti-inflammatory effect during the allergic response in the lung through the inhibition of prostaglandin immune response.[4]

Anti-asthmatic activity

The effects of Nigella as a bronchodilatory agent were studied in comparison with dexamethasone, a commonly prescribed steroid. The two substances were compared in a mouse model of allergic asthma. For the study, the mice were sensitized intraperitoneally and challenged intratracheally with conalbumin. The study group was treated with Nigella 24 hours after the first intratracheal challenge. Dexamethasone treated and untreated mice served as controls.[5] Post-experimental measurements indicated that Nigella sativa significantly reduced peripheral blood eosinophil count, IgG1 and IgG2a levels, cytokine profiles, and inflammatory cells in lung tissue. These effects were equivalent to the effects of dexamethasone except in the case of the unchanged IFN-y level. Nigella sativa reduced inflammation and showed immunoregulatory effect which may be useful for treatment of allergic asthma. The anti-inflammatory effect of thymoquinone from Nigella seeds was studied in a further mouse model of allergic asthma. Mice sensitized and challenged with ovalbumin antigen had an increased amounts of leukotriene B4 and C4, Th2 cytokines, and eosinophils in bronchoalveolar lavage fluid. A marked increase in lung tissue eosinophilia and goblet cell numbers also was observed. Administration of thymoquinone prior to the OVA challenge inhibited 5-lipoxygenase and significantly reduced the levels of LTB4 and LTC4. This was accompanied by a marked decrease in Th2 cytokines and BAL fluid and lung tissue eosinophilia, all of which are characteristics of airway inflammation. These results demonstrate the anti-inflammatory effect of thymoquinone in experimental asthma.[6]

In double blind randomized trial Nigella sativa seed aqueous extract on respiratory and pulmonary function test on chemical wars victims was been evaluated. Results of the study showed that all respiratory symptoms, chest wheezing, and pulmonary function test (PFT) values in the study group significantly improved in the second and third visits, compared to the first visit ($p < 0.05$ to $p < 0.001$). In addition, further improvement of chest wheezing and some PFT values on the third visit were observed compared to the second visit in this group ($p < 0.05$ to $p < 0.001$). In the third visits, all PFT values and most symptoms in the study group were significantly different from those of the control group ($p < 0.01$ to $p < 0.001$). The control group, however, showed only small improvements in some parameters in the second and third visits. At the end of the study, the use of inhaler and oral beta-agonists and oral corticosteroid in the study group decreased, while there were no obvious changes in use of the drugs in the control subjects. The authors concluded that this study suggests a prophylactic effect of Nigella sativa on chemical war victims and warrants further research regarding this effect.[7]

Research data from four studies were presented on the clinical efficacy of Nigella sativa in allergic diseases.[8] In these studies, a total of 152 patients with allergic diseases (allergic rhinitis, bronchial asthma, atopic eczema) were treated with Nigella sativa oil, given in capsules at doses of 40 to 80 mg/kg/day. The patients scored the subjective severity of target symptoms using a predefined scale. The following laboratory parameters were investigated: IgE, eosinophil count, endogenous cortisol in plasma and urine, ACTH, triglycerides, total cholesterol, LDL, and HDL cholesterol, and lymphocyte subpopulations. The score of subjective feeling decreased over the course of treatment with Nigella oil in all four studies. A slight decrease in plasma triglycerides and a discrete increase in HDL cholesterol occurred, while the lymphocyte subpopulations, endogenous cortisol levels and ACTH release remained unchanged. Authors concluded that Nigella oil to be an effective adjuvant for the treatment of allergic diseases. Another study investigated the effects of Nigella sativa seed supplementation on symptom levels, polymorphonuclear leukocyte (PMN) functions, lymphocyte subsets and hematological parameters of allergic rhinitis.[9] Twenty-four patients randomly selected from an experimental group of 31 (mean age 34 years) sensitive to house dust mites with allergic rhinitis and a control group of 8 healthy volunteers (mean age 23 years) were treated with allergen-specific immunotherapy in conventional doses for 30 days. After a month of immunotherapy, 12 of the 24 patients and the 8 healthy volunteers were given Nigella sativa seed supplementation (2 g/day orally) for 30 days. The remaining 12 patients continued only on immunotherapy during the same period. The other 7 patients were given 0.1 ml saline solution subcutaneously once a week as a placebo. The symptom scores, PMN functions, lymphocyte subsets, and other hematological parameters were evaluated before and after all treatment periods. There was a statistically significant increase in the phagocytic and intracellular killing activities of PMNs of patients receiving specific immunotherapy, especially after the addition of Nigella sativa seed. The CD8 counts of patients receiving specific immunotherapy plus Nigella sativa seed supplementation significantly increased, compared to the patients receiving only specific immunotherapy. PMN functions of the healthy volunteers increased significantly after Nigella sativa seed supplementation compared to baseline. Thus, Nigella sativa seed supplementation during specific immunotherapy of allergic rhinitis may be considered a potential adjuvant therapy. In previous studies, the relaxant anticholinergic (functional antagonism) and antihistaminic effects of Nigella sativa were demonstrated on guinea pig tracheal chains. In one study, the prophylactic effect of thymoquinone (one of the constituents of Nigella sativa) on tracheal responsiveness and white blood cell (WBC) count in lung lavage of sensitized guinea pigs was examined.[10] Four groups of guinea pigs sensitized to ovalbumin (OA) were given drinking water alone (group S), drinking water containing low or high concentrations of thymoquinone (S + LTQ and S + HTQ groups), or inhaled fluticasone propionate (FP 250 microg) twice a day (positive control group) (n = 7, for all groups). The tracheal responses of the control and four groups of sensitized animals to methacholine at an effective concentration causing 50% of maximum response (EC(50) M) were measured. The tracheal responses to 0.1 % ovalbumin, relative to contraction induced by 10 microM methacholine also were examined. Total WBC and its differential count in lung lavage also were measured. The tracheal responsiveness to methacholine, ovalbumin, and WBC of S guinea pigs was significantly higher than those of the controls ($p < 0.001$ for all cases). Tracheal responsiveness in S + LTQ, S + HTQ, and FP groups to both methacholine ($p < 0.05$ to $p < 0.001$) and OA ($p < 0.001$ for all cases) was significantly decreased compared to that of the S group. Total WBC also was decreased in all experimental groups compared to that of the S group ($p < 0.001$ for all groups). There was an increase in eosinophils and a decrease in neutrophils, lymphocytes, and monocytes in the S animals compared to the controls ($p < 0.001$ for all cases). Treatment with concentrations of both thymoquinone and FP variably improved differential WBC count changes compared to the S animals (nonsignificant to $p < 0.001$). The improvements in tracheal responsiveness, total WBC, eosinophils, and lymphocytes changes in the S animals treated with both concentrations of thymoquinone were significantly greater than those of FP ($p < 0.05$ to $p < 0.001$). These results showed a preventive effect of thymoquinone, one constituent of Nigella sativa, on tracheal responsiveness and inflammatory cells of lung lavage of the sensitized guinea pigs, which was comparable to or even greater than that of the inhaled steroid.

Anti-cancer activity

Anti-oxidants have been found to be quite successful in arresting the progress of some cancers. Anti-oxidants protect the body by neutralizing free radicals, thus ending the scavenger reaction. Thymoquinone is a primary active component of Nigella known for its inhibition of oxidative stress. Compared to a chemotherapeutic drug of choice, Nigella has demonstrated remarkable chemotherapeutic responses.

A study was conducted to evaluate and compare the effects of Nigella extracts on colon cancer cells. Cell viability, cell number, cellular morphology, and cellular metabolism were compared for the control and treatment groups. The results evidenced a significant decrease in the numbers of cancer cells in the groups treated with the extract, comparable to the results obtained with chemotherapeutic agents. The reduced cell numbers suggest that Nigella extracts may have important chemotherapeutic effects.[11]

Researchers at the Kimmel Cancer Center in Philadelphia found that thymoquinone blocked pancreatic cancer cell growth and killed the cells by enhancing the process of programmed cell death, or apoptosis. These findings suggest that thymoquinone could be used as a preventative strategy in patients who have been through surgery and chemotherapy or in individuals at high risk of developing cancer.[12]

Studies have attempted to elucidate the molecular targets by which Nigella exerts its anti-cancerous activity. High molecular weight glycoprotein mucin 4 (MUC4) is aberrantly expressed in pancreatic cancer and contributes to the regulation of differentiation, proliferation, metastasis, and the chemoresistance of pancreatic cancer cells. The absence of its expression in the normal pancreatic ductal cells makes MUC4 a promising target for novel cancer therapeutics.

Researchers evaluated the effect of thymoquinone on pancreatic cancer cells, and specifically investigated its effect on MUC4 expression. The MUC4-expressing pancreatic cancer cells FG/COLO357 and CD18/HPAF were incubated with thymoquinone, and in-vitro functional assays were conducted. The results indicate that treatment with thymoquinone (TQ) downregulated MUC4 expression through the proteasomal pathway and induced apoptosis in pancreatic cancer cells by the activation of c-Jun NH(2)-terminal kinase and p38 mitogen-activated protein kinase pathways. In agreement with previous studies, the decrease in MUC4 expression correlated with an increase in apoptosis, decreased motility, and decreased migration of pancreatic cancer cells. MUC4 transient silencing studies showed that c-Jun NH(2)-terminal kinase and p38 mitogen-activated protein kinase pathways are activated in pancreatic cancer cells, indicating that the activation of these pathways by TQ is directly related to the MUC4 downregulation induced by the drug. Overall, TQ has the potential for the development of novel therapies against pancreatic cancer.[13,14]

An herbal preparation including Nigella sativa seeds has been recommended for cancer patients by traditional medical practitioners in Sri Lanka. Investigations demonstrated that short-term treatment with the herbal decoction significantly inhibited diethylnitrosamine mediated expression of Glutathione S-transferase in rat liver.[15]

An investigation was conducted to determine whether longer-term treatment with the decoction would be successful in blocking the progress of overt tumors or histopathological changes leading to tumor development. Male Wistar rats were injected intraperitoneally with the tumor-producing agent diethylnitrosamine. Twenty-four hours later, the herbal decoction was orally administered to one group of rats, while the control animals were given distilled water. The rats' livers were examined at the end of nine-month and 16-month periods of treatment. The observed results of this animal study indicate that protection against carcinogenic changes in rat liver can be achieved by long-term treatment with a decoction of Nigella sativa seeds.[16]

Studies have indicated that cytokines can enhance immunogenicity and promote tumor regression, but the means for modulating cytokine production have not been investigated fully. Research was conducted to assess the effects of an herbal melanin extracted from Nigella sativa on the production of three cytokines-tumor necrosis factor alpha, interleukin 6, and vascular endothelial growth factor evidenced in human monocytes, total peripheral blood mononuclear cells, and THP-1 cell line. The cells were treated with variable concentrations of melanin, and the expression of cell lysates and secretion of proteins in the supernatants were detected.[17] On the protein level, melanin significantly induced TNF-alpha and IL-6 protein production and inhibited VEGF production by monocytes and peripheral blood mononuclear cell (PBMC). In the THP-1 cell line, melanin induced production of all three cytokine proteins. These observations support the use of Nigella-based melanin for treatment of diseases associated with imbalanced cytokine production, and possibly for enhancing other immunotherapies. Breast cancer is the second leading cause of cancer death in women, and the third most common cancer worldwide. In an effort to increase understanding of the molecular basis of this fatal disease, the therapeutic effect of Nigella sativa against mammary cancer in laboratory animals was studied.[18] The research animals that received injections of an extract including Nigella sativa in addition to a known carcinogenic substance showed a reduced rate of formation of mammary tumors, compared to the control animals, in which the carcinogen was administered without the herbal extract. These results suggest a protective role of Nigella against mammary cancer; however, the underlying mechanisms of these effects await further investigation. Another study showed that administration of Nigella sativa oil or thymoquinone can lower cyclophosphamide CTX-induced toxicity, as shown by an upregulation of anti-oxidant mechanisms. This, indicated a potential clinical application for these agents to minimize the toxic effects of treatment with anti-cancer drugs.[19]

Neuroprotective activity

A study was conducted to investigate the effects of Nigella sativa in comparison to methylprednisolone on experimental spinal cord injury in rats. After receiving spinal cord injuries, the laboratory rats were neurologically tested 24 hours after trauma, and spinal cord tissue samples were harvested for both biochemical and histopathological evaluation. The spinal cord injury significantly increased the spinal cord tissue malondialdehyde (MDA) and protein carbonyl (PC) levels; however, the injury decreased superoxide dismutase, glutathione peroxidase, and catalase enzyme activities compared to the control.[20] Treatment with Nigella extract significantly decreased tissue MDA and PC levels and prevented inhibition of SOD, GSH-Px, and CAT enzymes in the animal tissues. These results suggest that Nigella might be beneficial in treating damage to spinal cord tissue, and that its potential for clinical implications should be investigated further.

Hepatoprotective activity

To investigate the effects of Nigella sativa on lipid peroxidation, anti-oxidant enzyme systems, and liver enzymes, male Wistar albino rats received injections of Nigella extract in addition to CCl(4) twice a week for 60 days. Blood samples for the biochemical analysis were taken by cardiac puncture at the beginning and on the 60th day of the experiment. CCl(4) treatment for 60 days increased the lipid peroxidation and liver enzymes, and also decreased the anti-oxidant enzyme levels. The Nigella treatment decreased the elevated lipid peroxidation and liver enzyme levels, and also increased the reduced anti-oxidant enzyme levels, suggesting that Nigella decreases lipid peroxidation and liver enzymes, and increase the anti-oxidant defense system activity.[21]

Endotoxemia caused by lipopolysaccharide (LPS) produced an inflammatory condition contributing to multiple organ failure. Study was carried out to investigate the effects of thymoquinone (TQ), against LPS-induced hepatotoxicity. LPS markedly depleted liver reduced glutathione (GSH) and significantly increased the level of malondialdehyde (MDA) and the activity of caspase-3 enzyme in the liver. Serum tumor necrosis factor-alpha (TNF-alpha) and bilirubin levels and the activities of alkaline phosphatase (ALP) and gamma-glutamyl transferase (gamma-GT) enzymes were markedly increased in LPS-treated rats. TQ supplementation resulted in normalization of liver GSH and decreases in the levels of MDA and caspase-3 activity in the liver with reduction of serum TNF-alpha, serum total bilirubin and the activities of ALP and gamma-GT enzymes. Histopathological examination revealed that TQ administration improved LPS-induced pathological abnormalities in liver tissues.[22]

Gastroprotective activity

Thymoquinone was studied in ethanol induced gastric mucosal lesions in male Wistar albino rats.[23] Thymoquinone protected gastric mucosa against the injurious effect of absolute alcohol and promote ulcer healing, as evidenced from the ulcer index values. Nigella prevented an alcohol-induced increase in thiobarbituric acid-reactive substances, an index of lipid peroxidation. Nigella also increased gastric glutathione content, enzymatic activities of gastric superoxide dismutase and glutathione S-transferase. Likewise, Thymoquinone protected against the ulcerating effect of alcohol and mitigated most of the adverse biochemical effects induced by alcohol in gastric mucosa, but to a lesser extent than Nigella. Neither substance affected catalase activity in the gastric tissue. Nigella and Thymoquinone can partly protect gastric mucosa from acute alcohol-induced mucosal injury, and that these gastroprotective effects might be induced, at least partly by their radical scavenging activity.

A large number of diseases are ascribed to Helicobacter pylori (H. pylori), particularly chronic active gastritis, peptic ulcer disease, and gastric cancer. Successful treatment of H. pylori infection with antimicrobial agents can lead to regression of H. pylori-associated disorders. Antibiotic resistance against H. pylori is increasing, and it is necessary to find effective new agents. Nigella sativa seed , a commonly used herb, possesses in vitro anti-helicobacter activity.

A study was undertaken to evaluate the efficacy of Nigella seeds in eradicating H. pylori infection in non-ulcer dyspeptic patients. The study was conducted on 88 adult patients attending King Fahd Hospital of the University, Al-Khobar, Saudi Arabia, from 2007 to 2008, with dyspeptic symptoms and were found positive for H. pylori infection by histopathology and urease testing. The patients were randomly assigned to four groups, receiving i) triple therapy composed of clarithromycin, amoxicillin, omeprazole [n= 23], ii) 1 g NS + 40 mg omeprazole (OM) [n= 21], iii) 2 g NS + OM [n= 21] or iv) 3 g NS + OM [n= 23]. A negative H. pylori stool antigen test 4 weeks after the end of treatment was considered as eradication. H. pylori eradication was 82.6, 47.6, 66.7 and 47.8% with TT, 1 g NS, 2 g NS and 3 g NS, respectively. Eradication rates with 2 grams of NS and triple therapy were statistically not different from each other, whereas H. pylori eradication with other doses was significantly less than that with triple therapy (P < 0.05). Dyspepsia symptoms improved in all groups to a similar extent.

Nigella sativa seeds showed clinically important activity against H. pylori infection, comparable to triple therapy.[24]

In another study, 30 rats were divided into three groups: sham (group 1), control (group 2), and Nigella sativa (NS)treatment (group 3). All of the rats underwent intestinal ischemia for 60 minutes, followed by a 60-minute period of reperfusion. Rats were intraperitoneally infused only 0.9% saline solutions in group 2. Rats in the group 3 received NS (0,2 mL/ kg) intraperitoneally, before ischemia and before reperfusion. Total anti-oxidant capacity (TAC), catalase (CAT), total oxidative status (TOS), oxidative stress index (OSI), and myeloperoxidase (MPO) in ileum tissue were measured. Also, ileum tissue histopathology was evaluated using a light microscope. The levels of liver enzymes in group 3 were significantly lower than those in group 2 (p <.01). TAC and CAT activity levels in ileum tissue were significantly higher in group 3 than in group 2. Total oxidative stress, oxidative stress index, and myeloperoxidase in ileum tissue were significantly lower in group 3 than group 2 (p <.05 for TOS and MPO; p < .01 for OSI). Histological tissue damage was milder in the Nigella sativa treatment group than in the control group. The results suggest that Nigella sativa treatment protected the rats' intestinal tissue against intestinal ischemia-reperfusion injury.[25]

Cardioprotective activity

The effects of aqueous extracts of Nigella sativa on heart rate and contractility of the isolated hearts of guinea pigs were examined. Heart rates and contractility were measured in the presence of four concentrations of aqueous and macerated extracts from Nigella sativa and diltiazem, a calcium channel blocker, in two different groups of experiments. The study results showed a potent inhibitory effect of both extracts from Nigella sativa on heart rate and contractility of guinea pig heart that was comparable and even higher than that of diltiazem. The results may be attributable to calcium channel inhibitory or an opening effect for the plant on potassium channels of the isolated heart.[26]

A randomized, double-blind, placebo trial evaluated the use of Nigella with patients having mild hypertension. The subjects were randomized into three groups: a placebo and two test groups that received 100 and 200 mg of Nigella Seed extract, respectively, twice a day. After 8 weeks, systolic blood pressure (SBP) values in both case groups were found to be significantly reduced compared to the baseline values for each group. In addition, the decrease in SBP in the two case groups was statistically significant relative to the placebo group ($P < 0.05$-0.01). Meanwhile, diastolic blood pressure (DBP) values in the case groups were found to be significantly reduced from the baseline, and a significant reduction also was observed in these groups ($P < 0.01$) compared to the placebo group. In addition, extract administration reduced both SBP and DBP in a dose-dependent manner. Nigella sativa extract caused a significant decline in the level of total and low-density-lipoprotein (LDL)-cholesterol relative to baseline data.[27]

Some other studies did not have statistically significant results. The study, however, had a small sample size, the conclusion was that for future trials, a large sample size would be needed for assessing the efficacy of a given substance.[28]

A study was undertaken to examine the possible protective effects of propolis (a resinous hive product collected by honeybees from various plant sources) and thymoquinone on serum lipid levels and early atherosclerotic lesions in hypercholesterolemic rabbits. New Zealand rabbits were fed on either standard chow or atherogenic diet during four weeks and concomitantly received either propolis or thymoquinone. At the end of experiment period, serum samples were collected to determine lipid profile, kidney functions and anti-oxidant status. Tissues from the aorta, pulmonary artery and kidney were taken for histopathological examination. The cholesterol enriched diet induced a significant increase in serum TC, triglycerides, LDL-C, thiobarbituric acid reactive substances concentrations and a significant decrease in high density lipoprotein-cholesterol and in reduced glutathione levels compared to control group.[29] Administration of propolis or thymoquinone with the cholesterol-enriched diet significantly ($p < 0.05$) reduced TC, LDL-C, triglycerides, and thiobarbituric acid-reactive substances concentrations, while increased high density lipoprotein-cholesterol concentration, as well as glutathione content., Kidney function parameters were significantly affected by the cholesterol diet, and both propolis and thymoquinone counter regulated the cholesterol-induced changes. Histopathologically, early atherosclerotic changes were observed in the high cholesterol control group represented by endothelial damage and thickened foam cells, while propolis or thymoquinone provided protection against the high cholesterol-induced damage. anti-oxidant mechanism.

Analgesic activity

Extracts from the seeds of Nigella sativa are used as a spice or remedy for the treatment of various inflammatory diseases. A study was conducted to examine the analgesic effects of Nigella's polyphenols. The Nigella polyphenols were prepared, and analgesic and anti-inflammatory effects were studied in mice and rats using the acetic acid-induced writhing, formalin, light tail flick, carrageenan-induced paw edema, and croton oil-induced ear edema tests.[30] In the acetic acid-induced writhing test, oral administration of Nigella sativa polyphenols decreased the number of abdominal constrictions. Both oral and intraperitoneal administration significantly suppressed the nociceptive response in the early and late phases of the formalin test.

Pre-treatment with naloxone failed to reverse the analgesic activity of Nigella in this test. Nigella did not produce significant analgesia in the light tail flick test in mice. Oral administration of Nigella did not produce a significant reduction in carrageenan-induced paw edema. When injected intraperitoneally, however, Nigella inhibited paw edema in a dose-dependent manner. When applied topically, Nigella failed to reduce croton oil-induced ear edema.

These results suggest that polyphenols derived from Nigella sativa have analgesic and anti-inflammatory effects. The lack of analgesic effect of Nigella in the light tail flick test, as well as the failure of naloxone to reverse the analgesia in the formalin test reveal that mechanisms other than stimulation of opioid receptors are involved. A comparative, parallel, randomized, double-blind, placebo-controlled study with a treatment period of 7 days was conducted to examine the clinical effectiveness of Nigella sativa and Phyllanthus niruri extract (NSPN extract) in tonsillopharyngitis patients. Of the 200 enrolled patients, 186 completed the study, 12 withdrew, and 2 were principally screened as failure but were included inadvertently. NSPN capsules, each containing 360 mg Nigella sativa and 50 mg Phyllanthus niruri extracts, were administered orally (one capsule 3 times daily) for 7 days. At hour 5 or 6 of the first dosing of the study medication, the sore throat, assessed as pain and difficulty swallowing, was markedly alleviated in the NSPN group. In line with the significant alleviation of pain, from days 0 to 2 of treatment, subjects in the NSPN group also needed significantly less analgesic therapy (paracetamol tablets) than those in the placebo group. At the end of treatment (day 7), the sore throat was completely relieved in a significantly greater proportion of patients in the NSPN group than in the placebo group. NSPN extract also was found to be safe and well tolerated in acute tonsillopharyngitis patients. This study proved significant benefits of NSPN extract in the treatment of acute tonsillopharyngitis compared to the placebo.[31]

Anti-addiction

Opioid dependence is one of the major social and psychiatric problem in society. Unfortunately, no non-opiate treatment is available. This study was conducted to find non-opiate treatment for opiate withdrawal. The study included a total of 35 known opiate addicts. This study was based on DSM-IV criteria for opioid dependence. The study demonstrated that non-opioid treatment for opioid addiction decreased the withdrawal effects significantly. It further demonstrated no changes in physiological parameters (blood pressure, pulse rate, etc.) of the subjects during treatment. The subjects had increased appetite but no significant weight gain.[32] Nigella sativa can be effective in long-term treatment of opioid dependence. It not merely cures the opioid dependence but also cures the infections and weakness from which the majority of addicts suffer.

AYURVEDIC PROPERTIES

Nigella is a vata and kapha suppressant and pitta aggravator. Because of its rough and sharp properties, it helps to reduce body fats, and because of its hot potency, it is helpful in suppressing pain and inflammation. It helps to normalize the digestive tract, as it is light in nature. Its pungent taste is helpful in suppressing infection in the body. It also acts as diuretic in nature. Finally, the hot potency promotes sweating (diaphoretic).

Guna (properties): laghu (light), tikshan (sharp) and ruksh (dry)
Rasa (taste): katu (pungent) and tickta (bitter)
Vipak: Katu
Virya (potency): ushan (hot)

Safety Profile

No toxic effects have been determined for Nigella when it is in normal dosages.

Research suggests that Nigella (Black cumin seed) significantly inhibited CYP2D6 and CYP3A4 mediated metabolism of dextromethorphan. Drugs cleared by CYP2D6 and CYP3A4 substrates may be effected.[33]

Dosage

The usual recommended dosage is between 50 and 75 mg of a supplement made from standardized extracts.

Whole seeds powder 1-2 gram twice a day.

Notes

1. Akhtar MS, Riffat S. Field trial of Saussurea lappa roots against nematodes and Nigella sativa seeds against cestodes in children. J Pak Med Assoc. 1991 Aug;41(8):185-7.

2. M. M. Azza, M.M. Nadia, and S.M. Sohair, "Sativa seeds against *Schistosoma mansoni* different stages," *Mem. Inst. Oswaldo. Cruz. Rio de Janeiro*, 2005, 100(2):205–211.

3. I. Tekeoglu, A. Dogan, and L. Demiralpty? I am not sure what this means"Effects of thymoquinone (volatile oil of black cumin) on rheumatoid arthritis in rat models," *Phytotherapy Research*, Sept. 2007, 21(9):895–897.

4. El Mezayen R, El Gazzar M, Nicolls MR, Marecki JC, Dreskin SC, Nomiyama H. Effect of thymoquinone on cyclooxygenase expression and prostaglandin production in a mouse model of allergic airway inflammation. Immunol Lett. 2006 Jul 15;106(1):72-)

5. A.T. Abbas, M.M. Abdel-Aziz, K.R. Zalata, Abd Al-Galel Tel-D., "Effect of dexamethasone and Nigella sativa on peripheral blood eosinophil count, IgG1 and IGG2a, cytokine profiles and lung inflammation in murine model of allergic asthma," *Egypt J. Immunol,*, 2005, 12(1):95–102.

6. M. El Gazzar, R. El Mezayen, M.R. Nicolls, J.C. Marecki, and S.C. Dreskin, "Downregulation of leukotriene biosynthesis by thymoquinone attenuates airway inflammation in a mouse model of allergic asthma," *Biochim Biophys Acta.*, July 2006, 1760(7):1088-95. Epub March 31, 2006.

7. M.H. Boskabady and J. Farhadi, "The possible prophylactic effect of Nigella sativa seed aqueous extract on respiratory symptoms and pulmonary function tests on chemical war victims: A randomized, double-blind, placebo-controlled trial," *Journal of Alternative and Complementary Medicine*, Nov.. 2008, 14(9):1137--1144.

8. U. Kalus, A. Pruss, J. Bystron, M. Jurecka, A. Smekalova, J.J. Lichius, and H. Kiesewetter, "Effect of Nigella sativa (black seed) on subjective feeling in patients with allergic diseases," *Phytotherapy Research*. Dec.2003, 17(10):1209–1214.

9. H. Işik, A. Cevikbaş, U.S. Gürer, B. Kiran, Y. Uresin, P. Rayaman, E. Rayaman, B. Gürbüz, and S. Büyüköztürk, "Potential adjuvant effects of Nigella sativa seeds to improve specific immunotherapy in allergic rhinitis patients," *Med Princ Pract.*, 2010, 19(3):206–211.

10. R. Keyhanmanesh, M.H. Boskabady, M.J. Eslamizadeh, S. Khamneh, and M.A. Ebrahimi, "The effect of thymoquinone, the main constituent of Nigella sativa on tracheal responsiveness and white blood cell count in lung lavage of sensitized guinea pigs," *Planta Med.*, Feb. 2010, 76(3):218–222.

11. A. A. Norwood, M. Tan, M. May, M. Tucci, and H. Benghuzzi, "Comparison of potential chemotherapeutic agents, 5-fluoruracil, green tea, and thymoquinone on colon cancer cells (School of Health Related Professions, University of Mississippi Medical Center)," *Biomed Sci Instrum.* 2006, 42:350–356.

12. Chehl N, Chipitsyna G, Gong Q, Yeo CJ, Arafat HA. Anti-inflammatory effects of the Nigella sativa seed extract, thymoquinone, in pancreatic cancer cells. HPB (Oxford). 2009 Aug;11(5):373-

13. M.P. Torres, M.P. Ponnusam, S. Chakraborty, L. M. Smith , S. Das, H.A. Arafat, and S.K. Batra, "Effects of thymoquinone in the expression of mucin 4 in pancreatic cancer cells: Implications for the development of novel cancer therapies," *Mol Cancer Ther.*, May 2010, 9(5):1419–1431.

14. S. Banerjee, A.O. Kaseb, Z. Wang, D. Kong, M. Mohammad, S. Padhye, F.H. Sarkar, and R.M. Mohammad, "Antitumor activity of gemcitabine and oxaliplatin is augmented by thymoquinone in pancreatic cancer," *Cancer Res.*, July 1, 2009, 69(13):5575–5583. Epub June 23, 2009. .

15. Iddamaldeniya SS, Thabrew MI, Wickramasinghe S, Ratnatunge N, Thammitiyagodage MG. A long-term investigation of the anti-hepatocarcinogenic potential of an indigenous medicine comprised of Nigella sativa, Hemidesmus indicus and Smilax glabra. J Carcinog 2006;5:d

16. S.S. Iddamaldeniya, M.I. Thabrew, S.M. Wickramasinghe, N. Ratnatunge, and M.G. Thammitiyagodage, "A long-term investigation of the anti-hepatocarcinogenic potential of an indigenous medicine comprised of Nigella sativa, Hemidesmus indicus and Smilax glabra," *J Carcinog.*, May 9, 2006, 5:11.

17. A. El-Obeid, S. Al-Harbi, N. Al-Jomah, and A. Hassib, "Herbal melanin modulates tumor necrosis factor alpha (TNF-alpha), interleukin 6 (IL-6) and vascular endothelial growth factor (VEGF) production," *Phytomedicine*, May 2006, 13(5):324–333. Epub Sept. 19, 2005.

18. MA. el-Aziz, H.A. Hassan, M.H. Mohamed, A.R. Meki, S.K. Abdel-Ghaffar, and M.R. Hussein, "The biochemical and morphological alterations following administration of melatonin, retinoic acid and Nigella sativa in mammary carcinoma: an animal model," *Int J Exp Pathol.* Dec. 2005, 86(6):383–396.

19. F. Q, Alenzi, Yel-S. El-Bolkiny, and M.L. Salem, "Protective effects of Nigella sativa oil and thymoquinone against toxicity induced by the anticancer drug cyclophosphamide," *Br J Biomed Sci.* 2010, 67(1):20–28.

20. M. Kanter, O. Coskun, M. Kalayci, S. Buyukbas, and F. Cagavi, "Neuroprotective effects of Nigella sativa on experimental spinal cord injury in rats," *Hum Exp Toxicol.*, March 2006, 25(3):127–133.

21. M. Kanter, O. Coskun, and M. Budancamanak, "Hepatoprotective effects of Nigella sativa L and Urtica dioica L on lipid peroxidation, anti-oxidant enzyme systems and liver enzymes in carbon tetrachloride-treated rats," *World J Gastroenterol.*, Nov. 14, 2005, *11*(42):6684–6688.

22. G. K Helal, "Thymoquinone supplementation ameliorates acute endotoxemia-induced liver dysfunction in rats," *Pak J Pharm Sci.*, April 2010, 23(2):131–137.

23. M. Kanter, H. Demir, C. Karakaya, and H. Ozbek, "Gastroprotective activity of Nigella sativa L oil and its constituent, thymoquinone against acute alcohol-induced gastric mucosal injury in rats," *World J Gastroenterol.*, Nov. 14, 2005, 11(42):6662–6666.

24. E.M Salem, T. Yar, A.O. Bamosa, A. Al-Quorain, M.I. Yasawy, R.M. Alsulaiman, and M.A. Randhawa, "Comparative study of Nigella Sativa and triple therapy in eradication of Helicobacter pylori in patients with non-ulcer dyspepsia," *Saudi J Gastroenterol.*, July–Sept. 2010, 16(3):207–214.

25. A. Terzi, S. Coban, F. Yildiz, M. Ates, M. Bitiren, A. Taskin, and N. Aksoy, "Protective effects of Nigella sativa on intestinal ischemia-reperfusion injury in rats. J Invest Surg. 2010 Feb;23(1):21-7.

26. M. H. Boskabady, M.N. Shafei, and H. Parsaee, "Effects of aqueous and macerated extracts from Nigella sativa on guinea pig isolated heart activity," *Pharmazie.*, Dec. 2005, *60*(12):943–948.

27. F.R. Dehkordi and A.F. Kamkhah, "Antihypertensive effect of Nigella sativa seed extract in patients with mild hypertension," *Fundam Clin Pharmacol.*, Aug. 2008, 22(4):447–452.

28. W. Qidwai, H.B. Hamza, R. Qureshi, and A. Gilani, "Effectiveness, safety, and tolerability of powdered Nigella sativa (kalonji) seed in capsules on serum lipid levels, blood sugar, blood pressure, and body weight in adults: results of a randomized, double-blind controlled trial,." *J Altern Complement Med.*, June 2009;15(6):639–644.

29. M.A. Nader, D.S. el-Agamy, and G.M. Suddek, "Protective effects of propolis and thymoquinone on development of atherosclerosis in cholesterol-fed rabbits," *Arch Pharm Res.*, April 2010, 33(4):637–643.

30. A. Ghannadi, V. Hajhashemi, and H. Jafarabadi, "An investigation of the analgesic and anti-inflammatory effects of Nigella sativa seed polyphenols," *J. Med Food.*, Winter 2005, 8(4):488–493.

31. M. Dirjomuljono, I. Kristyono, R.R. Tjandrawinata, and D.Nofiarny, "Symptomatic treatment of acute tonsillo-pharyngitis patients with a combination of Nigella sativa and Phyllanthus niruri extract," *Int J Clin Pharmacol Ther.*, June 2008, 46(6):295–306.

32. S. Sangi, S.P.Ahmed, M.A. Channa, M. Ashfaq, and S.M. Mastoi, "A new and novel treatment of opioid dependence: Nigella sativa 500 mg." *J Ayub Med Coll Abbottabad.*, April–June 2008, 20(2):118–124.

33. F.I Al-Jenoobi, A.A. Al-Thukair, F.A. Abbas, M.J. Ansari, K.M. Alkharfy, A.M. Al-Mohizea, S.A. Al-Suwayeh, and S. Jamil. "Effect of black seed on dextromethorphan O- and N-demethylation in human liver microsomes and healthy human subjects," *Drug Metab Lett.*, Jan. 2010, 4(1):51–55.

34. H. Demir, M. Kanter, O. Coskun, Y.H. Uz, A. Koc, and A. Yildiz, "Effect of black cumin (Nigella sativa) on heart rate, some hematological values, and pancreatic beta-cell damage in cadmium-treated rats," *Biol Trace Elem Res..* May 2006, 110(2):151–162.

28

Ocimum sanctum

Introduction

Ocimum sanctum, known as Tulsi in Hindi and Surasa in Sanskrit, is an aromatic plant in the family Lamiaceae. Tulsi is native throughout the Old World tropics and is widespread as a cultivated plant and an escaped weed.[1] It is cultivated for religious and medicinal purposes and for its essential oil. Two main varieties are cultivated in India: green leaved or Lakshmi Tulsi and purple-leaved Krishna tulsi.[2] Tulsi has been used for thousands of years in Ayurveda for its diverse healing properties. It is mentioned by Charaka in the Charaka Samhita,[3] an ancient Ayurvedic text. Tulsi is considered to be an adaptogen,[4] balancing different processes in the body, and helping it adapt to stress.[5] Marked by a strong aroma and astringent taste, it is regarded in Ayurveda as a kind of "elixir of life" and is believed to promote longevity.[6] Tulsi's extracts are used in Ayurvedic remedies for common colds, headaches, stomach disorders, inflammation, heart disease, various forms of poisoning, and malaria. Traditionally, Tulsi is taken in many forms—as an herbal tea, a dried powder, fresh leaf, or mixed with ghee. Essential oil extracted from Tulsi is used mainly for medicinal purposes and in herbal cosmetics, and is widely used in skin preparations because of its anti-bacterial activity. For centuries, the dried leaves of Tulsi have been mixed with stored grains to repel insects.[7]

Studies suggest that Tulsi may be a COX-2 inhibitor, like many modern painkillers, because of its high concentration of eugenol (1-hydroxy-2-methoxy-4-allylbenzene). One such study showed Tulsi to be an effective treatment for diabetes by reducing blood glucose levels.[8] The same study showed significant reduction in total cholesterol levels with Tulsi.

Another study revealed that Tulsi's beneficial effect on blood glucose levels is due to its antioxidant properties.[9] Tulsi also shows some promise for protection from radiation poisoning [10] and cataracts.[11] The leaves are used in Ayurveda as a demulcent, a diaphoretic and an expectorant to treat bronchitis, cough, cold, and fever. Tulsi is an insecticide, an antihelmintic, a deodorizer, and also has been used as a laxative, a stimulant, an anti-inflammatory, a cardiotonic, and a blood purifier in hepatic disorders. Finally, it can be used to treat indigestion, and diminished appetite.

Synonymous Names

English: Sacred basil, holy basil
Hindi: Tulsi, tulasi
Sanskrit: Surasa, vrinda

Habitat

Ocimum sanctum grows wild throughout India and other tropical areas, to an elevation of 1800 meters.

Botanical Characteristics

Tulsi is an erect, much-branched annual herb that reaches a maximum height of 1.5 meters. The plant has simple, opposite green or purple leaves that are strongly scented, with hairy stems. They are elliptical, oblong, acute or obtuse, and pubescent on both sides. The leaves have petioles, up to 5 cm. long, and are usually somewhat toothed. Tulsi flowers are very small, purplish or crimson, occurring in long racemes in close whorls. The fruits or nutlets are small, subglobose or broadly ellipsoid, pale brown or reddish with small markings.[12]

Chemical Composition

Essential oil: Tulsi's leaf and flower contain an essential oil composed of eugenol, eugenal, carvacrol, methyl chavicol, linalool, caryophyllene, elemene and others.[13] Fatty acids: Stearic, myristic, palmitic, oleic, linoleic and linolenic acids[14] and their methyl esters.

Triterpenes and sterols: Ursolic acid, campesterol, cholesterol, stigmasterol, p-sitosterol and others.[15] Flavonoids and polyphenols: Vicenin-2, rosmarinic acid, galuteolin, cirsilineol, gallic acid, gallic acid methyl and ethyl esters, protocatechuic acid, vanillic acid, 4-hydroxybenzoic acid, vanillin, 4-hydroxybenzaldehyde, caffeic acid, chlorogenic acid and phenylpropane glucosides.[16]

Pharmacological Activity

Anti-microbial activity

Investigations were conducted to determine the effect on innate immunity of a tea fortified with five herbs selected from Indian traditional medicine (Ayurveda) for their putative immunoenhancing effect—Withania somnifera, Glycyrrhiza glabra, Zingiber officinale, Ocimum sanctum, and Elettaria cardamomum.[17] Ex-vivo natural killer (NK) cell activity was assessed after consumption of fortified tea compared to regular tea in two independent double-blind intervention studies. Both studies were conducted in India with healthy volunteers (age >or= 55 years) selected for a relatively low baseline NK cell activity and a history of recurrent coughs and colds. In a pilot study conducted with 32 volunteers, the consumption of tea significantly improved the NK cell activity of the volunteers in comparison with a population consuming regular tea. These results were validated in an independent crossover study with 110 volunteers. Data from these two studies indicate that regular consumption of the tea fortified with Ayurvedic herbs enhanced NK cell activity, which is an important aspect of the (early) innate immune response to infections.

Ocimum oils of various species were studied for their effectiveness on in-vitro activity against Propionibacterium acnes. An agar disc diffusion method was employed for screening antimicrobial activity of the essential oils of Ocimum basilicum L. (sweet basil), Ocimum sanctum L. (holy basil) and Ocimum americanum L. (hoary basil) against Propionibacterium acnes. Minimum inhibitory concentration (MIC) values of the basil oils were determined using an agar dilution assay.[18] The results indicated that the MIC values of sweet basil and holy basil oils were 2.0% and 3.0%, respectively, whereas hoary basil oil did not show activity against Propionibacterium acnes at the highest concentration tested. According to the disc diffusion assay, the formulations containing sweet basil oil exhibited higher activity against Propionibacterium acnes than those containing holy basil oil, and the thickened formulations tended to give a lower activity against Propionibacterium acnes than the non-thickened formulations. The prepared micro-emulsions were stable after being tested by a heat–cool cycling method for five cycles. These findings indicate the possibility of using Thai sweet and holy basil oil in suitable formulations for acne skin care.

Anti-oxidant activity

The anti-oxidant capacity of essential oils obtained by steam hydrodistillation of five species of the genus Ocimum was evaluated using a high-performance liquid chromatography-based hypoxanthine/xanthine oxidase and the DPPH assays. Strong anti-oxidant capacity was evident in all of the oils. Anti-oxidant capacity was correlated positively with a high proportion of compounds possessing a phenolic ring such as eugenol, while a strong negative correlation with other major volatiles was observed.[19] These correlations were confirmed to a large extent in the DPPH assay. The results of a 24-hour experiment with Ocimum sanctum showed that the anti-oxidant capacity factor reached a threshold between 10 and 12 hours, corresponding to maximum sunlight intensity and exhibited a clear diurnal variation. The data generated with these Ocimum species indicates that essential oils obtained from various herbs and spices may have an important role to play in cancer chemoprevention, functional foods, and in the preservation of pharmacologic products.[20] The mice used in this study were divided randomly into groups of six animals each. They were treated either with an intraperitoneal injection of saline or cocaine hydrochloride or with an oral feeding of oil of Ocimum sanctum, ascorbic acid or verapamil, or both (ascorbic acid and verapamil), and were evaluated for a respiratory burst of macrophages, superoxide, and nitric oxide (NO) production, estimation of TNF-alpha in the serum, and supernatant of cultured macrophages, estimation of lipid peroxidation (malondialdehyde- MDA) in the serum, and superoxide dismutase activity in the erythrocytes.

Unstimulated respiratory burst as well as superoxide production was enhanced after treatment with cocaine, and all three drugs were found to attenuate this enhancement.[21] The bactericidal capacity of macrophages decreased significantly upon exposure to chronic cocaine, as it was associated with decreased respiratory burst and superoxide production. There was a significant decrease in NO production by macrophages on chronic exposure to cocaine, and all the test drugs were found to restore nitrite formation to a normal level. There was an increase in the malondialdehyde (MDA) level and a decrease in the superoxide dismutase level upon chronic exposure to cocaine, and all three drugs effectively decreased the MDA level and increased the superoxide dismutase level. There was an increase in serum TNF-alpha upon chronic cocaine exposure, which was decreased significantly by ascorbic acid and verapamil. Ocimun sanctum, ascorbic acid, and verapamil were equally effective in improving the macrophage function and reducing oxidative stress. The effects of Ocimum sanctum leaf extract on the changes in the concentrations of serum triiodothyronine, thyroxine serum cholesterol and on the changes in the weight of the sex organs were investigated. Although the plant extract at the dose of 0.5 g kg-1 body weight for 15 days significantly decreased serum T4 concentrations, hepatic lipid peroxidation and glucose 6-phosphate G-6-P activity, the activities of the endogenous anti-oxidant enzymes superoxide dismutase SOD and catalase CAT were increased by the drug. However, no marked changes were observed in serum T3 level, T3/T4 ratio, and the concentration of serum cholesterol.[22]

Anti-inflammatory activity

The fixed oil extracted from Ocimum leaves exhibited significant anti-inflammatory activity against carrageenan induced paw edema in rats. Using various inflammation models, it was inferred that the anti-inflammatory activity was attributable to inhibition of both the cyclooxygenase and lipoxygenase pathways of arachidonic acid metabolism. The active principle responsible was found to be linolenic acid.[23,]

Anti-asthmatic activity

A 50% hydroalcoholic extract and the volatile oil extracted from fresh Ocimum leaves were evaluated against histamine- and acetylcholine-induced pre-convulsive dyspnea in pigs. Both the extract and the oil exhibited significant dose-dependent anti-asthmatic activity, with the percentage protection shown by 200 mg/kg of ethanol extract of fresh leaves equivalent to 0.5 ml of volatile oil. The volatile constituents of the fresh leaves were thought to be the main factor responsible for this activity.[25]

Anti-carcinogenic activity

The essential oil of Ocimum showed a significant inhibition of benzopyrene-induced squamous cell carcinoma in the stomach of Swiss mice. The chemopreventive potential of the oil was studied by assessing its effect on the carcinogen detoxifying enzyme, glutathione-S-transferase, and 3,4-benzopyrene-induced neoplasia in Swiss mice.[26] Another study was designed to evaluate the chemopreventive effects of ethanolic Ocimum sanctum leaf extract on cell proliferation, apoptosis, and angiogenesis during N-methyl-N'-nitro-N-nitrosoguanidine (MNNG)-induced gastric carcinogenesis.[27] The study animals were divided into four groups of ten each. The rats in group one were given MNNG (150 mg/kg body weight) by intragastric intubation three times, with a two-week interval between treatments. The rats in group two were administered MNNG as in group one, but in addition, they received intragastric intubation of ethanolic Ocimum extract (300 mg/kg body weight) three times per week, starting on the day following the first exposure to MNNG. The intubation of ethanolic Ocimun sanctum extract continued until the end of the experimental period. The rats in group three were given ethanolic Ocimum leaf extract only. The group four rats served as controls. All of the rats were killed after an experimental period of 26 weeks.

Intragastric administration of MNNG-induced well-differentiated squamous cell carcinomas that showed increased cell proliferation, and angiogenesis with evasion of apoptosis, as revealed by the upregulation of proliferating cell nuclear antigen, glutathione S-transferase-pi, Bcl-2, cytokeratin (CK) and vascular endothelial growth factor and with downregulation of Bax, cytochrome C, and caspase 3 protein expression. Administration of ethanolic Ocimum leaf extract reduced the incidence of MNNG-induced gastric carcinomas. This was accompanied by decreased expression of PCNA, GST-pi, Bcl-2, CK, and VEGF, and overexpression of Bax, cytochrome C, and caspase 3. This study provides evidence that in MNNG-induced gastric carcinogenesis, the key proteins involved in the proliferation, invasion, angiogenesis, and apoptosis are viable molecular targets for chemoprevention using ethanolic Ocimum leaf extract.[28]

The antitumor mechanism of ethanol extracts of Ocimum sanctum (EEOS) was elucidated in human non-small cell lung carcinoma (NSCLC) A549 cells in-vitro and the Lewis lung carcinoma (LLC) animal model. Ocimum extract exerted cytotoxicity against A549 cells, increased the sub-G1 population, and exhibited apoptotic bodies in A549 cells. Further, Ocimum extract cleaved poly(ADP-ribose) polymerase (PARP), released cytochrome C into cytosol, and simultaneously activated caspase-9 and -3 proteins. Also, Ocimum extract increased the ratio of proapoptotic protein Bax/antiapoptotic protein Bcl-2 and inhibited the phosphorylation of Akt and extracellular signal regulated kinase (ERK) in A549 cancer cells. In addition, it was found that Ocimum extract can suppress the growth of LLC inoculated onto C57BL/6 mice in a dose-dependent manner. Overall, these results demonstrate that Ocimum extract induces apoptosis in A549 cells via a mitochondria caspase- dependent pathway and inhibits the in-vivo growth of LLC, suggesting that Ocimum extract can be applied to lung carcinoma as a chemopreventive candidate.[29]

Cardioprotective activity

The effects of Curcuma longa and Ocimum sanctum on myocardial apoptosis and cardiac function were studied in an ischemia and reperfusion model of myocardial injury.[30] Wistar albino rats were divided into four groups and were orally fed saline, Curcuma, or Ocimum for a one-month period. On the 31st day, LAD occlusion was undertaken for 45 minutes, and reperfusion was allowed for 1 hour. The hemodynamic parameters mean arterial pressure, heart rate, left ventricular end-diastolic pressure, left ventricular peak positive and negative levels were monitored at pre-set points throughout the experimental duration, and subsequently the animals were sacrificed for immunohistopathological and histopathological studies. Chronic treatment with Curcuma longa significantly reduced TUNEL positivity, Bax protein, and upregulated Bcl-2 expression in comparison to the control group. In addition, Curcuma demonstrated mitigating effects on several myocardial injury induced hemodynamic and histopathological perturbations. The Ocimum treatment resulted in modest modulation of the hemodynamic alterations but failed to demonstrate any significant antiapoptotic effects or prevent the histopathological alterations compared to the control group.

In further research, Ocimum was investigated for its cardiac activity. Myocardial infarction was induced in rats with 85, 200, and 300 mg/kg of isoproterenol administered subcutaneously twice at an interval of 24 hours. Shifts in anti-oxidant parameters and lactate dehydrogenase, together with morphological and histopathological changes, were investigated.[31] A dose of 200 mg/kg ISO was selected for this study, as this dose offered a significant alteration in biochemical parameters along with moderate necrosis in the heart. The effect of pre- and co-treatment of hydroalcoholic extract of Ocimum sanctum at different doses (25, 50, 75, 100, 200, and 400 mg/kg) was investigated against ISO (200 mg/kg) induced myocardial infarction in rats. Modulation of various biochemical parameters and membrane integrity was studied. Ocimum at doses of 25, 50, 75 and 100 mg/kg significantly enhanced glutathione, superoxide dismutase, and LDH levels. It also inhibited lipid peroxidation, as observed by the reduced levels of thiobarbituric acid reactive substances. These results show that Ocimum at the dose of 50 mg/kg demonstrated the maximum cardioprotective effect. The results were further confirmed by histopathological findings. Thus, it was concluded that Ocimum may be of therapeutic and prophylactic value in the treatment of myocardial infarction.

In another study, administration of Ocimum leaf extract resulted in a fall of both diastolic and systolic pressure to normal levels, with no adverse side effects.[32] Cardioprotective activity of a combined treatment of Ginkgo biloba phytosomes (GBP) and Ocimum sanctum extract (Os) in isoproterenol (ISO)-induced myocardial necrosis in rats was studied.[33] The results showed significant myocardial necrosis, depletion of the endogenous anti-oxidants superoxide dismutase (SOD), catalase (CAT), glutathione peroxidase (GPx), glutathione reductase (GR), and glutathione (GSH), and increases in the serum marker enzymes aspartate aminotransferase (AST), lactate dehydrogenase (LDH), and creatine phosphokinase (CPK) in ISO-treated rats, compared to normal rats. Co-administration of Ginkgo biloba phytosome (100 mg per kg) with Ocimum sanctum at two doses (50 and 75 mg per kg) for 30 days to rats treated with ISO (85 mg per kg, sc) on the 29th and 30th days demonstrated a significant decrease in ISO-induced serum marker enzyme elevations and significant attenuation of the ISO-elevated myocardial lipid peroxidation marker malondialdehyde (MDA). A significant restoration of ISO-depleted activities and levels of AST, LDH, CPK, GSH, SOD, CAT, GPx, and GR in the hearts of the treatment groups was observed. The combination of Ocimum sanctum 75 mg per kg and Ginkgo biloba phytosome 100 mg/kg elicited greater protection than the combination of Ocimum 50 mg per kg and Ginkgo 100 mg per kg. However, the combined treatment failed to enhance cardioprotective activity of either herb when used alone.

Hypolipidemic activity

Orimum sanctum leaf powder at a level of 1% was fed to normal and diabetic rats for one month. A significant reduction in cholesterol and triglyceride levels in the liver, a reduction of total lipids in the kidney and a fall in total cholesterol and phospholipids in the heart were observed.[34]

Hypoglycemic activity

A study was conducted to determine if oral administration of the aqueous extract of the whole Ocimum plant protects against development of insulin resistance in fructose-fed rats. Male Wistar rats were randomly divided into four groups of eight animals each: group-S (starch diet), group-F (fructose diet), group-F+OS (fructose diet along with Ocimum extract at a dose of 200 mg/kg), and group-S+OS (starch diet along with Ocimum).[35] During the experimental period of 60 days, body weight, plasma glucose, insulin, and triglycerides were measured at an interval of 15 days. Insulin sensitivity was assessed at the end of experimental period by measuring the glucose-insulin index, which is the product of the areas under the curve of glucose and insulin during the oral glucose tolerance test. The nontoxic nature of Ocimum was revealed by unaltered body weight, plasma glucose, insulin, and triglyceride levels in group-S+OS compared to group-S. Significant gains in body weight, hyperglycemia, hyperinsulinemia, hypertriglyceridemia, and insulin resistance were observed in group-F compared to group-S. Ocimum treatment prevented the observed fructose-induced alterations in group-F+OS. These results suggest that oral administration of Ocimum aqueous extract could delay the development of insulin resistance in rats and may be used as an adjuvant therapy for treating diabetic patients with insulin resistance.

Ethanol extract and five partition fractions of Ocimum sanctum leaves were studied on insulin secretion together with an evaluation of their mechanisms of action.[36] The ethanol extract and each of the aqueous, butanol, and ethylacetate fractions stimulated insulin secretion from perfused rat pancreas, isolated rat islets, and a clonal rat beta-cell line in a concentration-dependent manner. The stimulatory effects of ethanol extract and each of these partition fractions were potentiated by glucose, isobutylmethylxanthine, tolbutamide, and a depolarizing concentration of KCl. Inhibition of the secretory effect was observed with diazoxide, verapamil, and Ca^{2+} removal. In contrast, the stimulatory effects of the chloroform and hexane partition fractions were associated with decreased cell viability and were unaltered by diazoxide and verapamil. The ethanol extract and the five fractions increased intracellular Ca^{2+} in clonal BRIN-BD11 cells, partly attenuated by the addition of verapamil. These findings indicate that constituents of Ocimum sanctum leaf extracts have stimulatory effects on physiological pathways of insulin secretion which may underlie its reported anti-diabetic action.

Radioprotective activity

The radioprotective effect of a leaf extract of Ocimum sanctum with WR-2721 was evaluated on bone marrow of adult Swiss mice. The mice were injected intraperitoneally with the extract (10 mg/kg daily for 5 consecutive days) or 100–400 mg/kg WR-2721 (single dose) or a combination of the two, after which the whole body of the mouse was exposed to γ-irradiation. Significant free radical scavenging activity in-vitro was observed with the leaf extract and WR-2721, which was further enhanced by combining the two, and resulted in greater bone marrow protection. Significant protection of chromosomes was obtained by a combination of leaf extract and WR-2721, with a reduction in the toxicity of the latter at higher doses, indicating that the combination may have promise for radioprotection in humans.[37]

Analgesic activity

Tulsi's fixed oil was shown to have marked analgesic activity in mice, measured using the acetic acid-induced writhing test. This suggests a possible mechanism of action related to the peripheral system.[38] A study was aimed at investigating the ameliorative effect of Ocimum sanctum in sciatic nerve transection (axotomy)-induced peripheral neuropathy in rats.

Sciatic nerve transection-induced axonal degeneration was assessed histopathologically. Paw pressure, Von Frey Hair, tail cold-hyperalgesia, and motor in-coordination tests were performed to assess the extent of neuropathy. Biochemical estimations of thiobarbituric acid reactive species (TBARS), reduced glutathione (GSH), and total calcium levels also were performed. A methanolic extract of Ocimum sanctum was administered at different doses (50, 100, and 200mg/kg p.o.) for 10 consecutive days starting from the day of surgery. Administration of Ocimum sanctum attenuated sciatic nerve transection-induced axonal degeneration and reduced the nociceptive threshold and motor in-coordination. Moreover, it attenuated an axotomy-induced rise in TBARS and total calcium and a decrease in GSH levels in a dose-dependent manner.

Anti-oxidant and calcium attenuating actions may be responsible for observed ameliorative effects of Ocimum sanctum in axotomy-induced neuropathy.[39]

Immunomodulatory activity

An ethanolic extract of the leaves of Ocimum sanctum was evaluated utilizing activities of the enzymes cytochrome P450, cytochrome B5, and aryl hydrocarbon hydroxylase in the liver and glutathione-S-transferase and reduced glutathione levels in the liver, lung, and stomach of the mouse. Administration of the extract at doses of 400 and 800 mg/kg for 15 days significantly increased these activities, all of which are important in the detoxification of both carcinogens and mutagens. An increase in extrahepatic glutathione-S-transferase and reduced glutathione levels in the liver, lung and stomach tissues also was observed.[40] An increase in cellular immunological response, represented by E-rosette formation and lymphocytosis, was seen with the methanolic extract (100 and 250 mg/kg) and an aqueous suspension (500 mg/kg) of Ocimum sanctum leaves in rats.[41] An in-vitro test produced a significant inhibition of antigen-induced histamine release from the peritoneal mast cells of sensitized rats and showed an increase in the anti-SRBC hemagglutination titer and the IgE antibody titer. These results indicated that Ocimum modulated the humoral immune responses by acting at various levels in the immune mechanism such as antibody production, release of mediators of hypersensitivity reactions, and tissue response to the mediators in the target organs.[42]

Anti-stress activity

Ocimum sanctum has been studied for its role in generalized anxiety disorder (GAD) in hospital-based clinical set-ups. Hamilton's brief psychiatric rating scale (BPRS) and thorough clinical investigations were used to screen the subjects. Thirty-five subjects (21 male and 14 female; average age 38.4 years) were medicated with the plant extract in a fixed-dose regime (500 mg/capsule, twice daily, p.o. after meal). They were thoroughly investigated clinically and using standard questionnaires based on different psychological rating scale at baseline (day 0), mid-term (day 30), and final (day 60). The observations exhibited that O. sanctum significantly ($p<0.001$) attenuated generalized anxiety disorders and also attenuated the correlated stress and depression. It further significantly ($p<0.001$) improved the willingness for adjustment and attention in humans. Ocimum sanctum could be useful in the treatment of GAD in humans and may be a promising anxiolytic agent.[43] An ethanolic extract of Ocimum leaves prevented changes in plasma levels of corticosterone induced by exposure to both acute and chronic noise stress in rats. The plant extract also exhibited anti-stress activity by improving SDH levels in albino rats.[44] Ocimum also showed a marked protective and inhibitory effect on stress induced gastric ulcers in albino rats. Microscopic and histopathological findings, such as congestion, erosion, discrete and multiple hemorrhages, ulcers and perforation in the control group of rats served as a measure for scoring the intensity.[45]

In another study, fresh leaves of Ocimum sanctum were evaluated for anti-stress activity against experimentally induced oxidative stress in albino rabbits. Animals in the test group received a supplement of 2 grams of fresh leaves of Ocimum per rabbit for 30 days. Anemic hypoxia was induced chemically by injecting the rabbits with 15 mg sodium nitrite per 100 g body weight intraperitoneally. Ocimum administration blunted the changes in cardiorespiratory parameters in response to stress. A significant decrease in blood sugar level was observed after 30 days of dietary supplementation of Ocimum leaves. A significant increase in levels of enzymatic (superoxide dismutase) and nonenzymatic (reduced glutathione) anti-oxidants was observed in the test group after the treatment with Ocimum. Oxidative stress led to a lesser depletion of reduced glutathione and plasma superoxide dismutase in the treated rabbits, suggesting the potential anti-stressor activity of Ocimum sanctum is partly attributable to its anti-oxidant properties.[57]

Anti-gonorrhea activity

In view of the widespread emergence of resistant isolates, an attempt was made to isolate and identify the components of Ocimum sanctum with activity against Neisseria gonorrheae. After a bioassay-guided purification of the hexane extract of leaves of Ocimum was carried out, eugenol was identified as the active compound. The anti-gonorrheal efficacy of eugenol was better against multi-resistant strains. In view of its efficacy and lower toxicity, eugenol may be a potentially suitable molecule to be developed clinically in response to emerging resistant isolates of N. gonorrheae.[47]

Wound-healing activity

Oxidative stress and free radicals have been implicated in the impaired healing of wounds. Ocimum sanctum possesses anti-inflammatory and anti-oxidant properties. A study was undertaken to assess the potential of alcoholic and aqueous extracts of Ocimum for wound healing in Wistar albino rats. For this study, the rats were divided into five groups of six animals each. The first group consisted of a normal wounded control. The other four groups were treated with two different doses each of alcoholic and aqueous extract of Ocimum. The wound-healing parameters were evaluated by using incision, excision, and dead-space wounds in the extract-treated rats and controls. The doses of alcoholic and aqueous Ocimum extract both were found to significantly increase wound-breaking strength, hydroxyproline, hexuronic acid, hexosamines, superoxide dismutase, and catalase, and to reduce glutathione and significantly decrease the percentage of wound contraction and lipid peroxidation compared to the control group. Ocimum sanctum has anti-oxidant properties that may be responsible and favorable for faster wound healing, and that this plant extract may be useful in managing abnormal healing and hypertropic scars.[48]

Anti-genotoxic activity

The anti-genotoxic effect of Ocimum extract was studied against the genotoxic effect induced by a synthetic progestin cyproterone acetate on human lymphocytes using chromosomal aberrations, mitotic index, sister chromatid exchanges, and a replication index as parameters. About 30 microM of cyproterone acetate was treated with Ocimum sanctum infusion. A clear dose-dependent decrease in the genotoxic damage of cyproterone acetate was observed, suggesting a possible modulating role of the plant infusion. Results of this study suggest that Ocimum infusion alone does not have genotoxic potential but that it can modulate the genotoxicity of cyproterone acetate on human lymphocytes in-vitro.[49]

Anti-psychotic activity

Use of typical anti-psychotics such as haloperidol in treating schizophrenia carries with it a high incidence of side-effects. In rodents, administration of haloperidol leads to the development of a behavioral state called catalepsy, in which the animal is not able to correct an externally imposed posture. A study was undertaken to evaluate the anti-cataleptic efficacy of a polyherbal formulation containing bioactives of several Ayurvedic herbs, including Ocimum, in mice.[50] Five groups of male albino mice were used in the study. Catalepsy was induced by administering haloperidol. The degree of catalepsy was measured as the time the animal maintained an imposed posture. The anti-cataleptic efficacy of the polyherbal formulation was compared with that of scopolamine. The superoxide dismutase level in brain tissue also was estimated to correlate the levels of oxidative stress and degree of catalepsy in the animal. A significant reduction in the cataleptic scores was observed in all of the groups treated with the formulation.

Anti-dementia activity

Dementia is an age-related mental problem and a characteristic symptom of various neurodegenerative disorders including Alzheimer's disease. Certain drugs, such as diazepam, barbiturates, and alcohol, disrupt learning and memory in animals and humans. And a new class of drugs known as nootropic agents now is used in situations where there is organic disorder in learning abilities.

A study was undertaken to assess the potential of Ocimum extract as a nootropic and an anti-amnesic agent in mice. An aqueous extract of the dried whole plant of Ocimum sanctum ameliorated the amnesic effect of scopolamine, diazepam, and aging-induced memory deficits in mice. Elevated plus maze and passive avoidance paradigms served as the behavioral models. The Ocimum sanctum extract significantly decreased transfer latency and increased step-down latency compared to the control, scopolamine, and aged groups of mice. Ocimum preparations could be beneficial in the treatment of cognitive disorders such as dementia and Alzheimer's disease.[51]

Anti-ulcer activity

The standardized methanolic extract of leaves of Ocimum sanctum, given in doses of 50-200 mg/kg orally twice daily for five days, showed a dose-dependent ulcer-protective effect against cold-restraint stress induced gastric ulcers. The optimal effective dose of the extract produced significant ulcer protection against ethanol and pyloric ligation-induced gastric ulcers but was ineffective against aspirin-induced ulcers. Ocimum significantly healed ulcers induced by 50% acetic acid after 5 and 10 days of treatment, significantly inhibited the offensive acid–pepsin secretion and lipid peroxidation, and increased the gastric defensive factors such as mucin secretion, cellular mucus, and the lifespan of mucosal cells. The Ocimum extract had an anti-oxidant effect but did not induce mucosal cell proliferation. Ocimum have effects on both offensive and defensive mucosal factors.[52]

Anti-cataract activity

Research was conducted to study the effect of Ocimum sanctum on selenite-induced morphological and biochemical changes in isolated rat lenses, as well as the incidence of cataracts in rat pups.[53] The transparent rat lenses were divided into normal, selenite only, and four treated groups. The selenite-only and the treated group lenses were subjected to oxidative stress in-vitro by incorporating sodium selenite in the culture medium. The effect of Ocimum was studied for levels of reduced glutathione and thiobarbituric acid- reacting substances in the selenite-challenged lenses. The lowest concentration of Ocimum offering significant modulation on these two parameters was determined. Subsequently, the effect of prior and co-treatment with the lowest effective concentration of Ocimum was studied on lens anti-oxidant enzymes such as superoxide dismutase, glutathione peroxidase, catalase, and glutathione-S transferase. Changes in lens protein profiles under different incubation conditions were analyzed by SDS gel-electrophoresis. In-vivo, cataract was induced by a single subcutaneous injection of sodium selenite to 9-day-old rat pups. The anti-cataract effect of Ocimum injected intraperitoneally 4 hours prior to the selenite challenge was evaluated by the presence of lens nuclear opacity in the rat pups on the 16th postnatal day. Insolubilization of lens proteins post-selenite injection was monitored for 4 days.

As a result, the lenses in the selenite-only group developed cortical opacities in 24 hours. Ocimum showed different degrees of positive modulation in selenite-induced morphological as well as biochemical changes. The lowest effective dose of Ocimum that significantly modulated glutathione and thiobarbituric acid-reacting substances was found to be 140 microg/ml. At this dose, a significant increase in anti-oxidant enzyme levels and preservation of normal lens protein profile was observed. Ocimum at the dose of 70 microg/ml did not show any significant protection with respect to either morphology or biochemistry of lenses. In-vivo, 5 and 10 mg/kg of Ocimum reduced the incidence of selenite cataract by 20% and 60%, respectively, and prevented protein insolubilization as well.

This study indicates that aqueous extracts of Ocimum possesses potential anti-cataract activity against selenite-induced experimental cataractogenesis. The protective effect was supported by restoration of the anti-oxidant defense system and inhibition of protein insolubilization of rat lenses as well.

Ethnoveterinary Usage

All parts of Ocimum sanctum are used in veterinary medicine to treat conditions including glossitis, ulcers, maggots in wounds, anthrax, pneumonia, indigestion, tympanitis, pain in the abdomen, constipation, stoppage of urination, liver flukes, loss of appetite, stomach pain, dog bite, cold and cough, cannabis poisoning, opacity of cornea, swelling of lungs, tachycardia, sprains, and sore eyes. The leaves are used to treat bleeding, coughs and colds, eye disease, udder infection, and wound-healing in ruminants.

Dr. Sodhi's Experience

When considering treatment with Holy basil, the practitioner should consider the following:

- Is there an infection of any type—viral, bacterial, fungal, parasitic?
- Is there an allergic response?
- Is the eosinophil count high?
- Is excess stress present?
- Is immune modulation desirable?
- Is there dysregulation in sugar metabolism?

Ocimum sanctum is known as "Holy Basil" for good reason. Traditionally, Holy Basil is planted at the center of every Indian home. Older homes in India were constructed to be balanced astrologically. A central area in the home was kept open with a Tulsi plant growing in the middle. The primary reason was that the plant repels insects. Also, its pleasant smell and stress adaptogenic properties benefit the entire household. Many Hindi saints wear beads made of Tulsi because of its stress-relieving effects; the plant's oil is absorbed through the skin from the beads around their neck.

The essential oil of Tulsi has anti-bacterial, anti-viral, anti-fungal, and anti-parasitic properties, and even can be used to treat tuberculosis. A traditional Indian remedy for fever, flu, and body aches is a tea infusion from Tulsi, in which the lid is kept on the teapot to retain the essential oils. The fresh leaves also may be crushed, made into a paste, and eaten with honey. Tulsi leaves also are sometimes smoked in a small, enclosed pipe to treat various lung conditions, including asthma.

Tulsi is an excellent herb to take when there is an allergic response, and for eosinophilia. As an immune modulator, it can be used for any condition in which the immune system is weak. Because of this, it can be used as an important adjunct therapy in the treatment of cancer.

Tulsi also lowers blood sugar and often is used to treat dysglycemia, including diabetes. Although it is not the most important herb in treating diabetes, it has an additive effect if used with Gymnema sylvestre (shardunika), Pterocarpus marsupium (Vijjasaar), and Azadirachta indica (Neem), enhancing the effects of formulations with these herbs synergistically. For this reason, it usually is used in formulas rather than by itself.

Case History

Our clinic donated several months' supply of an immune-modulating formula, which we had developed, to a cancer treatment center in Seattle for use with their patients. The center used it as an adjunct to chemotherapy with its patients for 3 months, monitoring the white blood cell count and rates of infection during the entire period. None of the patients who received the immune-modulating formulation developed infections during this treatment, and their white blood cell counts did not drop.

The formulation used in the study contained the following:

Emblica officinalis (amalaki), Ocinum sanctum (tulsi), Terminalia bellerica (bibhihtaki) extracts, 200 mg each

Tinospora cordifolia (guduchi), and Glycyrrhiza glabra (yastsimadhu) extracts, 100 mg. each

Terminalia chebula (haritaki) and Adhatoda vasica (vasaka), 50 mg each.

Safety Profile

The patients who received moderate doses of powdered Ocimum leaves for 3 months reported few side-effects except constipation. Large doses of the leaf extract were shown to induce an antispermatogenic effect in animals. The maximum tolerated dose of the 50% hydroalcoholic leaf extract was 1000 mg/kg body weight in albino rats.[54]

Dosage

Leaf infusion: 4–12 ml
Decoction: 28–56 ml
Seed powder: 1.5–2g
Extract : 5:1 100 to 300 mg three times per day

Ayurvedic Properties

Rasa: Katu (pungent), tikta (bitter)
Guna: Laghu (light), ruksha (dry)
Veerya: Ushna (hot)
Vipaka: Katu (pungent)
Dosha: Pacifies kapha and vata

Notes

1. G. Staples and M.S. Kristiansen, *Ethnic Culinary Herbs* (: University of Hawaii Press, 1999), p. 73. Please delete the City

2. S. K. Kothari and A.K. Bhattacharya, et al., "Volatile constituents in oil from different plant parts of methyl eugenol-rich Ocimim tenuiflorum L.f. (syn. O. sanctum L.) grown in South India," *Journal of Essential Oil Research*, Nov/Dec 2005.

3. M. Kuhn and D. Winston, *Winston & Kuhn's Herbal Therapy & Supplements: A Scientific and Traditional Approach* (ity: P Lippincott Williams & Wilkins, 2007), p. 260.

4. H. S Puri, *Rasayana: Ayurvedic Herbs for Longevity and Rejuvenation* (CRC Press, 2002), pp. 272–280.

5. N. P. Biswas and A.K. Biswas, "Evaluation of some leaf dusts as grain protectant against rice weevil Sitophilus oryzae (Linn.)," *Environment and Ecology*, 2005), 23(3), 485–488. [6] P. Prakash and N. Gupta, "Therapeutic uses of Ocimum sanctum Linn (Tulsi) with a note on eugenol and its pharmacological actions: A short review, Indian J Physiol Pharmacol. 2005 Apr;49(2):125-31.[7] Looks like former note 54 (now 5), not Note 56. Are these two reversed? I am confused about this query. I think note 5 is wrong. It is not about stress I think they got reversed. Correct this according to you.

6. Rai, U.V. Mani, and U.M. Iyer, "Effect of Ocimum sanctum leaf powder on blood lipoproteins, glycated proteins, and total amino acids in patients with non-insulin-dependent diabetes mellitus," *Journal of Nutritional & Environmental Medicine*, June 1, 1997, 7(2):113–118.

7. J. Sethi, S. Sood, S. Shashi, and A. Talwar, "Evaluation of hypoglycemic and anti-oxidant effect of Ocimum sanctum," *Indian Journal of Clinical Biochemistry*, 2004, 19(2) 152–155.

8. P. U. Devi and A. Ganasoundari, "Modulation of glutathione and anti-oxidant enzymes by Ocimum sanctum and its role in protection against radiation injury," *Indian Journal of Experimental Biology*, March 1999, 37(3): 262–268.

9. P. Sharma, S. Kulshreshtha, and A.L.Sharma, "Anti-cataract activity of Ocimum sanctum on experimental cataract," *Indian Journal of Pharmacology*, 1998, 30(1),16–20.

10. P. K. Warrier, *Indian Medicinal Plants* (Orient Longman, 1995), p. 168.

11. H. Skaltsa-Diamantidis, O. Tzakou, A. Loukis, and N. Argyriadou, "Analysis of essential oil of Ocimum sanctum L. New results," *Plant Medicine and Phytotherapy*, 1990, 24(2):79.

12. S. Singh, D.K. Majumdar, and M.R. Yadav, "Chemical and pharmacological studies on fixed oils of Ocimum sanctum," *Indian Journal of Experimental Biology*, 1996, 34(12):1212.

13. M Skaltsa, M. Couladi, S. Philianos, and M. Singh, "Phytochemical study of the leaves of Ocimum sanctum," *Fitoterapia*, 1987, 58(4):286.

14. H. Norr and H. Wagner, "New constituents from Ocimum sanctum," *Planta Medica*, 1992, 58(6):547.

15. J. Bhat, A. Damle, P.P. Vaishnav, R. Albers, M. Joshi, and G. Banerjee, "In vivo enhancement of natural killercell activity through tea fortified with Ayurvedic herbs," *Phytother Res.*, Jan. 2010, 24(1), 129–135.

16. J. Viyoch, N. Pisutthanan, A. Faikreua, K. Nupangta, K. Wangtorpol, and J. Ngokkuen, "Evaluation of in vitro antimicrobial activity of Thai basil oils and their micro-emulsion formulas against Propionibacterium acnes," *J. Int J Cosmet Sci.* April 2006, 28(2):125–133.

17. M.T Trevisan, M.G. Vasconcelos Silva, B. Pfundstein, B. Spiegelhalder, and R.W. Owen, "Characterization of the volatile pattern and anti-oxidant capacity of essential oils from different species of the genus Ocimum," *J Agric Food Chem.*, June 14, 2006, 54(12):4378–4382.

18. See Note 19.

19. S.K. Bhattacharya, N. Rathi, P. Mahajan, A.K.Tripathi, K.R. Paudel, G.P. Rauniar, and B.P. Das, "Effect of Ocimum sanctum, ascorbic acid, and verapamil on macrophage function and oxidative stress in mice exposed to cocaine," *Indian J Pharmacol.*, June 2009, 41(3):134–139.

20. S. Panda and A. Kar, "Ocimum sanctum leaf extract in the regulation of thyroid function in the male mouse," *Pharmacol Res.*, Aug. 1998, 38(2):107–110.

21. S. Singh, D.K. Majumdar, and H.M. Rehan, "Evaluation of anti-inflammatory potential of fixed oil of Ocimum sanctum (Holy Basil) and its possible mechanism of action," *Journal of Ethnopharmacology*, 1996, 46(3):195.

22. S. Singh and D.K. Majumdar, "Evaluation of anti-inflammatory activity of fatty acids of Ocimum sanctum fixed oil," *Indian Journal of Experimental Biology*, 1997, 35(4):380.

23. S. Singh and S.S. Agrawal, "Anti-asthmatic and anti-Inflammatory activity of Ocimum sanctum," *International Journal of Pharmacognosy*, 1991, 29(4):306.

24. K. Aruna and V.M. Sivaramakrishnan, "Amicarcinogenic effects of the essential oils from cumin, poppy and basil," *Phytotherapy Research*, 1996, 10:577.

25. P. Manikandan, P. Vidjaya Letchoumy, D. Prathiba, and S. Nagini, "Proliferation, angiogenesis and apoptosis-associated proteins are molecular targets for chemoprevention of MNNG-induced gastric carcinogenesis by ethanolic Ocimum sanctum leaf extract," *Singapore Med J.*, July 2007, 48(7):645–651.

26. See Note 27.

27. V. Magesh, J.C. Lee, K.S. Ahn, H.J. Lee, H.J. Lee HJ, E.O. B.S. H.J. Jung, J.S. Kim, D.K. Kim, S.H. Choi, K.S. Ahn, and S.H. Kim, "Ocimum sanctum induces apoptosis in A549 lung cancer cells and suppresses the in vivo growth of Lewis lung carcinoma cells," *Phytother Res.* Oct. 2009,23(10):1385–1391.

28. I. Mohanty, D.S. Arya, and S. K.Gupta, "Effect of Curcuma longa and Ocimum sanctum on myocardial apoptosis in experimentally induced myocardial ischemic-reperfusion injury," *BMC Complement Altern Med.*, Feb. 19, 2006, 6:3.

29. M. Sharma, K. Kishore, S.K.Gupta, S. Joshi, and D.S. Arya, "Cardioprotective potential of ocimum sanctum in isoproterenol induced myocardial infarction in rats," *Mol Cell Biochem.* Sept. 2001, 225(1):75-83.

30. G. Subbulakshmi and S.R. Sarvaiya, "Hypotensive effect of Ocimum sanctum," *Bombay Hospital Journal*, 1991 33(1):39-43.

31. Panda VS, , " Evaluation of cardioprotective activity of Ginkgo biloba and Ocimum sanctum in rodents," *Altern Med Rev.*, June 2009, 14(2):161–171.

32. V Rai, U. Lyer, and U. V. Mani, "Effect of Tulsi (Ocimam sanctum) leaf powder supplementation on blood sugar levels, serum Hpids and tissue lipids in diabetic nits," *Plant Foods and Human Nutrition*, 1997, 50(1):9.

33. S. S Reddy, R. Karuna, R. Baskar, and D. Saralakumari, "Prevention of insulin resistance by ingesting aqueous extract of Ocimum sanctum to fructose-fed rats," *Horm Metab* Res, Jan 2008, 40(1):44–49. Epub Dec 18, 2007.

34. J.M Hannan, L. Marenah, L. Ali, V. Rokeya, P.R. Flatt, and Y.H. Abdel-Wahab, "Ocimum sanctum leaf extracts stimulate insulin secretion from perfused pancreas, isolated islets and clonal pancreatic beta-cells, *J Endocrinol*. April 2006, 189(1):127–136.

35. A. Ganasoundari, P.U. Devi, and B.S. Rao, "Enhancement of bone marrow radioprotection and reduction of WR-2721 toxitity by Odmum sanctum," *Mutation Research,* 1998, 397(2}:303.

36. S Singh and D.K. Majumdar, "Analgesic activity of Ocimum sanctum and its possible mechanism of action," *International Journal of Pharmacognosy*, 1995, 33(3):188-192

37. A. Muthuraman, V. Diwan, A.S. Jaggi, N. Singh, and D. Singh, "Ameliorative effects of Ocimum sanctum in sciatic nerve transection-induced neuropathy in rats," *J Ethnopharmacol.*, Oct. 30, 2008, 120(1):56–62.

38. S. Banerjee, R. Prashar, and Rao A. R. Kumar, "Modulatory influence of alcoholic extract of Ocimum leaves on carcinogen metabolizing enzyme activities and reduced glutathione levels in mouse," *Nutrition and Cancer*, 1996, 25(2):205.

39. S. Godhwani, J.L. Godhwani, and D.S. Vyas, "Ocimum sanctum: A preliminary study evaluating its immunoregulatory profile in albino rats," *Journal of Ethnopharmacology*, 1988, 24:193.

40. P.K. Mediratta, V. Dewan, S.K. Bhattacharya, V.S. Gupta, P.C. Maiti, and P. Sen, "Effect of Ocimum sanctum Linn, on humoral immune responses," *Indian Journal of Medical Research*, 1988, 87:384.

41. D. Bhattacharyya, T.K. Sur, U. Jana, and P.K. Debnath, "Controlled programmed trial of Ocimum sanctum leaf on generalized anxiety disorders," *Nepal Med Coll J.*, Sept. 2008, 10(3):176–179.

42. K. Sembulingam, P. Sembulingam, and A. Namasivayam, "Effect of Ocimum sanctum Linn, on noise induced changes in plasma corticosterone level," *Indian Journal of Physiology and Pharmacology*, 1997, 41(2):139.

43. U. Roy, S. Mukhopadhyay, M.K. Poddar, and B.P. Mukherjee, "Evaluation of antistress activity of Indian medicinal plants, Withania somnifera and Ocimum sanctum with special reference to stress induced stomach ulcer in albino rats." Proceedings of an International Seminar on Traditional Medicine, Calcutta, India, Nov.7–9, 1992.

44. 46

45. P. Shokeen, M. Bala, M. Singh, and V. Tandon, "In vitro activity of eugenol, an active component from Ocimum sanctum, against multiresistant and susceptible strains of Neisseria gonorrhoeae," *Int J Antimicrob Agents*, June 17, 2008.

46. S. Shetty and L. Udupa, "Evaluation of anti-oxidant and wound healing effects of alcoholic and aqueous extract of Ocimum sanctum Linn in Rats: Evid based complement," *Alternat Med.*, March 2008, 5(1):95–101.

47. Siddique YH, Ara G, Beg T, Afzal M. Acta Biol Hung. 2007 Dec;58(4):397-409. Anti-genotoxic effect of Ocimum sanctum L. extract against cyproterone acetate induced genotoxic damage in cultured mammalian cells.

48. V. Nair, A. Arjuman, P. Dorababu, H.N. Gopalakrishna, Rao U. Chakradhar, and L. Mohan, "Effect of NR-ANX-C (a polyherbal formulation) on haloperidol induced catalepsy in albino mice," *Indian J Med Res.*, Nov. 2007, 126(5):480–484.

49. H. Joshi and M. Parle, "Evaluation of nootropic potential of Ocimum sanctum Linn. in mice," *Indian J Exp Biol.*, Feb. 2006, 44(2):133–136.

50. R. K Goel, K. Sairam, M. Dorababu, T. Prabha and Rao,C V "Effect of standardized extract of Ocimum sanctum Linn. on gastric mucosal offensive and defensive factors," *Indian J Exp Biol.*, Aug. 2005, 43(8):715–721.

51. S.K. Gupta, D. Srivastava,. Trivedi, S. Joshi, and N. Halder, "Ocimum sanctum modulates selenite-induced cataractogenic changes and prevents rat lens opacification," *Curr Eye Res.*, July 2005, 30(7):583–591.

Phyllanthus amarus

Introduction

Phyllanthus amarus is an important herb in the Ayurvedic tradition. It has been used therapeutically in Ayurveda for more than 2000 years and is known to have particular value in treating liver disorders including jaundice and hepatitis. The active constituents in Phyllanthus are believed to block DNA polymerase, the enzyme needed for the hepatitis virus to reproduce.[1] Known in Sanskrit as Bahupatra, Phyllanthus amarus has medicinal applications throughout Central and Southern Asia. The whole plant is used to treat indigestion, dyspepsia, bronchial conditions, diabetes, asthma, gonorrhea, dropsy, influenza, indigestion, colic, and disorders of the urogenital system and kidneys. The whole plant also is used to treat gonorrhea, menorrhagia, and other genital affections.

The young shoots and leaves of the low-growing Phyllanthus shrub are used to treat ulcers and dysentery. The decoction of the plant is a remedy for intermittent fevers and spleen and liver ailments.

Phyllanthus, which is extremely bitter in taste, is valued in Ayurveda for its astringent, stomachic, diuretic, febrifugal, and antiseptic properties. In modern medical applications, Phyllanthus has been observed for its hepatoprotective, anti-viral, hypoglycemic, chemoprotective, anti-cancer, anti-inflammatory and anti-oxidant properties.

Phyllanthus has been used as a liver protector and detoxifier in many areas of the world, including China, the Philippines, Cuba, Nigeria, Guam, Africa, the Caribbean, and Latin America. In more recent years, its applications have been most successful in liver conditions such as jaundice and hepatitis B. A tincture of the plant's extract is applied externally for scabies, ulcers, and wounds. The extract also is used in ophthalmology.

Synonymous Names

Latin: Phyllanthus amarus
Sanskrit: Bhumayaamalaki
Hindi: Jar-Amla

Habitat

Phyllanthus amarus grows widely in the tropical parts of all continents except Australia. It grows mainly as a weed in wastelands, agricultural lands, and riverbanks. Phyllanthus grows abundantly during the rainy season and occurs as a winter weed throughout the hotter parts of India, particularly on cultivated land.

Botanical Characteristics

Phyllanthus amarus is an annual, low-growing shrub that reaches a maximum height of 60 centimeters. It has an erect stem, slender and naked below, with spreading, leafy branches above. The numerous leaves are sub-sessile, pale green, glaucous below, and ellpitic to oblong in shape. The flowers bud in the leaf axis, and are numerous. The male flowers grow in clusters, and the females are solitary. Phyllanthus' seeds are three-lobed and rounded, with longitudinal regular parallel ribs on the back.

Chemical Composition

Dried leaves of Phyllanthus consist of 0.4% of the toxic bitter principle phyllanthin; traces of the tasteless substance hypophyllanthin, and about 5% of a colorless wax made up mostly of esters of long-chain fatty acids and alcohols, free fatty acids, and hydrocarbons. The leaves are rich in potassium, which is considered to be responsible for the herb's powerful diuretic effect. The stem contains saponins.[2]

Pharmacological Activity

Hepatoprotective activity

Several in-vitro studies have demonstrated inactivation of the hepatitis B virus by inhibiting DNA polymerase, which is required by the hepatitis B virus for replication. An in-vivo study on woodchucks confirmed this activity.[3] The results using human subjects have provided inconclusive results.

One study used 600 mg/day of Phyllanthus leaf on carriers of hepatitis B virus. After 15 to 20 days of treatment, 59% of the treated subjects had lost the virus, compared to 4% of the placebo subjects. Nine months later the hepatitis had not returned.[4]

A case of cirrhosis of the liver stemming from chronic infection by hepatitis B virus and hepatitis C virus was treated with two herbs—Phyllanthus amarus and milk thistle (Silybum marianum). The symptoms resolved, liver function tests approached normal, and the subject seroconverted to a negative antigen state within 5 weeks.[5] A study was undertaken to investigate the protective effects and possible mechanisms of an aqueous extract from Phyllanthus amarus on ethanol-induced rat hepatic injury.[6] In the in-vitro study, Phyllanthus increased the MTT reduction assay and decreased the release of transaminases in the rats' primary cultured hepatocytes being treated with ethanol. The hepatotoxic parameters studied in vivo included serum transaminases, serum triglyceride, hepatic triglyceride, and tumor necrosis factor alpha, interleukin 1 beta, together with histopathological examination.

In an acute toxicity study, single doses of Phyllanthus, or silymarin, a reference hepatoprotective agent administered 24 hours before ethanol lowered the ethanol-induced levels of transaminases. Treatment of rats with Phyllanthus for 7 days after 21 days with ethanol enhanced liver cell recovery by bringing the transaminase levels back to normal. Histopathological observations confirmed the beneficial role of Phyllanthus against ethanol induced liver injury in rats. The possible mechanism may involve Phyllanthus' anti-oxidant activity.[7] An ethanolic extract of Phyllanthus was studied for its hepatoprotective effect on aflatoxin B(1)-induced liver damage in mice using different biochemical parameters and histopathological studies. Aflatoxin was administered orally to the mice in each group except the control group. The extract of Phyllanthus amarus was given to all the groups (except the control group) after 30 minutes of administration of aflatoxin. The study was continued in this manner for 3 months.[8] Phyllanthus amarus showed a hepatoprotective effect by lowering the content of thiobarbituric acid reactive substances and enhancing the reduced glutathione level and activities of anti-oxidant enzymes, glutathione peroxidase, glutathione-S-transferase, superoxide dismutase, and catalase. Histopathological analyses of liver samples confirmed the hepatoprotective value and anti-oxidant activity of the ethanolic extract of the herb, which was comparable to the standard anti-oxidant, ascorbic acid. These data indicate that Phyllanthus possesses a potent protective effect against aflatoxin induced hepatic damage. The main mechanism for this action could be Phyllanthus' strong capability to reduce the intracellular level of reactive oxygen species, by enhancing the levels of both enzymatic and non-enzymatic anti-oxidants.

A controlled clinical trial studied the effects of Phyllanthus extract on 123 patients with chronic hepatitis B. The patients receiving the Phyllanthus extract were more likely to lose detectable hepatitis B e-antigen from their serum and also more likely to seroconvert hepatitis B e-antibody status from negative to positive. None of the patients changed their status with respect to hepatitis B s-antigen.[9] In a randomized controlled clinical trial, 55 patients with chronic viral hepatitis B were given Phyllanthus amarus compound for three months. A control group received recombinant human interferon alpha-1b for the same time period. The normalization rates of three critical indicators—ALT, A/G, and SB—in the Phyllanthus group were significantly higher than those of the control group. These results show that Phyllanthus has a remarkable effect in treating chronic viral hepatitis B for recovery of liver function and inhibition of the replication of HBV.[10]

In a clinical trial, hepatitis B virus carriers were given Phyllanthus amarus for one month. At the end of the study period, 60% of the carriers had lost the hepatitis B virus.[11]

Cardioprotective activity

Nine mildly hypertensive patients were treated with Phyllanthus amarus for 10 days. At the end of this period, the subjects showed significant increases in urine and serum sodium levels. A significant reduction in systolic blood pressure in non-diabetic hypertensive and female subjects was noted. Blood glucose also was reduced significantly in the treated group.[12]

Anti-viral activity

An active constituent in Phyllanthus, repandusinic acid, has been shown to have anti-viral properties in-vitro, inhibiting HIV and HTLV-I replication and HIV reverse transciptase activity.[13]

Anti-inflammatory activity

Studies have shown that the extracts obtained from Phyllanthus amarus, and some of the lignans isolated from it, exhibit anti-inflammatory properties. A study was undertaken to assess whether the anti-inflammatory actions of these lignans could be mediated by interaction with a platelet-activating factor receptor or interference with the action of this lipid. Extracts of Phyllanthus decreased the specific binding of the activating factor in mouse cerebral cortex membranes sites. These findings suggest that Phyllanthus exhibits anti-inflammatory and anti-allodynic actions that probably are mediated through its direct antagonistic action on the receptor binding sites.[14] Phyllanthus also has been shown to inhibit angiotensin-converting enzyme.[15] Another study assessed the anti-inflammatory effect of the extracts and purified lignans obtained from Phyllanthus. Given orally, the hexane extract, the lignan-rich fraction, or the lignans phyltetralin, nirtetralin, niranthin, but not hypophyllanthin or phyllanthin, inhibited carrageenan-induced paw edema and neutrophil influx. The hexane extract, the lignan-rich fraction, or nirtetralin also inhibited the increase of IL1-beta tissue levels induced by carrageenan. These results show that the hexane extract, the lignan-rich fraction, and the lignans niranthin, phyltetralin, and nirtetralin exhibited marked anti-inflammatory properties. The results also suggest that these lignans seem to be the main active principles responsible for the anti-inflammatory properties reported for the Phyllanthus extract.[16, 17]

Anti-diabetic activity

The effect of the aqueous leaf and seed extracts of Phyllanthus at a range of oral doses was investigated for their anti-diabetic and anti-lipidemic potentials. The extract produced a dose-dependent decrease in the fasting plasma glucose and cholesterol, and reduction in weight in the treated mice. The results suggest that the extract could be enhancing peripheral utilization of glucose, but the mechanisms on how this works remain unclear.[18] Extracts of six selected Malaysian plants with a reputation for usefulness in treating diabetes were examined for alpha-amylase inhibition using an in-vitro model.[19] Inhibitory activity studied by two different protocols (with and without pre-incubation) showed that the Phyllanthus amarus hexane extract had alpha-amylase inhibitory properties. Extraction and fractionation of Phyllanthus amarus hexane extract led to the isolation of dotriacontanyl docosanoate, triacontanol, and a mixture of oleanolic acid and ursolic acid. All of the compounds were tested in the alpha-amylase inhibition assay. The results revealed that the oleanolic acid and ursolic acid mixture was a potent alpha-amylase inhibitor, and that it contributed significantly to the alpha-amylase inhibition activity of the extract. Three pure pentacyclic triterpenoids—oleanolic acid, ursolic acid, and lupeol—were shown to inhibit alpha-amylase. The glycemic response to pancakes was monitored in 21 non-insulin-dependent diabetic patients while on oral hypoglycemic, after a 1-week washout period and after a 1-week, twice-daily treatment with 100 mL of an aqueous extract from 12.5 grams of powdered aerial parts of Phyllanthus amarus. The results showed that treatment with the aqueous extract of Phyllanthus amarus was ineffective in lowering both FBG and postprandial blood glucose in the untreated patients.[20]

Anti-cancer activity

A study was conducted to examine the anti-mutagenic and anti-carcinogenic potential of Phyllanthus amarus, using the bacterial pre-incubation mutation assay and an in-vivo alkaline elution method for DNA single-strand breaks in hamster liver cells.[21] The aqueous extract of the entire Phyllanthus plant showed an anti-mutagenic effect against induction by 2-aminofluorene, 2-aminoanthracene, and 4-nitroquinolone-1-oxide in Salmonella typhimurium strains, and in Escherichia coli. All of the results were dose-dependent; however, inhibition of N-ethyl-N-nitrosoguanidine-induced mutagenesis was observed only with S. typhimurium. The extract also exhibited activity against 2-nitrofluorene and sodium azide-induced mutagenesis with Salmonella typhimurium. When the alkaline elution method was used, the plant extract prevented in-vivo DNA single-strand breaks caused by dimethylnitrosamine in hamster liver cells. When the extract was administered 30 minutes prior to administration of DMN, the elution rate constant decreased more than 2.5 times compared to that of the control. These results indicate that Phyllanthus amarus possesses anti-mutagenic and anti-genotoxic properties.

The chemopreventive activity of Phyllanthus amarus extract was studied with regard to chemically induced stomach cancer in Wistar rats.[22] Administration of the extract significantly reduced the incidence of gastric neoplasms in the rats (44%), as well as their numbers. Moreover, elevated levels of enzymes in the stomach were found to be reduced after administration of Phyllanthus. For example, gamma-glutamyl transpeptidase activity was decreased to almost normal levels by 750 mg/kg body weight of the extract. Similarly, glutathione S-transferase activity and glutathione reductase levels in the treated group were found to be lowered, while reduced glutathione was increased. AgNOR dots and clusters, indicators of cellular proliferation, which were increased by treatment, became near to normal in Phyllanthus-treated animals. The aqueous extract of Phyllanthus amarus exhibited potent anti-carcinogenic activity against 20-methylcholanthrene-induced sarcoma development and increased the survival of tumor-harboring mice. Administration of the extract also was found to prolong the lifespan of Dalton's lymphoma ascites and Ehrlich ascites carcinoma-bearing mice, and reduced the volume of transplanted solid tumors.

The extract inhibited aniline hydroxylase, a P-450 enzyme. Phyllanthus extract was found to inhibit DNA topoisomerase II of Saccharomyces cerevisiae mutant cell cultures and inhibited cell cycle regulatory enzyme cdc25 tyrosine phosphatase. The anti-tumor and anti-cancer activities of Phyllanthus may be connected to the inhibition of metabolic activation of carcinogens, as well as the inhibition of cell-cycle regulators and DNA repair.[23] The effect of administering Phyllanthus amarus extract after inducing hepatocellular carcinoma by N-nitrosodiethylamine was studied in Wistar rats.[24] Administration of an aqueous extract of Phyllanthus amarus was found to significantly increase the survival of hepatocellular carcinoma-harboring animals. All of the untreated rats died from the tumor by about 34 weeks. Administration of Phyllanthus extract after tumor development increased the survival of animals to an average of 52 weeks. The effect of 75% methanolic extract of the plant Phyllanthus amarus was studied against cyclophosphamide induced toxicity in mice. Administration of CTX for 14 days produced significant myelosuppression, as seen from the decreased white blood cell count and bone marrow cellularity.

Phyllanthus significantly reduced the myelosuppression and improved the blood count and bone marrow cellularity, as well as the number of maturing monocytes.[25] The CTX treatment also reduced activity of the glutathione system and increased activity of phase I enzyme that metabolize CTX to its toxic side products. Phyllanthus was found to decrease the activity of the phase I enzyme. Phyllanthus also increased the cellular glutathione and glutathione-S-transferase, thereby decreasing the effect of toxic metabolites of CTX on the cells. Administration of Phyllanthus amarus did not reduce the tumor-reducing activity of CTX. In fact, there was a synergistic action of CTX and Phyllanthus in reducing the solid tumors in mice. The results indicated that administration of Phyllanthus can significantly reduce the toxic side effects of CTX without interfering with the anti-tumor efficiency of CTX.

Multi-drug resistance constitutes the major obstacle to the successful treatment of cancer. Multi-drug resistance is thought to be mediated by the super expression of P-glycoprotein, which extrudes drugs from the cells, therefore reducing their cytotoxicity. It is believed that inhibiting this activity may reverse the multi-drug resistance phenotype.

A study was undertaken to evaluate the possible cytotoxic effect and multi-drug resistance reversing properties of the extract and compounds isolated from Phyllanthus amarus.[26] For this purpose, two human leukemia cell lines were employed: K-562, and its vincristine-resistant counterpart Lucena-1, a P-glycoprotein-overexpressing subline. Lucena-1 was found to be significantly more resistant to the cytotoxicity of Phyllanthus amarus derivatives. The hexane extract, the lignans-rich fraction, and the lignans nirtetralin, niranthin, or phyllanthin exerted cytotoxic effects on the leukemia cells. These results suggest a potential action of Phyllanthus derivatives as multi-drug resistant reversing agents, mainly because of their ability to synergize with the action of conventional chemotherapeutics.

Anti-ulcer activity

A methanolic extract of Phyllanthus amarus significantly inhibited gastric lesions induced by the intragastric administration of absolute ethanol. Mortality, increased stomach weight, ulcer index, and intraluminal bleeding were reduced significantly by administration of Phyllanthus amarus. A biochemical analysis indicated that reduced glutathione of gastric mucosa produced by ethanol administration was significantly elevated by treatment with Phyllanthus amarus extract.[27]

Anti-fertility activity

The anti-fertility effects of an alcohol extract of Phyllanthus amarus were investigated in cyclic adult female mice. The results revealed no significant change in absolute body weight and organ weight in the extract-fed animals, indicating no alteration in general metabolic status. Further, the feeding had no effect on hematological and clinical biochemical tests reflecting its non-toxicity. Similarly, uterine and ovarian biochemical tests showed no change. Cohabited females with normal male mice were unable to become pregnant. These factors are related to a change in the hormonal milieu that governs female reproductive function. Upon withdrawal of feeding for 45 days, these effects were reversed. Thus, this extract manifests a definite contraceptive effect in female mice.[28]

Safety Profile

Chromatographic fractions obtained from Phyllanthus amarus were tested for toxicity on the serum biochemistry of rats. The results revealed that some fractions of Phyllanthus amarus had potentially deleterious effects on the blood. Therefore, caution should be exercised in using Phyllanthus as a medicinal plant.[29] Other sources have reported that Phyllanthus may have a hypoglycemic effect.[30]

But these side effects can be mitigated use this herb in combination with Eclipta alba, Eblica officinalis and Terminalia chebula.

Dosage

- Tincture 1:2; sig 0.3-2 ml TID (higher end of dosage scale for acute states)
- The usual dose of Phyllanthus is 600 to 900 mg daily.
- Extract 5:1 100 -250 mg three times per day

Notes

1. S. P. Thyagarajan, S.Subramanian, T. Thirunalasundari, et al., "Effect of Phyllanthus amarus on chronic carriers of hepatitis B virus," *Lancet*, 1988, 2(8614):764–766.

2. J.B. Calixto, A.R. Santos, V. Cechinel Filho, and R.A. Yunes, "A review of the plants of the genus Phyllanthus: Their chemistry, pharmacology, and therapeutic potential," *Med Res Rev.*, July 1998, 18(4):225–258.

3. Venkateswaran PS, Millman I, Blumberg BS. Effects of an extract from Phyllanthus niruri on hepatitis B and woodchuck hepatitis viruses: in vitro and in vivo studies. Proc Natl Acad Sci U S A. 1987 Jan;84(1):274-8

4. See Note 1.

5. J.M. McPartland, "Viral hepatitis treated with Phyllanthus amarus and milk thistle (Silybum marianum): A case report," *Complementary Medicine International*, March 1, 1996, 3(2): 40–42.

6. P. Pramyothin, C. Ngamtin, S. Poungshompoo, and C. Chaichantipyuth, "Hepatoprotective activity of Phyllanthus amarus Schum. et. Thonn. extract in ethanol treated rats: in vitro and in vivo studies," *J Ethnopharmacol.*, Nov 1, 2007, 114(2):169–173.

7. See note 6

8. F. Naaz, S. Javed, and M.Z. Abdin, "Hepatoprotective effect of ethanolic extract of Phyllanthus amarus Schum. et Thonn. on aflatoxin B1-induced liver damage in mice," *J Ethnopharmacol.*, Sept. 25, 2007, 113(3):503–509. Epub July 20. 2007.

9. M. Wang, H. Cheng, Y. Li, et al., "Herbs of the genus Phyllanthus in the treatment of chronic hepatitis B: Observations with three preparations from different geographic sites," *J Lab Clin Med*, 1995, 126(4):350–352.

10. V, Thamlikitkul, S. Wasuwat, and P. Kanchanapee, "Efficacy of Phyllanthus amarus for eradication of hepatitis B virus in chronic carriers," *J Med Assoc Thai*, 1991, 74(9):381–385.

11. B. S Blumberg, I. Millman, P.S. Venkateswaran, et al., "Hepatitis B virus and primary hepatocellular carcinoma: treatment of HBV carriers with Phyllanthus amarus," *Vaccine*, 1990, Supp 8:S86–92.

12. S. Mills and K. Bone, *Principles and Practice of Phytotherapy*. (New York, NY: Churchhill Livingstone, 2000), p. 220.

13. F. Notka, G. Meier, and R. Wagner, "Concerted inhibitory activities of Phyllanthus amarus on HIV replication in vitro and ex vivo," *Anti-viral Res.*, Nov. 2004, 64(2):93–102.

14. C. A Kassuya, A. Silvestre, O. Menezes-de-Lima Jr, D.M. Marotta, V.L. Rehder, and J.B. Calixto, "Antiinflammatory and antiallodynic actions of the lignan niranthin isolated from Phyllanthus amaru:. Evidence for interaction with platelet activating factor receptor, *Eur J Pharmacol.*, Sept. 2006, 28,546(1-3):182–188.] It is e-pub publication. We can delete it

15. S.P. Thyagarajan, S. Jayaram, V. Gopalakrishnan, R. Hari, P. Jeyakumar, and M.S. Sripathi, "Herbal medicines for liver diseases in India," *J Gastroenterol Hepatol.*, Dec. 2002, 17, Suppl 3:S370–376.

16. C. A Kassuya, D.F. Leite, L.V. de Melo, V.L. Rehder, and J.B. Calixto, "Anti-inflammatory properties of extracts, fractions and lignans isolated from Phyllanthus amarus," *Plant Medica*, Aug 1, 2005, 71(8): 21–726.

17. A.K Kiemer, T. Hartung, C. Huber, and A.M. Vollmar, "Phyllanthus amarus has anti-inflammatory potential by inhibition of iNOS, COX-2, and cytokines via the NF-kappaB pathway," *J Hepatol.*, March 2003, 38(3):289–297.

18. A. A. Adeneye, O.O. Amole, and A.K. Adeneye, "Hypoglycemic and hypocholesterolemic activities of the aqueous leaf and seed extract of Phyllanthus amarus in mice," *Fitoterapia*, Dec. 2006, 77(7–8):511–514. July 15, 2006.

19. H. Ali, P.J. Houghton, and A. Soumyanath, "Alpha-Amylase inhibitory activity of some Malaysian plants used to treat diabetes; with particular reference to Phyllanthus amarus," *J Ethnopharmacol.*, Oct. 11, 2006, 107(3):449–455.. This is for e-pub ahead publication. We can just delete it.

20. M.J. Moshi, J.J. Lutale, G.H. Rimoy, Z.G. Abbas, R.M. Josiah, and A.B. Swai, "The effect of Phyllanthus amarus aqueous extract on blood glucose in non-insulin dependent diabetic patients," *Phytother Res.*, Nov. 2001, 15(7):577–580.

21. B. Sripanidkulchaia, U. Tattawasartb, P. Laupatarakasemb, U. Vinitketkumneunc, K. Sripanidkulchaib, C. Furihatad, T. Matsushimae. Antimutagenic and anticarcinogenic effects of Phyllanthus amarus," *Phytomedicine*, 9(1), 26–32.

22. K. R. Raphael, M. Sabu, K.H. Kumar, and R. Kuttan, "Inhibition of N-Methyl N'-nitro-N-nitrosoguanidine (MNNG) induced gastric carcinogenesis by Phyllanthus amarus extract," *Asian Pac J Cancer Prev.*, April–June 2006, 7(2):299–302.

23. N.V. Rajeshkumar, K.L Joy, G. Kuttan, R.S. Ramsewak, M.G. Nair, and R. Kuttan, "Antitumour and anticarcinogenic activity of Phyllanthus amarus extract," *J Ethnopharmacol.*, June 2002, 81(1):17–22.

24. N.V. Rajeshkumar and R. Kuttan, "Phyllanthus amarus extract administration increases the life span of rats with hepatocellular carcinoma," *J Ethnopharmacol.*, Nov. 2000, 73(1–2):215–219.

25. K.B. H. and B. Kumar, "Chemoprotective activity of Phyllanthus amarus against cyclophosphamide induced toxicity in mice," *Phytomedicine,* June 15, 2005, 12 (6–7):494–500.

26. D.F. Leite, C.A. Kassuya, T.L. Mazzuco, A. Silvestre, L.V. de Melo, V.L. Rehder, V.M. Rumjanek, and J.B. Calixto, "The cytotoxic effect and the multidrug resistance reversing action of lignans from Phyllanthus amarus," *Plant Medica*, Dec 1, 2006, 72(15): 1353–1358.

27. K. R Raphael and R. Kuttan, "Inhibition of experimental gastric lesion and inflammation by Phyllanthus amarus extract," *J Ethnopharmacol.*, Aug. 2003, 87(2–3):193–197.

28. M. V Rao and K.M. Alice, "Contraceptive effects of Phyllanthus amarus in female mice," *Phytother Res.*, May 2001, 15(3):265–267.

29. A. A Adedapo, M. O. Abatan, S. O, Idowu and O.O.Olorunsogo, "Toxic effects of chromatographic fractions of Phyllanthus amarus on the serum biochemistry of rats," *Phytother Res.*, Sept. 2005, 19(9):812–815.

30. F. Brinker, *Herb Contraindications and Drug Interactions.* (Sandy, OR: Eclectic Medical Publications, 1998). p. 166.

30

Phyllanthus emblica

Introduction

Phyllanthus emblica, also known as Emblica officinalis, or Amla, is one of the most frequently used of the Ayurvedic herbs. A member of the family Euphorbiaceae, the plant grows to become a medium-sized tree. The fruit is similar in appearance to the common gooseberry, which is botanically unrelated to Amla. Because of these similarities, however, Amla often is called "Indian gooseberry."

Amla also is valued as a natural anti-oxidant and a rich natural source of Vitamin C derivatives. The fruit is acrid, cooling, refrigerant, diuretic, and laxative. The dried fruit is useful in treating hemorrhage, diarrhea, and dysentery. The plant is anti-bacterial, and its astringent properties prevent infection and aid in the healing of ulcers. Amla also is used as a laxative, and in the treatment of leucorrhea and artherosclerosis.[1]

The fruits of Amla are one of three "myrobalans" (a term derived from the Greek word for "acorns"), all of which have astringent properties. Because of their high concentrations of tannins, the fruits of these three species have long been used in tanning leather. They also are the principal ingredients in the popular Ayurvedic remedy Triphala, a rejuvenating rasayana that accounts for well over half of the sales in the Ayurvedic medicine industry.[2] According to accounts in the Caraka Samhita, by consuming a rasayana made with Amla as the main ingredient, a person will "live for a hundred years without any sign of decrepitude."[3]

Even though it is just a diminutive inch in diameter, one Amla fruit has the same ascorbic acid content as two oranges. Thus, Amla fruit juice, sediment, and residue have powerful anti-oxidant properties. Amla also is a carminative and stomachic and is used to treat respiratory problems. Amla is used in Ayurveda as an aphrodisiac, antipyretic, anti-diabetic, anabolic, and cerebral tonic. It raises the total protein level and increases body weight because of its positive nitrogen balance.[4]

Synonymous Names

English: Emblic myrobalan, Indian gooseberry
Hindi: Amla
Sanskrit: Amlaki

Other names in various other languages include nelli in Sinhala, nellikka in Malayalam, amlakhi in Assames, usirikai in Telugu, nellikkaai in Tamil and Kannada, as well as aonla, aola, ammalaki, dharty, aamvala, aawallaa, emblic, Emblic myrobalan, Malacca tree, nillika, and nellikya.

Chemical Composition

The major chemical constituents of Amla are polyphenols. The fruit and most other parts of the plant contain gallic acid, phyllemblin, phyllemblic acid, emblicol, ellagic acid, chebulagic acid, glucogallin, corilagin, 3,6-digalloyl glucose, putranjivin A, emblicanin A and B, punigluconin, pedunculagin, ascorbigen A, ascorbigen B and quercetin. Amla contains Ascorbigen A and Ascorbigen B, gamma lactone and is not same as Ascorbic acid. Ascorbic acid can be liberated from this. As a convenience these are often grouped together as Ascorbic acid. The key point difference is that Ascorbigen are more stable than Ascorbic acid. The tannins from Amla help further protect the Ascorbigen just like shock absorbers. They themselves trap the free radicals before oxidation of Ascorbigen can occur.

The cytokinins zeatin, zeatin riboside and zeatin nucleotide have been isolated from the Amla fruit. The fatty acids arachidic and behenic acids have been isolated from the seed oil.[6]

Habitat

Amla is native to the plains in the lower mountainous regions of the Indian subcontinent. It grows at elevations of 200 to nearly 2000 meters above sea level. Amla's natural habitat extends from Burma on the east to Afghanistan in the west, and from Deccan in south India to the foothills of the Himalayan range.

Botanical Characteristics

The Amla tree is small to medium in size, reaching 8 to 18 meters in height, with a crooked trunk and spreading branches. The branchlets are glabrous or finely pubescent, 10 to 20 centimeters long, and usually deciduous. The leaves are simple, subsessile, and closely set along the branchlets. The leaves are light green, and the flowers are greenish-yellow. The fruit is nearly spherical, light greenish-yellow, smooth, and hard, with six vertical stripes or furrows. The taste is sour, bitter, and astringent. It is quite fibrous.

Pharmacological Activity

The traditional uses of Amla in Ayurveda include the following:

- For digestive system disorders including dyspepsia, gastritis, hyperacidity, constipation, colic, colitis, and hemorrhoids.
- For bleeding disorders including bleeding hemorrhoids, hematuria, menorrhagia, bleeding gums, and ulcerative colitis.
- For metabolic disorders including anemia, diabetes, and gout.
- For lung disorders such as cough and asthma.
- For disorders related to aging such as osteoporosis, premature graying of hair, and weak vision
- For neurasthenia—fatigue, mental disorders, vertigo, and palpitations.

A review to determine glucosinolates in 19 Chinese medicinal herbs concluded that the highest contents of cancer-protective compounds were found in the seeds of Raphanus sativus L. (glucoraphenin), Sinapis alba (sinalbin) and Phyllanthus emblica L. (sinigrin).[5]

Anti-viral activity

The methanolic extract of Amla fruit has been shown in laboratory research to significantly inhibit the activity of HIV reverse transcriptase. Putranjivin A, di-O-galloyl-D-glucose, and digallic acid isolated from the fruit were also shown to have anti-viral activity.[6] Coxsackie virus B3 (CVB3) is believed to be a major contributor to viral myocarditis, as virus-associated apoptosis plays a role in the pathogenesis of experimental myocarditis. A study investigated the in-vitro and in-vivo anti-viral activities of Phyllaemblicin B, the main ellagitannin compound isolated from Phyllanthus emblica, against CVB3. It was found that Phyllaemblicin B inhibited CVB3-mediated cytopathic effects on HeLa cells with an IC(50) value of 7.75+/-0.15microg/mL. In an in-vivo assay, treatment with 12mgkg(-1)d(-1) Phyllaemblicin B reduced cardiac CVB3 titers, decreased the activities of LDH and CK in murine serum, and alleviated pathological damages of cardiac muscle in myocarditic mice. Phyllaemblicin B clearly inhibited CVB3-associated apoptosis effects both in-vitro and in-vivo. These results show that Phyllaemblicin B exerts significant anti-viral activities against CVB3. Phyllaemblicin B may represent a potential therapeutic agent for viral myocarditis.[7]

Anti-bacterial activity

The anti-bacterial properties of Amla have been investigated against 345 bacterial isolates belonging to six genera of Gram-negative bacterial populations. The Amla extracts demonstrated anti-bacterial properties against Escherichia coli, Klebsiella pneumoniae, Klebsiella ozaenae, Proteus mirabilis, Pseudomonas aeruginosa, Salmonella typhi, Salmonella paratyphi A, Salmonella paratyphi B, and Serratia marcescens, isolated from urine specimens.[8] In one study the chloroform soluble fraction of the methanolic extract of Phyllanthus emblica exhibited significant anti-microbial activity against some Gram-positive and Gram-negative pathogenic bacteria and strong cytotoxicity having a LC50 of 10.257 +/- 0.770 microg mL(-1).[9] Amla, which is a good source of vitamin C derivatives, has been shown to be beneficial to the immune system, coupled with its tonifying and anti-ageing effect. A study was conducted to evaluate the effect of Emblica officinalis feeding on the susceptibility of experimental mice to respiratory tract infection induced by Klebsiella pneumoniae. The effect of short- (15 days) and long- (30 days) term feeding of Amla in mice on the course of Klebsiella pneumoniae ATCC43816 infection in lungs was studied, in terms of bacterial colonization, macrophage activity, malondialdehyde (MDA) and nitrite production in broncheoalveolar lavage fluid (BALF).[10] The tumor necrosis factor (TNF)-alpha level in serum also was assessed. Though bacterial colonization decreased after short-term feeding, it was not significant. However, the decrease in bacterial load was significant ($P < 0.05$) after long term feeding.

The operative mechanisms in terms of lipid peroxidation, phagocytosis, and nitrite production were studied by estimating their levels in broncheoalveolar lavage fluid (BALF). A maximum decrease in malondialdehyde (MDA) levels and an increase in phagocytic activity and nitrite levels were seen on long-term feeding. These results suggest that dietary supplementation with Amla protects against bacterial colonization of lungs after long-term feeding in the experimental model. Further studies have to be conducted to understand the actual mechanism involved.[11]

A published review summarized the anti-viral and anti-bacterial properties of Amla.

A polyherbal cream has been formulated using diferuloylmethane (curcumin), purified extracts of Emblica officinalis (Amla), purified saponins from Sapindus mukorossi, Aloe vera, and rose water, along with approved excipients and preservatives.[12] Polyherbal cream inhibits the growth of strains and clinical isolates of Neisseria gonorrheae, including those resistant to penicillin, tetracycline, nalidixic acid, and ciprofloxacin. It has pronounced inhibitory action against Candida glabrata, Candida albicans, and Candida tropicalis isolated from women with vulvovaginal candidiasis, including three isolates resistant to azole drugs and amphotericin B. Polyherbal formula displayed a high virucidal action against human immunodeficiency virus HIV-1NL4.3 in CEM-GFP reporter T and P4 (Hela-CD4-LTR-betaGal) cell lines with a 50% effective concentration (EC50) of 1:20000 dilution and nearly complete (98-99%) inhibition at 1:1000 dilution. It also prevented entry of the HIV-1(IIIB) virus into P4-CCR5 cells (EC50 approximately 1:2492). Two ingredients, aloe and Amla, inhibited transduction of the human papillomavirus type 16 (HPV-16) pseudovirus in HeLa cells at concentrations far below those that are cytotoxic and those used in the formulation.

This formulation was found to be totally safe according to pre-clinical toxicology carried out on rabbit vagina after application for 7 consecutive days or twice daily for 3 weeks. This polyherbal formulation has the potential of regressing vulvovaginal candidiasis and preventing Neisseria gonorrhoeae, HIV, and HPV infections.

Hypocholesterolemic activity

In a human pilot study, blood cholesterol levels were reduced in both normal and hypercholesterolemic men. In this clinical study, the diet of normal and hypercholesterolemic men aged 35–55 years was supplemented with raw Amla fruit for 28 days. The men in both study groups showed decreases in total serum cholesterol levels. When the Amla supplements were discontinued, the subjects' cholesterol levels reverted to near their initial values after 2 weeks.[13] The effects of Amla on low-density lipoprotein oxidation and cholesterol levels were studied in-vitro and in-vivo. Low-density lipoprotein oxidation was induced in the study animals by feeding them a high-cholesterol diet. Amla extract was shown to inhibit cholesterol at a higher level than the anti-cholesterol drug Probucol.[14] Rats that were fed Amla extract along with a high cholesterol diet for 20 days showed significantly reduced levels of total, free and LDL cholesterol. Oxidized LDL levels in the animals' blood serum also was reduced by the Amla extract. Serum TBA-reactive substance levels decreased after oral administration of Amla. These results suggest that Amla may be effective for treating hypercholesterolemia and preventing atherosclerosis.

The lipid-lowering and anti-atherosclerotic actions of Amla fruits were evaluated in rabbits fed a high cholesterol diet. The fresh juice of Amla fruits for 60 days at a dose of 5 ml/kg per rabbit per day for 60 days lowered serum cholesterol, triglycerides, phospholipids, and low-density lipoprotein levels. The concentration of lipids in animal tissues decreased significantly, along with levels of aortic plaque. Analysis of the animals' urine showed increased amounts of cholesterol and phospholipids, suggesting that Amla may have affected the mode of absorption.[15]

A separate study revealed that Amla also reduces serum, aortic, and hepatic cholesterol in rabbits.[16]

Anti-carcinogenic activity

In animal studies, Amla has been shown to decrease carcinogenic responses, to reverse histopathological changes, and to reduce liver concentrations of gamma-GT-positive foci. Pre-treatment with defatted methanolic Amla fruit extract caused significant partial recovery of pathological manifestations in animals with laboratory-induced tumors. Amla extract was shown to suppress tumor formation by multiple carcinogenic agents, and at a variety of dosages.[17] Study explored the effect of gallic acid extracted from leaves of Phyllanthus emblica on the apoptosis of hepatocellular carcinoma BEL-7404 cells. A MTT assay was applied to detect the influence on proliferation in-vitro. An inverted microscope was utilized to observe the morphological changes after BEL-7404 cells were treated with gallic acid. The Annexin V/PI double-label method was used to detect earlier period apoptosis cells, and Tunel was restrained the BEL-7404 cell proliferation at different levels in a time- and concentration-dependent manner. The typical morphological changes of apoptosis were observed after the BEL-7404 cells were treated with gallic acid. The Annexin The V/PI double label method and the Tunel method showed that the viable apoptotic cell and apoptosis rates increased as the action time was prolonged. Thus, gallic acid can restrain BEL-7404 cell proliferation and induce apoptosis, and its effect on apoptosis is time dependent.[18] Osteoclasts are involved in several pathologies associated with bone loss— including rheumatoid arthritis, osteoporosis, bone metastasis of myeloma, osteosarcoma, and breast cancer. Crude extracts of Emblica officinalis are able to induce specifically programmed cell death of mature osteoclasts without altering the process of osteoclastogenesis. Emblica officinalis specifically increased the expression levels of Fas, a critical member of the apoptotic pathway.

Gel shift experiments on Emblica officinalis extracts demonstrate that it specifically competes with the binding of a transcription factor involved in osteoclastogenesis NF-kappaB to its specific target DNA sequences. This might explain the observed effects of Emblica officinalis on the expression levels of IL-6, an NF-kappaB-specific target gene. The application of natural products is suggested as an alternative tool for therapy applied to bone diseases.[20]

The radioprotective effect of Emblica officinalis extract was studied in mice.[21] The Swiss albino mice were exposed to gamma rays (5 Gy) in the absence (control) or presence (experimental) of Emblica officinalis, orally 100 mg/kg body weight, once daily for 7 consecutive days. A specimen of small intestine (jejunum) was removed from the mice and studied at different autopsy intervals from 12 hours to 30 days. In the control animals, crypt cell population, mitotic figures, and villus length were markedly reduced on day 1; these later started to increase progressively but did not attain the normal level, even at the last autopsy interval. The animals receiving Emblica officinalis prior to irradiation had a higher number of crypt cells and mitotic figures compared to the non-drug-treated control at all the autopsy intervals. Irradiation of animals resulted in a dose-dependent elevation in lipid peroxidation and a reduction in glutathione, as well as catalase concentration in the intestine at 1-hour post-irradiation. In contrast, Emblica officinalis treatment before irradiation caused a significant depletion in lipid peroxidation and an elevation in glutathione and catalase levels.

Amla extract was studied if it could reduce oxidative stress in patients with uremia.[22] The findings show that supplementation with Amla extract for 4 months reduced the plasma oxidative marker, 8-iso-prostaglandin, (M0 vs. M4 = 1415 +/- 1234 pg/ml vs. 750 +/- 496 pg/ml, $p < 0.05$) and increased plasma total anti-oxidant status (TAS) (M0 vs. M4 = 2.32 +/- 0.14 mM vs. 2.55 +/- 0.24 mM, $p < 0.05$) in uremic patients. No significant differences were observed in liver function (GOP and GPT), renal function (creatinine, blood urea nitrogen and uric acid), diabetic index (plasma glucose and adiponectin), and atherogenic index (LDL/HDL ratio, total cholesterol, and homocysteine) in the patients treated with Amla for 4 months. Ayurvedic medicine uses poly-pharmacy, single herb may not achieve same results as combination of herbs can achieve.

Anti-diabetic activity

Researchers investigated the effects of Amla on fructose-induced metabolic syndrome using a rat model.[23] Male Wistar rats were fed a high-fructose (65%) diet or standard chow for 1 week, and were treated with an ethyl acetate extract of Amla, a polyphenol-rich fraction, at 10 or 20 mg/kg body weight per day, or vehicle, for 2 weeks. Serum glucose, triglycerides, total cholesterol, and blood pressure levels of the high-fructose diet-fed rats were increased compared to those of the normal rats (P

< 0.001). The extract of Amla, ameliorated the high fructose-induced metabolic syndrome, including hypertriacylglycerolemia and hypercholesterolemia. Elevated levels of hepatic triglycerides and total cholesterol in rats receiving the high-fructose diet were reduced significantly, by 33.8% and 24.6%, respectively (P < 0.001), after administration of the extract of Amla at the dose of 20 mg/kg with the regulation of the sterol regulatory element-binding protein (SREBP)-1 expression. The protein levels of PPAR-alpha and SREBP-2 were not affected by feeding the high fructose diet with extract of Amla. Amla extract at the dose of 20 mg/kg significantly inhibited the increased serum and hepatic mitochondrial thiobarbituric acid-reactive substance levels (21.1% and 43.1 %, respectively; P < 0.001). Amla extract inhibited the increase of cyclo-oxygenase-2 with regulation of NF-kappaB and bcl-2 proteins in the liver, while the elevated expression level of bax was decreased significantly, by 8.5% and 10.2 % at the doses of 10 and 20 mg/kg body weight per day, respectively.[40]

In another study, Amla and Curcuma longa in a combined extract caused a marked reduction in blood sugar levels in both normal fasting and alloxan-induced diabetic rats, with a good response in the glucose tolerance test.[24]

Protection against toxicity

In a study, administration of an extract of Amla fruit reduced toxicity induced by lead nitrate, aluminum sulphate, nickel chloride, cesium chloride, and 3,4-benzo(a)pyrene. Reductions in the clastogenic effects of all four compounds also were observed.[25] Another study compared the capabilities of Amla extract and synthetic ascorbic acid to modify the adverse effects of environmental toxins. Amla extract was shown to be effective in counteracting genotoxicity induced by both aluminum and lead. Amla also proved to be effective against clastogenicity and carcinogenicity induced by nickel. The more potent effect of the extract was attributed to a synergistic action between the naturally occurring compounds present.[26]

Hepatoprotective activity

The activities of Amla and its flavonoid quercitin were assessed for their hepatoprotective action. Liver damage was induced in albino rats and mice using country-made liquor and paracetamol. The research results indicated that the possible mechanism of action for Amla's hepatoprotective activity is in decreasing glutathione depletion and preventing stimulation of cytochrome P450. Because quercetin alone was more effective than the Amla extract, it is thought to be the active principle. Toxic effects induced by lead nitrate and aluminum sulphate also were counteracted by administration of Amla extract and ascorbic acid in albino rats.[27,28] The protective effect of Emblica officinalis was investigated for its effects on the liver mitochondria of ethanol-administered rats.[29] Oxidative stress and reactive oxygen species-mediated toxicity are considered to be two of the key underlying mechanisms responsible for alcohol-induced liver injury and mitochondrial dysfunction. The alcohol administered rats showed a significant elevation of plasma transaminases (aspartate and alanine aminotransferases), alkaline phosphatase, and gamma-glutamyl transferase compared to the control rats. However, activities of hepatic mitochondrial anti-oxidant enzymes, superoxide dismutase, glutathione peroxidase, and reduced glutathione, were significantly lower. Chronic alcohol feeding also increased lipid peroxide levels, protein carbonyl content, and overproduction of nitric oxide followed by lowered activities of NADH dehydrogenase, succinate dehydrogenase (SDH), and cytochrome c oxidase and content of cytochromes.

Administration of Emblica officinalis fruit extract at a dose of 250 mg/kg of body weight/day to alcoholic rats offers protection by simultaneously lowering the carbonyl content and lipid peroxidation and elevating the anti-oxidant enzyme activities, SDH, NADH dehydrogenase, and cytochrome c oxidase activities, and the content of cytochromes in hepatic mitochondria. Emblica officinalis can provide protection for chronic alcohol consumption.

Anti-pancreatitis activity

Acute pancreatitis was induced in the animals through the injection of a mixture of trypsin, bile, and blood into the duodenal opening of the pancreatic duct. Animals in the experimental group were pre-treated with 28 mg of Amla extract, given orally for 15 days before the pancreatitis was induced. For experimental purposes, the control group was not treated. At the end of the study period, serum amylase, cell damage and inflammation were evaluated in both groups. The control group showed a significant rise in serum amylase, whereas the group treated with Amla extract did not. A microscopic examination revealed that cell damage and inflammation in the Amla-treated group was lower than the untreated pancreatitis group.[30]

Immunomodulatory activity

In laboratory experimentation with mice, an aqueous Amla extract enhanced natural killer cell activity and antibody-dependent cellular cytotoxicity, resulting in an increase in lifespan of 35% in the mice with tumors. The drug's anti-tumor action may be the result of its ability to augment natural cell-mediated cytotoxicity. A functional NK cell or K cell population was essential for the activity to take place.[31]

Antidyspepsia activity

Amla has long been used in Ayurveda to treat dyspepsia and other gastric complaints. Research has confirmed its effectiveness in the treatment of dyspepsia.[32]

Anti-oxidant activity

Phyllemblin, a polyphenol isolated from Amla, has demonstrated a number of direct pharmacological actions, including mild stimulation of an isolated frog heart, mild cerebral depressant action, spasmolytic activity, and potential adrenaline and barbiturate sedation, similar to that of rutin. It was concluded that phyllemblin, a powerful anti-oxidant, may be acting in the same manner.[33,34] A study was undertaken to explore the possible ameliorative effect of Emblica officinalis on ochratoxin-induced lipid peroxidation in the kidney and liver of mice. Adult male albino mice were orally administered 50 micrograms (LD, low dose) and 100 micrograms (HD, high dose) of ochratoxin/0.2 ml of olive oil/animal/day for 45 days.[35] The results revealed a significant ($p < 0.05$), dose-dependent increase in lipid peroxidation, as well as decreased activity of enzymatic anti-oxidants (superoxide dismutase, catalase, glutathione peroxidase, glutathione reductase, and glutathione transferase) and non-enzymatic anti-oxidants (glutathione and total ascorbic acid) in both the organs, as compared to the findings for olive oil-treated control group. Administration of Emblica officinalis aqueous extract (2 mg/animal/day) and ochratoxin for a period of 45 days caused a significant amelioration of the ochratoxin-induced lipid peroxidation in the mouse liver and kidney.

The authors of the above study carried out another study to evaluate the spermatotoxic effect of ochratoxin and its amelioration by Emblica officinalis aqueous extract.[36] When male albino mice were treated with ochratoxin (50 and 100 microg/0.2 mL of olive oil/animal/day for 45 days, orally), alterations in various reproductive parameters (sperm count, sperm motility, sperm viability, and fertility rate) were recorded when treated further with the aqueous extract of Emblica officinalis (2 mg/animal/day for 45 days) amelioration was noted in the ochratoxin-induced spermatotoxic effect. Oral administration of ochratoxin for 45 days, compared to the vehicle control (Group 2), caused a dose-dependent significant ($p < 0.05$) reduction in cauda epididymal sperm count, sperm motility, sperm viability, and fertility rate (Groups 4 and 5). Oral administration of aqueous extract of Emblica officinalis alone did not cause any significant changes in the above-mentioned parameters (Group 3). However, Emblica officinalis aqueous extract along with ochratoxin treatment resulted in significant recovery in all of the sperm parameters, as well as in fertility rate (Groups 6 and 7) in comparison to the ochratoxin-alone treated animals (Groups 4 and 5). Amelioration was higher in the high-dose ochratoxin plus extract-treated animals than that for the respective low dose. When normal human sperm cell suspension was treated with ochratoxin (in-vitro), various morphological alterations were observed. These were mitigated further, when treated with aqueous extract of Emblica officinalis.

Diabetic neuropathic pain is an important microvascular complication of diabetes mellitus, and oxidative stress plays a vital role in the associated neural and vascular complications. A study investigated the ethyl acetate:methanol fraction of Emblica officinalis (10 mg/kg), in type II diabetes (high fat diet fed/low dose streptozotocin) induced diabetic neuropathy in male Sprague-Dawley rats.[37] The diabetic rats exhibited significant hyperalgesia (nociception) compared to the control rats. Treatment with Emblica officinalis extract and quercetin in the diabetic rats showed a significant increase in tail-flick latency in the hot immersion test and the pain threshold level in the hot plate test compared to the control rats. Changes in lipid peroxidation status and anti-oxidant enzymes (superoxide dismutase and catalase) levels observed in the diabetic rats were significantly restored by Emblica officinalis extract and quercetin treatment. Both Emblica officinalis extract and quercetin attenuated diabetic-induced axonal degeneration. This study provides experimental evidence of the preventive and curative effect of Emblica officinalis on nerve function and oxidative stress in an animal model of diabetic neuropathy. Emblica officinalis may be used for preventive therapy in diabetic patients at the risk of developing neuropathy.

Arsenic, an important human toxin, is naturally occurring in groundwater and its accumulation in plants and animals have assumed a menacing proportion in a large part of the world, particularly Asia. Epidemiological studies have shown a strong association between chronic arsenic exposure and various adverse health effects, including cardiovascular diseases, neurological defects, and cancers of the lung, skin, bladder, liver, and kidney.

The protective role of the fruits of Emblica officinalis (500 mg/kg b.wt.) was studied in adult Swiss albino mice against arsenic-induced hepatopathy.[38] The arsenic-treated group ($NaAsO(2)$, 4 mg/kg b.wt.) showed a significant increase in serum transaminases and lipid peroxidation (LPO) content in the liver, whereas significant decreases were recorded in hepatic superoxide dismutase (SOD), catalase (CAT), glutathione-S-transferase (GST), and serum alkaline phosphatase activity. The combined treatment of Emblica and arsenic (pre- and post-) reduced the serum transaminases and LPO content in the liver, whereas a significant increase was noticed in SOD, CAT, GST and serum alkaline phosphatase activities. The liver histopathology showed that Emblica fruit extract had reduced karyolysis, karyorrhexis, necrosis, and cytoplasmic vacuolization induced by $NaAsO(2)$ intoxication.

Connective tissue activity

During wound-healing, the wound site is rich in oxidants, such as hydrogen peroxide, contributed mostly by neutrophils and macrophages. Ascorbic acid and tannins of low molecular weight— namely, emblicanin A (2,3-di-O-galloyl-4,6-(S)-hexahydroxydiphenoyl-2-keto-glucono-delta-lactone) and emblicanin B (2,3,4,6-bis-(S)-hexahydroxydiphenoyl-2-keto-glucono-delta-lactone)—present in Emblica officinalis have been shown to exhibit a strong anti-oxidant action. Researchers have proposed that the addition of these anti-oxidants to the wound microenvironment would support the repair process.

An investigation was undertaken to determine the efficacy of emblica on dermal wound-healing in vivo.[39] Full-thickness excision wounds were made on the back of the rat, and topical application of emblica accelerated wound contraction and closure. Emblica increased cellular proliferation and cross-linking of collagen at the wound site, as evidenced by an increase in the activity of extracellular signal-regulated kinase 1/2, along with an increase in DNA, type III collagen, acid-soluble collagen, aldehyde content, shrinkage temperature, and tensile strength. Higher levels of tissue ascorbic acid, alpha-tocopherol, reduced glutathione, superoxide dismutase, catalase, and glutathione peroxidase support the conclusion that emblica application promotes anti-oxidant activity at the wound site. As part of an ongoing search for the novel pharmacological activities of Phyllanthus emblica, a study has shown its type I collagen promoting and anti-collagenase effects on primary mouse fibroblast cells. At a concentration of 0.1 mg/ml, emblica extract significantly increased the type I pro-collagen level up to 1.65-fold, and 6.78-fold greater than that of an untreated control, determined by immunocytochemistry and Western blot analysis, respectively. Emblica extract caused an approximately 7.75-fold greater type I pro-collagen induction compared to the known herbal collagen enhancer asiaticoside at the same treatment concentration (0.1 mg/ml). Emblica extract inhibited collagenase activity in a dose-dependent manner. Maximal inhibition was observed (78.67 +/- 3.51%) at a concentration of 1 mg/ml. Emblica extract has a promising pharmacological effect that benefits collagen synthesis and protects against its degradation and could be used as a natural anti-aging ingredient.[40,44]

Researchers used aqueous extracts of unprocessed Emblica officinalis fruit powder (powder A), and the powder obtained after hot water extraction and drying of powder A (powder B).[41] Chondroprotection was measured in three different assay systems. First, the effects of both fruit powders were tested on the activities of the enzymes hyaluronidase and collagenase type 2. Second, an in-vitro model of cartilage degradation was set up with explant cultures of articular knee cartilage from osteoarthritis patients. Cartilage damage was assayed by measuring glycosaminoglycan release from explants treated with and without the Emblica officinalis fruit powders. Aqueous extracts of both fruit powders significantly inhibited the activities of hyaluronidase and collagenase type 2 in-vitro. Third, in the explant model of cartilage matrix damage, extracts of glucosamine sulphate and powder B (0.05 mg/ml) exhibited statistically significant, long-term chondroprotective activity in cartilage explants from 50% of the patients tested. This result is important because glucosamine sulphate is the leading nutraceutical for osteoarthritis. Powder A induced a statistically significant, short-term chondroprotective activity in cartilage explants from all of the patients tested. This study identified and quantified new chondroprotective activities of Emblica officinalis fruits.

Amla extract also is known to provide protection for human dermal fibroblasts against oxidative stress and, therefore, is thought to be useful for natural skin care. A study investigated the effects of Amla extract on human skin fibroblasts, especially for production of procollagen and matrix metalloproteinases (MMPs) in-vitro.[42] The mitochondrial activity of human skin fibroblasts was measured using WST-8 assay. Quantification of procollagen, MMPs, and tissue inhibitor of metalloproteinase-1 (TIMP-1) released from human skin fibroblasts was performed using the immunoassay technique. Amla extract stimulated proliferation of fibroblasts in a concentration dependent manner, and also induced the production of procollagen in a concentration- and time-dependent manner. Conversely, MMP-1 production from fibroblasts was decreased dramatically, but there was no evident effect on MMP-2. TIMP-1 was significantly increased by Amla extract. Amla extract appears to work effectively in therapeutic, and cosmetic applications through control of collagen metabolism.

Anti-inflammatory and anti-pyretic activity

Extracts of Amla leaves inhibit polymorphonuclear leucocyte and platelet activity, supporting their anti-inflammatory and anti-pyretic action. The most relevant cause of morbidity and mortality in cystic fibrosis patients is the lung pathology characterized by chronic infection and inflammation sustained mainly by Pseudomonas aeruginosa. Innovative pharmacological approaches to control the excessive inflammatory process in the lungs of cystic fibrosis patients are thought to be beneficial to reduce extensive damage to the airway tissue.

The Emblica officinalis extracts were tested in IB3-1 CF bronchial epithelial cells exposed to the Pseudomonas aeruginosa laboratory strain PAO1.[43] Emblica officinalis strongly inhibited the PAO1-dependent expression of the neutrophil chemokines IL-8, GRO-alpha, GRO-gamma, of the adhesion molecule ICAM-1, and of the pro-inflammatory cytokine IL-6. Pyrogallol, one of the compounds extracted from Emblica, inhibited the Pseudomonas aeruginosa-dependent expression of these pro-inflammatory genes similarly to the whole Emblica extract, whereas a second compound purified from Emblica, namely 5-hydroxy-isoquinoline, had no effect. Emblica officinalis may provide a novel treatment in cystic fibrosis patients.[44]

Protective effect in myocardial necrosis

An ethanolic extract of Amla given orally at a dose of 1 g/kg for two consecutive days was found to protect against isoproterenol-induced myocardial necrosis.[45, 46]

Ethnoveterinary Usage

Amla fruits are eaten, and its seeds are applied to wounds in ruminants. Other parts of the plant are used to cure cold and cough, burns, wounds, maggots in wounds, mastitis, hematuria, general poisoning (and particularly datura poisoning particular), ringworm, sprained hoof, abscess, diarrhea, bloody dysentery, E. coli bacillosis, indigestion, glossitis, tympanitis, lumbar fracture and stoppage of urine.[47]

Dr. Sodhi's Experience

When considering treatment with Amla, the practitioner should consider the following:

- Is there any type of weakness? Cancer? HIV? Viral infections?
- Is there disturbance in the gastrointestinal tract?
- Is vaginal tissue affected?
- Are the eyes affected?
- Are there respiratory problems, especially if accompanied by great debility, like cystic fibrosis, HIV and tuberculosis?
- Is the prostate involved?
- Are the liver, spleen, or pancreas affected?
- Is cholesterol high?
- Is there heavy metal toxicity?
- Is there an excess of kapha?

Amla is one of the most important adaptogens in Ayurveda. An old saying in India is, "If you eat

Amla, your wisdom will increase as you age." The father of one of my co-workers in India died at the age of 107. Almost up until the time of his death, he still walked three to five miles a day, he had all of his own teeth, his eyes were only slightly refracted, he had never had surgery, and he recognized everyone who came to see him. His secret? He ate Amla every day!

Amla has many beneficial qualities. It is one of the richest sources of natural vitamin C available and provides powerful immune support. We use Amla at our clinic with great success to treat dyspepsia, gastritis, flatulence, and peptic ulcers. It also revitalizes and nourishes vaginal tissues, as either a douche or a suppository. Amla has a therapeutic effect on the eyes, as well, because it strengthens collagen. It protects the eyes from cataracts and helps with macular degeneration and other eye conditions. It also heals mucus membranes and promotes hair growth. Amla supports the healing of lung and sinus conditions, especially in cases of extreme debility. For example, in advanced AIDs patients, when the body becomes weak and depleted, it increases body mass and rebuilds strength and vitality.

In male health conditions, Amla can be used for prostatitis, benign prostate hypertrophy, and prostate cancer. As an adjunct to chemotherapy and/or radiation for cancer patients, Amla reduces side-effects and enhances the effects of the treatments. Amla supports the health of the spleen, liver, and pancreas. It helps to lower cholesterol, supports the liver during heavy metal detoxification, and has been used with success in the treatment of acute pancreatitis.

Case Histories

Peptic ulcers

A Russian female nurse with a peptic ulcer came to our clinic after having been given the drug Nexium. She reported although the Nexium helped with her symptoms, she was concerned about long-term use, and she had been told that she would have to take it for the rest of her life. This patient had a typical pitta-vaata constitution and personality, with symptoms commonly associated with a pitta imbalance, such as anger and irritability, in addition to inflammation, which in her case was affecting her digestive tract.

We gave her a pitta-pacifying diet and an herbal formulation including 1/2 teaspoon of Amla extract (equal to about 2000 mg of whole fruit) and Asparagus racemosus (Shataavari) (500 mg three times a day). In just a week, the patient was able to stop taking the Nexium. She is continuing the herbs, and as long as she stays on the pitta-pacifying diet, she is symptom-free. Her ulcer is gone, but if she deviates from the diet for a significant period of time, symptoms of hyperacidity do reoccur. Luckily, since the stomach lining heals quickly, she is able to relieve her symptoms relatively quickly by simply returning to a pitta-pacifying diet.

Corneal ulcers

A 70-year-old female patient from Florida came to our clinic with diabetes and corneal ulcers. Her conditions were not improving with any conventional treatment protocols. We worked to get her blood sugar under control with Gymnema sylvestre and Neem prepration and prescribed Amla eye washes, prepared by soaking one tablespoon Amla powder in sterile water overnight and then straining the decoction through a coffee filter. She was also taking Amla preparation one teaspoon three times per day of with following herbs. Emblica officinalis (amalaki), Aegle marmelos (biva), Quercus infectoria (mayaphal), Piper longum (pipli), Centella asiatica (brahmi), Ellettaria cardomomum (ela), Myristica fragrans (jatipala), Cinnamomum zeylanicum (twak), Nambusa arundinacia, Santalum album (chandana), Asparagus racemosus (shataavari), Withania somnifera (ashwagandha), Tribulus terristris (gokshura), Terminalia chebula (haritaki),

Adhatoda vesica (vasaka), Leptadenia reticulate (dori), Aquilaria agallocha (agru), Desmostachya bipinnata (kush), Cyperus rotundus (motha), Gmelina arboreta (gambhari), Uraria picta (prasniparni), Clitoria ternatea (aparajita), Imperata cylindrical (koshtaki), Oraxylum indicum (shiyonak), Trapa bispinosa (shringatak), Curcumin longum (Curcuma), Pueraria lobata (kudzu), Gymnema auranticum (meda), Boerhaavia diffusa (purnanava), Panax ginseng (kudju), Premna mucronata (arni), Phaseolus trilobus (mudgaparni), Desmodium gangeticum (shalaparni), castor root, Solanum nigrum (kakmachi), clarified butter, dehydrated sugar cane, and honey.

Within the next 9 months, the patient's corneal ulcers healed, her vision cleared up, and no new ulcers formed.

Pancreatitis

Having just read a report of Amla's use in treating acute pancreatitis in dogs, the family of a woman suffering from pancreatitis called me. The patient had been in the hospital for 3 months. She was vomiting continually, couldn't keep food in her stomach, and had lost a considerable amount of weight. She also was taking antibiotics, but so far these had had no effect on her symptoms.

My options were limited, as the patient was still in the hospital, but I provided Amla extract in a 2-ounce dropper bottle, and instructed the hospital staff to put a few drops in her mouth when no one was looking. I assured them that because Amla is a fruit, it would do no harm and would not interfere with any of the medications she was taking already. Within 2 days, the patient began to eat normally, eventually she recovered fully and discharged from the hospital.

Prostatitis

A 26-year-old male cyclist with acute prostatitis came to see me. He had been given three rounds of antibiotics with no change in his symptoms.

Cyclists are prone to prostate infections, so we recommended that he get a saddle that did not put pressure on the prostate, and we put him on Amla extract at a dose of 500 mg three times a day, along with one teaspoon of Amla paste, also three times a day. Amla paste is a traditional herbal paste made from a base of Amla extract to which many other herbs are added, to produce a powerful formulation for enhancing the immune system, protecting the body from oxidative damage, accelerating tissue repair and regeneration, and protecting against chromosomal damage from heavy metals and environmental pollutants.

The enhanced formula we use at the clinic contains standardized extracts of the following herbs: Emblica officinalis (amalaki), Aegle marmelos (biva), Quercus infectoria (mayaphal), Piper longum (Pippli), Centella asiatica (brahmi), Ellettaria cardomomum (ela), Myristica fragrans (jatipala), Cinnamomum zeylanicum (twak), Nambusa arundinacia, Santalum album (chandana), Asparagus racemosus (shataavari), Withania somnifera (ashwagandha), Tribulus terristris (gokshura), Terminalia chebula (haritaki), Adhatoda vesica (vasaka), Leptadenia reticulate (dori), Aquilaria agallocha (agru), Desmostachya bipinnata (kush), Cyperus rotundus (motha), Gmelina arboreta (gambhari), Uraria picta (prasniparni), Clitoria ternatea (aparajita), Imperata cylindrical (koshtaki), Oraxylum indicum (shiyonak), Trapa bispinosa (shringatak), Curcumin longum (Curcuma), Pueraria lobata (kudzu), Gymnema auranticum (meda), Boerhaavia diffusa (purnanava), Panax ginseng (kudju), Premna mucronata (arni), Phaseolus trilobus (mudgaparni), Desmodium gangeticum (shalaparni), castor root, Solanum nigrum (kakmachi), clarified butter, dehydrated sugar cane, and honey.

In the first week after beginning the protocol, the cyclist's symptoms had vanished. He stayed on the protocol for 2 months, to prevent a state of chronic infection from developing, as prostatitis can easily become chronic.

Herbal Protocols

For chronic ulcers:

Chronic ulcers differ from acute ulcers in that the lining of the stomach thickens, and it often takes longer for the stomach to repair itself completely. In this case, Piper longum (Pippli), 500 mg three times a day, may be given, in addition to Shataavari and Amla (as in the case above) for up to 6 months.

For leucorrhea and bacterial vaginosis:

In women with leucorrhea, especially if they have an underlying pathology such as yeast, bacteria, or fungi leading to bacterial vaginosis, Amla douches allows the tissue to slough off, eliminating the infection and rejuvenating the area by supporting the growth of new tissue. To prepare a douche, add 1/2 tseaspoon Amla extract (equal to 2000 mg whole fruit) to 1/2 cup of water, or soak 1 tablespoon of the whole herb powder in 1/2 cup of water overnight, and filter before use.

For hair growth and conditioning:

Amla extract may be soaked in coconut oil, applied directly to the hair in the evening, and massaged well into the scalp. Then the patient can sleep with the mixture in the hair by covering the hair with a scarf to avoid soiling the bed sheets. In the morning, the Amla should be washed out with water only; shampoo should not be used. After washing the hair, a simple rinse of Amla extract dissolved in water improves hair growth and also reduces the amount of gray hair.

For eye care, including cataracts:

To make an eye wash, place one teaspoon of Amla extract in a glass of water and leave overnight. After filtering through a coffee filter, this solution is effective as an eye wash for almost any eye condition.

For heavy metal toxicity:

Triphala (equal parts Terminalia bellerica, Terminalia chebula, Emblica officinalis), 500 mg extract three times a day, should be given with one teaspoon of Amla (also three times a day), preferably in a compound formula such as that described in the case of prostatitis. The anti-oxidant power of this combination is much stronger than that of vitamin E, an anti-oxidant commonly used in Western medicine.

For high cholesterol:

For high cholesterol, Amla (500 mg extract), may be taken alone or in combination with Triphala (also 500 mg extract). Both should be taken three times a day. Better results are obtained when Amla is used as part of a formulation. If HDL is low, Amla should be given with Guggulu (Commiphora mukul), and ghee. Organic ghee can increase HDL by as much as 10 points, as long as consumption is limited to no more than three teaspoons a day.

Safety Profile

Amla fruits are considered a food, and no toxicity has been noted.

Dosage

>Fresh fruit: As required
>Infusion: 10–15 ml powder: 36 grams
>Extract 50:1 100 to 500 mg three times per day

Ayurvedic Properties

>Rasa (taste): sour and astringent are dominant, but the fruit has five tastes, including sweet, bitter, and pungent
>Veerya (nature): cooling
>Vipaka (taste developed through digestion): sweet
>Guna (qualities): light, dry

Doshas (effect on humors): pacifies all three doshas: vata, kapha, pitta, especially effective for pitta

Because of its cooling nature, Amla is a common ingredient in treatments for burning sensations anywhere in the body and for many types of inflammation and fever; these are manifestations of pitta (fire) agitation.

Notes

1. Author? *Selected Medicinal Plants of India* (Chemexcil, Mumbai: Ministry of Health and Family Welfare,1989). It's compilation so no authors have been listed. I checked all the refernces and it is referenced as above

2. Dharmananda Subhuti [which is first and last name?], *Amla— Key Herb of Ayurvedic Medicine* (City: Publisher, date).Please see this http://books.google.com/books/about/Emblic_Myrobalans_AMLA_Key_Herb_of_Ayurv.html?id=0fyuPgAACAAJ

3. A.C. Kaviratna and P. Sharma (translators), <u>Caraka-Samhita</u>, *Vol. 3,* 2nd ed. rev (Delhi, India: Indian Books Centre, 1996).

4. Government of India, *Ayurvedic Pharmacopoeia of India* (New Delhi: Sairam TV, 1999).

5. Y. Hu, H. Liang, Q. Yuan, and Y. Hong "Determination of glucosinolates in 19 Chinese medicinal plants with spectrophotometry and high-pressure liquid chromatography," *Nat Prod Res.*, Aug. 2010, 24(13):1195–1205.

6. S. El-Mekkawy, M.R. Meselhy, I.T. Kusumoto, S. Kadota, M. Hattori, and T. Namba, "Inhibitory effects of Egyptian folk medicines on human immunodeficiency virus (HIV) reverse transcriptase," *Chemical and Pharmaceutical Bulletin*, 1995, 43(4):641.

7. Y.F, Wang, X.Y. Wang, Z. Ren, C.W. Qian, Y.C. Li, K. Kaio, Q.D. Wang, Y. Zhang, L.Y. Zheng, J.H. Jiang, C.R. Yang, Q. Liu, Y.J. Zhang, and Y.F. Wang, "Phyllaemblicin B inhibits Coxsackie virus B3 induced apoptosis and myocarditis," *Anti-viral Res.*, Nov. 2009, 84(2):150–158.

8. S. Saeed and P. Tariq, "Anti-bacterial activities of Emblica officinalis and Coriandrum sativum against Gram negative urinary pathogens Pak," *J Pharm Sci.*, Jan. 2007, 20(1):32–35.

9. S. Rahman, M.M. Akbor, A. Howlader, and A. Jabbar, "Antimicrobial and cytotoxic activity of the alkaloids of Amlaki (Emblica officinalis)," *Pak J Biol Sci.*, Aug. 2009, 15;12(16):1152–1155.

10. A. Saini, S. Sharma, and S. Chhibber, "Protective efficacy of Emblica officinalis against Klebsiella pneumoniae induced pneumonia in mice," *Indian J Med Res.*, Aug. 2008, 128(2):188–193.

11. See Note 10.

12. G. P. Talwar, S.A. Dar, M.K. Rai, K.V. Reddy, D. Mitra, S.V. Kulkarni, G.F. Doncel, C.B. Buck, J.T. Schiller, S. Muralidhar, M. Bala, S. S. Agrawal, K. Bansal, and J.K. Verma, "A novel polyherbal microbicide with inhibitory effect on bacterial, fungal and viral genital pathogens," *Int J Antimicrob Agents*, Aug. 2008, 32(2):180–185.

13. A. Jacob, M. Pandey, S. Kapoor, and R. Saroja, "Effect of the Indian gooseberry (amla) on serum cholesterol levels in men aged 35–55 years," *Eur J Clin Nutr.*, Nov. 1988, 42(11):939–944.

14. H. J. Kim, T. Yokozawa, H.Y. Kim, C. Tohda, T.P. Rao, and L.R. Juneja, "Influence of amla (Emblica officinalis Gaertn.) on hypercholesterolemia and lipid peroxidation in cholesterol-fed rats," *J Nutr Sci Vitaminol* (Tokyo), Dec. 2005, 51(6):413–418.

15. R. Mathur, A. Sharma, V.P. Dixit, and M. Varma, "Hypolipidaemic effect of fruit juice of Emblica offitinalis in cholesterol-fed rabbits," *Journal of Ethnopharmacology*, 1996, 50:6.

16. C.P. Thakur, "Emblica offitinalis reduces serum, aortic and hepatic cholesterol in rabbit," *Experientia*, 1985, 41(3):423.

17. S. Sultana, S. Ahmed, and T. Jahangir, "Emblica officinalis and hepatocarcinogenesis: A chemopreventive study in Wistar rats," *J Ethnopharmacol.*, June 19,118(1):1-6. Epub March 30, 2008.

18. Z. G, Zhong, J.L. Huang, H. Liang, Y.N. Zhong, W.Y. Zhang, D.P. Wu, C.L. Zeng, J.S. Wang, and Y.H. Wei, "The effect of gallic acid extracted from leaves of Phyllanthus emblica on apoptosis of human hepatocellular carcinoma BEL-7404 cells," *Zhong Yao Cai.*, July 2009, 32(7):1097–1101.

19. R. Piva, L. Penolazzi, M. Borgatti, I. Lampronti,E. Lambertini, E. Torreggiani, and R. Gambari, "Apoptosis of human primary osteoclasts treated with molecules targeting nuclear factor-kappaB. Ann," *N Y Acad Sci.*, Aug. 2009, 1171:448–456.

20. See Note 19.

21. A. Jindal, D. Soyal, A. Sharma, and P.K. Goyal,. "Protective effect of an extract of Emblica officinalis against radiation-induced damage in mice," *Integr Cancer Ther.,* March 2009, 8(1):98–105.

22. T. S. Chen, S.Y. Liou, and Y.L. Chang Y, "Supplementation of Emblica officinalis (Amla) extract reduces oxidative stress in uremic patients," *Am J Chin Med.*, 2009, 37(1):19–25.

23. H.Y. Kim, T. Okubo, L.R. Juneja, and T. Yokozawa, "The protective role of amla (Emblica officinalis Gaertn.) against fructose-induced metabolic syndrome in a rat model, *Br J Nutr.*, Feb. 2010, 103(4):502–512.

24. Maroli, S., S. Shahani, S. Pawaand N.D. Moulic. Hypoglycemic effect of Curcuma longa and Phyllanthus emblica combination in NIDDM. Indian Journal of Pharmacology 1996; 28, 1, 44--45

25. K. Agarwal, H. Dhir, A. Sharma, and G. Talukder, "The efficacy of two species of Phyllanthus in counteracting nickel clastogenicity," *Fitoterapia*, 1992, 63(1):49.

26. A. Ghosh, A. Sharma, and G. Talukder, "Comparison of the protection afforded by a crude extract of Phyllanthus emblica fruit and an equivalent amount of synthetic ascorbic acid against the cytotoxic effects of cesium chloride in mice," *International Journal of Pharmacognosy*, 1993p. Vol. 31, No. 2 , Pages 116-120

27. R.K. Gulati, S. Agarwal, and S.S. Agrawal, "Hepatoprotective studies on Phyllanthus emblica Linn, and quercetin," *Indian Journal of Experimental Biology*, 1995, 33(4):261.

28. A. K Roy, H. Dhir, A. Sharma, and G. Talukder, "Phyllanthus emblica fruit extract and ascorbic acid modify hepatotoxic and renotoxic effects of metals in mice," *International Journal of Pharmacognosy*, 1991, 29(2):117.

29. V.D. Reddy, P. Padmavathi, and NCh. Varadacharyulu, "Emblica officinalis protects against alcohol-induced liver mitochondrial dysfunction in rats," *J Med Food*, April 2009, 12(2):327–233.

30. S.P. Thorat, N.N. Rege, A.S. Naik, et al., "Emblica qfficinalis: A novel therapy for acute pancreatitis—an experimental study," *Hepatic, Pancreatic and Biliary Surgery*, 1995 9(1):25.

31. L Ganju, D. Karan, S. Chanda, K.K. Srivastava, R.C. Sawhney, and W. Selvamurthy, "Immunomodulatory effects of agents of plant origin," *Biomed Pharmacother.*, Sept 2003, 57(7):296–300.

32. Y.K. Chawla, P. Dubey, R. Singh, S. Nundy, and B.N. Tandon, "Treatment of dyspepsia with Amalaki (Emblica officinalis Linn.)— an Ayurvedic drug," *Indian Journal of Medical Research,*1982, 76:895.

33. K. Tarwadi and V. Agte, "Anti-oxidant and micronutrient potential of common fruits available in the Indian subcontinent," *Int J Food Sci Nutr.*, Aug. 2007, 58(5):341–349.

34. M.R.R. Rao and H.H. Siddqui, "Pharmacological studies on Emblica officinalis Gaertn.," *Indian Journal of Experimental Biology*, 1964, 2:29.

35. D. Chakraborty and R. Verma, "Ameliorative effect of Emblica officinalis aqueous extract on ochratoxin-induced lipid peroxidation in the kidney and liver of mice," *Int J Occup Med Environ Health*, 2010, 23(1):63–73.

36. D. Chakraborty and R. Verma, "Spermatotoxic effect of ochratoxin and its amelioration by Emblica officinalis aqueous extract," *Acta Pol Pharm.*, Nov.–Dec. 2009, 66(6):689–695.

37. N.P. Kumar, A.R. Annamalai, and R.S. Thakur, "Antinociceptive property of Emblica officinalis Gaertn (Amla) in high fat diet-fed/low dose streptozotocin induced diabetic neuropathy in rats," *Indian J Exp Biol.*, Sept. 2009, 47(9):737–742.

38. A. Sharma, M.K. Sharma, and M. Kumar, "Modulatory role of Emblica officinalis fruit extract against arsenic induced oxidative stress in Swiss albino mice," *Chem Biol Interact.*, June 15, 2009, 180(1):20–30.

39. M. Sumitra, P. Manikandan, V.S. Gayathri, P. Mahendran, and L. Suguna L., "Emblica officinalis exerts wound healing action through up-regulation of collagen and extracellular signal-regulated kinases (ERK1/2)," *Wound Repair Regen.*, Jan–Feb 2009, 17(1):99–107.

40. P. Chanvorachote, V. Pongrakhananon, S. Luanpitpong, B. Chanvorachote, S. Wannachaiyasit, and U. Nimmannit, "Type I pro-collagen promoting and anti-collagenase activities of Phyllanthus emblica extract in mouse fibroblasts," *J Cosmet Sci.*, July-Aug., 2009, 60(4):395–403.

41. V.N. Sumantran, A. Kulkarni, R. Chandwaskar, A. Harsulkar, B. Patwardhan, A. Chopra, and U.V. Wagh, "Chondroprotective Potential of Fruit Extracts of Phyllanthus emblica in Osteoarthritis," *Evid Based Complement Alternat Med.*, Sept. 2008, 5(3):329–335.

42. T. Fujii, M. Wakaizumi, T. Ikami, and M. Saito, "Amla (Emblica officinalis Gaertn.) extract promotes procollagen production and inhibits matrix metalloproteinase-1 in human skin fibroblasts," *J Ethnopharmacol.*, Sept. 2, 2008, 119(1):53–57.

43. A. Ihantola-Vormisto, J. Summanen, H. Kankaanranta, H. Vuorela, A.M. Asmawi, and E. Moilanen, "Anti-inflammatory activity of extracts from leaves of Phyllanthus emblica," *Planta Medica*, 1997, 63(6):518.

44. E. Nicolis, I. Lampronti, M.C. Dechecchi, M. Borgatti, A. Tamanini, N. Bianchi, V. Bezzerri, I. Mancini, M.G. Giri, P. Rizzotti, R. Gambari, and G. Cabrini G., "Pyrogallol, an active compound from the medicinal plant Emblica officinalis, regulates expression of pro-inflammatory genes in bronchial epithelial cells," *Int Immunopharmacol.*, Dec. 2008, 10;8(12):1672–1680.

45. M. Tariq, S.J. Hussain, M. Asif, and M. Jahan, "Protective effects of fruit extracts of Emblica officinalis Gaertn. and Terminalia chebula in experimental myocardial necrosis in rats," *Indian Journal of Experimental Biology*, 1977, 15:485.

46. K.R Shanmugasundaram, P. G, Seethapathy, and E.R. Shanmugasundaram, "Anna Pavala Sindhooram—an antiatherosclerotic Indian drug," *Journal of Ethnopharmacology*, 1983, 7(3):247.

47. Government of India, *Ayurvedic Pharmacopoeia of India*, New Delhi: SairamTV, 1999 (5):363-365.

31

PICRORHIZA KURROA

INTRODUCTION

Picrorhiza kurroa is a small perennial herb that is well-known in the Ayurvedic system of medicine. It traditionally has been used to treat disorders of the liver and upper respiratory tract, to reduce fevers, and to treat dyspepsia, chronic diarrhea, and scorpion sting. Picrorhiza's active constituents are obtained from its root and rhizomes. The plant is self-regenerating; however, unregulated over-harvesting has threatened it to near extinction. Research on Picrorhiza has focused on its hepatoprotective, anticholestatic, anti-oxidant, and immune-modulating activity.[1,2]

Ancient Ayurvedic literature mentions Picrorhiza kurroa as an important remedy,[3,4,5] and describes it as useful in jaundice, nausea anorexia, dyspepsia, and periodic fevers.[6] The Indian and colonial addendum of 1901 to the 1897 *British Pharmacopeia* included Picrorhiza as an official drug.[7] In Ayurveda, Picrorhiza is considered to be a kapha and pitta suppressant. It helps in regulating peristaltic movements, and also tones up the digestive tract because of its light properties. It also is a good anti-worm agent because of its bitter taste. It has positive activity on the cardiovascular system, and helps in improving the heart condition.

Picrorhiza curbs infection in the body and also expels mucus in the respiratory tract. It helps to tone the urinary tract because of its light property. It is highly effective in skin-related ailments because of its cold potency. The rhizome of Picrorhiza traditionally has been used to treat ailments affecting the liver, including hepatitis and jaundice.

SYNONYMOUS NAMES

English: Picrorhiza
Botanical Name: Picrorhiza Kurroa
Sanskrit: kutkia
Hindi: Kutki, Kuru

HABITAT

Picrorhiza is found in the Himalayan region, growing at elevations of 3,000 to 5,000 meters. In India it is found in Himachal Pradesh and Kashmir.

BOTANICAL CHARACTERISTICS

A small, perennial shrub, Picrorhiza has a long, creeping rootstock that is bitter in taste, and grows in rock crevices and moist, sandy soil. The leaves of Picrorhiza are flat, oval, and sharply serrated. The leaves measure 2 to 4 inches long and have a circular shape and sharp apex. The flower stalk is 2 to 4 inches long and bears white or purple flowers. The fruit is ½ inch long and oval in shape. The plant flowers in the summer and bears fruit in the rainy season.

Chemical Composition

Kutkin, the active principle of Picrorhiza kurroa, is composed of kutkoside and the iridoid glycoside picrosides I, II, and III. Other identified active constituents are apocynin, drosin, and nine cucurbitacin glycosides.[8,9] Apocynin is a catechol that has been shown to inhibit neutrophil oxidative burst in addition to being a powerful anti-inflammatory agent,[10] and the curcubitacins have been shown to be highly cytotoxic and possess anti-tumor properties.[11]

Pharmacological Activity

Many investigators have studied Picrorhiza kurroa and several other Ayurvedic drugs as hepatoprotective agents.[12,13] Experimentally, Picrohiza has been shown to have the following pharmacodynamic and biodynamic actions: choleretic effects in rats and dogs,[14] anti-necrotic effect in carbon tetrachloride-induced damage in rats and rabbits, reduction of fatty infiltration and lipid deposits in galactosamine-induced liver damage, reduction of paracetamol-induced hepatic damage,[15] reversal of loss in body weight in alcohol-treated rats and also improved food intake in CCL 4-induced liver-damage,[16] enhancement in the levels of DNA, RNA, protein, and cholesterol post-partial hepatectomy, an increase in mitotic index, scavenging of super-oxide anions and inhibition of lipid peroxidation, anti-viral effects on vaccinia viruses,[17] and anti-inflammatory effects in carrageenan edema, and inhibition of experimental passive cutaneous anaphylaxis.[18] This large number of diverse effects of Picrorhiza indicates that picrosides may be acting at some fundamental level in cell homeostatic controls.

Published literature and ongoing work show the efficacy and safety of Picrorhiza in treating acute viral hepatitis, treating drug-induced liver damage, and long-term prophylactic use in bronchial asthma.[19,20,21] In the form of fine root powder, Picrorhiza is a widespread remedy in India for fevers, anorexia, and jaundice, and as an adaptogen. Standardized extracts offer fresh opportunities for its use in viral hepatitis and alcohol- or drug-induced liver damage.

The hepatoprotective action of Picrorhiza kurroa is not fully understood but may be attributed to its ability to inhibit the generation of oxygen anions and to scavenge free radicals.[22] Its antioxidant effect has been shown to be similar to that of superoxide dismutase, it is metal-ion chelators, and xanthine oxidase inhibitors.[23] In rats infected with malaria, Picrorhiza restored depleted glutathione levels, thereby enhancing detoxification and anti-oxidation and helping maintain a normal oxidation-reduction balance.[24] In this same animal model, Picrorhiza demonstrated an anti-lipid peroxidative effect.[25] Picrorhiza has been shown to stimulate liver regeneration in rats, possibly via stimulation of nucleic acid and protein synthesis.[26]

Picrorhiza's anti-inflammatory action is attributed to the apocynin constituent, which has been shown to have potent anti-inflammatory properties in addition to inhibiting oxidative burst in neutrophils.[27] Although the mechanism is unclear, animal studies indicate that Picrorhiza's constituents exhibit strong anticholestatic activity against a variety of liver-toxic substances and appear to be even more potent than silymarin. Picrorhiza also exhibits a dose-dependent choleretic activity, evidenced by an increase in bile salts and acids, and bile flow.[28]

Hepatoprotective activity

Numerous animal studies, primarily using rats, have demonstrated that the active constituents of Picrorhiza are effective at preventing liver toxicity and the subsequent biochemical changes caused by numerous toxic agents. In one study, hepatocytes damaged by exposure to galactosamine, thiocetamide, and carbon tetrachloride were incubated with Picrorhiza constituents. A concentration-dependent restorative effect was observed in regard to normal hepatocyte function.[29]

A similar effect was seen when 25 mg/kg/day oral Picrorhiza extract was administered to rats poisoned by exposure to aflatoxin B1. Picrorhiza kurroa significantly prevented the biochemical changes induced by aflatoxin B1.[30] In galactosamine induced liver injury in rats, Picrorhiza significantly reduced liver lipid content, GOT, and GPT.

When given at a dose of 3 to12 mg/kg orally for 45 days, Picrorhiza extract was effective in reversing ethanol-induced liver damage in rats.[31] In another animal model of hepatic ischemia, rats administered Picrorhiza orally at 12 mg/kg daily for 7 days prior to induced ischemia demonstrated improved hepatocyte glycogen preservation and reduced apoptosis, compared to the control animals.[32] Picrorhiza principles also were effective in treating Amanita mushroom poisoning in an in-vivo animal model.[33] And in an in-vitro study Picrorhiza's anti-oxidant activity was demonstrated by subjecting human Glioma and Hep 3B cells to a hypoxic state. Picrorhiza treatment reduced the cellular damage cause by hypoxia, indicating that Picrorhiza constituents may protect against hypoxia/re-oxygenation-induced injuries.[34] Liver injury was induced in rats by subcutaneous injection of 500 mg/kg of galactosamine hydrochloride dissolved in normal saline. Group 1 received 200 mg/kg of Picrorhiza extract at 24, 4 and 0 hours before galactosamine. Group 2 received 50 mg/kg at same time intervals. The control groups received only 5% gum arabic. The animals were sacrificed 24 hours later. Blood was taken to determine transaminases, glutamate dehydrogenase, alkaline phosphatase, and bilirubin. Liver lipids also were measured.[35] The experimental results showed the effects of Picrorhiza on galactosamine-induced liver injury in the rat. At the small dose of the root powder 50 mg/kg given three times at 24th, 4th and/or before galactosamine, only a directional change was seen in GPT and GLDH, but at 200 mg/kg po a significant reduction ($p<0.05$) was observed in liver lipid content, GOT, and GPT. GLDH showed a directional reduction, but alkaline phosphatase and bilirubin were not reduced significantly.

Activity against viral hepatitis

Studies indicate that Picrorhiza extracts may be of therapeutic value in treating viral hepatitis. An in-vitro study that investigated anti-hepatitis B-like activity of Picrorhiza found it to have promising anti-hepatitis B surface antigen activity.[36, 38]

In a randomized, double-blind, placebo-controlled trial of 33 patients diagnosed with acute viral hepatitis, 375 mg Picrorhiza root powder was administered three times daily for 2 weeks. The treatment group was composed of 15 patients; the remaining 18 subjects were controls and received the placebo. Bilirubin, SGOT, and SGPT values were significantly lower in the treatment group, and the time required for bilirubin values to drop to 2.5 mg/dL was 27.4 days in the treatment group versus 75.9 days for the placebo group.[37]

In a double-blind trial, an herbal preparation with Picrorhiza as the principal ingredient was shown to significantly reduce serum bilirubin and transaminases in patients with viral hepatitis.[39] Further research has been carried out in research centers in India and many other countries.

Picrorhiza root powder was administered in a randomized double-blind manner to patients diagnosed with acute viral hepatitis. The patients received three capsules of Picrorhiza or a placebo three times a day for 2 weeks.[40] The results showed statistically significant differences in values between the placebo and Picrorhiza groups. Therapy-induced changes in the symptoms and signs of viral hepatitis were observed in both groups. Picrorhiza induced a more marked and early relief of anorexia, nausea, and malaise. No side-effects were observed from the experimental doses, although the larger doses had a laxative effect.

Anti-asthmatic, anti-allergic activity

In-vivo studies of bronchial obstruction indicate that the drosin constituent of Picrorhiza kurroa prevented allergen- and platelet activating factor-induced bronchial obstruction when given to guinea pigs via inhalant and oral routes. In vitro histamine release was also inhibited by the plant extract.[41] Picrorhiza extract given orally at 25 mg/kg to mice and rats resulted in a concentration-dependent decrease in mast cell degranulation. Induced bronchospasm was not prevented, however, indicating a lack of direct post-synaptic histamine receptor blocking activity.[42]

Anti-oxidant activity

Accumulation of advanced glycation end products (AGEs) or advanced oxidation protein products (AOPPs) has been identified as a risk factor for accelerated atherosclerosis seen in diabetes and chronic kidney disease. Little is known, however, about the intervention for atherogenesis associated with these oxidized proteins.

A study was performed to test the hypothesis that ethanol extraction of Picrorhiza scrophulariiflora may improve AGEs- or AOPPs-induced accelerated atherosclerosis in vivo.[43] Hypercholesterolemic or normal rabbits were assigned randomly to eight groups treated with an intravenous injection of AGEs- or AOPPs-modified rabbit serum albumin (AGEs-RSA or AOPPs-RSA), unmodified RSA, or the vehicle in the presence or absence of (10 mg/kg/2 days) gavage for 10 weeks. Compared to the hypercholesterolemic rabbits without Picrorhiza treatment, the Picrorhiza administration significantly decreased the aortic plaque volume and oxidized low density lipoprotein (Ox-LDL) deposition in the hypercholesterolemic animals. This was accompanied by significant histological improvement, including a decrease in intimal and smooth muscle cell proliferation and macrophage influx in the affected areas. Picrorhiza administration almost completely abolished the accelerated atherosclerosis induced by chronic treatment of AGEs- or AOPPs-RSA in both the hypercholesterolemic and the normal rabbits. Picrorhiza administration significantly restored the AGEs- or AOPPs-induced redox imbalance and inflammation, evidenced by a decrease in plasma Ox-LDL, thiobarbituric acid reactive substances, and TNF-alpha, and an increase in glutathione peroxidase activity.

Evidence indicates that inflammatory processes are involved in the development and/or progression of diabetic nephropathy. Effective treatment for inflammation in the kidneys of diabetic is practically unknown, however. The rhizomes of Picrorhiza scrophulariiflora are a traditional medication long used to treat inflammatory diseases.

The aim of one study was to test the hypothesis that the ethanol extract of Picrorhiza may reduce inflammation in patients with diabetic kidneys.[44] The streptozotocin-induced diabetic rats were randomly assigned to two groups treated with a gavage of either Picrorhiza or the vehicle. A group of non-diabetic control rats was treated concurrently. Compared to the vehicle-treated diabetic rats, the Picrorhiza-treated animals displayed a significant decrease in renal macrophage infiltration and overexpression of chemokine (C-C motif) ligand 2 (CCL2) and TGFB1. This was associated with attenuation of the structural and functional abnormalities of early diabetic nephropathy, such as glomerular hypertrophy, mesangial expansion, and albuminuria. Administration of Picrorhiza significantly reduced NADPH oxidase-dependent superoxide generation and decreased expression of malondialdehyde and advanced oxidation protein products in diabetic kidney. These data suggest that

Picorrhiza might improve diabetic nephropathy, probably through inhibition of redox-sensitive inflammation.

Anti-cancer activity

Picrorhiza kurroa, is used traditionally to treat fever, asthma, hepatitis, and other inflammatory conditions. The exact mechanism of its therapeutic action, however, is still unknown. Because nuclear factor-kappaB (NF-kappaB) activation plays a major role in inflammation and carcinogenesis, it is postulated that Picrorhiza must interfere with this pathway by inhibiting the activation of NF-kappaB mediated signal cascade.

An electrophoretic mobility shift assay showed that pre-treatment with Picrorhiza abrogated tumor necrosis factor (TNF)-induced activation of NF-kappaB. The glycoside also inhibited NF-kappaB activated by carcinogenic and inflammatory agents, such as cigarette smoke condensate, phorbol 12-myristate 13-acetate, okadaic acid, hydrogen peroxide, lipopolysaccharide, and epidermal growth factor. When examined for the mechanism of action, Picrorhiza inhibited activation of Ikappa-B-alpha kinase, leading to inhibition of phosphorylation and degradation of Ikappa-B alpha. It also inhibited phosphorylation and nuclear translocation of p65.[45]

Further studies revealed that Picrorhiza directly inhibits the binding of p65 to DNA, which was reversed by the treatment with reducing agents, suggesting a role for a cysteine residue in interaction with Picrorhiza.[46] Mutation of Cys(38) in p65 to serine abolished this effect of Picrorhiza. NF-kappaB inhibition by Picrorhiza leads to suppression of NF-kappaB-regulated proteins, including those linked with cell survival (inhibitor of apoptosis protein 1, Bcl-2, Bcl-xL, survivin, and TNF receptor-associated factor 2), proliferation (cyclin D1 and cyclooxygenase-2), angiogenesis (vascular endothelial growth factor), and invasion (intercellular adhesion molecule-1 and matrix metalloproteinase-9). Suppression of these proteins enhanced apoptosis induced by TNF. Overall, the results show that Picrorhiza inhibits the NF-kappaB activation pathway, which may explain its anti-inflammatory and anti-carcinogenic effects.

Many natural products have been used as immunomodulators either as immunosuppressants or as immunostimulators. A lab successfully isolated a 1,6-di-O-caffeoyl-beta-D-glucopyranoside, monomer named caffeoyl glycoside from the roots of Picrorhiza scrophulariiflora (Kutki). In this study, researchers evaluated the effects of this compound on immunomodulation in-vitro. The results showed that caffeoyl glycoside stimulated cell proliferation of splenocytes and peritoneal macrophages, and significantly enhanced the cytotoxicity of natural killer (NK) cells. Caffeoyl glycoside also increased CD4 and CD8 cell populations, also found to have immunomodulatory activity by regulating expression of Th1 and Th2 related cytokines. Taken together, these results indicated that caffeoyl glycoside might have potential effects in regulating the immune system, and this compound might be a useful immunotherapeutic agent in treating various immunity-related diseases.[47]

Kidney protection

A study investigated the effect of the ethanol extract of Picrorhiza scrophulariiflora on renal function and tissue damage in a rat remnant kidney model. Rat models of chronic kidney disease induced by 5/6 nephrectomy (5/6 Nx) were randomly assigned to two groups for treatment with a gavage of either Picrorhiza or a vehicle for 9 weeks. The rats in the control group received only a sham operation. Compared with the vehicle-treated 5/6 Nx rats, the Picrorhiza-treated rats displayed significantly decreased urinary excretion of malondialdehyde, serum levels of AGEs, and AOPPs, and increased serum SeGSHPx activities. These changes were associated with attenuated urinary protein excretion, glomerular sclerosis, and interstitial fibrosis.

Picrorhiza improved the renal functions and renal pathologies in rats with chronic kidney disease probably by inhibiting the oxidative stress.[48]

The hypoglycemic effect of an aqueous extract of Picrorrhiza on diabetic nephropathy was investigated. The body weight of each of eight rats per group was measured 7 days after streptozotocin (STZ) treatment. The blood glucose levels 3 days after STZ treatment and the changes in body weight, kidney weight, blood glucose levels, and serum blood urea nitrogen (BUN) also were measured, and the histopathology of the kidney was examined. Body weight decreases and increases of kidney weight, blood glucose levels, and serum BUN and creatinine levels were detected in the diabetic control with histopathological changes related to diabetic nephropathy in the kidney. The level of hyperglycemia, however, was lowered significantly in all groups that received the Picrorhiza extract. In addition, the changes related to diabetic nephropathy with the body weight also were significantly lower in the captopril, ACE inhibitor and all Picrorhiza extract-dosing groups than in the diabetic control. In conclusion, an aqueous extract of Picrorhiza has relatively good inhibitory effects on STZ-induced diabetes with early diabetic nephropathy with an efficacy similar to and equal to ACE inhibitor.[49]

Dr. Sodhi's Experience

When considering treatment with Kutki, the practitioner should consider the following:

- Is the liver in need of protection/support?
- Is something needed for immune modulation or autoimmune disease?
- Is cancer present?
- Is the patient a child with asthma?
- Is there a pitta-aggravation?
- Is there the need for a bitter herb?

Kutki is one of a group of bitter herbs known as mahatika, which are widely used in Ayurveda to treat the liver. Kutki in particular has powerful hepatoprotective properties. Both Kutki and Eclipta alba (bhringaraj) also are used extensively in traditional Chinese medicine, in which they are said to "increase the disease free state" (arogyavardhani).

These claims have been supported by many different experimental models, in which Kutki has been shown to normalize liver enzymes. It also is used for immune modulation in patients with lupus, psoriatic arthritis, and rheumatoid arthritis, especially when standard protocols for these autoimmune diseases do not completely resolve all symptomology.

Case History

A female patient with rheumatoid arthritis came to our clinic for treatment and did not respond to our usual protocol for the disease. In an attempt to find a better treatment plan, I initiated a complete panchakarma series, to which I added Picrorhiza, 500 mg three times a day. She responded much more favorably to this treatment. Her pain improved, the swelling decreased, and she was able to return to work.

Safety Profile

Picrorhiza is not readily water-soluble and, therefore, is not usually taken as a tea. Although it is ethanol soluble, its bitter taste makes tinctures unpalatable, so it typically is administered as a standardized, encapsulated powder extract. Picrorhiza root extracts are widely used in India with no report of adverse effects.[50] Loose stools and colic have been reported when unprepared Picrorhiza rhizomes are used as medicine. Extracts in alcohol, however, have shown much less tendency to cause such effects. Although the use of the herb is not discouraged in India during pregnancy and breast-feeding, little information is available to support the safety of Picrorhiza use by pregnant and nursing women.

Dosage

The typical adult dosage of Picrorhiza is 400 to 1500 mg/day, with dosages up to 3.5 g/day sometimes recommended for fever. Generally, 3 to 4 grams of the drug are given as an anti-periodic and 0.6–1.2 g as a bitter tonic.

Picrorhiza extract : 100-200 mg three times per day

Ayurvedic Properties

In Ayurveda, Picrorhiza is a kapha and pitta suppressant. According to Ayurveda, its properties are:
Gunna: ruksha (dry) and laghu (light)
Rasa: madhur (sweet)
Virya: sheet (cold)

Notes

1. C. K. Atal, M.L. Sharma, A. Kaul, and A. Khajuria, "Immunomodulating agents of plant origin. I: preliminary screening," *J Ethnopharmacol*, 1986;18:133–141.
2. B. P Subedi, "Plant profile: Kutki (Picrorhiza scrophulariiflora)," *Himalayan Bioresources* 2000:4.
3. Kashyap-Samhita or Vriddha-JivakiyaTantra. Trans IGM Shastri, Bombay Sastu Sahitya; 1970, pp 757.
4. Charak-Samhita. Jamnagar: Gulabkunvarba Ayurvedic Society; 1949, pp 1600–1607
5. Vagbhattacharya, Rasa-Ratna Samucchaya. Varanasi: Chow Oumbha Sanskrit Series; 1976. ???
6. S. D. Pade, *Arya-Bhishak* (Ahmedabad: Sastu Sahitya, 1957), p. 135.
7. E. White and J. Humphrey, *Pharmacoepia* (London: Henry Kimpton, 1901), p. 557.
8. K. Weinges, P. Kloss, and W.D. Henkels, "Natural products from medicinal plants. XVII. picroside-II, a new 6-vanilloyl-catapol from Picrorhiza kuroa Royle and Benth," *Justus Liebigs Ann Chem,*,1972, 759:173–182.
9. H. Stuppner and H. Wagner, "New cucurbitacin glycosides from Picrorhiza kurroa," *Planta Med*, 1989,55:559–563.
10. J.M. Simons, B.A. Hart, T.R. Ip Va?Ching, et al., "Metabolic activation of natural phenols into selective oxidative burst agonists by activated human neutrophils," *Free Radic Biol Med*, 1990, 8:251–258. This what it says in pubmed Please see the note 29 http://www.ncbi.nlm.nih.gov/pmc/articles/PMC2834342/
11. P. C Verma, V. Basu, V. Gupta, G. Saxena, and L.U. Rahman, "Pharmacology and chemistry of a potent hepatoprotective compound Picroliv isolated from the roots and rhizomes of Picrorhiza kurroa royle ex benth (kutki)," *Curr Pharm Biotechnol.*, Sept. 2009, 10(6):641–649.
12. A.B Vaidya, C.K. Bhatia, J.M. Mehta, and U.K. Sheth, "Therapeutic potential of Luffa echinata Roxb in viral hepatitis," *Ind J Pharmacol* 1976, 243–246.
13. S.S. Handa, A. Sharma, and K.K. Chakravarti, "Natural products and plants as liver protective drugs," *Fitoterapia*, 1986, 57:307–312.

14. V.N. Pandey and G.N. Chaturvedi, Effect of indigenous drug kutaki on bile after producing bibary fistula in dogs," *J Res Ind Med*, 1970, 5:1–24.

15. K. Mogre, K. Vora, and U.K. Sheth, "Effect of Picrorhiza kurroa and Eclipta alba on Na+ K+ T Pase in hepatic injury by hepatotoxic agents," *Ind J Pharmac* 1981, 13:252–259.

16. P.D. Pilankar, "A study of hepatoprotective effects of some indigenous plants in experimental animals," Ph.D. thesis, University of Bombay, India, 1981.

17. N. Singh, N. Misra, S.P. Singh, R.P. Kohli, and K.P. Bhargava, "Protective effect of Picrorhiza kurroa against cutaneous vaccinial (viral) infection in guinea pigs," *J Res Ay Sid* 1982, 33:162–171.

18. S. S. Mahajan and R.D. Kulkarni, "Effect of disodium cromoglycate and Picrorhiza kurroa toot powder in sensitivity of guinea pigs to histamine and sympathomimetic amines," *Intern Arch All Appl Immunol*, 1976; 53:137–144.

19. V.N. Pandey, "Clinical and experimental studies on certain liver diseases with special references to indigenous drug Kutaki (Picrorhiza kurroa) in the treatment of jaundice (Kamala Roga), D Ay M thesis, Varanasi, Banaras Hindu University, 1966. This is fine. It's a thesis submission and degree

20. R.A. Ansari, S.C.Tripathi, G.K. Patnaik, and B.N. Dhawan, "Antihepatotoxic properties of picroliv and other fractions from rhizome of Picrorhiza kurroa," *J Ethno-pharmacol*, 1991, 34:61–69.

21. D. Ralaram, "A preliminary trial of Picrorhiza kurroa in bronchial asthma," *Ind J Pharmac*, 1975, 7:95–96.

22. A. Russo, A.A. Izzo, V. Cardile, et al., "Indian medicinal plants as antiradicals and DNA cleavage protectors," *Phytomedicine*, 2001, 8:125-132.

23. R. Chander, N.K. Kapoor, and B.N. Dhawan, "Picroliv, picroside-I and kutkoside from Picrorhiza kurroa are scavengers of superoxide anions," *Biochem Pharmacol* 1992, 44:180–183.

24. R. Chander, N.K. Kapoor, and B.N. Dhawan, "Effect of picroliv on glutathione metabolism in liver and brain of Mastomys natalensis infected with Plasmodium berghei," *Indian J Exp Biol* 1992, 30:711–714.

25. R. Chander, K. Singh, P.K. Visen, et al., "Picroliv prevents oxidation in serum lipoprotein lipids of Mastomys coucha infected with Plasmodium berghei," *Indian J Exp Biol*, 1998,36:371–374.

26. V. Singh, N. K, Kapoor, and B.N. Dhawan, "Effect of picroliv on protein and nucleic acid synthesis," *Indian J Exp Biol*, 1992, 30:68–69.

27. See Note 10.

28. B. Shukla, P.K. Visen, G.K. Patnaik, et al., "Choleretic effect of picroliv, the hepatoprotective principle of Picrorhiza kurroa," *Planta Med*,1991,57:29–33.

29. P.K. Visen, B. Saraswat, and B.N. Dhawan, "Curative effect of picroliv on primary cultured rat hepatocytes against different hepatotoxins: An in vitro study," *J Pharmacol Toxicol Methods*, 1998, 40:173–179.

30. R. Rastogi, A.K. Srivastava, and A.K. Rastogi, "Biochemical changes induced in liver and serum aflatoxin B1-treated male Wistar rats: Preventive effect of picroliv," *Pharmacol Toxicol* 2001, 88:53–58.

31. B. Saraswat, P.K. Visen, G.K. Patnaik, and B.N. Dhawan, "Ex vivo and in vivo investigations of picroliv from Picrorhiza kurroa in an alcohol intoxication model in rats," *J Ethnopharmacol* 1999, 66:263–269.

32. A.K Singh, H. Mani, and P. Seth, "Picroliv preconditioning protects the rat liver against ischemia-reperfusion injury," *Eur J Pharmacol*, 2000, 395:229–239.

33. Y. Dwivedi, R. Rastogi, N.K. Garg, et al., "Effects of picroliv, the active principle of Picrorhiza kurroa, on biochemical changes in rat liver poisoned by Amanita phalloides," *Chung Kuo Yao Li Hsueh Pao*,1992,13:197–200.

34. J.P. Gaddipati, S. Madhavan, G.S. Sidhu, et al., Picroliv—a natural product protects cells and regulates the gene expression during hypoxia/reoxygenation," *Mol Cell Biochem*, 1999, 194:271–281.

35. A.B.Vaidya, D.S. Antarkar, J.C. Doshi, et al., "Picrorhiza kurroa (Kutaki) Royle ex Benth as a hepatoprotective agent experimental and clinical studies," *J Postgrad Med* 1996, 42:105–108

36. R. Mehrotra, S. Rawat, D.K. Kulshreshtha, et al., "In vitro studies on the effect of certain natural products against hepatitis B virus," *Indian J Med Res*, 1990, 92:133–138.

37. See Note 35

38. See Note 35

39. D. S, Antarkar, A.B. Vaidya, J.C. Doshi, A.V. Athavale, K. Vinchoo, M.R. Natekar, P.S. Tathed, R. Vijaya, N. Kale, et al. A double-blind chinical trial of Arogyawardhani: An Ayurvedic drug—in acute viral hepatitis," *Ind J Med Res*, 1980; 72:588.

40. A.B Vaidya, D.S. Antarkar, A.V. Athhavale, R. Vijaya, A.J. Baxi, and J.C. Doshi, "Treatment of acute viral hepatitis with Picrohiza kurroa," *Assn Phys Ind* (Abstracts), 1981.

41. W. Dorsch and H. Wagner, "New antiasthmatic drugs from traditional medicine?" *Int Arch Allergy Appl Immunol*, 1991,94:262–265.

42. C.C. Baruah, P.P. Gupta, A. Nath, et al., "Anti-allergic and anti-anaphylactic activity of picroliv—a standardised iridoid glycoside fraction of Picrorhiza kurroa," *Pharmacol Res,* 1998, 38:487–492.

43. Z.J. Guo, F.F. Hou, S.X. Liul, J.W. Tian, W.R. Zhang, D. Xie, A.M. Zhou, A.Q. Liu, and X. Zhang, "Picrorhiza scrophulariiflora improves accelerated atherosclerosis through inhibition of redox-sensitive inflammation," *Int J Cardiol.*, Aug. 21, 2009, 136(3):315–324.

44. L.J. He, M. Liang, F.F. Hou, Z.J., **check** and X. Zhang, "Ethanol extraction of Picrorhiza scrophulariiflora prevents renal injury in experimental diabetes via anti-inflammation action," *J Endocrinol.*, March 2009, 3:347–355.

45. P. Anand, A.B. Kunnumakkara, K.B. Harikumar, K.S. Ahn, V. Badmaev, and B.B., "Aggarwal modification of cysteine residue in p65 subunit of nuclear factor-kappaB (NF-kappaB) by picroliv suppresses NF-kappaB-regulated gene products and potentiates apoptosis," *Cancer Res.*, Nov. 1, 2008, 68(21):8861–8870.

46. See note 45

47. S. Zeng, D. Wang, Y. Cao, N. An, F. Zeng, C. Han, Y. Song, and X. Deng, "Immunopotentiation of caffeoyl glycoside from Picrorhiza scrophulariiflora on activation and cytokines secretion of immunocyte in vitro," *Int Immunopharmacol.*, Dec.10, 2008, 8(12):1707–1712.

48. J.X. Feng, H.Y. Li, Z.Q. Liu, Z.M. Zhou, J.W. Tian, and M. Liang, "Effect of the ethanol extract of Picrorhiza scrophulariiflora on the progression of chronic kidney disease in a rat remnant kidney model," *Nan Fang Yi Ke Da Xue Xue Bao*, July 2010, 30(7):1505–1508.

49. H.S. Lee and S.K. Ku, "Effect of Picrorrhiza rhizoma extracts on early diabetic nephropathy in streptozotocin-induced diabetic rats," *J Med Food*, June 2008, 11(2):294–301.

50. Council for Scientific and Industrial Research, *Annual Report* India: Regional Research Laboratory, 1989–1990).

Piper longum

Introduction

Piper longum, known in English as long pepper and by its Sanskrit name Pippli, is one of the most noted of all Ayurvedic herbs. It is highly prized for its therapeutic effect on the digestive system. Along with black pepper and ginger, Pippli is part of the famous Ayurvedic digestive formula known as Trikatu.

Ancient Ayurvedic texts list Pippli as one of the most powerful rasayana herbs, which means that it is a valuable enhancer of longevity. It also is considered to be a purifying herb, with soothing qualities that improve the quality of sleep. Ancient texts and contemporary studies point to the wide ranging effectiveness of Pippli in respiratory, liver, digestive, metabolic, parasitic, and malignant conditions.

Long pepper has long been used in medicine and as a culinary spice throughout the Indian sub-continent, Sri Lanka, Middle Eastern countries, and the Americas. It also is used in Europe and parts of Africa, where it was introduced by traders from India. It is said that the Roman emperors valued long pepper even more highly than black pepper.

The dried fruit spikes of Piper longum are widely used for flavoring a variety of foods. They are considered to have stimulant, carminative, laxative and stomachic properties. The berries are also given with honey for asthma, coughs and sore throats. The root is a stimulant and is also used in treating gout, rheumatism and lumbago. The whole plant is considered by tribal people in India to be useful in treating disorders of the spleen, cholera, dysentery, asthma, cough and bronchitis.

Synonymous Names

Latin: Piper longum
Sanskrit: Pippli
Hindi: Pippli
English: Long pepper, dried catkins

Habitat

Long pepper is native to southern Asia and is wild as well as cultivated throughout the hotter parts of India from central to the northeastern Himalayas. The herb also grows wild in Malaysia, Singapore, Bhutan, Myanmar, and elsewhere in tropical climate.

Botanical Characteristics

Piper longum is a slender, aromatic climbing vine with perennial woody roots. Its stems are jointed. Its leaves are ovate and cordate, with broad rounded lobes at the base, entire and glabrous. The flowers are cylindrical spikes; the male spikes are larger and more slender than the female spikes. The fruits are small, ovoid berries, shiny greenish black in color, and embedded in fleshy spikes.

Chemical Composition

Alkaloids and amides

The berries of Piper longum contain a large number of alkaloids and related compounds, the most abundant of which is the active element piperine. Also present are methyl piperine, pipernonaline, piperettine, asarinine, pellitorine, piperundecalidine, piperlongumine, piperlonguminine, retrofractamide A, pergumidiene, brachystamide-B, a dimer of desmethoxypiplartine, N-isobutyl-decadienamide, brachyamide-A, brachystine, pipercide, piperderidine, longamide, dehydropipernonaline piperidine and tetrahydropiperine. Piperine, piperlongumine, tetrahydropiperlongumine, trimethoxy cinnamyolpiperidine and piperlonguminine have been found in the root."[1]

Lignans

Sesamin, pulviatilol, fargesin, and others have been isolated from the fruits.[2,3,4,5]

Esters

The fruits contain tridecyl-dihydro-p-coumarate, eicosanyl-(E)-p-coumarate and Z-12-octadecenoic-glycerol-monoester.[6]

Volatile oil

The essential oil of the fruit is a complex mixture, the three major components of which are (excluding the volatile piperine) caryophyllene and pentadecane (both about 17.8%) and bisaboline (11%). Others include thujine, terpinoline, zingiberine, p-cymene, p-methoxyacetophenone and dihydrocarveol.[7,8]

Pharmacological Activity

Anti-cancer activity

The tumor-reducing activity of extracts of eight common spices, including Pippli, were studied in mice. Before administering the herbal extracts, the animals were transplanted intraperitoneally with tumorous tissue. The extracts of black pepper, asafoetida, Pippli, and garlic increased the lifespan in these mice by 64.7%, 52.9%, 47% and 41.1%, respectively. These results indicate the potential use of spices as anti-cancer agents as well as anti-tumor promoters.[9]

Immunomodulatory activity

Research has verified the immunostimulatory effects of Pippli.[10] Tests such as hemagglutination titer, macrophage migration index, and phagocytic index in mice have demonstrated the immunostimulatory action of Piper longum fruits to be both specific and non-specific. The effect was more prominent at lower doses (225 mg/kg) and was marginally reduced when the dose was increased. In another study, Piper longum offered protection against externally induced stress.[11] Pippli rasayana was tested in mice infected with Giardia lamblia. The herbal preparation produced significant activation of macrophages, as shown by an increased MMI and phagocytic activity.[12]

Stimulant effects

A petroleum ether extract antagonized pentobarbitone in anaesthetised dogs and morphine induced respiratory depression in mice.[13]

Isolated piperine showed a central stimulant action in frogs, mice, rats, and dogs and increased the hypnotic response in mice. It also antagonized respiratory depression induced by morphine or for effects against morphine-induced respiratory depression and analgesia. Both substances were found to reverse depression but, unlike nalorphine, piperine did not antagonize morphine-induced analgesia in rats.[14]

Anti-asthmatic activity

Studies have been carried out to validate the traditional claims of Ayurveda for Piper longum's anti-asthmatic activity. An extract of Long pepper fruits in milk reduced passive cutaneous anaphylaxis in rats, and protected guinea pigs against antigen induced bronchospasm.[15]

Bioavailability enhancement

Piperine has been shown to enhance the bioavailability of structurally and therapeutically diverse drugs, possibly by modulating membrane dynamics, because of its easy partitioning and increasing permeability.[16] The effect of Trikatu, a compound preparation in which Piper longum is a major ingredient, was tested in combination with other drugs. The results showed that Trikatu increased bioavailability either by promoting rapid absorption from the gastrointestinal tract or by protecting the drug from being metabolized during its first passage through the liver after being absorbed, or by a combination of both mechanisms.

Hepatoprotective activity

Studies have shown that Pippli inhibits liver fibrosis in animals. This provides support for the traditional use of Pippli in alcoholic liver disease and chronic hepatitis.

Piperine was evaluated and found to exert significant protection against tertiary butyl hydroperoxide and carbon tetrachloride-induced hepatotoxicity, by reducing both in vitro and in vivo lipid peroxidation. A fruit extract was assessed in rodents for its hepatoprotective action against CCL_4-induced acute, chronic and reversible damage and chronic irreversible damage, using morphological, biochemical and histopathological assessment parameters. The extract was shown to improve the regeneration process by restricting fibrosis, but offered no protection against acute damage or against cirrhotic changes.[18, 19]

Hypocholesterolemic activity

Methyl piperine significantly inhibited the elevation of total serum cholesterol, and the total cholesterol to HDL-cholesterol ratio in rats that were fed a high-cholesterol diet. The unsaponifiable fraction of the oil of Piper longum also significantly decreased total serum cholesterol and hepatic cholesterol in hypercholesterolemic mice.[20]

Anti-inflammatory activity

Pippli's anti-inflammatory and analgesic effects may be equal to that of Ibuprofen, according to one animal study.[21] Another study showed anti-inflammatory activity of a decoction of Piper longum fruits using carrageenan-induced rat edema.[22]

Anti-amoebic activity

Pippli has been shown to have anti-amoebic action against Entamoeba histolytica. Piper longum fruits were tested for their efficacy against Entamoeba histolytica in-vitro and experimental amoebiasis in vivo. Both the ethanolic extract and isolated piperine produced an improvement of 90% and 40% respectively, in rats with amoebiasis.[23]

Anti-bacterial activity

The essential oil of Piper longum showed anti-bacterial action against a number of bacterial strains, although a 50% ethanolic extract of the fruits did not show any effect. The active agent piperlonguminine was found to have potent activity against Bacillus subtilis, and piperine was more effective against Staphylococcus aures.[24, 25]

Anti-mutagenicity activity

Using Salmonella typhimurium strains TA 100 and TA 1535, the mutagenicity and anti-mutagenicity of extracts of several spices were checked. Spices including pepper, Pippli, ginger, and mustard increased the number of revertants, indicating their mutagenic potential. Conversely, garlic extract was found to inhibit the mutagenicity produced by direct acting mutagens such as N-methyl N'-nitro-N-nitrosoguanidine and sodium azide. Asafoetida and turmeric extract were found to inhibit microsomal activation dependent mutagenicity of 2-acetamidofluorene. Similar results were obtained using curcumin and eugenol, which are phenolics present in turmeric and clove, respectively. These results indicated that some of the spices may ameliorate the effect of environmental mutagens present in the food.[26]

Ethnoveterinary Usage

A decoction of the roots is given for swellings of the joints of cattle in the northwestern Himalayan regions.

Dr. Sodhi's Experience

Before treatment with Piper longum, the practitioner should consider the following:

- Is there hypochlorhydria?
- Is there parasitic condition?
- Are there food/environmental allergies?
- Is there a need to improve/enhance absorption of another medication, natural or synthetic?
- Is there a lack of IgA?
- Is there an upper respiratory infection?

Pippli is used in Ayurveda principally to enhance absorption of medications, facilitating transport throughout the body. It also is often used as a digestive adaptogen, or rasayana. Great success has been achieved in treating childhood asthma with Pippli in India. In some cases, the patients forget that they ever had the disease! For this reason, many believe that Pippli could be a promising new treatment for cystic fibrosis, a debilitating illness.

In Ayurveda, Pippli promotes what is known as pachaka pitta, or heat in the small intestines, with increased production of mucus. For individuals with low secretory IgA, Pippli can be especially helpful, increasing digestion and immunity while enhancing IgA secretion. Pippli also promotes full digestion of food without intermediate molecules such as fatty acids, disaccharides, and phenols. When foods are digested fully, there is less antigenic load on the body. This characteristic may account for Pippli's anti-allergic effects.

Pippli also is hepatoprotective and aids the absorption of prescription liver medications, reducing the amount of time necessary for them to become effective. It also may enhance absorption of steroids, making it possible to achieve equal effects with reduced doses.

Case Histories

Candidiasis

A 50-year old nurse from New York, diagnosed with systemic candidiasis, had been taking Hydrochloric acid and Nyastatin for one year with no significant improvement in her symptomology. We assessed her secretory IgA and found that she had none. We decided to use the following protocol:

For increased digestive fluids and medicinal absorption: Pippli extract, 1000 mg three times a day. We had her put the extract powder directly into hot water, as tasting it can stimulate the digestive process in the mouth.

For improved digestion and elimination:
Triphala (equal parts Terminalia chebula, Terminalia bellerica, and Emblica officinalis), 500 mg extract three times a day.

For fungal infection:
Azadirachta indica (Neem), 300 mg extract, in a proprietary blend of Emblica officinalis (amalaki), Terminalia chebula (haritaki), Terminalia bellerica (bahera), Tinospora

cordifolia (guduchi), and Rubia cordifolia (manjistha).

For maintenance of proper intestinal flora: 100 B mixed probiotic organisms, one three times per day

Protocols

For childhood asthma:

The success rate in treating childhood asthma with Pippli is so great in India that many patients forget they have the condition. The usual dose is 500–1000 mg Pippli extract, taken in honey. Depending upon the symptoms and the source of the allergy, the following herbs may be added:

When eosinophilic count is high, add Boswellia serrata (salai)

When toxic substances or environmental pollutants, such as insecticides, plastics exposure, etc. are triggering the symptoms, add Curcumin (Curcuma).

For upper respiratory infections:

Pippli extract, 500 mg, along with a combination immune support formulation such as 200 mg each of Emblica officinalis (amalaki), Ocinum sanctum (tulsi), Terminalia bellerica (bibhihtaki), with 100 mg. each Tinospora cordifolia (guduchi), and Glycyrrhiza glabra (yastsimadhu), plus 50 mg each Terminalia chebula (haritaki) and Adhatoda vasica (vasaka).

For decreased white blood cell count:

Use 500 mg Pippli, Withania somnifera (ashwagandha), and/or Bacopa monniera (indriay brahmi) extracts. For patients on chemotherapy, these herbs will increase immune response. For deficiencies in white blood cell count in the following circumstances, use the following protocols:

Chemotherapy: Withania somnifera (ashwagandha)

Upper respiratory infection: Pippli

Nervous system weakness, multiple sclerosis: Bacopa monniera

Insufficient secretory IgA: Pippli

To prevent influenza:

Take 500 mg Pippli with an immune support formula such as 200 mg each Emblica officinalis (amalakiki), Ocinum sanctum (tulsi), Terminalia bellerica (bibhihtaki), with 100 mg. each Tinospora cordifolia (guduchi), and Glycyrrhiza glabra (yastsimadhu), plus 50 mg each Terminalia chebula (haritaki), and Adhatoda vasica (vasaka) herbal extracts throughout the season.

For lung weakness and COPD:

Take Pippli with amla, 500 mg extract of each.

For gastrintestinal disturbances, including flatulence, bloating, irregular bowel movements, and constipation:

Take Pippli with triphala, i.e. equal parts Terminalia chebula (haritaki), Terminalia bellerica (bibhitaki), Emblica officinalis (amalaki).

For parasitic infections:

Take Pippli with Asparagus racemosus (shataavari), and an antiparasitic formulation such as: Azadirachta indica (Neem), Embelia ribes (vidang), Piper longum (Pippli), Aegle marmelos (bilva), Mormordica charantia (kaviilak), Berberis aristata (daaruhaldi), Holarrhena antidysenterica (kutaj), Ocimum santum (tulsi) in a base of 15 mg magnesium malate.

For dyspepsia and gastric inflammation:

Take Pippli with Curcumin longum (Curcuma).

For heliobacter pylori:

500 mg Asparagus racemosus (shataavari), 500 mg of an antiparasitic formulation: Azadirachta indica (Neem), Embelia ribes (vidang), Piper longum (Pippli), Aegle marmelos (bilva), Momordica charantia (karela), Berberis aristata (daaruhaldi), Holarrhena antidysenterica (kutaj), Ocimum santum (tulsi) in

a base of 15 mg magnesium malate. Take for 3 to 4 months with a probiotic, 10 billion mixed organisms.

For food allergies:

500 mg Pippli with food for 2 months, then switch to Curcumin (Curcuma) or an immune support formulation, 500 mg three times a day for 2 months.

For hypochlorhydria:

Pippli 500 mg before each meal for 2 to 3 months, with or without trikatu (equal parts Piper longum, Piper nigrum, Zingiber officinale).

For severe hypochlorhydria, or if you are allergic to many foods, Pippli vardhman (vardh, meaning "increase," man meaning "measure") is often helpful. The dose of Pippli is increased gradually in increments each day for 40 days, then decreased in reverse order in the same increments for another 40 days::

Days	MG	Days	MG
1 + 80	500	21 + 60	10500
2 + 79	1000	22 + 59	11000
3 + 78	1500	23 + 58	11500
4 + 77	2000	24 + 57	12000
5 + 76	2500	25 + 56	12500
6 + 75	3000	26 + 55	13000
7 + 74	3500	27 + 54	13500
8 + 73	4000	28 + 53	14000
9 + 72	4500	29 + 52	14500
10 + 71	5000	30 + 51	15000
11 + 70	5500	31 + 50	15500
12 + 69	6000	32 + 48	16000
13 + 68	6500	33 + 48	16500
14 + 67	7000	34 + 47	17000
15 + 66	7500	35 + 46	17500
16 + 65	8000	36 + 45	18000
17 + 64	8500	37 + 44	18500
18 + 63	9000	38 + 43	19000
19 + 62	9500	39 + 42	19500
20 + 61	10000	40 + 41	20000

Safety Profile

Pippli should not be used for long periods of time as it can cause kapha aggravation, leading to excess mucous production, or pitta aggravation, creating extra heat in the body. To avoid these side-effects, Pippli may be used for months, and then repeated after a few months of rest. Because of its heating nature, it should be used with caution in inflammatory diseases such as ulcerative colitis.

Piper longum is used widely in cooking and traditional medicine, so it is generally assumed to be safe in moderate doses. However, as the fruits are reported to have contraceptive activity in experimental models, its use during pregnancy and lactation should be avoided.

Piperine may interfere with enzymatic drug biotransformations, resulting in the inhibition of hepatic arylhydrocarbon hydroxylase and UDP glucuronyltransferase, and may alter the pharmacokinetic parameters of barbiturates and phenytoin. A single oral dose of 3 g/kg body weight in experimental animals, and chronic toxicity studies with 100 mg/kg body weight for 90 days, revealed no undesirable effects.[26, 27]

In the evaluation of anti-fertility activity, long pepper at a dose of 1 g/kg body weight was found to be an effective contraceptive agent without toxic or teratogenic effects.[29]

Dosage

Powdered fruits and roots: 500 milligram to 1 gram

Extract 5:1 100 -200 mg per day

Ayurvedic Properties

Rasa: Katu (pungent)
Guna: Laghu (light), snigdha (unctuous), tikshna (sharp)
Veerya: Anushnashita (slight hot)
Vipaka: Madhur (sweet)
Dosha: Pacifies kapha and vata

Notes

1. V.S. Parmar, S.C. Jain, S. Gupta, et al., "Polyphenols and alkaloids from *Piper* species," *Phytochemistry* 1998, 49(4):1069.
2. W. Tabuneng, H. Bando, and T. Amiya, " Studies on the constituents of the crude drug Piper Longi Fructus," *Chemical and Pharmaceutical Bulletin*, 1983, 31(10):35–62.
3. N.B. Shankaracharya, L.J. Rao, J.P. Naik, and S. Nagalakshmi, "Characterization of chemical constituents of Indian Long Peper *(Piper longum* L.)," *Journal of Food Science and Technology*, 1997, 34(1):73.
4. R. K Sharma, Y.K.S. Rathore, and S. Kumar, "Chemical examination of dried fruits of Pippli (*Piper longum* Linn)," *Journal of Scientific Research into Plant Medicines*, 1983, 4(4):63.
5. C.K. Atal, R.N. Girotra, and K.L. Dhar, ":Occurrence of sesamin in *Piper longum* Linn.," *Indian Journal of Chemistry*, 1966, 4:252.
6. B. Das, A. Kashinathan, and P. Madhusudhan, "Long chain esters and alkamides from *Piper longum*," *Bolletino Chimico Farmaceutico*,1998, 137(8):319.
7. S. S. Nigam and C. Radhakrishnan, "Chemical examination of the essential oil derived from the berries *of Piper longum*," *Bulletin of the National Institute of Science of India*, 1968, 37:189.
8. K.L. Handa, M.L. Sharma, and N.C. Nigam, "The essential oil *of Piper longum*, properties of the components and isolation of two monocyclic sesquiterpenes," *Parfume Kosmetik*, 1963, 44(9):233.
9. M.C. Unnikrishnan and R. Kuttan, "Tumor-reducing and anticarcinogenic activity of selected spices," *Cancer Lett.*, May 1990, 15;51(1):85–89.
10. D. M Tripathi, N. Gupta, V. Lakshmi, K.C. Saxena, and A.K. Agarwal, "Antigiardial and immunostimulatory effect *of Piper longum* on giardiasis due to *Giardia lamblia*," *Phytotherapy Research*, 1999, 13(7):561.
11. N. N. Rege, U.M. Thatte, and S.A. Dhanukar, "Adaptogenic properties of six rasayana herbs used in Ayurvedic medicines," *Phytotherapy Research*, 1999, 13(4):275.
12. A.K. Agarwal, M. Singh, N. Gupta, et al., "Management of giardiasis by an immunomodulatory herbal drug 'Pippli Rasayana', *Journal of Ethnopharmacology*, 1994, 44(3): 143.

13. N. Singh, V.K. Kulshreshta, R.K. Srivastava, and R.P. Kohli, "Analeptic activity of some *Piper longum* alkaloids," *Journal of Research into Indian Medicine*, 1973, 8(1):1.

14. Singh, N., V.K. Kulshrestha, R.K. Srivastava, R.P. Kohli A comparative evaluation of piperine and nalorphine against morphine induced respiratory depression and analgesia. JRIM 1973: 8, 4, 21—26.

15. S. A. Dhanukar, A. Zha, and S.M. Karandikar, "Antiallergic activity *of Piper longum*," *Indian Journal of Pharmacology*, 1981, 13:122.

16. C.K Atal, U. Zutshi, and P.G. Rao, "Scientific evidence on the role of Ayurvedic herbals on bioavailability of drugs," *Journal of Ethnopharmacology*, 1981, 4(2):229.

17. Kumar S, Kamboj J, Suman, Sharma S. Overview for various aspects of the health benefits of Piper longum linn. fruit. J Acupunct Meridian Stud. 2011 Jun;4(2):134-40.

18. I. B Koul and A. Kapil, "Evaluation of the hepatoprotective potential of piperine, an active principle of black and long peppers," *Planta Medica*, 1993, 59(5):413.

19. N. Rege, S. Dhanukar, and S.M. Karandikar, "Hepatoprotective effects of P. *longum* against carbon tetrachloride induced liver damage, *Indian Drugs*, 1984, 21:569.

20. Y. Li, H. Wang, E. Wu, and W. Su, "Effect of methyl piperate on rat serum cholesterol level and its mechanism of action," *Zhonggacayao*, 1993, 24(1):27.

21. Venkatesh S, Durga KD, Padmavathi Y, Reddy BM, Mullangi R. Influence of piperine on ibuprofen induced antinociception and its pharmacokinetics. Arzneimittelforschung. 2011;61(9):506-9.

22. Mujumdar AM, Dhuley JN, Deshmukh VK, Raman PH, Naik SR. Anti-inflammatory activity of piperine. Jpn J Med Sci Biol. 1990 Jun;43(3):95-100.

23. S. Ghosal, K. Prasad, and V. Lakshmi, "Anti-amoebic activity *of Piper longum* against *Entamoeba histolytica in vitro* and *in vivo,*" *Journal of Ethnopharmacology*, 1996, 50(3):167.

24. R.H. Singh, K.L. Khosa, and B.B. Upadhyaya, "Anti-bacterial activity of some Ayurvedic drugs," *Journal of Research into Indian Medicine*, 1974, 9(2):65.

25. Kumar A, Khan IA, Koul S, Koul JL, Taneja SC, Ali I, Ali F, Sharma S, Mirza ZM, Kumar M, Sangwan PL, Gupta P, Thota N, Qazi GN. Novel structural analogues of piperine as inhibitors of the NorA efflux pump of Staphylococcus aureus. J Antimicrob Chemother. 2008 Jun;61(6):1270-6

26. Soudamini KK, Unnikrishnan MC, Sukumaran K, Kuttan R. Mutagenicity and anti-mutagenicity of selected spices. Indian J Physiol Pharmacol. 1995 Oct;39(4):347-53.

27. C.K Atal, R.K. Dubey, and J. Singh, "Biochemical basis of enhanced drugs bio-availability by piperine: Evidence that piperine is a potent inhibitor of monoxygenase system," *Indian Journal of Pharmacology*, 1984, 16:52.

28. A.H Shah, A.H. Al-Shareef, A.M. Ageel, and S. Qureshi, "Toxicity studies in mice of common spices, *Cinnamomum zeylanicum* bark and *Piper longum* fruits," *Plant Foods and Human Nutrition*, 1998, 52(3):231.

29. P.C. Das, A.K. Sarkar, and S. Thakur, ":Studies on animals of a herbo-mineral compound for long acting contraception," *Fitoterapia*, 1987, 58(4):257.

33

Piper nigrum

Introduction

Piper nigrum is a flowering vine in the family Piperaceae, universally valued for its fruit, which usually is dried and used as a spice and seasoning. In Ayurveda, Piper nigrum is an important healing spice, and along with Long pepper and ginger, is a component of the preparation Trikatu, renowned for its ability to enhance the bioavailability and efficacy of other medicines.[1]

Piper nigrum is native to India and has been used as an ingredient in Indian cooking since at least 2000 BC. In modern Ayurveda, Piper nigrum is used to treat digestive disorders, because of its anti-inflammatory, antimicrobial and anti-spasmodic properties. Used externally, Piper nigrum helps to alleviate neuralgia, scabies, piles, and various skin disorders. It is used as an aromatic stimulant in treating cholera, to relieve weakness following fevers, for vertigo, and as an antiperiodic for malaria and arthritic disease. Piper nigrum also possesses cleansing and anti-oxidant properties, enhancing oxygen flow to the brain, aiding digestion and circulation, stimulating the appetite, and maintaining respiratory and joint health.

Ancient texts as early as the Fifth Century describe Piper nigrum as an antidote for constipation, diarrhea, earache, gangrene, heart disease, hernia, hoarseness, indigestion, insect bite, insomnia, joint pain, liver problems, lung disease, oral abscess, sunburn, and toothache.[2] In Chinese medicine, Piper nigrum is used to improve the appetite and to treat colds, influenza, abdominal pain, diarrhea, and epilepsy.

The alkaloid piperine is the chemical constituent responsible for Piper nigrum's spiciness. In its dried form, the fruit is referred to as a peppercorn. The widely-used spice black pepper is produced from the still-green unripe berries of Piper nigrum.

Synonymous Names

English: Black pepper
Hindi: Golmirch, kalimirch
Sanskrit: Maricha
Tamil: Milagu
Kannada: MeNasu
Malayalam: Kuru Mulaku
Telugu: Miriyam
Konkani: Miriya Konu

Habitat

Although Piper nigrum is native to southern Thailand and Malaysia, its most important habitat is the tropical regions of India, particularly the Malabar Coast.[3] Piper nigrum is cultivated in many areas, including Sri Lanka, China, and parts of Africa.

Black pepper grows best in moist, well-drained soil that is rich in organic matter.

Botanical Characteristics

Piper nigrum is a perennial woody vine that spreads over trees, or on poles or trellises for support. Wherever the vine's stout, trailing stems touch the ground, new roots are readily formed. The plant grows to an average height of 12 feet (4 meters). Its pale green leaves are glossy and about 12 cm in length and 8 cm wide.

The small flowers appear in its leaf nodes on spikes that lengthen as the fruit matures. The female flower bears two anthers, and the male a single pistil. The fruit is a small, dark red berry about 5 mm in diameter, containing a single round seed, which is white and hollow. In its dried form, Piper nigrum's berry is the aromatic, pungent black peppercorn.

Cultivation

The Piper nigrum vine is propagated using cuttings about 40 to 50 cm in length, which are tied to trees, poles, or trellises at intervals of about 6 feet (2 meters). Trees with rough bark provide the best support for the climbing vine. For cultivation of Piper nigrum, competing undergrowth is cleared away, leaving only enough trees to provide shade and adequate ventilation.

Piper nigrum plants bear fruit beginning in the fourth or fifth year, and typically continue to bear fruit for 7 years. A single plant will bear 20 to 30 fruiting spikes. The fruit is harvested when the majority of the berries are full-grown and hard, but still mostly green. If the berries are allowed to ripen on the vine, they lose pungency. For harvesting, the spikes are collected and allowed to dry, then the peppercorns are stripped off the spikes.

Chemical Composition

Following are the chemical constituents of Piper nigrum:[4,5,6,7,8,9]

Volatile oil: A number of volatile oils, including sabinene (15-25%), caryophyllene, a-pinene, p-pinene, 3-ocimene, 8-guaiene, farnesol, 8-cadinol, guaiacol, 1-phellandrene, 1,8 cineole, p-cymene, carvone, citronellol, cc-thujene, cc-terpinene, bisabolene, dl-limonene, dihydrocarveol, camphene, and piperonal, have been isolated from Piper nigrum's dried fruits.

Alkaloids and amides: Alkaloids and amides are the main pungent principles of Piper nigrum. Piperine, piperylin, piperolein A and B, cumaperine, piperanine, piperamides, pipericide, guineensine, and sarmentine have been identified as the principle alkaloids. Others include chavicine, piperidine and piperettine, methyl caffeic acid, piperidide, (3-methyl pyrroline, and a series of vinyl homologues of piperine and their stereoisomers.

Amino acids: Dried peppercorns are rich in p-alanine, arginine, serine, threonine, histidine, lysine, cystine, asparagines, and glutamic acid, in combination with y-aminobutyric acid and pipecolic acid.

Vitamins and minerals: Piper nigrum is rich in vitamins and minerals including ascorbic acid, carotenes, thiamine, riboflavin, and nicotinic acid, as well as the minerals potassium, sodium, calcium, magnesium, iron, phosphorus, copper, and zinc.

Pharmacological Activity

Anti-cancer activity

Investigation into Piper nigrum's anti-cancer effects has yielded encouraging results, especially in experimental colon cancer. Ingestion of Piper nigrum caused increased activity of p-glucuronidase in the distal colon, and mucinase levels in the colon and feces were decreased to near normal. Researchers hypothesized that Piper nigrum may inhibit hydrolysis of glucuronide conjugates, causing toxins to be freed and mucinase to be degraded. This activity may protect against hydrolysis of protective mucins in the colon.[10]

In research using Swiss albino mice, the alkaloid piperine was evaluated for its effect on the mitochondrial tricarboxylic acid cycle and phase I and glutathione-metabolizing enzymes in chemically induced lung carcinogenesis. Treatment with piperine caused significant decreases in the activities of the mitochondrial enzymes isocitrate dehydrogenase, ketoglutarate dehydrogenase, succinate dehydrogenase, and malate dehydrogenase in cancerous lung tissue, and significantly increased NADPH cytochrome reductase, cytochrome P450 (cytp450), and cytochrome b5(cyt-b5). These results indicate that piperine may enhance and increase mitochondrial energy production.[11]

Over-expression of P-glycoprotein, multidrug resistance protein 1(MRP1) and breast cancer resistance protein (BCRP) in tumor cells is one of the important mechanisms leading to multidrug resistance (MDR), which impairs the efficacy of chemotherapy. P-glycoprotein, MRP1 and BCRP are ABC (ATP-Binding Cassette) transporters, which can expel a variety of lipophilic anti-cancer drugs and protect tumor cells. Piperine can potentiate the cytotoxicity of anti-cancer drugs in resistant sublines, such as MCF-7/DOX and A-549/DDP. Piperine reverses the resistance to doxorubicin many folds. It also re-sensitized cells to mitoxantrone 6.98 folds. The combination of mitoxantrone and prednisone is used as a second-line treatment for metastatic hormone-refractory prostate cancer. Piperine can reverse multidrug resistance protein by multiple mechanisms.[12]

Phosphatidylinositol 3-kinases (PI 3K), protein kinase (AKT), mammalian target of rapamycin (mTOR), rRibosomal protein S6 kinase beta-1 (S6K1), and mitogen activated protein kinase (MAPK), signaling that cascades play an important role in cell proliferation, survival, angiogenesis, and metastasis of tumor cells. β-caryophyllene oxide, a isolated from essential oils from guava (Psidium guajava), oregano (Origanum vulgare), cinnamon (Cinnamomum spp.), clove (Eugenia caryophyllata), and black pepper (Piper nigrum.) inhibited the PI3K/ AKT/mTOR/S6K1 and MAPK activation pathways in human prostate and breast cancer cells. Not only did beta-caryophyllene oxide inhibit the constitutive activation of PI3K/AKT/mTOR/S6K1 signaling cascade; but also caused the activation of extracellular-signal-regulated kinases (ERK), c-Jun amino-terminal kinases (JNK), and P38 mitogen-activated protein kinases (p38 MAPK in tumor cells).[13]

β-caryophyllene oxide increased reactive oxygen species (ROS) generation from mitochondria, which is associated with the induction of apoptosis as characterized by positive Annexin V binding and TUNEL staining, loss of mitochondrial membrane potential, release of cytochrome c, activation of caspase-3, and cleavage of PARP. Inhibition of ROS generation by N-acetylcysteine (NAC) significantly prevented β-caryophyllene oxide -induced apoptosis. Subsequently, β-caryophyllene oxide also down-regulated the expression of various downstream gene products that mediate cell proliferation (cyclin D1), survival (bcl-2, bcl-xL, survivin, IAP-1, and IAP-2), metastasis (COX-2), angiogenesis (VEGF), and increased the expression of p53 and p21.

β-caryophyllene oxide can significantly potentiate the apoptotic effects of various pharmacological PI3K/AKT inhibitors when employed in combination in tumor cells. Overall, these findings suggest that β-caryophyllene oxide can interfere with multiple signaling cascades involved in tumorigenesis and can be used as a potential therapeutic candidate for both the prevention and the treatment of cancer.[13]

The synergistic administration of piperine and docetaxel significantly improved the anti-tumor efficacy of docetaxel in a xenograft model of human castration-resistant prostate cancer. Docetaxel is the treatment approved by the FDA for castration resistant prostate cancer, yet its administration only increases median survival by only 2--4 months. Docetaxel is metabolized in the liver by hepatic CYP3A4 activity. Piperine inhibits the CYP3A4 enzymatic activity and increases docetaxel efficacy.[14]

Piperine inhibited the lung metastasis induced by B16F-10 melanoma cells in C57BL/6 mice. Simultaneous administration of the piperine with tumor induction produced a significant reduction (95.2%) in tumor nodule formation.[15]

Antimicrobial activity

Piper nigrum has been shown to be effective against a variety of common microbes. Extracts of the plant inhibited aflatoxin production in cultures of Aspergillus parasticus.[16]

Both the ethanol and the aqueous extracts of the dried fruits of Piper nigrum were found to have significant activity against a penicillin G-resistant strain of Staphylococcus aureus. The extracts also were toxic to cultures of Escherichia coli, Staphylococcus fecalis, Staphylococcus albus, Corynebacterium diphtheria, Salmonella dysenteriae, and Salmonella sonnei. Piper nigrum's volatile oil also exhibited significant antimicrobial activity against animal pathogens and various organisms responsible for food poisoning.[17,18,19]

Enhanced Bioavailability

Piperine has been shown to enhance bioavailability by increasing the permeability of intestinal cells. As a result, absorption of nutrients in the intestines is increased. Piperine enhanced the oral bioavailability of carbamazepine, phenytoin, propranolol, rifampicin, and theophylline, possibly by decreasing the elimination and/or by increasing its absorption.[20,21,22]

This action is believed to be the result of increased lipid peroxidation and the stimulation of γ-glutamyl transpeptidase enzyme activity. An aqueous extract of Piper nigrum increased acid secretion in anesthetized rats, an action believed to be the result of cholinergic activity.[23]

A Study in Gaddi goats, Trikatu (a combination of piper nigrum, piper longum and zingiber officinalis) showed significant reduction the elimination half-life of pefloxacin, belonging to the 3rd generation of quinolones, suggesting better penetration of the drug.[24]

In another study, piperine, isolated from Piper nigrum significantly enhanced the bioavailability of beta lactam antibiotics, amoxicillin trihydrate, and cefotaxime sodium significantly in rats. The improved bioavailability is reflected in various pharmacokinetic parameters.[25]

Trikatu has been shown to enhance the bioavailability of drugs like such as vasicine and indomethacin. But Trikatu significantly decreased the serum levels of diclofenac sodium, but the anti-inflammatory effects of the combination was more than diclofenac sodium alone.[26]

Anti-convulsant activity

Piperine was assessed for its effectiveness as an anticonvulsant. The alkaloid and its derivatives interfered with laboratory-induced convulsive activity in animals. In additional research, piperine reduced convulsions produced by intra-cerebroventricular injections of kainite.[27]

Thermogenic activity

Animal studies have demonstrated Piperine to be an effective thermogenic agent. Piperine caused increased oxygen uptake when administered to the perfused hind limbs of experimental rats. For purposes of the study, vascular resistance of oxygen uptake was blocked by glyceryl nitrate.[28]

Hepatoprotective activity

Piper nigrum was shown to stimulate the production of various detoxification enzymes, including glutathione S-transferase, cytochrome b5, cytochrome P450, acid-soluble sulfhydryl content, and malondialdehyde, in a dose-dependent manner.

Piperine protected the liver against the toxic effects of tert-butyl hydroperoxide and carbon tetrachloride by reducing lipid peroxidation, preventing enzymatic leakage of GPT and AP, and inhibiting GSH depletion and total thiols.[29]

Anti-oxidant activity

Piper nigrum's rich content of phenolic amides makes it an excellent anti-oxidant. The herb's anti-oxidant properties exceed those of a-tocopherol and are roughly the same as the synthetic anti-oxidants butylatedhydroyanisole (BHA) and butylated droxytoluene (BHT).[30]

Anti-inflammatory activity

Piperine depresses the acute inflammatory process, possibly by stimulating the pituitary adrenal axis. In laboratory models of inflammation including carrageenan-induced paw edema and cotton pellet and croton oil-induced granuloma pouch, piperine exhibited significant anti-inflammatory activity.[31]

Cognitive function activity

The effect of piperine on the central nervous system has been investigated with encouraging results. Male Wistar rats were administered piperine at a variety of doses ranging from 5, 10, and 20 mg/kg body weight daily for a 4-week period. The animals were evaluated for neuropharmacological changes on a weekly basis. Piperine showed anti-depression activity at all dosages evaluated, indicating that Piper nigrum may have potential in improving cognitive function.[32]

Anti-spasmodic activity

A research investigation was conducted to assess the anti-spasmodic effects of an aqueous extract of Piper nigrum on animal tissue. The extract reduced the contractions of rat ileum tissue induced by KCl or carbachol in a dose-dependent manner. The extract's spasmolytic effect was not attenuated by either glibenclamide or tetraethylammonium, suggesting that the effect was possibly mediated via Ca2+ influx.[33]

Antihypertensive action

Intravenous administration of piperine caused a dose-dependent (1 to 10 mg/kg) decrease in mean arterial pressure in normotensive anesthetized rats. The next higher dose (30 mg/kg) did not cause any further change in mean arterial pressure. In Langendorrf's rabbit heart preparation, piperine caused partial inhibition where as verapamil caused complete inhibition of force and rate of ventricular contractions and coronary flow. Piperine was shown to be a Ca2+ channel blocker. In the rat aorta, piperine demonstrated an endothelium independent vasodilator effect and was more potent against high K+ precontractions than phenylephrine, again suggesting that piperine. In bovine coronary artery preparations, piperine inhibited high K+ precontractions completely. All these finding suggests that piperine possesses a blood pressure-lowering effect mediated possibly through calcium channel blockers.[34]

Ethnoveterinary Usage

The dried fruit of Piper nigrum is used in veterinary medicine to treat respiratory conditions in ruminants, and as a galactogogue, increasing milk production.

It also is useful in cases of placental retention in swine, and in the treatment of fowl pox. Also, in combination with other herbs, Piper nigrum is used in treating mastitis, fever, bloat, diarrhea, and foot-and-mouth disease in animals.[35, 36]

Dr. Sodhi's Experience

Questions to consider when using Piper nigrum:
- Is digestion is weak?
- Is hydrochloric acid low in the stomach?
- Do you need to stimulate thermogenesis?
- Is bioavailability enhancing needed?
- Do you need to enhance detoxification?

Piper nigrum alone or in combination with piper longum and Zingiber officinalis, called Trikatu, is used to stimulate digestive juices. You will start the treatment with 1/8 teaspoon powder, taken with warm water before every meals. Then the dose is slowly increased to ¼ teaspoon, then ½ teaspoon, ¾ teaspoon, and one teaspoon, increasing in increments of ¼ teaspoon. This is repeated until you start to feel a burning sensation in the stomach. At this is stage, you start the reversed order. The protocol is very helpful in when digestion is weak, suffering with low hydrochloric acid in the stomach, as well as thermogenesis and detoxification.

Safety Profile

The safety of Piper nigrum is well-established because of its widespread use for many centuries as a culinary spice. As a caution, nursing women should avoid excess amounts of Piper nigrum, because metabolites of the spice are excreted into breast milk.

Piper nigrum will enhance the effects of carbamazepine, phenytoin , propranolol, rifampicin, and theophylline. The piperine constituent of pepper seems to inhibit p-glycoprotein in- vitro. Drugs that might be affected include some chemotherapeutic agents (etoposide, paclitaxel, vinblastine, vincristine, vindesine), antifungals (ketoconazole, itraconazole), protease inhibitors (amprenavir, indinavir, nelfinavir, saquinavir), H2 antagonists (cimetidine, ranitidine), some calcium channel blockers (diltiazem, verapamil), digoxin, corticosteroids, erythromycin, cisapride (Propulsid), fexofenadine (Allegra), cyclosporine, loperamide (Imodium), and quinidine.[37]

Piper nigrum will enhance the effects of carbamazepine, phenytoin , propranolol, rifampicin and theophylline.

The plant also is a known enzyme inducer. And it may reduce blood levels of some medications, if consumed in large amounts over a long period of time.

Dosage

Dried fruit: 300–600 mg
Oleoresin: 15–20 mg

Ayurvedic Properties

Piper nigrum is considered to be a warming spice in Ayurveda, contributing a pungent taste. It is excellent for pacifying kapha and vata and increases pitta.
Rasa: Katu (pungent)
Guna: Laghu (light), tikshna (sharp)
Veerya: Ushna (hot)
Vipaka: Katu (pungent)
Dosha: Pacifies vata and pitta

Notes

1. R.K. Johri and RK,U. Zutshi, U 1992" An Ayurvedic formulation Trikatu and its constituents.," *Journal of Ethnopharmacology*, 1992, 37(2):85.

2. J. Turner, *Jack (2004).Spice: The History of a Temptation* (City: . Vintage Books, 2004), .p. 171.

3. J. Innes Miller, *The Spice Trade of the Roman Empire* (Oxford: Clarendon Press, 1969), p. 80.

4. I.P. Kapoor IP, B. Singh B, G. Singh G, C.S. De Heluani CS, M.P. De Lampasona MP, and C.A. Catalan CA, " Chemistry and in vitro anti-oxidant activity of volatile oil and oleoresins of black pepper (Piper nigrum)," . *Journal of Agriculture Food Chemistry*,. 2009; June 24, 2009, 24;57(12): 5358--5364.

5. Z. Lin Z, J.R. Hoult JR, D.C. Bennett DC, and A. Raman, "A1999 sStimulation of mouse melanocyte proliferation by Piper nigrum fruit extract and its main alkaloids, pPiperine,". *Planta Medica*, 1999, 65(7):600.

6. U. Topal U, M. Sasaki M, M. Goto M, and S. Otles, S. "Chemical composition and anti-oxidant properties of Essentila oil from nine species of Turkish plants obtained by supercritical carbon dioxide extraction and steam distillation," .*International Journal of Food Science and Nutrition*,. Nov–Dec 2008 Nov-Dec;; 59(7--8);, 619--634.

7. E.M. Williamson EM,and F.J. Evans, *FJ 1988 Potter's Nnew Ccyclopedia of Bbotanical Ddrugs and Ppreparations* . (City: Publisher: CW Daniel, Saffron Walden, 1988).

8. N. Nakatani N, R. Inatani R, H. Ohta H, and A. Nishioka, " A1986 Chemical constituents of pPeppers (Piper spp.) and application to food preservation: Nnaturally occurring antioxidative compounds," . *Environmental Health Perspectives*, 1986, 67:135.

9. I. Lavilla I, A.V. Filgueiras, and C. AV, Bendicho, "C 1999 Comparison of digestion of trace and minor metals in plant samples,". *Journal of Agricultural and Food Chemistry*, 1999, 47(12):5072. 50–72?

10. N. Nalini N, K. Sabitha K, P. Viswanathan P, and V.P. Menon VP, "1998 Influence of spices on the bacterial (enzyme) activity in experimental colon cancer,". *Journal of Ethnopharmacology*, 1998, 62(1):15.

11. K. Selvendiran K, C. Thirunavukkarasu C, J.P. Singh JP, R. Padmavathi R, and D. SakthisekaranD, ".Chemopreventive effect of piperine on mitochondrial TCA cycle and phase-I and glutathione-metabolizing enzymes in benzo(a) pyrene induced lung carcinogenesis in Swiss albino mice," *Mol Cell Biochem*,. March 2005, Mar;271(1--2):101--106.

12. S. Li S, Y. Lei Y, Y. Jia Y, N. Li N, M. Wink M, and Y. Ma Y, "Piperine, a piperidine alkaloid from Piper nigrum re-sensitizes P-gp, MRP1 and BCRP dependent multidrug resistant cancer cells," *Phytomedicine*,. Dec. 15, 2011 Dec 15;, 19(1):83--87.

13. K.R. Park KR, D. Nam, H.M. D, Yun HM, S.G. Lee SG, H.J. Jang HJ, G. Sethi G, S.K. Cho SK, and K.S. Ahn KS, "β-Caryophyllene oxide inhibits growth and induces apoptosis through the suppression of PI3K/AKT/mTOR/S6K1 pathways and ROS-mediated MAPKs activation," .*Cancer Lett.*, Dec 22, 2011 Dec 22, ;312(2):178--188.

14. P. Makhov P, K. Golovine K, D. Canter D, A. Kutikov A, J. Simhan, J, M.M. Corleww MM, R.G. Uzzo RG, and V.M. Kolenko VM, "Co-administration of piperine and docetaxel results in improved anti-tumor efficacy via inhibition of CYP3A4 activity," .*Prostate.*, July 17, 2011 Jul 27.

15. C.R. Pradeep CR and, G. Kuttan G, "Effect of piperine on the inhibition of lung metastasis induced B16F-10 melanoma cells in mice," .*Clin Exp Metastasis*,. 2002, ;19(8):703--708.

16. H.J. Dorman and S.G.HJ, Deans, " SG 2000 Antimicrobial agents from plants: Anti-bacterial activity of plant volatile oils,." *Journal of Applied Microbiology*, 2000, 88(2):308.

17. S.R. Jain and A SR, Kar, " A1971 Anti-bacterial activity of some essential oils and their combinations,". *Planta Medica*, 1971, 20:118.

18. C.S.S. Rao and S.S.CSS, Nigam SS, "1976 Antimicrobial activity of some Indian essential oils," . *Indian Drugs*, 1976, 14:62.

19. S.R. Jain SR and M.R. Jain, " MR 1972 Antifungal studies on some indigenous volatile oils and their combinations," .*Planta Medica* , 1972, 22:136.

20. S. Pattanaik S, D. Hota D, S. Prabhakar S, P. Kharbanda P, and P. Pandhi P, "Pharmacokinetic interaction of single dose of piperine with steady-state carbamazepine in epilepsy patients," .*Phytother Res.*, Sept. 2009, Sep;23(9):1281--1286.

21. R.K. Bhardwa, H. j RK, Glaeser, L. H, Becquemont, U. L, Klotz, U, S.K. Gupta SK, and M.F. Fromm MF, "Piperine, a major constituent of black pepper, inhibits human P-glycoprotein and CYP3A4.J," *Pharmacol Exp Ther.*, Aug. 2002, Aug;302(2):645--650.

22. G. Bano G, R.K. Raina RK, U. Zutshi U, K.L. Bedi KL, R.K. Johri RK, and S.C. Sharma SC, "Effect of piperine on bioavailability and pharmacokinetics of propranolol and theophylline in healthy volunteers," *Eur J Clin Pharmacol.*, 1991, ;41(6):615--617.

23. R.K. Johri RK, N. Thusu N, A. Khajuria, and U. A, Zutshi, " U 1992 Piperine-mediated changes in the permeability of rat intestinal epithelial cells. The status of gamma-glutamyltranspeptidase activity, uptake of amino acids and lipid peroxidation,". *Biochemistry and Pharmacology* 1992, 1,43(7):1401.

24. M.S. Dama, MS,C. Varshneya C, M.S. Dardi MS, and V.C. Katoch VC, "Effect of trikatu pretreatment on the pharmacokinetics of pefloxacin administered orally in mountain Gaddigoats,. *J Vet Sci.,* March 2008, Mar;9(1):25--29.

25. A.R. Hiwale, AR, J.N. Dhuley JN, and S.R. Naik SR, "Effect of co-administration of piperine on pharmacokinetics of beta-lactam antibiotics in rats," .*Indian J Exp Biol.*, March 2002, Mar;40(3):277--281.

26. L.G. Lala LG, P.M. D'Mello, and S.R. PM, Naik SR, "Pharmacokinetic and pharmacodynamic studies on interaction of "Trikatu" with diclofenacsodium," ,*J Ethnopharmacol,.* April 2004, Apr;91(2--3):277--280.

27. R. D'Hooge R, Y.I..Q. Pei YQ, A. Raes A, P. Lebrun P, P.P. Bogaert PP, and P.P.de Deyn, PP "1996 Anticonvulsant activity of Piperine on seizures induced by excitatory amino acid receptor agonists,". *Arzneimittelforschung*, 1996,; 46(6):557.

28. T.P. Eldershaww TP, E.Q. Colguhoun EQ, K.L. Bennett KL, K.A Dora KA, and M.G. Clark MG,. "Resiniferatoxin and piperine; capsaicin like stimulators of oxygen uptake in perfused rat hindlimbs,". *Life Science*, 1994, ;55(5):389--397.

29. I. B. Koul IB and A., Kapil, A "1993 Evaluation of the liver protective potential of pPiperine, an active principle of black and long peppers,". *Planta Medica*, 1993, 59(5):413.

30. Nakatami, Note 8.

31. A.M. MujumdarAM, J.N. DhuleyJN, V.K. DeshmukhVK, P.H. Raman PH, and S.R. Naik, " SR1990 Anti-inflammatory activity of pPiperine,". *Japanese Journal of Medical Science and Biology*, 1990, 43(3):95.

32. J. Wattanathorn J, P. Chonpathompikunlert P, S. Muchimapura S, A. Priprem A, and O. Tankamnerdthai, " O.Piperine, the potential functional food for mood and cognitive disorders,". *Food Chem Toxicol.*, Sept. 2008 Sep;, 46(9):3106--3110.

33. M.K.Naseri MK, and H. Yahyavi, H. "Antispasmodic effect of Piper nigrum fruit hot water extract on rat ileum,". *Pak J Biol Sci.*, June 1, 2008, Jun 1;11(11):1492--1496.

34. S.I. Taqvi, SI A.J., Shah AJ, and A.H. Gilani, AH. "Blood pressure lowering and vasomodulator effects of piperine,". *J. Cardiovasc Pharmacol.*, Nov. 2008, Nov;52(5):452--458.

35. International Institute of Rural Reconstruction, *1994 Ethnoveterinary Mmedicine in Asia. An Iinformation Kkit on Ttraditional Aanimal Hhealth Ccare Ppractices* (. IIRR, Silang, Philippines: IIRR, 1994).

36. E. Mathias E, D.V. Rangnekar DV, and C.M. McCorkle, CM 1988 Ethnoveterinary Mmedicine: aAlternative for Llivestock Ddevelopment. Proceedings of an International Conference, BAIF Development Research Foundation, Pune, India, 1988.

37. R.K. Bhardwaj RK, H. Glaeser H, and L. Becquemont L, et al., " Piperine, a major constituent of black pepper, inhibits human P-glycoprotein and CYP3A4," *J Pharmacol Exp Ther*, 2002, ;302:645--650.

34

Pterocarpus marsupium

Introduction

Pterocarpus marsupium is a moderately large deciduous tree commonly found in the hills of south and central India. The golden heartwood of Pterocarpus, known in Ayurvedic tradition as Vijaysar, is widely considered to be of value in treating diabetes and other glycemic disorders. In folkloric tradition, diabetic patients often are treated by drinking water that has been stored in wooden tumblers made from the heartwood of Pterocarpus marsupium. The effectiveness of this traditional use has been corroborated in clinical trials.[1]

The gum, which is obtained from incisions in Pterocarpus bark, is astringent and is used to treat leucoderma, diarrhea, pyrosis, and toothache. Bruised leaves are applied externally for boils, sores, and various skin diseases. Vijaysar also is believed to enhance the complexion. Its flowers are to treat fever, and indigenous communities use various parts of the tree to treat burns, syphilis, stomach ache, cholera, dysentery, and menorrhagia.

The Pterocarpus marsupium tree yields one of the most important timbers of India. Its sapwood is pale-yellow to white, and the heartwood is golden yellow brownish in color, which stains yellow when moist. The yellow color is believed to be the result of the flavonoid content of the wood.

An aqueous infusion of Pterocarpus wood is used as an astringent and, along with the alcoholic extract, is widely known to have a hypoglycemic action. Researchers postulate that Vijaysar's anti-diabetic activity is the result of its ability to reduce glucose absorption from the gastrointestinal tract, which leads to improved insulin and pro-insulin levels in the blood.

Vijaysar also has been documented to aid in regeneration of pancreatic B cells. Modern research studies have investigated the cardiotonic, cholesterol reducing, and anti-inflammatory actions of this important medicinal plant.

Synonymous Names

English: Indian Malabar Kino, Indian Kino, Gummy Kino
Hindi: Vijaysar kaashtha
Sanskrit: Pitasala Asana, Beejak
Telugu: Paiddagi Chekka
Marathi: Biyala lakda
Tamil: Vegaimaram chakkal
Trade name: Bijaisaar Kaashtha
Ayurvedic name: Bijasar or Vijaysar

Habitat

Pterocarpus marsupium is native to India, Nepal, and Sri Lanka, where it occurs in parts of the Western Ghats. [2,3]

Botanical Description

Pterocarpus marsupium is a medium-to-large, deciduous tree that can grow up to 30 meters in height. It bears compound leaves that have three to seven oblong leaflets, 3 to 5 inches in length, with wavy margins. Pterocarpus' fragrant yellow flowers occur in large pannicles. Its seed pods are orbicular, flat, and winged.

The bark of the Pterocarpus marsupium tree is rough, gray, longitudinally fissured, and scaly. Older trees exude a blood-red gum resin. The tree's heartwood is golden yellow, while its sapwood is pale yellow to white in color.

Chemical Constituents

The primary chemical components of Pterocarpus are liquiritigenin, isoliquiritigenin, pterosupin, epicatechin, pterostilbene, kinotannic acid, beta-eudesmol, marsupol, carpusin, marsupinol, kinoin and kino-red.

From an aqueous extract of the heartwood of Pterocarpus marsupium, five new flavonoid C-glucosides were isolated: [4] 6-hydroxy-2-(4-hydroxybenzyl)-benzofuran-7-C-beta-d-glucopyranoside, (2) 3-(alpha-methoxy-4-hydroxybenzylidene)-6-hydroxybenzo-2(3H)-furanone-7-C-beta-d-glucopyranoside, 2-hydroxy-2-p-hydroxybenzyl-3(2H)-6-hydroxybenzofuranone-7-C-beta-d-glucopyranoside (4) (3) & (4), 8-(C-beta-d-glucopyranosyl)-7,3',4'-trihydroxyflavone, and 1,2-bis(2,4-dihydroxy,3-C-glucopyranosyl)-ethanedione.

Pharmacological Activity

Anti-diabetic activity

Pterocarpus marsupium demonstrates unique pharmacological properties, which include beta cell protective and regenerative properties, as well as blood glucose-lowering activity. These effects have been reproduced in numerous animal and human trials conducted over the past 50 years. The animal studies have used various species including rats, dogs, and rabbits with induced diabetes and subsequent treatment with various extracts of Pterocarpus marsupium. In all of these studies, Pterocarpus marsupium was found to reverse the damage to the beta cells and actually repopulate the islets, causing a nearly complete restoration of normal insulin secretion. [1-3, 5-7]

In various animal studies, test animals that did not receive any type of treatment either remained severely hyperglycemic at the end of the study or did not survive during the testing period. Compared to the control groups, significant percentages of the animals treated with Pterocarpus marsupium did not become diabetic or hyperglycemic. [8,9]

On the basis of the data gleaned from studies such as these, researchers have concluded that Pterocarpus marsupium extract will not only repair or regenerate beta cells in animals but also may act in a protective manner, preventing beta cells from destruction by nullifying the effects of a toxic exposure. This ability to offer protection to beta cells may have particular benefit to newly diagnosed Type I diabetics who are still experiencing an autoimmune activity.

One such animal study investigated the effect of an aqueous infusion of Vijaysar against the acute hyperglycemic response caused by anterior pituitary extract in glucose-fed albino rats, alloxan-induced diabetic rats, alloxan-diabetic rabbits, and normal rabbits. The aqueous extract of Pterocarpus was found to be more active than the alcoholic extract, and was also found to be active in both acute and chronic experiments in normal rabbits.[10] Aqueous extract of Pterocarpus also showed a more potent hypoglycemic effect than two other Ayurvedic herbs used in diabetic treatment - Gymnema sylvestre and Centella indica. Administration of aqueous extract of Pterocarpus for a period of 15 days resulted in reduced glucose absorption from the gastrointestinal tract, which was attributed to the action of tannates.

Pterostilbene from Vijaysar, when administered intravenously to dogs, led to a fall in blood sugar of 10 mg/kg, whereas higher doses led to an initial hyperglycemia followed by hypoglycemia. The substance also caused a fall in the blood pressure of anesthetized dogs and was found to be toxic at 30 mg/kg. The flavonoid fraction and the pure component (-)-epicatechin of Pterocarpus marsupium was shown to cause regeneration of the beta cells of the pancreas, which was considered to explain its hypoglycemic action.[11]

Additional in-vitro studies have shown that (-)-epicatechin enhances insulin release by increasing the conversion of proinsulin to insulin. This effect was found to be more pronounced in immature rat islets. Marsupin and pterostilbene administered intraperitoneally to streptozotocin-hyperglycemic rats significantly lowered blood glucose levels, with an effect comparable to that of metformin.[12]

Aqueous extracts of Pterocarpus marsupium, Ocimum sanctum leaves and Trigonella foenum graecum seeds have been shown to exert hypoglycemic and antihyperglycemic effects in experimental as well as clinical settings. As no work has been carried out so far to assess the effect of these herbs on fructose-induced hyperglycemia, hyperinsulinemia and hyper-triglyceridemia, a study was conducted to assess whether these extracts attenuate the metabolic alteration induced by fructose-rich diet in rats. Forty animals; five groups of eight, were fed the following experimental diets: chow diet, 66% fructose diet, 66% fructose diet + Pterocarpus leaves extract (1 g/kg/day), 66% fructose diet + Ocimum sanctum leaves extract (200 mg/kg/day) and 66% fructose diet + Trigonella foenumgraecum (Fenugreek) seeds extract (2 g/kg/day) for 30 days.[13]

Fructose feeding to normal rats for 30 days significantly increased serum glucose, insulin, and triglyceride levels in comparison to control feeding. Treatment with all the three plant extracts for 30 days significantly lowered the serum glucose levels in comparison to the control group; however, only Pterocarpus extract substantially prevented hyper-triglyceridemia and hyperinsulinemia, while the other two herbal extracts had no significant effect on these parameters.[13]

These results, taken together with the clinical benefits of Pterocarpus revealed in previous studies, suggest the usefulness of Pterocarpus marsupium bark in treating insulin resistance. These benefits are presumed to be the result of several antidiabetic principles (-epicatechin, pterosupin, marsupin and pterostilbene), which have been identified in Pterocarpus.

Another property displayed by Pterocarpus marsupium in the research environment is an insulin-like activity that appears to be distinct from its stimulation of insulin production from the repair of beta cells.[14,15] It is extrapolated that Pterocarpus marsupium may lower blood sugar through an pathway unrelated to insulin. There seem to be different cellular binding sites for insulin and for Pterocarpus marsupium. Thus, glucose-lowering activity may occur regardless of the presence of insulin.

This property of Pterocarpus marsupium would make it valuable in the treatment of both Type I and Type II diabetes. In patients with Type II diabetics, (those that suffer primarily from insulin resistance), Pterocarpus would completely bypass the normally ineffective insulin pathway, allowing for glucose uptake. In treating those with Type I diabetes (in which insulin is absent), Pterocarpus could supplement in part the treatment of the absence of insulin.

In clinical studies using human subjects, Pterocarpus marsupium has shown remarkable anti-diabetic action, similar to the results seen in animal studies. In two clinical trials, diabetic patients were given no treatment other than administration of an extract of Pterocarpus marsupium.

The first study evaluated both newly diagnosed and untreated Type II diabetics. Ninety-seven patients were given varying doses of an extract of Pterocarpus marsupium ranging from 2 to 4 grams a day over a period of 12 weeks.[16] At the end of the study period, parameters were evaluated for all patients. The results showed that 67% of the patients were able to reduce and maintain glucose levels by using various amounts of Pterocarpus marsupium extract. Of this group, 73% showed stabilized glucose levels at a daily dose of 2 grams of Pterocarpus extract, whereas 16% required 3 grams a day and 10% stabilized at 4 grams per day. All of the patients showed a significant decrease in both fasting and postprandial glucose levels. The average fasting blood sugar fell from 151mg/dl to 119mg/dl, and postprandial glucose dropped from 216mg/dl to 171mg/dl. The study participants also experienced a reduction in mean glycosylated hemoglobin from 9.8% to 9.4%. The study participants treated with Pterocarpus extract also demonstrated improvements in common diabetic symptoms without any adverse side-effects reported during the treatment period.

In the second study using human subjects, 22 diabetics, mostly with Type II diabetes, ranging in age from 29 to 70 years old were given a decoction of either 2 or 4 ounces three times daily, made from 36 or 72 grams of dry bark of Pterocarpus marsupium respectively, for 7 days.[17] Four parameters were monitored during this study: (1) fasting blood sugar, (2) glucose tolerance, (3) urine sugar content, and (4) diabetic symptoms. The subjects were separated into two group: Group A with 10 participants and Group B with 12 participants. Group A received a decoction of 2 ounces three times a day, and Group B received 4 ounces three times a day. Of the subjects in Group A, 3 of 10 patients showed an improvement in only one area of testing— glucose tolerance. In contrast, 9 of the 12 patients in Group B experienced benefits in all testing areas. These patients showed a significant improvement in glucose tolerance and glucose uremia, and also a decrease in fasting blood sugar and amelioration of some diabetic symptoms. No undesirable side effects were noted during the course of the study.

A small clinical trial was carried out with 10 patients, who were given 200 ml of the water, which was stored in the Pterocarpus marsupium tumbler overnight, twice a day for one month, taken after lunch. After dinner they drank water stored for the entire day. Reduction of blood sugar from the second week of treatment was encouraging, and this hypo-glycemic activity continued as long as the heartwood was given.

In an open trial with two groups, patients were administered either 500 mg of Sassurea lappa twice a day or 100 ml of Pterocarpus marsupium decoction twice a day after meals for 30 days. Both drugs were found effective in the management of diabetes and no side effects were observed. There was a decrease in the mean postprandial blood sugar from the initial 283 mg percent to 241 mg percent after the treatment period, in patients treated with Pterocarpus marsupium. There was only a slight decrease in cholesterol levels.[18]

Long-term complications frequently encountered in diabetes mellitus patients are extremely difficult to treat. One of these complications is the effect of diabetes on the eyes, one manifestation of which is the development of cataracts. A study was undertaken to assess the effect of three antidiabetic plants on the development of cataract in rats. An aqueous extract of Pterocarpus marsupium bark, Ocimum sanctum Linn leaves, and an alcoholic extract of Trigonella foenum-graecum Linn seeds were given to alloxan diabetic rats until cataracts developed. Serum glucose and body weight were monitored at regular intervals, and cataracts were examined by observation with the naked eye, as well as with a slit lamp at 75, 100 and 115 days after administration of alloxan. Administration of all three plant extracts exerted a favorable effect on body weight and blood glucose. The effects were best with Pterocarpus extract, followed by Trigonella and Ocimum sanctum. During the course of cataract development, Pterocarpus exerted an anti-cataract effect, evidenced by a decreased opacity index.[19]

Cardiotonic activity

Pterocarpus marsupium has been shown to have a strong antihyperlipidemic activity, in addition to its antihyperglycemic activity. Research has showed that it causes significant reduction of serum triglyceride, total cholesterol, and LDL and VLDL cholesterol levels without any effect on the level of HDL-cholesterol.[20] Further study demonstrated that Pterocarpus marsupium may lower blood lipid levels. Pterocarpus bark extract produced a reduction in serum triglycerides, total cholesterol and, low density lipoproteins (LDL) and very low density lipoproteins (VLDL) cholesterol.

A study was undertaken to evaluate the cardiotonic activity of the aqueous extract of heartwood of Pterocarpus marsupium. This plant species contains 5,7,2-4 tetrahydroxy isoflavone 6-6 glucoside, which is a potent anti-oxidants and is believed to prevent cardiovascular diseases.[21] The cardiotonic effect of the aqueous extract of heartwood of Pterocarpus marsupium was studied by using the isolated frog heart perfusion technique. A calcium-free Ringer solution was used as vehicle for administration of aqueous extract of Pterocarpus marsupium as a test extract and digoxin as a standard. A significant increase in height of force of contraction (positive inotropic effect) and a decrease in heart rate (negative chronotropic effect) at a very low concentration (0.25 mg/ml) was observed with the test extract compared to the same dose of a standard drug, digoxin. A significant increase in height of force of contraction with a decrease in heart rate was observed as the dose of test extract was increased. The test extract produced cardiac arrest at 4 mg/ml, a higher concentration, compared to the standard digoxin treatment (0.5 mg/ml). In contrast to digoxin, a drug with a narrow therapeutic window, Pterocarpus marsupium was shown to have a wide therapeutic window.

Anti-inflammatory activity

Pterocarpus marsupium also has shown strong potential for its anti-inflammatory activity. In this study, an extract of Pterocarpus marsupium containing pterostilbene was evaluated for its PGE2-inhibitory activity in LPS-stimulated PBMC. In addition, the COX-1/2 selective inhibitory activity of Pterocarpus marsupium extract was investigated.[22]

Biological activity, as well as the safety of Pterocarpus extract, was evaluated in healthy human volunteers. Pterocarpus extract, pterostilbene, and resveratrol inhibited PGE2 production from LPS stimulated human peripheral blood mononuclear cells (PBMC) with IC50 values of 3.2 +/- 1.3 microg/mL, 1.0 +/- 0.6 microM and 3.2 +/- 1.4 microM, respectively. When the pterostilbene content of Pterocarpus marsupium (PM) extract is calculated, PGE2 production inhibition of PM extract is comparable to PGE2 production inhibition of purified pterostilbene.

Further, in a COX-1 whole blood assay (WBA) Pterocarpus extract was not effective, while in a COX-2 whole blood assay (WBA), Pterocarpus extract decreased PGE2 production, indicating COX-2 specific inhibition. In healthy human volunteers, the oral use of 450 mg PM extract did not decrease PGE2 production ex vivo in a WBA. Pterostilbene levels in serum were increased but were five-fold lower than the observed IC50 for PGE2 inhibition in LPS-stimulated PBMC. No changes from baseline of the safety parameters were observed, and no extract-related adverse events occurred during the study. This study described the selective COX-2 inhibitory activity of a Pterocarpus marsupium extract. Moreover, the PGE2 inhibitory activity of Pterocarpus marsupium extract was related to its pterostilbene content.

In humans, 450 mg of Pterocarpus extract resulted in elevated pterostilbene levels in serum, which were below the active concentration observed in-vitro. In addition, short-term supplementation of 450 mg Pterocarpus marsupium extract is considered to be a safe dose, based on the long history of use, the absence of abnormal blood cell counts and blood chemistry values, and the absence of extract-related adverse events. This strongly argues for a dose-finding study of Pterocarpus marsupium extract in humans to corroborate the in-vitro observed inhibitory activity on PGE2 production to resolve the potential use of Pterocarpus marsupium extract in inflammatory disorders and/or inflammatory pain.[23]

Antimicrobial activity

The antimicrobial activity of Hemidesmus indicus, Ficus bengalensis and Pterocarpus marsupium was evaluated against pathogenic bacteria Staphylococcus aureus, Pseudomonas aeruginosa and Klebsiella pneumonia in an in vitro condition. Aqueous extracts from roots of Hemidesmus indicus and barks of Ficus bengalensis and Pterocarpus marsupium were tested for antimicrobial activity using the zone of inhibition method and also screened for phytochemicals. The aqueous extract of Pterocarpus marsupium inhibited growth of bacteria with the minimal inhibitory concentration ranging from 0.04 mg to 0.08 mg and extracts of Ficus bengalensis and Hemidesmus indicus showed inhibition at the range of 0.04 mg to 0.1 mg against the bacteria tested. The susceptibility of bacterial pathogens was in the order of S. aureus, K. pneumoniae and P. aeruginosa. The antimicrobial activity of plant extracts was synergistic with the antibiotics tested.[24]

Anti-cancer activity

Pterostilbene, a dimethyl ester derivative of resveratrol, may act as a cytotoxic and hence as an anti-cancer agent. This study was conducted to test the anti-cancer activity of pterostilbene purified from Pterocarpus marsupium on breast (MCF-7) and prostate (PC3) cancer cell lines. The purified pterostilbene was found to cause apoptosis in both of the cell lines, which was marked by DNA fragmentation, formation of apoptotic bodies, and membrane distortions. Apoptosis probably was a result of the production of reactive oxygen species in MCF-7 and nitric oxide over production in PC3 cells. Even the drug detoxifying anti-oxidant enzymes could not nullify the effect of pterostilbene as required by the cancer cells for survival. Pterostilbene was found to inhibit the cell-proliferating factors such as Akt, Bcl-2 and induced the mitochondrial apoptotic signals such as Bax, and the series of caspases. It also inhibited Matrix metalloproteinase 9 (MMP9) and alpha-methylacyl-CoA recemase (AMACR), two well known metastasis inducers. Pterostilbene has multiple target sites to induce apoptosis and after proper validation it can be used as a potential agent for the cure of breast and prostate cancer.[25]

Dr. Sodhi's Experience

When treating patients with Vijaysar, the practitioner should consider the following:

- Is diabetes present, especially with excessive weight gain or obesity?
- Is weight loss desirable?

- Is body-building desired?
- Are they excessive triglycerides?

Vijaysar is widely used for diabetes and weight loss. Because of its insulin-like action, it works to improve glycogen storage. For this reason, it is often used by body-builders, and by people with high levels of triglycerides. Vijaysar is also rich in bioflavonoids.

Ayurvedic Properties

Rasa : Katu, Tikta
Guna : Snigdha, Sara, Teekshna
Virya : Ushna
Vipaka : Katu
Prabhava : Medhya

Case History

A medical doctor called me seeking help for his daughter, who had insulin-dependent diabetes and was obese. He was hoping to find an herb that would help with both her diabetes and her weight gain, because every time her insulin had to be increased, she put on more weight.

We sent the doctor Vijayasar extract and instructed him to give his daughter 2 to 3 grams three times a day. A week later he called and reported excitedly that his daughter had been able to reduce her insulin intake to two or three units per day. A few years later I saw him at a medical conference. "You saved my daughter!" he told me, "She's lost so much weight! She's using minimal insulin, and we couldn't be more pleased."

Safety Profile

In clinical trials with Pterocarpus marsupium, no side effects have been noticed except loose stools and gastric upset. In small animals, extracts of Pterocarpus marsupium showed no untoward effect in doses used to elicit hypoglycemic effect.

Dosage

Decoction: 50 to 100 ml
Powder: 3 to 6 g
Extracted juice: 125 mg
Extract: 1-3 gram two three times per day

Notes

1. F. Ahmad, P. Khalid, M. M. Khan, M. Chaaubey, A. K. Rastogi, and J. R. Kidwai, "Hypoglycemic activity of Pterocarpus marsupium wood," *Journal of Ethnopharmacology*, 1991, 35:71–75.

2. B. K Chakravarthy, Saroj Gupta, and K.D Gode, "Functional beta cell regeneration in the islets of pancreas in alloxan induced diabetic rats by (-)-Epicatechin," *Life Sciences*, 1982, 31(24): 2693–2697.

3. M. Manickam, M. Ramanathan, M.A. Jahromi, J.P. Chansouria, and A.B. Ray, "Antihyperglycemic activity of phenolics from Pterocarpus marsupium," *J Nat Prod*, June 1997, 60(6):609–610.

4. Maurya R, Singh R, Deepak M, Handa SS, Yadav PP, Mishra PK.,**"Constituents of Pterocarpus marsupium: An ayurvedic crude drug,"** *Phytochemistry*, 2004, 65(7):915–920.

5. M.C Pandey, Demonstrator; P. V Sharma, "Hypoglycaemic effect of bark of pterocarpus marsupium roxb. (Bijaka) on alloxan induced diabetes," *Medicine & Surgery*, June 16, 1976: 9–11.

6. B.K Chakravarthy, Saroj Gupta, S.S Gambhir, K.D Gode, "Pancreatic Beta-cell regeneration in rats by (-)-epicatechin," *Lancet*, October 3, 1981: 759–760.

7. B.K Chakravarthy, Saroj Gupta, KD Gode, "Antidiabetic effect of (-)-Epicatechin," *Lancet*, July 31, 1982: 272–273. This is fine too

8. J. K. Grover, V. Vats, and S.S. Yadav, *Pterocarpus marsupium* extract (Vijayasar) prevented the alteration in metabolic patterns induced in the normal rat by feeding an adequate diet containing fructose as sole carbohydrate," *Diabetes, Obesity and Metabolism*, 7(4), July 2005, 414–420.

9. E.W Sheehan. D.D. Stiff, F. Duah, D.J. Slatkin, P.L. Schiff, Jr., and M.A. Zemaitis MA, "The lack of effectiveness of (-)epicatechin against alloxan induced diabetes in Wistar rats," *Life Sci*, 1983, 33:593.

10. See Pandey, Note 5.

11. F. Ahmad, P. Khalid, M. M. Khan, A. K. Rastogi, and J.R. Kidwai. "Insulin like activity in (-) epicatechin," *Acta Diabetol Lat*, Oct–Dec 1989, 26(4):291–300.

12. Ahmad F, Khan MM, Rastogi AK, Chaubey M, Kidwai JR. Effect of (-)epicatechin on cAMP content, insulin release and conversion of proinsulin to insulin in immature and mature rat islets in vitro. Indian J Exp Biol. 1991 Jun;29(6):516-20.

13. See Grover et al., Note 8.

14. See Ahmad et al., Note 11.

15. See Rizvi et al, Note 12.

16. Indian Council of Medical Research, "Flexible dose open trail of Vijayasar in cases of newly-diagnosed non insulin dependent diabetes mellitus, *Indian J Med Res*, July 1998, 108:24-29.

17. M. C Pandey and P.V. Sharma, "Hypoglycaemic effect of bark of pterocarpus marsupium roxb.," *Medicine & Surgery*, Nov. 15, 1975: 21–23.

18. M. Modak, P. Dixit, J. Londhe, S. Ghaskadbi, A. Paul, and T. Devasagayam, "Indian herbs and herbal drugs used for the treatment of diabetes," Journal of Biochemical Nutrition, May 2007, 40(3): 163–173

19. V. Vats, S. P. Yadav, N. R. Biswas, and J. K. Grover Anti-cataract activity of *Pterocarpus marsupium* bark and *Trigonella foenum-graecum* seeds extract in alloxan diabetic rats," *Journal of Ethnopharmacology*, August 2004, 93(2–3): 289–294.

20. M.A. Jahromi and A.B. Ray, "Antihyperlipidemic effect of flavonoids from pterocarpus marsupium," *J Nat Prod*, July 1993, 56(7):989–994.

21. N.C. Mohire, V.R. Salunkhe, S.B. Bhise, and A.V. Yadav, "Cardiotonic activity of aqueous extract of heartwood of Pterocarpus marsupium," *Indian J Exp Biol.*, June 2007, 45(6):532–537.

22. S. Hougee, J. Faber, A. Sanders, R.B. de Jong, W.B. van den Berg, J. Garssen, M.A/ Hoijer, and H.F. Smit, "Selective COX-2 inhibition by a Pterocarpus marsupium extract characterized by pterostilbene, and its activity in healthy human volunteers," *Planta Med.*, May 2005, 71(5):387–392.

23. ee Hougee et al, Note 24.

24. M. Gayathri and K. Kannabiran, "Antimicrobial activity of Hemidesmus indicus, Ficus bengalensis and Pterocarpus marsupium roxb.," *Indian J Pharm Sci.*, Sept. 2009, 71(5):578–581.

25. A. Chakraborty, N. Gupta, K. Ghosh, and P. Roy, "In vitro evaluation of the cytotoxic, anti-proliferative and anti-oxidant properties of pterostilbene isolated from Pterocarpus marsupium," *Toxicol In Vitro*, June 2010, 24(4):1215–1228.

35

Rubia cordifolia

Introduction

Rubia cordifolia, also known as Manjistha, or Madder, forms the basis for several widely used Ayurvedic preparations. The plant perhaps is best known as the source of a brilliant red dye. Dye-makers have used the root for centuries in many areas of the world to produce crimson, scarlet, mauve, and brown hues for cotton and woolen textiles.

Manjistha's sweet, bitter, acrid roots have a wide range of medicinal applications in Ayurveda. The herb is considered to be one of Ayurveda's best blood purifiers. Its biologically active constituents improve blood quality by increasing the hemoglobin in red blood cells, removing congestion, and improving circulation. Topical preparations made from Manjistha are used to treat skin conditions and improve the complexion.

Manjistha also is known for its therapeutic effect on urinary health. A key chemical component of the herb, ruberythic acid, helps to dissolve calcium containing stones in the urinary tract. Manjistha extract is given to treat rheumatism and inflammatory conditions of the chest. Clinical research has confirmed Manjistha's anti-oxidant and hepatoprotective properties. Manjistha is a rejuvenative tonic, increasing the body's natural resistance and helping to fight allergic reactions and infections.

Synonymous Names

English: Indian madder, Dyer's madder
Hindi: Manjit, Majeelh
Sanskrit: Manjistha, chitravalli

Habitat

Manjistha is a perennial climber found throughout the lower hills of the Indian Himalayas up to an altitude of 2500 meters. The plant also is found in Greece, Africa, China, Japan, Afghanistan, Vietnam, Malaysia, Indonesia, and Sri Lanka.

Botanical Characteristics

Manjistha is an herbaceous climbing plant, with long, twisted roots covered with thin, red bark. Manjistha's quadrangular stems are often many yards in length and are rough and grooved, becoming slightly woody at the base. The leaves grow in whorls of four to eight, with glabrous, shiny petioles having somewhat prickly angles. The smooth, shiny fruits, which become dark purple when ripe, are 4 to 6 millimeters in length.

Chemical Composition

Purpurin, munjistin, xanthopurpurin, and pseudopurpurin are the dominant chemical constituents of Manjistha.

Quinones:

A chemical analysis of Manjistha revealed the anthraquinone glycosides 1-hydroxy 2-methoxy anthraquinone, 1,4-dihydroxy-2-methyl-5-methoxy anthraquinone, 1,3-dimethoxy 2-carboxy anthraquinone and rubiadin.[1]

Iridoids: Manjistha's iridoids include 6-Methoxygeniposidic acid, along with manjistin, garancin and alizarin.[2]

Triterpenoids: The oleananes rubiprasin A, B and C, as well as arborane triterpenoids including rubiarbonol A, B, C, D, E and F have been isolated.[3,4]

Pharmacological Activity

Anti-inflammatory activity

The mechanism of Manjistha's anti-inflammatory action has been investigated in laboratory research. Researchers concluded that madder inhibits the lipoxygenase enzyme pathway and the production of cumene hydroperoxides, which are believed to be responsible for inflammatory responses in conditions such as asthma and arthritis. Mollugin is the active compound of Rubia cordifolia, which has been used as a traditional Chinese medicine for the treatment of various inflammatory diseases including arthritis and uteritis.

A study investigated for the first time the inhibitory effects and the mechanisms of action of mollugin (M1) and its synthetic derivatives (M2-M4) on tumor necrosis factor (TNF)-alpha-induced inflammatory responses in HT-29 human colon epithelial cells.[5] Treatment with M1 and its derivatives M2-M4 significantly inhibited TNF-alpha induced attachment of U937 monocytic cells to HT-29 cells, which mimics the initial phase of colon inflammation. TNF-alpha-induced mRNA induction of the chemokines, monocyte chemoattractant protein (MCP)-1 and interleukin (IL)-8, and the intercellular cell adhesion molecule (ICAM)-1, which are involved in adhesion between leukocytes and epithelial cells, was suppressed by M1-M4, and M1 was the most efficacious. In addition, M1-M4 significantly suppressed TNF-alpha-induced NF-kappaB transcriptional activity. Such NF-kappaB inhibitory activity of M1-M4 (20 microM) correlated with the ability to suppress TNF-alpha-induced chemokine expression and U937 monocytic cell adhesion to HT-29 colonic epithelial cells. Treatment of HT-29 cells with M1 and PDTC, a NF-kappaB inhibitor, synergistically suppressed both TNF-alpha-induced NF-kappaB activation and monocytic cell adhesion to HT-29 cells. M1-M4 inhibited TNF-alpha-induced expression of inflammatory molecules via NF-kappaB, and that M1, a potent NF-kappaB inhibitor, may be a valuable new drug candidate for the treatment of colon inflammation.

Anti-platelet activity

Conditions such as deep-vein thrombosis are believed to be aggravated by a phospholipid known as platelet activating factor (PAF). When animal experiments were conducted using 3H-labelled PAF, Manjistha extract inhibited the aggregation of platelets in a dose-dependent manner.[6]

Hepatoprotective activity

Manjistha offers protection against a variety of liver toxins. Quinone derivatives extracted from Manjistha interfered with the secretion of hepatitis B surface antigen in human hepatoma cells. This action indicates Manjistha may be effective against acute and chronic hepatitis caused by the hepatitis B virus (HBV).[7,8]

Anti-cancer activity

Cyclic hexapeptides and quinones extracted from Manjistha have shown potent anti-tumor activity against a variety of proliferating cells. These active agents inhibit aminoacyl-tRNA binding and peptidyl-tRNA translocation by binding to eukarytic SOS ribosomes. As a result, protein synthesis is arrested.[9,10,11]

Cisplatin is a powerful chemotherapeutic used in treating a wide range of cancers, but its usefulness is limited because of its toxicity to many normal tissues, including cells of the kidney proximal tubule. A study was undertaken to investigate whether the hydro-alcoholic extract of Manjistha could serve as adjunctive therapy to cisplatin in order to decrease the intensity of the toxic response. Cisplatin at a dose of 12 mg/kg was administered intraperitoneally to one group of Swiss albino mice. Another group of animals was given hydro-alcoholic extract of Manjistha at different doses along with the cisplatin injection. Various parameters, including serum creatinine and serum urea were analyzed.

Research results indicate that Manjistha extract could significantly decrease cisplatin-induced nephrotoxicity. The tissues of animals given Manjistha along with cisplatin showed a significant improvement in anti-oxidant status. A remarkable positive change was noted in serum creatinine and urea levels. Lipid peroxidation in the kidney and liver tissues was also considerably reduced in the animals treated with Manjistha extract. These results indicate that Manjistha could offer a useful adjunct to chemotherapy with cisplatin to ameliorate renal damage to patients.

In another study, exposure of Jurkat T cells to mollugin (15-30 microM), purified from the roots of Rubia cordifolia, caused cytotoxicity and apoptotic DNA fragmentation along with mitochondrial membrane potential disruption, mitochondrial cytochrome c release, phosphorylation of c-Jun N-terminal kinase (JNK), activation of caspase-12, -9, -7, -3, and -8, cleavage of FLIP and Bid, and PARP degradation, without accompanying necrosis. While these mollugin-induced cytotoxicity and apoptotic events, including activation of caspase-8 and mitochondria-dependent activation of caspase cascade, were completely prevented by overexpression of Bcl-xL, the activation of JNK and caspase-12 was prevented to much lesser extent. Pre-treatment of the cells with the pan-caspase inhibitor (z-VAD-fmk), the caspase-9 inhibitor (z-LEHD-fmk), the caspase-3 inhibitor (z-DEVD-fmk), or the caspase-12 inhibitor (z-ATAD-fmk) at the minimal concentration to prevent mollugin-induced apoptosis appeared to completely block the activation of caspase-7 and -8, and PARP degradation but failed to block the activation of caspase-9 and -3 allowing a slight enhancement in the level of JNK phosphorylation. Both FADD-positive wild-type Jurkat clone A3 and FADD-deficient Jurkat clone I2.1 exhibited a similar susceptibility to the cytotoxicity of mollugin, excluding involvement of Fas/FasL system in triggering mollugin-induced apoptosis. Normal peripheral T cells were more refractory to the cytotoxicity of mollugin than were Jurkat T cells. These results demonstrated that mollugin-induced cytotoxicity in Jurkat T cells was attributable mainly to apoptosis provoked via endoplasmic reticulum stress mediated activation of JNK and caspase-12, and subsequent mitochondria-dependent activation of caspase-9 and -3, leading to activation of caspase-7 and -8, which could be regulated by Bcl-xL.[12]

Anti-oxidant activity

Manjistha's anti-oxidant properties have been confirmed in laboratory research. Studies showed that Madder inhibited $FeSO_4$-induced lipid peroxidation and glutathione depletion, in an action believed to be the result of the presence of rubiadin, an active quinone.[13]

Anti-urolithiasis activity

A study was conducted to investigate the protective effect of the hydro-alcoholic extract of roots of Rubia cordifolia against ethylene glycol-induced urolithiasis and its possible underlying mechanisms, using male Wistar albino rats. The ethylene glycol feeding resulted in hyperoxaluria and hypocalciuria, as well as increased renal excretion of phosphate. Supplementation with hydro-alcoholic extract of Rubia cordifolia significantly prevented changes in urinary calcium, oxalate, and phosphate excretion dose-dependently. The increased calcium and oxalate levels and number of calcium oxalate crystals deposits in the kidney tissue of the calculogenic rats were reverted significantly by the Rubia cordifolia treatment and also prevented impairment of renal functions. Rubia cordifolia protected against ethylene glycol-induced urolithiasis, and prevented the growth of urinary stones. The mechanism underlying this effect is mediated possibly through an anti-oxidant, nephroprotection, and its effect on the urinary concentration of stone-forming constituents.[14]

Anti-psoriatic activity

Psoriasis is a skin disease associated with hyperproliferation and aberrant differentiation of keratinocytes. Studies have identified the root of Rubia cordifolia as a potent antiproliferative and apoptogenic agent in cultured HaCaT cells (IC(50) 1.4 microg/ml). Ethanolic extract of Radix Rubiae was fractioned sequentially with hexane, ethyl acetate, n-butanol and water. The ethyl acetate fraction was found to have the most potent antiproliferative action on HaCaT cells (IC(50) 0.9 microg/ml). The mechanistic study revealed that the ethyl acetate fraction induced apoptosis on HaCaT cells, as it was capable of inducing apoptotic morphological changes. The annexin V-PI staining assay also demonstrated that the ethyl acetate fraction significantly augmented HaCaT apoptosis. In addition, the ethyl acetate fraction decreased the mitochondrial membrane potential in a concentration- and time-dependent manner. The standardized ethyl acetate fraction was formulated into topical gel, and its keratinocyte-modulating action was tested on a mouse tail model. The ethyl acetate fraction dose-dependently increased the number and thickness of the granular layer and epidermal thickness on the mouse tail skin, indicative of the keratinocyte differentiation-inducing activity. Taking the in-vitro and in-vivo findings together, ethyl acetate fraction is a promising antipsoriatic agent.[15]

Lipid metabolism activity:

The naphthohydroquinone rubimaillin, which has an angular-type three cyclic skeleton, was isolated from Rubia cordifolia and was found to inhibit lipid droplet accumulation in mouse macrophages and to selectively inhibit cholesteryl ester synthesis (IC(50): 18 microM). The metabolism of cholesterol from lysosomes to lipid droplets was inhibited by the compound with a similar IC(50) (45 microM). Rubimaillin inhibited the acyl-CoA, cholesterol acyltransferase (ACAT1) activity in ACAT1-expressing cells (IC(50): 80 microM). Rubimaillin inhibited macrophage ACAT activity in order to decrease cholesteryl ester synthesis, leading to a reduction in the number of lipid droplets. Rubimaillin was found to inhibit the ACAT2 isozyme in ACAT2-expressing cells (IC(50): 22 microM). Rubimaillin found to be dual inhibitor of ACAT1 and ACAT2 but is more selective for the ACAT2 isozyme.[16]

Ethnoveterinary Usage

Manjistha is used in veterinary medicine to treat liver fluke, dysentery, maggots, wounds, land intestinal worms.[17]

Dr. Sodhi's Experience

When considering treatment with Manjistha, the practitioner should consider the following:

- Are there problems with the skin?
- Is hemorrhage occurring?
- Is dysmenorrhea present?
- Is there bleeding from a wound?

Manjistha is an excellent herb for the skin. It is good for the complexion, enhancing the quality and luster of the skin. Manjistha may be used to treat skin disorders including acne, blemishes, and darkened skin. It is a cooling herb, so it may be is used to treat all types of bleeding disorders, which are considered in Ayurveda to be caused by excess heat in the body. Petechial hemorrhages, intestinal hemorrhage, menorrhagia, and urinary tract bleeding all may be treated successfully with Manjistha. Because of its adaptogenic properties, Manjistha can be used to treat irregularities in normal conditions such as bleeding between menses, as well as for pathological bleeding conditions such as hemorrhage or traumatic wounds.

Case Histories

Spontaneous abortion

A 32-year-old woman who had experienced a spontaneous abortion came to our clinic for help. She had been treated previously with a dilation and curettage procedure and oral contraceptives to control her heavy bleeding, but she was still experiencing spotting between menstrual periods and her menses were extremely heavy. Her ultrasound results were unremarkable. After 3 or 4 months of this condition, she sought help from us.

After general testing, we found that her liver was inflamed. We discussed her diet and learned that she was eating a standard American diet including fried foods, pizza, and meat. We counseled her that this diet was placing a heavy burden on her system and that her excessive bleeding was her body's attempt to eliminate some of the congestion.

We advised that she follow a pitta-pacifying diet, and prescribed the following herbal protocol:

Manjistha powder: 5–10 grams in water

One capsule three times per day of the following herbal blend:

Saraca indica (Ashoka) extract: 200 mg, with 100 mg of pyridoxine-5-phosphate, and 50 mg of Centella asiatica (brahmi) extract, in a proprietary blend of Symplocus racemosus (lodh), bamboo manna, and Aloe vera (kumari) Asparagus racemosus extract 500 mg one capsule three times per day

We also advised her to increase her water intake, and to use calcium and magnesium supplements to support her normal clotting factors. We suggested that she increase her intake of vegetables to get more vitamin K in her diet, which also would support her clotting factors.

The patient returned to our clinic 2 weeks later and reported that she was not spotting as much, although her menses were still somewhat heavy. The bleeding had been reduced so she needed only seven pads per day, as opposed to the 15 pads she had needed previously. The next month, her menses had improved further so she needed only three or four pads per day. She had no clots and no bleeding between periods. After 3 months, her menstruation had fully normalized.

Safety Profile

Manjistha is generally recognized as being safe for use at the recommended dosages. No adverse effects have been reported. Individual ingredients versus whole-plant extract and different species, however, differ vastly in the profile of interactions and adverse reactions.

Madder color extracted from the roots of Rubia tinctorum (madder root) has been used as a food coloring in Japan. Studies revealed that Rubia has subchronic and chronic toxicity and potent carcinogenicity targeting the rat liver and kidney. A 2-year carcinogenicity study was conducted to further elucidate the long-term effects of Rubia and its target organs. Male and female F344 rats were fed a diet containing 0%, 2.5%, and 5.0% Rubia for 104 weeks. Incidence of hepatocellular adenomas and/or carcinomas was increased significantly with a dose-relation in the treated groups of both sexes. [18]

Dosage

Powdered root: 1–3 g
Decoction: 56–112 ml
Extract: 50 mg three times per day

Ayurvedic Properties

Rasa: Kashaya (astringent), tikta (bitter), madhur (sweet)
Guna: Guru (heavy), ruksha (dry)
Veerya: Ushna (hot)
Vipaka: Katu (pungent)
Doshas: Pacifies kapha and pitta

Notes

1. M.M.R. Guntupalli, V.R. Chandana, P. Palpu, and S. Annie, "Hepatoprotective effects of rubiadin, a major constituent of Rubia cordifolia Linn," *Journal of Ethnopharmacology*, Feb. 2006, 103(3): 484-490.

2. L.J. Wu, S.X. Wang, and H. Hua Metal, "6-Methoxygeniposidic acid, an iridoid glycoside from Rubia cordifolia," *Phytochemistry,* 1991, 30(5):1710.

3. H. Itokawa, Y.F. Qiao, K. Takeya, et al ."New triterpenoids from Rubia cordifolia var. pratensii (Rubiactac)," *Chemical and Pharmaceutical Bulletin* , 1989, 37(6):1670.

4. H. Itokawa, Y.F. Qiao, K. Takeya, and Y. litaka, "New triterpenoids from Rubia \cordifolia ," *Chemical and Pharmaceutical Bulletin*, 38(5):H35.

5. K.J. Kim, J.S. Lee, M.K. Kwak, H.G. Choi, C.S. Yong, J.A. Kim, Y.R. Lee, W.S. Lyoo, and Y.J. Park, "Anti-inflammatory action of mollugin and its synthetic derivatives in HT-29 human colonic epithelial cells is mediated through inhibition of NF-kappaB activation," *Eur J Pharmacol.*, Nov. 2009, 10, 622(1-3):52–57.

6. H. Itokawa, Z. Z lbraheim, Q. Ya-Fang, and K. Takeya, "Anthraquinones, naphthohydraquinones and naphthohydroquinone dimers from Rubia cortiifolia and their cytotoxic activity," *Chemical and Pharmaceutical Bulletin*, 1993, 41(10):1869.

7. A.H Gilai and K.H. Janba, "Effect of Rubia cordifolia extract on acraminophen and CCl,-induced hepatotoxicity," *Phytotherapy Research*, 1995, 9(5):372.

8. S. Pandey, M. Sharma, P. Chaturvedi, and Y.B. Tripathi, "Protective effect of Rubia cordifolia on lipid peroxide formation in isolated rat liver homogenate," *Indian Journal of Experimental Biology*, 1994, 32(3):180.

9. H. Morita, T. Yamamiya, K.Takeya, and H. Itokawa, "New anti-tumor bicyclic hexapeptides, RA-IX, XII, X1II and XIV from Rubia cordifolia," *Chemical and Pharmaceutical Bulletin*, 1992, 40(5):1352.

10. J. Joy and C.K. Nair, "Amelioration of cisplatin induced nephrotoxicity in Swiss albino mice by Rubia cordifolia extract," *J Cancer Res Ther.*, July–Sept. 2008, 4(3):111–115.

11. J.K. Son, S.J. Jung, J.H. Jung, Z. Fang, C.S. Lee, C.S. Seo, D.C. Moon, B.S. Min, M.R. Kim, and M.H. Woo, "Anticancer constituents from the roots of Rubia cordifolia L," Feb. 2008, 56(2):213–216.

12. S.M. Kim, H.S. Park, D.Y.Jun, H.J. Woo, M.H. Woo, C.H. Yang, and Y.H. Kim, "Mollugin induces apoptosis in human Jurkat T cells through endoplasmic reticulum stress-mediated activation of JNK and caspase-12 and subsequent activation of mitochondria-dependent caspase cascade regulated by Bcl-xL," *Toxicol Appl Pharmacol.*, Dec.1, 2009, 241(2):210–220.

13. Y.B Tripathi, S. Shukla, M. Sharma, and V.K. Shukla, "Anti-oxidant property of Rubia cordifolia extract and its comparison with Vitamin E and parabenzoquinone," *Phytotherapy Research*, 1995, 9(6):440.

14. K. Divakar, A.T. Pawar, S.B. Chandrasekhar, S.B. Dighe, and G. Divakar, "Protective effect of the hydro-alcoholic extract of Rubia cordifolia roots against ethylene glycol induced urolithiasis in rats," *Food Chem Toxicol.*, April 2010, 48(4):1013–1018.

15. Z.X. Lin, B.W. Jiao, C.T. Che, Z. Zuo, C.F. Mok, M. Zhao, W.K. Ho, W.P. Tse, K.Y. Lam, R.Q, Fan, Z.J. Yang, and C.H. Cheng, "Ethyl acetate fraction of the root of Rubia cordifolia L. inhibits keratinocyte proliferation in vitro and promotes keratinocyte differentiation in vivo: potential application for psoriasis treatment," *Phytother Res.*, July 2010, 24(7):1056–1064.

16. D. Matsuda, T. Ohshiro, M. Ohba, W. Jiang, B. Hong, S. Si, and H. Tomoda, "The molecular target of rubimaillin in the inhibition of lipid droplet accumulation in macrophages," *Biol Pharm Bull.*, Aug. 2009, 32(8):1317–1320.

17. Dosseh C, Tessier AM, Delaveau P. New quinones in Rubia cordifolia L. Roots, III. Planta Med. 1981 Dec;43(4):360-6. [18] K. Inoue, M. Yoshida, M. Takahashi, M. Shibutani, H. Takagi, M. Hirose, and A. Nishikawa, "Induction of kidney and liver cancers by the natural food additive madder color in a two-year rat carcinogenicity study," *Food Chem Toxicol.*, Jan. 2009, 47(1):184–191.

18. K. Inoue, M. Yoshida, M. Takahashi, H. Fujimoto, K. Ohnishi, K. Nakashima, M. Shibutani, M. Hirose, and A. Nishikawa, "Possible contribution of rubiadin, a metabolite of madder color, to renal carcinogenesis in rats," *Food Chem Toxicol.*, April 2009, 47(4):752-759. Epub Jan. 8, 2009.

36

Shilajit

Introduction

Although it is not from a plant source, Shilajit nevertheless is one of the most important preparations of Ayurvedic and various other medical traditions. In its raw form, Shilajit is a bituminous substance, composed of vegetable organic matter within a dark-red gummy matrix. It is bitter in taste and has a strong odor.

In Sanskrit, Shilajit means "conqueror of mountains and destroyer of weakness." It flows out from fissures in the rocks during the heat of the summer sun. When dry, it is hard, organic, humus-rich, and mineral-like, usually with a pale brown to brownish black color. Shilajit is found on rocks at high altitudes (1000 to 5000 meters) in the Himalayan regions of India.[1,2] The flora of the Himalayas is rich and varied, and for thousands of years, plant life has grown, absorbed nutrients from the soil, then died and decayed. The Shilajit found in the Himalayas is believed to be a fossilized form of thousands of years of accumulation of decomposing plant material, much like fossil fuels such as coal and oil. Shilajit is collected in the Himalayas during the summer months when the ice melts.

In Ayurveda, Shilajit is considered to be a rasayana herb and an adaptogen.[3] It has been found to contain at least 85 minerals in ionic form, as well as humic acid and fulvic acid.[4] Clinical research has been conducted to determine Shilajit's pharmacological activity, and the results have confirmed its traditional uses in treating impotence, sterility, and mental diseases,[5] and for improving memory and learning.[6] Shilajit also has been used to treat benign prostatic hypertrophy,[7] epilepsy, obesity, diabetes, anemia, inflammation, ulcers, wounds, fevers, asthma, bronchitis, diabetes, dyspepsia, arthritis, rheumatic pain, tuberculosis, jaundice, heart disease, gout, kidney stones, parasitic skin diseases, urinary problems, leprosy, and allergic disorders. [8, 9,10,11]

Synonymous Names

Latin: Asphaltum
English: Mineral pitch, asphalt C
Sanskrit: Shilajit, silajit, silaras
Hindi: Silajatu
Russian: Mumiyo

Habitat

In India, Shilajit is found in the Himalayas from Arunachal Pradesh in the east to Kashmir in the west. It also is found in Afghanistan, Bhutan, China, Nepal, Pakistan, Tibet, Uzbekistan, Russia, and Norway, where it is collected from steep rock faces at altitudes between 1000 and 5000 meters.

CHEMICAL COMPOSITION

Different samples from India, Nepal, Pakistan, Kazakhstan, Kyrgyzstan and Tibet show composition as follows:[12,13]

  pH of 1% aqueous solution: 6.2 to 8.2

  Relative % composition of low molecular weight extracts: 4.3 to 29.7

  Fulvic acid % composition: 15.4 to 21.4

  Relative % composition of humic constituents: 5.6 to 19.8

  and dibenzo-a-pyrones.

PHARMACOLOGICAL ACTIVITY

Shilajit has been used as a rejuvenator and an adaptogen for thousands of years in several traditional systems of medicine. Many therapeutic properties have been ascribed to it, a number of which have been verified by modern scientific evaluation.[14]

Shilajit has been shown to have pharmacological activity in the following areas:

  anxiolytic,[15]

  memory and learning enhancement,[16]

  anti-depressant,[17]

  gastric acid inhibiting,[18]

  anti-ulcerogenic (stress-induced and aspirin-induced ulcers),[19,20]

  anti-inflammatory,[21]

  anti-allergic,[22]

  lipid peroxidation-inhibiting (in -vitro),[23]

  macrophage/phagocytic stimulating (in-vitro),[24]

  anti-diabetic,[25]

  weight loss-attenuating,[26]

  hyperglycemia-inhibiting,[27]

  total cholesterol and triglyceride-lowering, and HDL-cholesterol-increasing,[28]

  pancreatic islet B cell superoxide dismutase (SOD) activity-protecting,[29]

  anticlastogenic,[30]

  and hepatoprotective.[31]

Cognitive activity

Administration of Shilajit (25 and 50 mg/ kg i.p. for 5 days) significantly lowers the levels of 5-Hydroxytryptophan (5HT) and 5-Hydroxyindoleacetic acid (5-HIAA) is the main metabolite of serotonin and increases the levels of dopamine, noradrenaline, and their metabolites, in the rat brain. These findings confirms its uses as an Ayurvedic rasayana (rejuvenator).[32] Sitoindosides VII-X, and withaferin-A, isolated from the aqueous methanol extract from the roots of cultivated varieties of Withania somnifera, as well as Shilajit, are used in Indian medicine to attenuate cerebral functional deficits, including amnesia, in geriatric patients. Acetylcholinesterase inhibitors are used as an intervention in Alzheimer's disease.

An investigation was conducted to assess whether the memory-enhancing effects of plant extracts from Withania somnifera and Shilajit resulted from neurochemical alterations of specific transmitter systems.[33] Histochemistry to analyze acetylcholinesterase activity, as well as receptor autoradiography to detect cholinergic, glutamatergic and GABAergic receptor subtypes, was performed in brain slices from adult male Wistar rats injected intraperitoneally daily with an equimolar mixture of sitoindosides VII-X and withaferin-A or with Shilajit, at doses of 40 mg/kg of body weight for 7 days.

Administration of Shilajit led to reduced acetylcholinesterase staining, restricted to the basal forebrain nuclei, including the medial septum and the vertical limb of the diagonal band. Systemic application of the defined extract from Withania somnifera, however, led to differential effects on

AChE activity in the basal forebrain nuclei, slightly enhanced AChE activity was found in the lateral septum and globus pallidus, whereas in the vertical diagonal band AChE activity was reduced following treatment with sitoindosides VII-X and withaferin-A.

These changes were accompanied by enhanced M1-muscarinic cholinergic receptor binding in the lateral and medial septum, as well as in the frontal cortices, whereas the M2-muscarinic receptor binding sites were increased in a number of cortical regions including the cingulate, frontal, piriform, parietal and retrosplenial cortex. Treatment with Shilajit or the extract from Withania somnifera affected neither GABA and benzodiazepine receptor binding nor NMDA(N-methyl-D-aspartate) and α-amino-3-hydroxy-5-methyl-4-isoxazolepropionic acid receptor (AMPA)glutamate receptor subtypes in any of the cortical or subcortical regions studied.

The data suggests that Shilajit and the extract of Withania somnifera preferentially affects events in the cortical and basal forebrain cholinergic signal transduction cascade. The drug induced increase in cortical muscarinic acetylcholine receptor capacity might partly explain the cognition-enhancing and memory-improving effects of extracts from Withania somnifera observed in animals and humans.

Anti-inflammatory; anti-ulcer activity

Shilajit was conducted to evaluate the possible anti-ulcerogenic and anti-inflammatory activities of Shilajit obtained from the rocky mountains of Zarlek, Badekshan, Afghanistan. The study results showed that Shilajit increased the carbohydrate/protein ratio and decreased gastric ulcer index, indicating an increased mucosal barrier. Shilajit was found to have significant anti-inflammatory effect in carrageenan-induced acute pedal edema, granuloma pouch and adjuvant-induced arthritis in rats. These results substantiate the use of Shilajit in treating peptic ulcers and inflammation.[34]

Anti-diabetic activity

In diabetic rats, Shilajit produced a significant reduction in blood glucose levels and also produced beneficial effects on the lipid profile. The maximum effect was observed with the 100 mg/kg/day dose of Shilajit. A combination of Shilajit (100 mg/kg) with glibenclamide (5 mg/kg/day) or metformin (0.5 gm/kg/day) enhanced the glucose-lowering ability and improved the lipid profile more significantly than any of these drugs given alone.[35] An herbomineral formulation, whose main ingredients are Shilajit, Gymnema sylvestre, Pterocarpus marsupium, Casearia esculanta, Eugenia jambolana, Ocimum sanctum, and Momordica charantia. The treatment showed a progressive and significant increase in liver glycogen at 2, 4, and 8 weeks, respectively. Streptozotocin induced a decrease in pancreatic islet cell superoxide dismutase, which was reversed by herbal treatment for a period of 8 weeks.[36]

Urinary function

Shilajit is used to improve kidney function. It is effective in treating painful urination and/or incontinence from an enlarged prostate or stones of the bladder or kidneys.

Sexual debility

Shilajit is used as an aphrodisiac in India, where it is known as the "Indian Viagra." The safety and spermatogenic activity of processed Shilajit were evaluated in oligospermic patients.[38] Initially, 60 infertile male patients were assessed, and those having total sperm counts below 20 million ml(-1) semen were considered oligospermic and enrolled in the study (n = 35). Shilajit capsule (100 mg) was administered twice daily after major meals for 90 days. Total semenogram and serum testosterone, luteinising hormone, and follicle-stimulating hormone were estimated before and at the end of the treatment. Malondialdehyde (a marker for oxidative stress), content of semen, and biochemical parameters for safety also were evaluated. Of the patients who completed the treatment, 28 showed significant (P < 0.001) improvement in oligospermia (+37.6%), total sperm count (+61.4%), motility (12.4-17.4% after different time intervals), normal sperm count (+18.9%), with a concomitant decrease in pus and epithelial cell count compared to the baseline value. A significant decrease of semen malondialhyde content (-18.7%) was observed. Serum testosterone (+23.5%; P < 0.001) and FSH (+9.4%; P < 0.05) levels increased significantly. HPLC chromatogram revealed Shilajit constituents in semen. Unaltered hepatic and renal profiles of patients indicated that Shilajit was safe at the given dose.

Another study examined the possibility of using Shilajit as a fertility agent.[39] The effects of Shilajit on spermatogenesis and ovogenesis were studied using male and female rats. Shilajit was administered orally to 7-week-old rats over a 6-week period. In the male rats, the number of sperm in the testes and epididymides were significantly higher than in the control. A histological examination revealed an apparent increase in the number of seminiferous tubular cell layers in the testes of the treated rats. However, there were no significant differences in the weights of heart, spleen, liver, kidney, brain, testes, and epididymides. In the female rats, the effect of Shilajit was estimated by the ovulation-inducing activity. Over a 5-day period, ovulation was induced in seven of nine rats in the Shilajit administration group and in three of nine rats in the control. Shilajit was estimated to have both a spermatogenic and an oogenic effect in mature rats.

Adaptogenic activity

A herbal formulation comprising of Withania somnifera, Ocimum sanctum, Asparagus racemosus, Tribulus terrestris, and Shilajit, all of which are classified in Ayurveda as rasayanas— which are reputed to promote physical and mental health, improve defense mechanisms of the body, and enhance longevity.

A study was undertaken to investigate the adaptogenic activity of this herbal preparation (ST) against chronic unpredictable, but mild, footshock stress-induced perturbations in behavior (depression), glucose metabolism, suppressed male sexual behavior, immunosuppression, and cognitive dysfunction in CF strain albino rats. Gastric ulceration, adrenal gland and spleen weights, ascorbic acid, and corticosterone concentrations of adrenal cortex and plasma corticosterone levels, were used as the stress indices. Panax ginseng was used as the standard adaptogenic agent for comparison. In addition, rat brain levels of tribulin, an endogenous endocoid postulated to be involved in stress, were assessed in terms of endogenous monoamine oxidase (MAO) A and MAOB inhibitory activity.[40]

Chronic unpredictable footshock induced marked gastric ulceration, and a significant increase in adrenal gland weight and plasma corticosterone levels, with concomitant decreases in spleen weight and concentrations of adrenal gland ascorbic acid and corticosterone. These effects were attenuated by herbal combination (50 and 100 mg/kg, p.o.) and Panax (100 mg/kg, p.o.), administered once daily over a period of 14 days, the period of stress induction. Chronic stress also induced glucose intolerance, suppressed male sexual behavior, and induced behavioral depression (using Porsolt's swim despair test and learned helplessness test) and cognitive dysfunction (attenuated retention of learning in the active and passive avoidance tests), and immunosuppression (leucocyte migration inhibition and sheep RBC challenged an increase in paw edema in sensitized rats).

All of these chronic stress-induced perturbations were attenuated, dose-dependently by herbal preparation (ST) (50 and 100 mg/kg, p.o.) and Panax (100 mg/kg, p.o.). A chronic stress-induced increase in rat brain tribulin activity also was reversed by these doses of ST and by PG. The results indicated that ST has significant adaptogenic activity, qualitatively comparable to Panax, against a variety of behavioral, biochemical, and physiological perturbations induced by unpredictable stress, which has been proposed to be a better indicator of clinical stress than acute stress parameters.

Anti-oxidant activity

Anti-oxidants can safely neutralize a free radical without becoming a free radical themselves. Shilajit is a powerful anti-oxidant that has the added benefit of being able to cross the blood-brain barrier.

Anti-anemia activity

Shilajit is a good source of trace minerals and iron. Shilajit's fulvic acids improve the bioavailability of iron. [41]

The anti-oxidant and anti-inflammatory properties of Shilajit help to decrease and relieve joint inflammation and pain. The effects on the neurotransmitters in the brain also seem to help relieve joint pain.[42]

Anti-choleseremic activity

Shilajit was found to lower serum cholesterol, liver cholesterol, serum triglycerides, and serum phospholipids in the test subjects fed a high-cholesterol diet.[43]

Miscellaneous activity

High-altitude problems such as hypoxia, acute mountain sickness, high-altitude cerebral edema, pulmonary edema, insomnia, tiredness, lethargy, lack of appetite, body pain, dementia, and depression may occur when a person residing in a lower altitude ascends to high-altitude areas.

Shilajit contains humus, organic plant materials, and fulvic acid (FA) as the main carrier molecules. It actively takes part in transporting nutrients into deep tissues and helps to overcome tiredness, lethargy, and chronic fatigue. Shilajit improves the ability to handle high altitudinal stresses and stimulates the immune system. Shilajit can be given as a supplement to people going to high-altitude areas so it can act as a "health rejuvenator" and help to overcome high-altitude related problems.[44] Extracts of Shilajit contain significant amounts of fulvic acid , and it has been suggested that it is responsible for many therapeutic properties of Shilajit.

Shilajit was fractionated using anion exchange and size-exclusion chromatography. One neutral (S-I) and two acidic (S-II and S-III) fractions were isolated, characterized, and compared with standardized fulvic acid samples. The most abundant fraction (S-II) was fractionated further into three sub-fractions (S-II-1 to S-II-3). Shilajit fractions are the products of polysaccharide degradation, and all fractions, except S-II-3 contained type II arabinogalactan. Shilajit fractions highly exhibited dose-dependent complement-fixing activity in-vitro. Further, a strong correlation was found between the complement fixing activity and carboxylic group content in the Shilajit fractions and other fulvic acid sources. These data provide a molecular basis to explain at least part of the beneficial therapeutic properties of Shilajit and other humic extracts.[45]

Safety Profile

Shilajit should not be taken by people who have low blood pressure, and should not be taken with prescription anti-depressants (SSRIs and MAO inhibitors) or anti-anxiety medications.[46] Its safety in infants and during pregnancy is unknown.

Dosage

The recommended dosage is 250–500 mg 2 times per day after meals.

Notes

1. S. Ghosal, et al., "Shilajit I: Chemical constituents," *J Pharm Sci.*, 1976, 65,772–773.
2. S. Ghosal, et al., "The core structure of shilajit humus," *Soil Biol Biochem.*, 1991, 23:673–680.
3. D. Winston and S. Maimes. *Adaptogens: Herbs for Strength, Stamina, and Stress Relief* (City: Healing Arts Press, 2007). Please see this http://www.amazon.com/Adaptogens-Strength-Stamina-Stress-Relief/dp/1594771588#
4. H. S. Puri, *Ayurvedic Minerals, Gems and Animal Products for Longevity and Rejuvenation* (Delhi, India: India Book House, 2006).
5. R. Schliebs, et al., "Systemic administration of defined extracts from Withania somnifera (Indian ginseng) and shilajit differentially affects cholinergic but not glutamatergic and GABAergic markers in rat brain," *Neurochem Int.*, 1997, 30:181–190.
6. S.Ghosal et al., "Effects of shalajit and its active constituents on learning and memory in rats," *Phytother Res.*, 1993, 7:29–34
7. B. Dash, *Ayurvedic Cures for Common Diseases* (Delhi, India: Hind Pocket Books Ltd, 1997), 150.
8. A.K. Nadkarni, *Indian Materia Medica* (Bombay, India: Popular Prakashan, 1976), pp. 23–32.
9. V. P Tiwari, et al., "An interpretation on Ayurvedic findings on silajatu," *J Res Indian Med.* 1973, 8:53–60.
10. Y.C Kong, et al., "Chemical studies on a Nepalese panacea shilajit I.," *Int J Crude Drug Res.*, 1987, 25:179–182.
11. S. Ghosal, et al., "Mast cell protecting effects of shilajit and its constituents," *Phytother Res.*, 1989, 3:249–252.
12. S. Ghosal, et al., "The need for formulation of shilajit by its isolated active constituents," *Phytother Res.*, 1991, 5:211–216.
13. S. Ghosal, et al., "Shilajit, Part 3: Antiulcerogenic activity of fulvic acids and 4-methoxy-6-carbomethoxybiphenyl isolated from shilajit," *Phytother Res.*, 1988, 2:187–191.
14. S.P. Agarwal, R. Khanna, R. Karmarkar, M.K. Anwer, and R.K. Khar, "Shilajit: A review," *Phytother Res.*, May 2007, 21(5):401–405.
15. A. K Jaiswal and S.K. Bhattacharya, "Effects of shilajit on memory anxiety and brain monoamines in rats," *Indian J Pharmacol.*, 1992, 24:12–17. *See also* Note 6.

16. See Notes 6 and 12.
17. See Note 12.
18. See Note 12.
19. R.K. Goel, R.S. Banerjee, and S.B. Acharya, "Antiulcerogenic and anti-inflammatory studies with Shilajit," *J Ethnopharmacol.*, April 1990, 29(1):95–103.
20. S.B. Acharya, et al., "Pharmacological actions of shilajit," *Indian J Exp Biol.*, 1988, 26:775–777.
21. See Note 13.
22. See Note 11.
23. Y. B. Tripathi, et al., "Antilipid peroxidative property of shilajit," *Phytother Res.*, 1996, 10:269–270.
24. S. Bhaumik, et al., "Effect of shilajit on mouse peritoneal macrophages," *Phytother. Res.*, 1993, 7:425–427.
25. P. Basnet, et al., "Shilajit, an ayurvedic drug, prevents diabetes in nonobese diabetic mice and in multiple low-dose streptozotocin treated rats," *Phytomedicine*, 2000;7(2):110–111. (abstract)
26. S.K. Bhattacharya, "Activity of shilajit on alloxan-induced hyperglycemia in rats," *Fitoterapia*, 1995, 66:328–332.
27. N.A. Trivedi, et al., "Effects of shilajit on blood glucose, lipid profile and vascular preparation in alloxan induced diabetic rats," *Indian J Pharmacol.*, 2001, 33:143. (abstract); S. Qureshi, et al., "Effect of salajeet treatment on biochemical and cytological changes induced by cyclophosphamide in mice," *Fitoterapia*, 1994, 65:137–140.
28. See Note 27.
29. See Note 26.
30. See Note 26.
31. I. Vaishwanar, et al., "Effect of two Ayurvedic drugs, shilajeet and eclinol, on changes in liver and serum lipids produced by carbon tetrachloride," *Indian J Exp Biol.*, 1976, 14:58–61.
32. S. K. Bhattacharya and S. Ghosal, "Effect of Shilajit on rat brain monoamines," *Phytotherapy Research*, Jan 11, 2006, 6(3):163–164.
33. R. Schliebs, A. Liebmann, S.K. Bhattacharya, A. Kumar, S. Ghosal, and V. Bigl, "Systemic administration of defined extracts from Withania somnifera (Indian Ginseng) and Shilajit differentially affects cholinergic but not glutamatergic and GABAergic markers in rat brain," *Neurochem Int.*, Feb. 1997, 30(2):181–190.
34. See Note 19.
35. N.A. Trivedi, B. Mazumdar, J.D. Bhatt, and K.G. Hemavathi, "Effect of shilajit on blood glucose and lipid profile in alloxan induced diabetic rats," *Indian Journal of Pharmacology* 36(6).
36. S.D. Anturlikar, S. Gopumadhavan, B.L. Chauhan, and S.K. Mitra, "Effect of D-400, a herbal formulation, on blood sugar of normal and alloxan-induced diabetic rats," *Indian Journal Physiol. Pharmacol.*, 1995, 39(2): 95–100.
37. Wilson E, Rajamanickam GV, Dubey GP, Klose P, Musial F, Saha FJ, Rampp T, Michalsen A, Dobos GJ. Review on shilajit used in traditional Indian medicine. J Ethnopharmacol. 2011 Jun 14;136(1):1-9.
38. T.K Biswas, S. Pandit, S. Mondal, S.K. Biswas, U. Jana, T.. Ghosh, P.C. Tripathi, P.K. Debnath, R.G. Auddy, and B.Auddy, "Clinical evaluation of spermatogenic activity of processed Shilajit in oligospermia," *Andrologia.* Feb. 2010, 42(1):48–56.
39. J.S. Park, G.Y. Kim, and K. Han, "The spermatogenic and ovogenic effects of chronically administered Shilajit to rats," *J Ethnopharmacol.*, Oct. 11, 2006, 107(3):349–353.
40. S. K. Bhattacharya, A. Bhattacharya, and A. Chakrabarti, "Adaptogenic activity of Siotone, a polyherbal formulation of Ayurvedic rasayanas," *Indian J Exp Biol.*, Feb. 2000, 38(2):119–128.
41. See Note 40.
42. See Note 19.
43. See Note 23.
44. H. Meena, H.K. Pandey, M.C. Arya, and Z. Ahmed, "Shilajit: A panacea for high-altitude problems," *Int J Ayurveda Res.*, Jan. 2010, 1(1):37–40.
45. A. Schepetkin, G. Xie, M.A. Jutila, and M.T. Quinn, "Complement-fixing activity of fulvic acid from Shilajit and other natural sources," *Phytother Res.*, March 2009, 23(3):373–384.

Sida cordifolia

Introduction

Sida cordifolia, or Bala, has been used in India for more than 2,000 years to treat ailments including bronchial asthma, headache, nasal congestion, aching joints and bones, cough, and edema. It is considered to have diaphoretic, diuretic, central nervous system stimulating, and anti-asthmatic properties.

Chemical analysis of Sida cordifolia in the early part of the twentieth century reported that one of the herb's alkaloids closely resembled ephedrine in its pharmacological action. More recent work revealed that, although this sympatho-mimetic alkaloid had activity similar to ephedra (now banned because of its deleterious effect on the cardiovascular system), it is actually chemically different in nature. Thus, the herb may provide a safe treatment for obesity.

Because of its stimulant effect, Bala is commonly used as a heart tonic. Concurrently, research has shown the herb to cause marked and persistent increases in blood pressure in anesthetized animals. The plant also has demulcent, emollient, and diuretic properties, and the seeds of the plant are considered to be an aphrodisiac.

According to Ayurvedic tradition, Sida cordifolia is tonic, astringent, emollient, and aphrodisiac. In India it is used to treat gonorrhea, debility, and rheumatism. In Europe it is used as an anti-tubercular agent. The expressed juice of the whole plant is useful to treat premature ejaculation, and the juice of the roots is applied to sores. A decoction of the root bark is applied to treat sciatica and rheumatism.

Synonymous Names

Latin: Sida cordifolia
English: Country mallow
Sanskrit: Bala, Vatya
Hindi: Bariyar, Kharethi
Other names: Arrow leaf Sida, Cuban jute, Indian hemp

Habitat

Sida cordifolia is found throughout the tropical and subtropical plains of India and Sri Lanka.

Botanical Characteristics

Sida cordifolia is an erect, perennial undershrub reaching up to 2 meters in height. The stem of this deeply rooted plant is ascending, terete or sulcate, softly villious, and densely stellate-pubescent throughout. The leaves are ovate and subacute at the apex. The flowers are yellow peduncles, axillary, jointed much above the panicles, with the upper flowers nearly sessile and fasciculate toward the tip of the branches, forming a subspicate inflorescence. The fruits are subdiscoid, 6–8 millimeters across, with 10 three-sided mericarps. The seeds are trigonous, glabrous, and tufted-pubescent near the hilum.

Chemical Composition

Sida cordifolia has been found to contain pseudoephedrine, beta-phenethylamine, vaccine, asparagin, ephedrine, hypaphorine, the alkaloids vasicinone, vasicine, and vasicinol; also, it contains phytosterols, mucin, gelatin, potassium nitrate, and rutin.

Pharmacological Activity

Anti-inflammatory and analgesic activity

The analgesic and anti-inflammatory activities of a new alkaloid isolated from Sida cordifolia were investigated in animal models. In the acetic-acid induced writhing model, the compound showed 25.4% and 52.43% inhibition of writhing response at doses of 25 and 50 mg/kg body weight, respectively. The alkaloid also produced a significant increase in the tail flick latency in the radiant heat tail-flick method. In Carrageenan-induced rat paw edema, the alkaloid produced 16.93% and 24.43% inhibition of paw edema at the doses of 25 and 50 mg/kg body weight, respectively, at the third hour of study.[1]

In laboratory research, extracts of the aerial and root parts of Sida cordifolia showed good analgesic, anti-inflammatory, and hypoglycemic activities. The ethyl acetate extract of the root showed anti-inflammatory activity comparable to indomethacin. The ethyl acetate extract possessed significantly higher activity than did the methanol extract of the root part. The ethyl acetate extract of both the root and the aerial parts of Sida cordifolia showed good central and peripheral analgesic activities at a dose of 600 mg/kg.[2]

Hepatoprotective activity

A study was conducted to assess the effects of the aqueous extract of Sida cordifolia leaves on liver regeneration.[3] For the research, 20 rats were divided into four groups, three of which received aqueous Bala extract at dosages of 100, 200, and 400 mg/kg, respectively, with the fourth group receiving water only, as a control. Twenty-four hours after administration of the extract, the animal's livers were removed and observed for hepatic regeneration. The study animals treated with Bala extract showed higher rates of liver regeneration than the controls did, indicating that the herbal extract stimulates liver regeneration after partial hepatectomy in rats.

Further research has shown that fumaric acid isolated from Sida cordifolia has hepatoprotective properties.[4]

Anti-obesity activity

The Ayurvedic herb Ephedra sinica is widely used in treating weight loss. Ephedra species are well known for their thermogenic activity resulting from the alkaloids ephedrine and norephedrine. Ephedrine and norephedrine assist weight loss by suppressing the appetite. Other alkaloids such as norpseudoephedrine are less potent than ephedrine and norephedrine and can cause serious side-effects. Therapy with norephedrine has been linked to stroke in young people. The U.S. Food and Drug Administration has restricted the use of norephedrine in the United States.[5]

Sida cordifolia seems to have an anti-obesity effect similar to that of Ephedra; however, studies have shown that Sida's anti-obesity effect is not limited to its ephedrine content; other constituents may play a synergistic role.

Hypoglycemic activity

The methanol extract of Sida cordifolia root has been found to possess significant hypoglycemic activity.[6]

Anti-pyretic and anti-ulcerogenic activity

The anti-pyretic and anti-ulcerogenic properties of the methanolic extract of Sida cordifolia were investigated in rats. An oral extract dose of 500 mg/kg significantly reduced pyrexia induced by the TAB vaccine. In addition, the extract exhibited a significant anti-ulcerogenic effect against aspirin and ethanol induced ulcers, with an effectiveness comparable to that of standard drugs.[7]

Cardiac activity

An animal study investigated the cardio-stimulant activity of the hydroalcoholic extract of Bala leaves. The extract was observed to induce hypotension and bradycardia in the study animals. The hypotensive response and bradycardia was completely abolished after administration of atropine, but enhanced by hexamethonium.[8] These results show that Sida cordifolia extract produces hypotension and bradycardia, mainly because of direct stimulation of the endothelial vascular muscarinic receptor and indirect cardiac muscarinic activation.

Hydroalcoholic extract of Sida cordifolia leaves were given in myocardial infarction (MI) in rats. The albino rats were administered Sida cordifolia extract (100 and 500 mg/kg) and propranolol (10 mg/kg) orally once daily for 30 days. At the end of treatment period, MI was induced by administering isoproterenol (ISO) or by subjecting the heart to ischemia reperfusion injury (IRI). Endogenous biomarkers (LDH and CK-MB) and anti-oxidants (SOD and catalase) were estimated in serum and heart tissue. The LDH and CK-MB activities were elevated in heart tissue and depleted in the Sida cordifolia extract and propranolol groups compared to the isoproterenol and icshemic reperfusion injury control. Further, both doses of Sida cordifolia were found to significantly increase endogenous anti-oxidants in heart tissue and biochemical findings were supported by histopathological observations.[9]

Central nervous system activity

A study was aimed at assessing the effects of ethanolic extract of Sida cordifolia root on quinolinic acid -induced neurotoxicity and to compare its effect with the standard drug Deprenyl (selegiline) in the rat brain.[10] The rats were divided into six groups: (1) control group, (2)quinolinic acid (55 microg/100 g bwt/day), (3) 50% ethanolic plant extract treated group (50 mg/100 g bwt/day), (4) Deprenyl (100 microg/100 g bwt/day), (5) quinolinic acid (55 microg/100 g bwt/day) + 50% ethanolic plant extract-treated group (50 mg/100 g bwt/day), and (6) quinolinic acid (55 microg/100 g bwt/day) + Deprenyl (100 microg/100 g bwt/day).

At the end of the experimental period, a status of lipid peroxidation products, protein peroxidation product, activities of the scavenging enzymes, and activities of the inflammatory markers were analyzed. The results revealed that the lipid peroxidation products decreased and the activities of the scavenging enzymes increased significantly in the brain of the plant extract treated group, the deprenyl-treated group, and also in the co-adminstered groups. The markers of inflammatory responses such as cyclooxygenase and lipoxygenase were found to be significantly increased in the quinolinic acid treated rats, and this was decreased upon administration of the plant extract and deprenyl. Study revealed that 50% ethanolic extract of Sida cordifolia has potent anti-oxidant and anti-inflammatory activity and the activity is comparable with the standard drug deprenyl.

Studies were done to evaluate the effect of Sida on stress-induced changes in cortisol, WBC, and blood glucose level in mice. Results of this study were encouraging.[11]

Another animal study was conducted to assess the toxicity of Bala and to observe its effect on the central nervous system. Toxicity results showed that the hydroalcoholic extract of Bala was toxic at a dosage of 5000 mg/kg. The extract demonstrated a depressive effect on the animals' central nervous systems, as observed in several behavior screening tests. In the motility test, Bala extract caused a significant reduction of spontaneous activity at a dose of 1000 mg/kg at 30 and 60 minutes. The same form of the extract also decreased the ambulation and rearing in open-field tests at 30, 60, and 120 minutes at a dose of 1000 mg/kg.[12]

Anti-cancer activity

Cryptolepine (5-methyl indolo (2,3b)-quiniine), an indoloquinoline alkaloid, from Sida cordifolia was isolated. Cryptolepine induced the expression of p21(WAF1/CIP1) with growth arrest in p53-mutated human osteosarcoma MG63 cells. Four micromolar of Cryptolepine completely inhibited the growth of MG63 cells and caused G2/M-phase arrest, up-regulated the expression of p21(WAF1/CIP1) at both mRNA and protein levels in a dose-dependent manner. Cryptolepine arrested the growth of MG63 cells by activating the p21(WAF1/CIP1) promoter through the specific Sp1 site in a p53-independent manner. In addition, cryptolepine-mediated cell cycle arrest was reduced by the knockout of the p21(WAF1/CIP1) gene in human colon cancer HCT116 cells, suggesting that the cell cycle arrest was at least partially mediated through the induction of p21(WAF1/CIP1) expression, may be a suitable chemotherapeutic agent for treatment of osteosarcoma.[13]

SAFETY PROFILE

Ayurvedic formulations containing Bala should not be prescribed in combination with cardiac glycosides, monoamine oxidase inhibitors, and similar alkaloids. Although no drug interactions have been reported with Sida cordifolia preparations, great care should be taken while prescribing the herb in combination with these medications because of the great variations in the active constituents.

DOSAGE

Powder: 1–3 grams

Notes

1. R.K. Sutradhar, A.M. Rahman, M. Ahmad, S.C. Bachar, A. Saha, and T.G. Roy, "Anti-inflammatory and analgesic alkaloid from Sida cordifolia linn Pak," *J Pharm Sci.*, July 2007, 29(3):185–188.

2. V.R. Kanth and P.V. Diwan, "Analgesic, anti-inflammatory and hypoglycemic activities Sida cordifolia," *Phytother Res.*, Feb. 1999, 13(1):75–77.

3. R.L Silva, G.B. Melo, V.A. Melo, A.R. Antoniolli, P.R. Michellone, S. Zucoloto, M.A. Picinato, C.F. Franco, A. Mota Gde, and C. Silva Ode, "Effect of the aqueous extract of Sida cordifolia on liver regeneration after partial hepatectomy," *Acta Cir Bras.*, 2006, 21 Suppl 1:37–39.

4. R.S. Kumra and S.H. Mishra, "Isolation and assessment of hepatoprotective activity of fumaric acid obtained for the first time from Sida cordifolia Linn," *Indian Drugs*, 1997, 34(12):702–706.

5. C.N. Boozer, J.A. Naseer, S.B. Hemsfield, et al., "An herbal supplement containing Ma Huang-Gurana for weight loss: A randomized, double-blind trial," *Int J Obes.*, 2001, 25(3):316–324.

6. See Note 2.

7. B.K. Philip, A. Muralidharan, B. Natarajan, S. Varadamurthy, and S. Venkataraman, "Preliminary evaluation of anti-pyretic and anti-ulcerogenic activities of Sida cordifolia methanolic extract," *Fitoterapia*, April 2008, 79(3):229–231.

8. I.A. Medeiros, M.R. Santos, N.M. Nascimento, and J.C. Duarte, "Cardiovascular effects of Sida cordifolia leaves extract in rats," *Fitoterapia*, Jan. 2006, 77(1):19–27.

9. J.B. Kubavat and S.M. Asdaq, "Role of Sida cordifolia L. leaves on biochemical and anti-oxidant profile during myocardial injury," *J Ethnopharmacol.*, July 6, 2009, 124(1):162–165.

10. S.S. Swathy, S. Panicker, R.S. Nithya, M.M. Anuja, S. Rejitha, and M. Indira, "Antiperoxidative and antiinflammatory effect of Sida cordifolia Linn. on quinolinic acid induced neurotoxicity," *Neurochem Res.*, Sept. 2010, 35(9):1361–1367.

11. M. Sumanth and S.S. Mustafa, "Antistress, adoptogenic activity of Sida cordifolia roots in mice," *Indian J Pharm Sci*, 2009, 71:323–324.

12. C.I. Franco, L.C. Morais, L.J. Quintans-Júnior, R.N. Almeida, and A.R. Antoniolli, "CNS pharmacological effects of the hydroalcoholic extract of Sida cordifolia L. leaves," *J Ethnopharmacol.*, April 26, 2005, 98(3):275–279.

13. T.A Matsui, Y. Sowa, H. Murata, K. Takagi, R. Nakanishi, S. Aoki, M. Yoshikawa, T. Kobayashi, T. Sakabe, T. Kubo, and T. Sakai T., "The plant alkaloid cryptolepine induces p21WAF1/CIP1 and cell cycle arrest in a human osteosarcoma cell line," *Int J Oncol.*, Oct. 2007, 31(4):915–922.

Solanum Nigrum

Introduction

Solanum nigrum, or black nightshade, is a widespread herb that bears oval, black berries. Although in large quantities the berries of Solanum nigrum may have adverse effects, the plant nonetheless has considerable medicinal value, particularly as a hepatoprotective agent, and also as a treatment for various skin disorders.

In Ayurvedic tradition, Solanum nigrum is known for its antiperiodic, antiphlogistic, diaphoretic, diuretic, emollient, febrifuge, and sedative properties. Its leaves, stems, and roots are used externally in the form of a poultice or wash to treat sores, boils, and wounds, and as a cosmetic. Extracts of Solanum nigrum are analgesic, anti-spasmodic, and anti-inflammatory. In infants, an infusion of Solanum can be used as an enema and to cure colic. The juice extract of the fresh herb is effective in treating fevers and toothaches.

The leaves of black nightshade are effective in treating digestive disorders. The raw juice of the leaves can be used alone or mixed with other juices or liquids, making a tonic for stomach disorders including flatulence, colitis, and peptic ulcers. This infusion also is used to treat dysentery, and Solanum helps to remove phlegm from the bronchial tubes of asthma patients.

Solanum is used extensively used to treat chronic skin conditions. The juice is applied externally to areas affected with acne, eczema, and psoriasis. Because of its pain-relieving properties, a decoction of the plant is used to wash inflamed areas of the body. A paste made from black nightshade often is applied over skin ulcers, burns, herpes, and ringworm, and on painful joints.

Synonymous Names

Botanical name: Solanum nigrum
English: Black nightshade
Hindi: Makoya, Makoy, Manathakkali
Sanskrit: Kakamachi
Bengali: Gurkkamai

Habitat

Solanum nigrum is common in tropical areas, growing in shady places up to an altitude of 1800 meters. The plant grows as a weed all over dry parts of India.

Botanical Characteristics

Solanum nigrum is an annual herb that grows to an average height of 1 meter. Its erect, angular, branching stem is covered with inward-bent hairs. The stem is rounded at the base and angular at its apex. The plant grows diffusely with several arching branches. Its taproot has few branches and the bark is thin, smooth, and pale-brown.

Solanum bears alternate, dark-green, toothed leaves that are egg-shaped. The flowers grow in clusters, which are white, cream, or violet in color. The fruit is pea-sized and many-seeded purple or blackberry.

Chemical Composition

Black nightshade's chemical constitution consists of 82% moisture, 5.9% protein, 1% fat, 2.1% minerals, and 8.9% carbohydrate. Minerals and vitamins include calcium, iron, phosphorus, riboflavin, niacin, and vitamin C.

Solanum's active chemical constituents are believed to be its glyco-alkaloids, which are solasodine, disogenin, and five steroidal glycosides SN-0 SN-1 SN-2 SN-3 and SN-4. Other constituents are palmitic acid, isochlorogenic acid, stearic acid, oleic and linoleic acid.

Pharmacological Activity

Anti-cancer activity

To explore the anti-tumor activity of the aqueous extract of Solanum nigrum and its possible mechanisms, its effects on tumor growth in-vivo was studied in mice. The study results showed that Solanum extract inhibited growth of cervical carcinoma tumors. Solanum nigrum arrested tumor growth in the G0/G1 phase and induced apoptosis of more transplanted tumor cells in a dose-dependent manner. These results indicated that Solanum extract may suppress the growth of cervical carcinomas by modulating the immune response of the tumor bearing mice and causing tumor cell cycle arrest in the G0/G1 phase, as well as inducing apoptosis with little toxicity to the animals.[1]

An additional study demonstrated that the total alkaloids isolated from Solanum nigrum inhibited the growth of human cervical cancer HeLa cells in a culture medium with much lower toxicity to normal human lymphocytes. The results further revealed that Solanum extract induced cell death by apoptosis. An immunohistochemical assay showed downregulation of the bcl-2 and p53 genes and no obvious change of the bax gene in the extract treated cells. Subcutaneous injection of HeLa cells induced tumor formation in mice, and Solanum extract showed a significant inhibitory effect on tumor formation. These results suggested that Solanum nigrum extract may be a potential, natural apoptosis-inducing agent in treating cervical cancer.[2]

In another study, the polyphenols and anthocyanidin in various parts of the Solanum nigrum plant were analyzed by HPLC. The leaves were found to be richer in polyphenols than were the stem and fruit. The leaves contained the highest concentration of gentisic acid, luteolin, apigenin, kaempferol, and m-coumaric acid. The anthocyanidin, however, existed only in the purple fruits. Cytotoxicity of the leaf, stem, or fruit extract was evaluated against cancer cell lines and normal cells. The results showed that the AU565 breast cancer cells were more sensitive to the extract. Further, the results demonstrated a significant cytotoxic effect of the Solanum nigrum leaf extract on AU565 cells, mediated via two different mechanisms depending on the exposure concentrations. A low dose of leaf extract induced autophagy but not apoptosis. Higher doses (>100 microg/mL) of leaf extract could inhibit the level of p-Akt and cause cell death from the induction of autophagy and apoptosis. These findings suggested that the Solanum nigrum leaf extract induced cell death in breast cells via two distinct antineoplastic activities, the abilities to induce apoptosis and autophagy, suggesting that it may provide a useful remedy to treat breast cancer.[3]

Solamargine, a steroidal alkaloid glycoside from Solanum nigrum has displayed a cytotoxicity superior to many human tumor cells. In human K562 leukemia cells solamargine could induce an early lysosomal rupture within 2 hours, as assessed by acridine-orange relocation and alkalinization of lysosomes. Intracellular lysosomal rupture was confirmed with the release of cathepsin B to cytosol detected by the Western Blot test. solamargine caused subsequent mitochondrial damage, including mitochondrial membrane permeabilization as detected by a decrease in membrane potential as well as the release of cytochrome c from mitochondria. The cellular Ca(2+) overload is more pronounced in solamargine treated cells. The cells exposed to 10muM solamargine for 30 minutes showed a maximum seven-fold increase in intracellular calcium concentration compared to the vehicle-treated controls. The down expression of Bcl-2, upregulation of Bax, caspase-3 and caspase-9 activities that the cytotoxicity of solamargine was involved in a lysosomal-mitochondrial death pathway.[4]

Anti-ulcer activity

Solanum nigrum is recommended in Ayurvedic medicine for the management of gastric ulcers. A study was undertaken to investigate the anti-ulcer effect of Solanum nigrum extract on cold restraint stress, indomethacin, pyloric ligation, and ethanol-induced gastric ulcer models and ulcer-healing activity on an acetic acid-induced ulcer model in rats. Treatment with Solanum extract at the higher dose significantly inhibited the gastric lesions induced by all the tested factors. A corresponding attenuation of gastric secretory volume, acidity, and pepsin secretion was observed in the ulcerated rats. In addition, the Solanum extract accelerated the healing of acetic acid-induced ulcers after 7 days of treatment. Solanum extract was shown to significantly inhibit $H^+K^+ATPase$ activity and decrease gastrin secretion in the alcohol-induced ulcer model. The severity of the reaction to ulcerogenics and the reduction of ulcer size by Solanum extract was evidenced by histological findings.[5]

Solanum extract possesses anti-ulcerogenic as well as ulcer healing properties, perhaps due to its antisecretory activity.

Hepatoprotective activity

Solanum nigrum has been used in many traditional medicine systems as a hepatoprotective agent. A study was conducted to investigate the effects of Solanum nigrum extract on thioacetamide-induced liver fibrosis in mice. Hepatic fibrosis was produced by thiocetamide (0.2 g/kg, i.p.) three times a week for 12 weeks. Mice in the three thiocetamide groups were treated daily with distilled water and Solanum extract via gastric feeding throughout the experimental period. The Solanum extract reduced the hepatic hydroxyproline and alpha-smooth muscle actin protein levels of the thiocetamide-treated mice. It also inhibited thiocetamide-induced collagen (alpha-1)(i) chain and transforming growth factor-beta1 (TGF-beta1) mRNA levels in the liver. Histological examination also confirmed that Solanum extract reduced the degree of fibrosis caused by thiocetamide treatment. These results suggests that oral administration of Solanum extract significantly reduces thiocetamide-induced hepatic fibrosis in mice, probably via the reduction of TGF-beta1 secretion.[6]

The protective effects of a water extract of Solanum nigrum extract against liver damage were evaluated in carbon tetrachloride induced chronic hepatotoxicity in rats. The rats were orally fed Solanum extract along with CCl4 for 6 weeks. The results of this study showed that the treatment with Solanum extract significantly lowered the CCl4-induced serum levels of key hepatic enzyme markers, superoxides, and hydroxyl radicals. The complete liver profile values for all markers were brought back to control levels by the extract supplement. Liver histopathology showed that Solanum extract reduced the incidence of liver lesions including hepatic cells' cloudy swelling, lymphocytes infiltration, hepatic necrosis, and fibrous connective tissue proliferation induced by CCl4 in rats.[7]

Solanum nigrum water extract prevented hepatic injury and hepatocarcinogenesis by 2-acetylaminofluorene, acetylaminofluorene and sodium nitrite. Solanum nigrum supplementation significantly alleviated acetylaminofluorene induced hepatic injury and early hepatocarcinogenesis, as well as the acetylaminofluorene and sodium nitrite-induced lethal hepatoma, which may result from the overexpression of glutathione S-transferase, nuclear factor (erythroid-derived 2)-like 2 (Nrf2), and anti-oxidant enzymes.[8]

Solanum nigrum fruit extract was investigated for its anti-oxidant and antihyperlipidemic activity against ethanol-induced toxicity in rats. The experimental animals were intoxicated with 20% ethanol (7.9 g/ kg/day) for 30 days via gastric intubation. Solanum nigrum fruits extract was administered at a dose of 250 mg/kg body weight along with the daily dose of ethanol for 30 days. As a result, the ethanol-induced rats showed a significant elevation in the levels of thiobarbituric acid reactive substances (TBARS), which lowered the anti-oxidant defense systems, such as reduced glutathione (GSH) and vitamins C and E, compared to the controls. In the lipid profiles, the levels of total cholesterol (TC), triglycerides (TG), low density lipoproteins (LDL), very low density lipoproteins (VLDL), free fatty acids (FFA), and phospholipids were elevated significantly in the ethanol-induced group, whereas the high density lipoproteins (HDL) were found to be reduced in the plasma, and the phospholipid levels were decreased significantly in the tissues. Supplementation with Solanum nigrum fruit extract improved the anti-oxidant status by decreasing the levels of TBARS and altering the lipid profiles to near normal. These activities were comparable to silymarin (25 mg/kg body weight).[9]

Dr. Sodhi's Experience

Thirty years ago, when I was very young doctor, a farmer came to me with acute low back pain. I prescribed him massage treatment and an anti-inflammatory protocol, even analgesic injections. His pain did not improve. I saw this patient one month later and asked him, "How is your back pain?" He replied, "Doctor, your treatment didn't work and I couldn't even move. My mother made a soup of the Solanum nigrum plant fresh from the farm. After two days, all my pain is gone." Later I learned that Solanum has a steroid-like structure and may play a role in getting inflammation under control. I have used Solanum nigrum in liver preparation with greater success in many kinds of liver diseases.

Safety Profile

Large doses of Solanum nigrum berries may be toxic in some people. The herb should not be given internally except under the supervision of a qualified professional.

Ayurvedic Properties

Guna: Sara, snigdha, laghu
Virya: Ushna
Vipaka: Katu
Dosha: Tridoshahara
Karma: Bhedana, Rasayana
Swarya, hrudya, vrishya, kushta nashaka, vajeekarana, ushna virya.

Notes

1. J Li, Q. Li, T. Feng, and K. Li, "Aqueous extract of Solanum nigrum inhibit growth of cervical carcinoma (U14) via modulating immune response of tumor bearing mice and inducing apoptosis of tumor cells," *Fitoterapia*, Dec..2008, 79(7–8):548–556.

2. J. Li , Q.W. Li, D.W Gao, Z.S Han, and K. Li, "Antitumor effects of total alkaloids isolated from Solanum nigrum in vitro and in vivo," *Pharmazie*, July 2008, 63(7):534–538.

3. H.C. Huang, K.Y. Syu, and J.K. Lin, "Chemical composition of Solanum nigrum Linn extract and induction of autophagy by leaf water extract and its major flavonoids in AU565 breast cancer cells," *J Agric Food Chem.*, Aug. 11, 2010, 58(15):8699–8708.

4. L Sun, Y. Zhao, X. Li, H. Yuan, A. Cheng, and H. Lou, "A lysosomal-mitochondrial death pathway is induced by solamargine in human K562 leukemia cells," *Toxicol In Vitro*,2010 Sep;24(6):1504-1

5. Jainu M, Devi CS. Antiulcerogenic and ulcer healing effects of Solanum nigrum (L.) on experimental ulcer models: possible mechanism for the inhibition of acid formation. J Ethnopharmacol. 2006 Mar 8;104(1-2):156-63

6. C.C Hsieh, H.L. Fang, and W.C. Lina, "Inhibitory effect of Solanum nigrum on thioacetamide-induced liver fibrosis in mice," *J Ethnopharmacol.*, Sept. 2, 2008, 119(1):117–121.

7. H.M Lin , H.C. Tseng, C.J. Wang, J.J. Lin, C.W. Lo, and F.P. Chou, "Hepatoprotective effects of Solanum nigrum Linn extract against CCl(4)-induced oxidative damage in rats," *Chem Biol Interact.*, Feb. 15, 2008, 171(3):283–293.

8. J. D. Hsu, S.H. Kao, C.C. Tu, Y.J. Li, and C.J. Wang, "Solanum nigrum L. extract inhibits 2-acetylaminofluorene-induced hepatocarcinogenesis through overexpression of glutathione S-transferase and anti-oxidant enzymes," *J Agric Food Chem*, Sept. 23, 2009, 57(18):8628–8634.

9. V. Arulmozhi, M. Krishnaveni, K. Karthishwaran, G. Dhamodharan, and S. Mirunalini, "Anti-oxidant and antihyperlipidemic effect of Solanum nigrum fruit extract on the experimental model against chronic ethanol toxicity" *Pharmacogn*, Jan. 2010, 6(21):42–50.

Swertia chirayita

Introduction

Swertia chirayita is an ancient Ayurvedic herb, also known as "Nepali Neem" because it is common in the forests of Nepal. The name sometimes refers to other gentian-like plants that are sold in Indian bazaars. It was introduced into Europe in 1839 and still is widely used there.

Swertia commonly is used to stimulate the appetite and relieve acidity and nausea and is highly valued as a tonic in debility and convalescence. It serves as a treatment for liver disorders, and is an alterative, a laxative, a vermifuge, and a sedative. It has been used to treat asthma, cough, bronchitis, and malaria.

Among the various species of Swertia reported in India, it is considered to be the most important for its medicinal properties. Swertia is a component in a variety of herbal preparations because of its antipyretic, hypoglycemic, anti-fungal, and anti-bacterial properties. Notwithstanding its value in the herbal industry, the plant still is collected from the wild.

Swertia is bitter in taste, cooling light and dry—characteristics that are considered to be therapeutic to the blood and liver. Its use has also been mentioned in Unani medicine.[1] A concoction of chirayita with cardamom, turmeric, and kutki (Picrorhiza) is given for gastrointestinal infections, and along with ginger, it is considered to be good for fever. When given along with Neem, manjishta (Rubia cordifolia) and gotu kola, Swertia serves as a cure for various skin problems. It is used in combination with other herbs for scorpion bite.

A slow-growing species, Swertia is harvested when it begins to flower in July–September. Seed setting commences around October–November, and the seeds germinate immediately after shedding. Sparsely cultivated, little effort has been directed toward developing proper agricultural techniques for commercial cultivation.

Only a few scattered reports in the literature suggest germination studies and nursery practices of Swertia chirayita.[2,3] After 3 C° chilling treatment for 15 days, 91% seed germination was reported.[4] Another study reported a maximum of 81% germination.[5] Some of the factors that discourage commercial cultivation of the plant are the low germination percentage and viability of the seeds, long gestation periods, and delicate field-handling.[6]

In our Ayush Farms we are cultivating and encouraging farmers to grow Swertia on buy back guarantee.

Synonymous Names

Latin: Swertia chirayita, Gentian chirayita
English: Chiretta
Hindi: Chirayita
Sanskrit: Kir-ata

Other names: Chirayata, Kirata-tikta, Kiryat-charayatah, Bhunimba, Bhuchiretta, Charayatah, Chiretta, Chiraita, Indian Gentian, Jwaran-thakah, Kirata, kiraita, Kiriath, Kiriyattu, Kiryat-charayatah, Mahatita, Nilavemu, Nila-vembu, Qasabuz-Zarirah

Habitat

Swertia is indigenous to the temperate Himalayas, where it is found at an altitude of 1200–3000 meters from Kashmir to Bhutan, and in the Khasi hills at 1200–1500 meters It may be cultivated in sub-temperate regions between 1500 and 2100 meters. The plant can tolerate a variety of soils with sandy loam that is rich in carbon and humus. It also is found in open ground areas and recently slashed and-burnt forests.

Some authors have described Chirayita as an annual,[7,8] and other authorities describe it as a biennial or pluri–annual plant.[9] It is not clear whether the plant behaves differently due to climatic conditions or varying genotypes.

Botanical Characteristics

Swertia has an erect stem, about 2 to 3 feet in length. The middle portion is round, and the upper is four angled with a prominent line at each angle. The stems are orange-brown or purplish in color and contain wide, continuous, yellowish pith. The root is simple, stout, tapering, and short, almost 7 centimeters long, and usually half an inch thick. The flowers appear in the form of numerous small, axillary, opposite, laxcymes arranged as short branches. The whole inflorescence is about 2 feet long.

The flowers are small, stalked, and greenish yellow, tinged with purple color, rotate and tetramerous. The corolla is twice as long as the calyx and is divided near the base into four ovate–lanceolate segments. The upper surface of the petal has a pair of nectaries covered with oblong scales and ending as fringes. The fruit a small, one-celled capsule with a transparent yellowish pericarp, which divides from above, septicidally into two valves. The seeds are numerous and tiny.

Chemical Composition

Swertia chirayita belongs to the botanical family Gentianaceae, the members of which are well-reputed to contain many important chemical constituents, namely iridoids, xanthones, mangiferin and C–gluco-flavones. Reviews detailing the chemical constituents of the Swertia genus have been reported.[10,11,12] The entire plant is used in traditional medicine; however, the root is considered to be the most powerful part.

Chirayita contains a yellow bitter acid, ophelic acid, two bitter glucosides, chiartin and amarogentin (one of the most bitter substances known), gentiopicrin, two yellow crystalline phenols, a neutral, yellow crystalline compound, and a new xanthone, swechirin. The herb contains swertanone, swertenol, episwertinol, chiratenol, gammacer-16-en-3ß-ol, 21-a-H-hop-22(29)-en-3ß-ol, taraxerol, oleanolic acid, ursolic acid, swerta-7,9(11)-dien-3ß-ol, and pichierenol, as well as ß-amyrin, y-taraxasterol, lupeol, and erythrodiol. It also yields, 1,3,6,7-tetrahydroxyxanthone-C-2-ß-D-glucoside (mangiferin), which have contributed a significant immunomodulatory potential.

A new xanthone, 1,5-dihydroxy-3,8-dimethoxyxanthone (chiratol)V— besides swerchirin and 7-O-Me swertiarin and monohydroxy terephthalic acid, and 2,5-dihydroxy terephthalic acid— was isolated from the herb. The herb also yields 1,5,8-trihydroxy-3-methoxyxanthone, 1-hydroxy-3,5,8-trimethoxyxanthone, 1-hydroxy-3,7,8-trimethoxy xanthone, 1,8-dihydroxy-3,5-dimethoxy-xanthone, 1,8-dihodroxy-3,7- dimethoxy xanthone, 1,3,6,7-tetrahydroxyxanthone C-2-ß-D-glucoside (mengiferin), 1,3,8-trihydroxy-5- methoxyxanthone, 1,3,5,8- tetrahydroxy xanthone and 1,3,7,8- tetrahydroxy xanthone, a novel dimeric xanthone (chiratanin), and the alkaloids gentianine, gentiocricine, and enicoflavine.[13]

Pharmacological Activity

Anti-leishmanicidal activity

Active principles from Swertia chirayita have been shown in laboratory research to inhibit the activity of Leishmania donovani. The glucoside Amarogentin, isolated from the methanolic extract of Swertia chirayita, exhibited potent inhibitory action against type I DNA topoisomerase from Leishmania donovani. Researchers hypothesized that the substance acts by preventing the formation of binary complex.[14]

Further evidence of this activity was seen in an animal model of experimental leishmaniasis. The liposomal and the niosomal forms of amarogentin both were found to be more effective inhibitors than was free amarogentin. Blood pathology, histological staining of tissues, and specific enzyme levels related to normal liver function revealed no toxicity.[15]

Anti-ulcerogenic activity

The intensity of experimentally induced gastric ulcers was reduced significantly by an ethanolic extract of Swertia chirayita. In ulcers induced by indomethacin and necrotizing agents in rats, depletion of ethanol-induced gastric wall mucus and restoration of the non-protein sulfhydryl content in the glandular stomachs were achieved by pretreating the rats with the extract. The extract also showed anti-cholinergic activity by inhibiting acetylcholine induced contraction of guinea pig ileum under experimental conditions.[16]

Central nervous system depressant activity

Swertia chirayita ethanolic extract reversed mangiferin-induced CNS stimulatory effects in albino mice and rats. Swertiamarin and mangiferin, both present in the same plant, were shown to antagonize each other in in-vivo studies.[17]
Anti-diabetic activity

A 95% ethanolic extract of Swertia was observed to lower blood glucose levels significantly in fed, fasted, and glucose-loaded albino rats. The hypoglycemic activity of tolbutamide was increased in healthy albino rats by administering Swertia chirayita extract orally.[18] Ethanolic extract of Swertia chirayita exhibits hypoglycemic activity. The hexane fraction containing swerchirin, the main hypoglycemic principle, induced a significant fall in blood sugar in albino rats. These results indicate that Swertia chirayita may have clinical application in control of diabetes.[19]

Hepatoprotective activity

The methanol extract of Swertia chirayita has been studied to determine its anti-hepatotoxic activity using paracetamol and galactosamine models. The extract was found to be active at a dose of 100 mg/kg and on fractionating. Swertia's activity was found to reside mainly in the chloroform fraction, which was most active at a dose level of 25 mg/kg. These two hepatotoxins induce hepatotoxicity by different mechanisms, suggesting a broad and non-specific protection of the liver for Swertia chirayita.[20]

The liver-protecting activity also was ascertained in carbon tetra-chloride-induced liver damage in albino rats over 16 days. Simultaneous administration of Swertia chirayita at a dose of 50 mg/kg produced improvement in both biochemical and histopathological parameters, and again the chloroform extract was the most active.[21]

Anti-microbial activity

Swertia chirayita also possesses anti-microbial activity against gram-negative and gram-positive bacteria. An herbal antiseptic and antifungal veterinary ointment is prepared from the herb.[22]

Anti-inflammatory activity

The extract of Swertia chirayita has exhibited a significant anti-inflammatory activity.[23]

The effect of aqueous extract of Swertia chirayita stem on the balance of pro- and anti-inflammatory cytokines in primary joint synovium of adjuvant induced arthritic mice was studied. The level of pro-inflammatory cytokines was found to be elevated in the joint synovium of arthritic mice in comparison to normal joints. Administration of Swertia chirayita extract in varying doses through the oral route did not modulate the pro-inflammatory cytokines on day 2. In contrast, by day 12, a dose-dependent reduction of tumor necrosis factor-alpha (INF-alpha) interleukin-1beta, (IL-beta) and interferon-gamma (IFN-gamma), and elevation of Interleukin-10 (IL-10) was observed in the joint homogenates of the arthritic mice. Interleukin-6 was not downregulated in the joint homogenate of the arthritic mice at the dose of 11.86 mg/kg but significant reduction was observed at higher doses. The aqueous extract was found to possess two polar compounds, amarogentin and mangiferin, but was devoid of swerchirin, chiratol, methyl swetianin, and swertanone. Mangiferin has been reported to possess potent anti-inflammatory property, and it is presumed that its presence in the aqueous extract of Swertia chirayita is responsible for reducing TNF-alpha, IL-1beta, IL-6, and IFN-gamma and/or elevating IL-10 in the joint homogenates of arthritic mice on day 12. Swertia chirayita may have significant use in reducing inflammation and in maintaining anti-inflammatory cytokine balance.

Anti-viral activity

Swertia chirayita showed anti-viral properties against Herpes simplex virus type-1.[24] The anti-viral activity of Swertia was tested against Herpes simplex virus (HSV) type-1, using multiple approaches at both the cellular and molecular levels. Cytotoxicity, plaque reduction, virus infectivity, antigen expression, and polymerase chain reaction assays were conducted to test the anti-viral activity of the plant extract. Swertia plant crude extract (1gm/mL) at 1:64 dilution inhibited HSV-1, plaque formation at more than 70% level. The HSV antigen expression and time kinetics experiments conducted by indirect immunofluorescence tests revealed a characteristic pattern of small foci of single fluorescent cells in the extract-treated HSV-1 infected cells at 4 hours post-infection dose, suggested drug inhibited viral dissemination. Infected cell cultures treated with Swertia extract at various time intervals, tested by PCR, failed to show amplification at 12, 24–72 hours. The HSV-1 infected cells treated with the anti-viral drug Acyclovir did not show any amplification by PCR.

Anti-cancer activity

Considerable attention has focused on plants that are sources of natural anti-oxidant compounds, because most of them have a modulatory effect on physiological function and biotransformation reactions involved in the detoxification process. Such compounds are likely to afford protection from cytotoxic, genotoxic, and metabolic actions of environmental toxicants, thereby reducing the risk for cancer.

A study was conducted to assess the anti-carcinogenic activity of Swertia chirayita. All four of the detoxification enzymes studied— GST, GPx, SOD, and CAT—were found to be activated to different degrees following treatment with infusion of Swertia chirayita, its crude extract, and a purified

Amarogentin rich extract. Activation of the enzymes was accompanied by a significant reduction in lipid peroxidation and inhibition of incidence, as well as multiplicity of Dimethylbenz(a) anthracene (DMBA) induced papillomas. The effect of Swertia chirayita on apoptosis and cell proliferation also was studied in mice skin exposed to DMBA. Both the crude and the purified extracts significantly inhibited cell proliferation and induced apoptosis. These observations suggest the chemopreventive potential of Swertia chirayita.[25]

Safety Profile

The drug normally produces no problems at recommended doses. The maximum tolerated dose of the 50% ethanolic extract of the whole plant is 1000 mg/kg IP in adult rats.

Dosage

Whole plant: 0.5-2 g
Liquid extract or tincture 1:1: 2–5 ml

Ayurvedic Properties

Rasa: Tikta (bitter)
Guna: Laghu (light), ruksha (dry)
Veerya: Ushna (hot)
Vipaka: Katu (pungent)
Dosha: Balances tridosha

Important Note: Swertia Chirayita and Swetia chirata is the same plant.

Notes

1. B. Mukherji (Ed.), *Indian Pharmaceutical Codex, Indigenous Drugs,* Vol. I (New Delhi: CSIR, 1953), pp. 64–65.
2. R. Raina, A. K. Johri, and L. J. Srivastava, "Seed germination studies in Swertia chirata L.," *Seed Res.,* 1994, 22:62–63.
3. D. B. Basnet, "Evolving nursery practices and method of cultivation of high value medicinal plant Swertia chirata Ham.," *Environ. Ecol.,* 2001, 19:935–938.
4. See Note 2.
5. See Note 3.
6. H. K. Badola and M. Pal, "Endangered medicinal plant species in Himachal Pradesh," *Curr. Sci.,* 2002, 83:97–798.
7. Anonymous, *The Wealth of India: Raw Materials: Publication and Information Directorate,* Vol. X (New Delhi: CSIR, 1982), pp. 78–81.
8. K. R. Kirtikar and B. D. Basu (Eds.), *Indian Medicinal Plants,* Vol. III (Allahabad, country ?,1984), pp. 1664–1666.
9. D. M. Edwards, "The marketing of non -timber forest product from the Himalayas: The trade between East Nepal and India," Rural Development Forestry Network, **where?** 1993, pp. 1–21.
10. R. Bentley, and H. Trimen (Eds.), *Medicinal Plants* (London: J and A Churchill, 1880), p. 183; K. M. Nandkarni (Ed.), *Indian Materia Medica*, Vol. I, (Bombay: Popular Prakashan, 1976), pp. 1184–1186.
11. A. K. Chakravarty, S. Mukhopadhyay, S. K. Moitra, and B. Das, "Syringareinol, a hepatoprotective agent and other constituents from Swertia chirayita," *Indian J. Chem.,* 1994, 33:405–408.
12. K. K. Purushothaman, A. Sarada, and V. Narayanaswami, "Chemical examination of Swertia chirayita," *Leather Sci.* (Madras), 1973, 20:132–134; K. K. Purushothaman, A. Sarada, and V. Narayanaswami, "Chemical examination of kiratatikta (Swertia chirayita)," *JRIM*, 1973, 8:23–28.
13. Rakesh K. Asthana, Narendra K. Sharma, Dinesh K. Kulshreshtha, Sunil K. Chatterjee A xanthone from Swertia chirayita *Phytochemistry,* 30(3), 1991:1037-1039.

14. S. Ray, H.K. Majumder, A.K. Chakravarty, S. Mukhopadhyay, R.R. Gil, and G.A. Cordell, "Amarogentin, a naturally occurring secoiridoid glycoside and a newly recognized inhibitor of topoisomerase I from Leishmania donovani," *J. Nat. Prod.*, 1996, 59:27–29.

15. S. Medda, S. Mukhopadhyay, and M.K. Basu, "Evaluation of the in vivo activity of and toxicity of amarogentin, an antileishmanial agent, in both liposomal and niosomal forms," *J. Anti Micro Chemother.*, 1999, 44:791–794.

16. S. Rafatullah, M. Tariq, J.S. Mossa, M.A. Al-Yahya, M.S. Al-Said, and A. M. Ageel, "Protective effect of Swertia chirayita against indomethacin and other ulcerogenic agent-induced gastric ulcers," *Exp. Clin. Res.*, 1993, 19:69–73.

17. Bhattacharya SK, Reddy PK, Ghosal S, Singh AK, Sharma PV. Chemical constituents of Gentianaceae XIX: CNS-depressant effects of swertiamarin. J Pharm Sci. 1976 Oct;65(10):1547-9.

18. S. K. Mitra, S. Gopumadhavan, and T. S. Muralidhar, "Effect of D-400, an ayurvedic herbal formulation on experimentally-induced diabetes mellitus," *Phytother. Res.*, 1996, 10:433.

19. B. Chandrashekar, M. B. Bajpai, and S.K. Mukherjee, " Hypoglycemic activity of Swertia chirayita (Roxb ex Flem) Karst," *Indian J. Exp. Biol.*, 1990, 28, 616–618.

20. See Note 11.

21. S. Mukherjee, A. Sur, and B. R. Maiti, "Hepatoprotective effect of Swertia chirayita on rats," *Indian J. Exp. Biol.* , 1997, 35, 384–388.

22. Alam KD, Ali MS, Parvin S, Mahjabeen S, Akbar MA, Ahamed R. In vitro antimicrobial activities of different fractions of Swertia chirayita ethanolic extract. Pak J Biol Sci. 2009 Oct 1;12(19):1334-7.

23. I.V. Kumar, B.N. Paul, R. Asthana, A. Saxena, S. Mehrotra, and G. Rajan, "Swertia chirayita mediated modulation of interleukin-1beta, interleukin-6, interleukin-10, interferon-gamma, and tumor necrosis factor-alpha in arthritic mice," *Immunopharmacol Immunotoxicol.* Nov. 2003, 25(4):573–583;

24. H. Verma, P.R. Patil, R.M. Kolhapure, and V. Gopalkrishna, "Anti-viral activity of the Indian medicinal plant extract *Swertia chirata* against herpes simplex viruses: A study by *in-vitro* and molecular approach," *Indian J Med Microbiol*, 2008, 26:322–326.

25. P. Saha, S. Mandal, A. Das, P.C. Das, and S. Das, "Evaluation of the anticarcinogenic activity of Swertia chirata Buch. Ham, an Indian medicinal plant, on DMBA-induced mouse skin carcinogenesis model," *Phytother-Res.*, :May 2004, 18(5): 373–378.

Terminalia bellerica

Introduction

Terminalia bellerica is a highly valued herb in Ayurveda, forming part of the renowned rasayana Triphala, which is widely believed to enhance longevity and act as a tonic for the whole body. The tree's Sanskrit name, Bibhitaki, refers to its capacity to keep a person healthy and free from disease. Terminalia bellerica has a strong purgative action. It is known to expel stones and other accumulations in the digestive, urinary, and respiratory tracts. It also is a strong rejuvenator, especially for the voice, vision, and hair. The preparation Triphala is widely prescribed for liver disorders and gastrointestinal problems.

Research has shown that Terminalia bellerica reduces levels of lipids throughout the body, and specifically lipid levels in the liver and heart. This shows a strong action in preventing heart and liver fat congestion, which can lower the disease risk associated with those organs. Other studies indicate that Terminalia bellerica has retroviral actions in inhibiting viral growth in leukemia patients. Another study indicates the strong inhibiting effect of Terminalia bellerica on the HIV virus.[1] The fruit of Terminalia bellerica historically has been used by several ethnic groups in India and neighboring countries to treat a variety of ailments. It is considered to be a tonic, hepatoprotective, anti-viral, purgative, hypolipidemic, astringent, and anti-diarrheal. It also is reputed to improve immunity and bodily resistance to infectious disease and, therefore, is used for coughs, sore throats, and eye and skin diseases such as conjunctivitis and leprosy.

Synonymous Names

English: Beleric myrobalan
Hindi: Bhaira, bahera
Sanskrit: Bibhitaki, vibeekaka, bibhitaki

Habitat

Terminalia bellerica is native to the forests of India, Sri Lanka, and other Asian countries, growing well in all but the most arid climates. It grows to an altitude of about 1200 meters. Also, it is cultivated in gardens and parks and at roadsides.

Botanical Characteristics

Terminalia bellerica is a large deciduous tree that may reach up to 30 meters in height. Its trunk and limbs are straight and are covered with a cracked, grayish-blue bark. The leaves are broadly elliptical, measuring about 10–25 centimeters in length and 5–8 centimeters in width, coriaceous, alternate, and directed mainly toward the apex of the branches. The flowers are in axillary spikes, pale greenish-yellow, and have an unpleasant odor. The fruits are globular, grey, hairy, and about 1–2 centimeters in diameter.

Chemical Composition

Triterpenoids:

Belleric acid, the glycoside saponins bellericoside and bellericanin, and sterols such as p-sitosterol have been isolated from Terminalia bellerica fruit.[2]

Polyphenols:

Phyllemblin, ellagic acid, gallic acid, ethyl gallate, chebulagic acid, and hexahydroxy diphenic acid ester are present.[3,4]

Fixed oil:

A fixed oil is extracted from Terminalia bellerica seed.

Pharmacological Activity

Anti-viral activity:

A bioactivity-guided fractionation of an extract of Terminalia bellerica fruit rind led to the isolation of two new lignans named (1) termilignan and (2) thannilignan, together with (3) 7-hydroxy-3',4'-(methylenedioxy)flavan and (4) anolignan B. All four of these compounds possessed demonstrable anti-HIV-1 activity in vitro.[5]

Anti-oxidant activity:

Free radical-induced cellular damage is involved in several pathological conditions including cancer, rheumatism, liver injury, ischemic heart disease, and aging. Triphala, which contains Terminalia bellerica, showed scavenging activity against mitochondrial lipid peroxidation, and the phenolic compounds present were credited for this anti-oxidant activity.[6]

Cardiovascular activity:

In-vivo and in-vitro studies have shown Terminalia bellerica's cardiovascular activity, including negative inotropic and chronotropic activity, as well as hypotensive effects. These actions were attributed to cholinergic activity.[7,8]

Hypolipidemic activity:

Terminalia bellerica reduces the levels of lipids throughout the body and specifically lowers lipid levels in the liver and heart. This shows a strong action in preventing heart and liver fat congestion, with a resulting decrease in the disease risk associated with these organs.

When Terminalia bellerica was administered to animals in which arteriosclerosis had been induced by feeding a cholesterol-rich diet, significant decreases in the cholesterol level of the liver and aorta were observed.[9,10,11]

Anti-microbial activity:

Anti-bacterial activity of Terminalia bellerica has been shown against a wide range of bacterial organisms. Triphala was active against Clostridium tetanus[12,13] and several viruses such as the vesicular stomatitis virus and a rotavirus.[14,15] The anti-salmonella activity of Terminalia bellerica, an ingredient of the Ayurvedic preparation Triphala, has been reported for treating digestive and liver disorders. The fruits of T. bellerica were extracted with petroleum ether, chloroform, acetone, alcohol, and water, and the efficacy of extracts against Salmonella typhi and Salmonella typhimurium was evaluated.[16] The alcoholic and water extracts of T. bellerica showed significant anti-salmonella activity, and MIC was 12.5 mg/ml against S. typhimurium. Aqueous extracts of Picrohiza kurroa and Vitits vinefera also showed low anti-Salmonella activity, whereas aqueous extracts of Asparagus racemosus and Zingiber officinale showed no anti-salmonella activity. Extracts of Terminalia bellerica, Picrohiza kurroa, and Vitits vinefera with other solvents, such as chloroform and petroleum ether, showed insignificant activity. Aqueous extract of Terminalia bellerica was bactericidal at high concentrations, whereas low concentrations showed bacteriostatic properties. In-vitro cellular toxicity studies showed no cytotoxicity associated with Terminalia bellerica extracts. Pre-treatment of mice with an aqueous extract of Terminalia bellerica conferred protection against experimental salmonellosis, and 100% survival of animals has been reported when challenged with lethal doses of Salmonella typhimurium.

In another study, Terminalia bellerica was found to be effective against cholera.[17] Similar results were realized by using Terminalia bellerica in combination with Emblica and Terminalia chebula in common bacterial infections among HIV patients [18]

Hepatoprotective activity

The fruit of Terminalia bellerica is hepatoprotective. This action is thought to be attributable to the presence of gallic acid.[19] When administered orally, it had a good protective effect against carbon tetrachloride-induced hepatotoxicity, as shown by an improvement in serum transaminase and bilirubin levels and a significant inhibition of microsomal lipid peroxidation and a reduction in triglyceride levels in the liver.[20] These results support the traditional use of Terminalia bellerica in the treatment of liver disease.

Anti-ulcer activity:

The fruit of Terminalia bellerica has been effective in reducing the total acidity and peptic activity and increasing mucin content, which suggests a role in ulcer management.[21] Triphala has been effective in treating ulcers induced by pylorus ligation, aspirin, and prednisolone.[22] A documented case of the preparation's action in healing a leg ulcer with subsequent generation of new tissue growth revealed its potential for managing other types of ulcers as well.[23] [19]

In one study, Terminalia bellerica, in combination with Emblica and Terminalia chebula, prevented the intestinal damage induced by administering methotrexate (MTX) to albino rats in a dose of 12 mg/kg, orally for 4 days.[24]

Anti-obesity activity:

Terminalia bellerica and Triphala have been shown to be anti-obesity agents, reducing weight, skinfold thickness, and circumference of the hips and waist in obese subjects. Clinical studies have revealed these preparations to be safe.[25,26,27]

Opthalmic activity:

Myopia and hypermetropia were controlled by Triphala ghee, an ancient Ayurvedic recipe that contains the fruit of Terminalia bellerica as one of the main ingredients in butter oil.[28] Triphala also has been recommended for the management of stye (hordeolum) in the eye.[29]

Anti-mutagenic activity:

The anti-mutagenic effect of Terminalia bellerica has been attributed to the polyphenols present in the fruit.[30]

Hypoglycemic activity:

The preparation Triphala has shown hypoglycemic activity.[31] The effect of continuous administration of dried 75% methanolic extract of fruits of Terminalia bellerica suspended in water was studied in alloxan-induced hyperglycemia and the anti-oxidant defense mechanism in rats.[32] Terminalia bellerica prevented alloxan-induced hyperglycemia significantly from the 6th day of administration, with a 54% reduction on the 12th day. Oxidative stress produced by alloxan was significantly lowered by administration of the Terminalia bellerica extract. This was evident from a significant decrease in thiobarbituric acid reactive substances, conjugated dienes, and hydroperoxides in the blood and liver, respectively. Similarly, a decreased glutathione level produced by alloxan was increased by administering the extract in the blood and liver, but the increase was not significant. Superoxide dismutase, which was decreased by alloxan, was significantly increased from the 9th day in the blood and liver of the Terminalia bellerica treated group. Similarly, there was a significant increase in the activity of catalase in the blood and liver. A decrease in glutathione peroxidase by administration of alloxan was found to be increased significantly in the blood and liver from the 9th day after the extract treatment. Glutathione reductase also was found to be increased in the blood and liver.

Anti-inflammatory effects and immune modulation:

The rasayana Triphala, which contains Terminalia bellerica, has been found to be useful in the treatment of rheumatic diseases.[33,34] The immunomodulatory activities of Triphala (Terminalia chebula, Terminalia bellerica, and Emblica officinalis) were assessed by testing various neutrophil functions including adherence, phagocytosis (phagocytic index and avidity index), and nitro blue tetrazolium (NBT) reduction in albino rats.[35] Much attention is being directed to the immunological changes that occur during stress. Noise (100 dB) stress for 4 hours/day for 15 days, was employed to alter the neutrophil functions. The neutrophil function tests and corticosterone levels were carried out in eight different groups of animals: control, Triphala, noise-stress, and corresponding immunized groups. Sheep red blood cells (SRBC $5 \times 10(9)$ cells per ml) were used to immunize the animals belonging to the immunized groups. In Triphala administration (1 g/kg/d for 48 d), avidity index was significantly enhanced in the Triphala group, while the remaining neutrophil functions and steroid levels were not altered significantly. The neutrophil functions, however were significantly enhanced in the Triphala immunized group, with a significant decrease in corticosterone level. Upon exposure to the noise-stress, the neutrophil functions were significantly suppressed, followed by a significant increase in corticosterone levels in both the noise stress and the noise-stress immunized groups. These noise-stress-induced changes were significantly prevented by Triphala administration in both the Triphala noise-stress and the Triphala noise-stress immunized groups. Oral administration of Triphala appeared to stimulate the neutrophil functions in the immunized rats and significantly prevented stress-induced suppression in neutrophil functions.

Anti-allergy activity:

Allergic rhinitis is an immunological disorder and an inflammatory response of the nasal mucosal membranes. Allergic rhinitis, a state of hypersensitivity, occurs when the body overreacts to a substance such as pollen or dust. A polyherbal formulation (Aller-7) has been developed for the treatment of allergic rhinitis using a unique combination of extracts from seven medicinal plants: Phyllanthus emblica, Terminalia chebula, Terminalia bellerica, Albizia lebbeck, Piper nigrum, Zingiber officinale, and Piper longum.

Because inflammation is an integral mechanistic component of allergy, a study aimed to determine the anti-inflammatory activity of Aller-7 in various in vivo models. The efficacy of Aller-7 was investigated in compound 48/80-induced paw edema both in Balb/c mice and Swiss Albino mice, carrageenan induced paw edema in Wistar Albino rats, and

Freund's adjuvant-induced arthritis in Wistar Albino rats.[36] The trypsin inhibitory activity of Aller-7 also was determined and compared with ovo-mucoid. At a dose of 250 mg/kg, Aller-7 demonstrated 62.55% inhibition against compound 48/80-induced paw edema in Balb/c mice, whereas under the same conditions, prednisolone at an oral dose of 14 mg/kg exhibited 44.7% inhibition. Aller-7 significantly inhibited compound 48/80-induced paw edema at all three doses of 175, 225 or 275 mg/kg in the Swiss albino mice, and the most potent effect was observed at 225 mg/kg. Aller-7 (120 mg/kg, p.o.) demonstrated 31.3% inhibition against carrageenan induced acute inflammation in the Wistar albino rats, while ibuprofen (50 mg/kg, p.o.) exerted 68.1% inhibition. Aller-7 also exhibited a dose-dependent (150–350 mg/kg) anti-inflammatory effect against Freund's adjuvant-induced arthritis in Wistar albino rats, and an approximately 63% inhibitory effect was observed at a dose of 350 mg/kg. The trypsin inhibitory activity of Aller-7 was determined using ovo-mucoid as a positive control. Ovomucoid and Aller-7 demonstrated IC50 concentrations at 1.5 and 9.0 microg/ml, respectively. These results demonstrate that this novel polyherbal formulation is a potent anti-inflammatory agent that can ameliorate the symptoms of allergic rhinitis.

HK-07 is a polyherbal formulation containing extracts of Curcuma longa, Zingiber officinale, Piper longum, Emblica officinalis, Terminalia bellerica, Ocimum sanctum, Adhatoda vasica, and Cyperus rotundus. The compound HK-07 was evaluated using Wistar rats and Duncan Hartley guinea pigs. The anti-anaphylactic activity was investigated in rats using the active anaphylaxis model. The effect on mast cell stabilization was performed by ex vivo challenge of antigen in sensitized rat intestinal mesenteries. Antihistaminic activity was studied in guinea pigs using histamine-induced bronchospasm where pre-convulsive dyspnea was used as an end point following exposure to histamine aerosol.[37] Treatment with HK-07 at 125, 250, and 500 mg/kg, p.o. showed a significant reduction in the signs and severity of symptoms ($P < 0.05$), onset ($P < 0.001$), and mortality rate ($P < 0.05$) following anaphylactic shock-induced bronchospasm. HK-07 also significantly reduced the serum IgE levels ($P < 0.001$) in these animals compared to the untreated controls. Treatment of sensitized animals with HK-07 at 500 mg/kg, p.o. for 2 weeks resulted in a significant reduction in the number of disrupted mast cells ($P < 0.001$) when challenged with an antigen (horse serum). HK-07 significantly prolonged the latent period of convulsion ($P < 0.008$) compared to control following exposure of guinea pigs to histamine aerosol.

Anti-asthmatic activity:

An investigation was carried out to determine the pharmacological basis for the medicinal use of Terminalia bellerica in hyperactive gastrointestinal and respiratory disorders.[38] A crude extract of Terminalia bellerica fruit was studied in-vitro and in-vivo. The extract caused relaxation of spontaneous contractions in isolated rabbit jejunum. The preparation also inhibited carbachol and potassium-induced contractions in a pattern similar to that of dicyclomine, but different from that of nifedipine and atropine. Terminalia bellerica shifted the calcium concentration-response curves to the right, as did nifedipine and dicyclomine. In the guinea-pig ileum, Terminalia bellerica produced a rightward parallel shift of acetylcholine-curves, followed by a non-parallel shift at the higher concentration, with suppression of maximum response similar to that of dicyclomine but different from that of nifedipine and atropine. Terminalia bellerica exhibited a protective effect against castor oil-induced diarrhea and carbachol-mediated bronchoconstriction in rodents. In the guinea-pig trachea, Terminalia relaxed carbachol-induced contractions and inhibited potassium contractions. Terminalia bellerica fruit possess a combination of anticholinergic and Ca(++) antagonist effects, which explain its folkloric use in treating colic, diarrhea and asthma.

Anti-cancer activity:

Triphala, a combination of fruit powder of three different plants: Terminalia chebula, Terminalia bellerica, and Emblica officinalis, showed cancer chemopreventive potential. Triphala in the diet significantly reduced the benzo(a)pyrene [B(a)P] induced forestomach papillomagenesis in mice.[39] In the short-term treatment groups, the tumor incidence was lowered to 77.77% by 2.5% and 5% of the Triphala mixed diet. In the case of long-term treatment, the incidence of tumors was reduced to 66.66% and 62.50%, respectively, in the 2.5% and 5% Triphala-containing diet. The tumor burden was 7.27 +/- 1.16 in the B(a)P treated control group, whereas it was reduced to 3.00 +/- 0.82 ($p < 0.005$) by 2.5% dose and 2.33 +/- 1.03 ($p < 0.001$) by the 5% dose of Triphala. In long-term studies, the tumor burden was reduced to 2.17 +/- 0.75 ($p < 0.001$) and 2.00 +/- 0.71 ($p < 0.001$) by the 2.5% and 5% diet of Triphala, respectively. It was important to observe that Triphala was more effective than its individual constituents in reducing the incidence of tumors. Triphala also significantly increased the anti-oxidant status of animals, which might have contributed to the chemoprevention. The concomitant use of multiple agents seemed to have high chemoprevention potential.

Ethnoveterinary Usage

Terminalia bellerica seeds are widely used to treat wounds in ruminants.[40]

Dr. Sodhi's Experience

Before beginning treatment with Terminalia bellerica (Bibhitaki), the practitioner should consider the following:

- Are there problems with digestion?
- Is there kapha aggravation?
- Is there damaged mucosal tissue?
- Is there congestion with poor or no expectoration?
- Is a gastrointestinal astringent needed?
- Is there a problem with bile secretion and/or liver function?
- Is there an infection with digestive symptoms?

Bibhitaki perhaps is best known as part of the traditional compound Triphala, a formulation that is referenced in almost every Ayuvedic textbook. Triphala is a powerful adaptogen, or rasayana, and is widely believed to enhance longevity. It also enhances digestion, acts as a mild diuretic, and is a powerful anti-oxidant.

Triphala is composed of equal parts of three fruits: bibhitaki, amalaki (Embilica officinalis), and haritaki (Terminalia chebula). Soothing to the gastrointestinal tract, bibhitaki can be used to treat ulcers, as it heals mucosal tissue throughout the body—in the eyes, nose, eyes, and vagina.

Bibhitaki is rich in tannins and has anti-histaminic, anti-fungal, yeast-inhibiting, and choleretic effects. It also stimulates bile secretions and is useful for treating many liver conditions. It is especially good for kapha imbalance, which usually is characterized by the excess production of bodily fluids such as mucus, and tissue, as in tumor formation. It can be used for bronchodilation in bronchitis, upper respiratory infections, and bronchial asthma.

Safety Profile

Terminalia bellerica is a safe and well-tolerated herb when used at recommended doses and in the form of Triphala. The fixed oil is purgative in large doses.[41]

Dosage

Powder: 1–3 grams

Ayurvedic Properties

Rasa: Kashaya (astringent), madhur (sweet)
Guna: Laghu (light), ruksha (dry)
Veerya: Ushna (hot)
Vipaka: Madhur (sweet)
Dosha: Pacifies tridosha

Notes

1. R. Valsaraj, P. Pushpangadan, U.W. Smitt, A. Adsersen, S.B. Christensen, A. Sittie, U. Nyman, C. Nielsen, and C.E. Olsen, "New anti-HIV-1, antimalarial, and antifungal compounds from Terminalia bellerica," *J Nat Prod.*, July 1997, 60(7):739–742.

2. A. K Nandy, G. Podder, N.P. Sahu, and S.B. Mahato, "Triterpenoids and their glycosides from Terminalia belerica," *Phytochemistry*, 1989, 28(10):27–69.

3. M. Ali and K.K. Bhutani, "Occurrence of hexahydroxydiphenic acid ester in Terminalia belerica fruits," *Indian Journal of Natural Products*, 1991, 7(1):16

4. L.R. Row and P.S. Murty, "Chemical examination of Terminalia bekrica Roxb," *Indian Journal of Chemistry*, 1970, 8:1047–1048.

5. See Note 1.

6. T. Vani, M. Rajani, S. Sarkar, and C.J. Shishoo, "Antioxidant properties of the Ayurvedic formulation Triphala and its constituents," *International Journal of Pharmacognosy*, 1997, 35(5):313.

7. R.D. Srivastava, S. Swivedi, K.K. Sreenivasan, and C.N. Chandrashekhar, "Cardiovascular effects of Terminalia species of plants," *Indian Drugs*, 1992, 29(4):144.

8. J. N Sharma, M.N. Rajpal, T.S. Rao, and S.K. Gupta, "Some pharmacological investigations on the alcoholic extract of Triphala alone and in combination with petroleum ether extract of oleogum resin of Commiphora mukul, *Indian Drugs*, 1988 25(6):220.

9. H.P. Shaila, S.L. Udupa, and A.L. Udupa, "Hypolipidemic activity of three indigenous drugs in experimentally induced atherosclerosis," *International Journal of Cardiology*, 1998, 67(2):119.

10. H.P Shaila, A.L. Udupa, and S.L. Udupa, "Preventive actions of Terminalia belerica in experimentally induced atherosclerosis," *International Journal of Cardiology*, 1995, 4(2):101.

11. C.P. Thakur, B. Thakur, S. Singh, P.K. Sinha, and S. K. Sinha, "The Ayurvedic medicines Haritaki, Amla, and Behera reduce cholesterol-induced atherosclerosis in rabbits," *International Journal of Cardiology*, 1998, 21(2):167.

12. I. Ahmad, Z. Mehmood, and F. Mohammad, "Screening of some Indian medicinal plants for their anti-bacterial properties," *Journal of Ethnopharmacology*, 1998, 62(2):183.

13. G.G. Kulkarni, S.D. Ravetkar, and P.H. Kulkarni, "Anti-bacterial properties of Ayurvedic preparations 'Bhallatakasava' and 'Sukshma Triphala', *Deerghayu International*, 1995, 11(42):3.

14. S. A. Bopegamage and A. Petrovicova, "Anti-viral effect of selected Ayurvedic preparations on vesicular stomatitis virus," in P.H. Kulkarn (Ed.), *Biorhythm* (City: Ayurved Acad. Pune, 1995), p. 20.

15. S.A. Bopegamage, A. Petrovicova, N.N. Nossik, and L.A. Lavrukina, "Compilation of the in-vitro and in-vivo anti-viral activities of some Ayurvedic products," in P.H. Kulkarn (Ed.), *Biorhythm*. (City: Ayurved Acad. Pune, 1995), p. 24.

16. Madani A, Jain SK. Anti-Salmonella activity of Terminalia belerica: in vitro and in vivo studies. Indian J Exp Biol. 2008 Dec;46(12):817-21..

17. A. Sharma, V.K. Patel, and A.N. Chaturvedi, "Vibriocidal activity of certain medicinal plants used in Indian folklore medicine by tribals of Mahakoshal region of central India," *Indian J Pharmacol.*, June 2009, 41(3):129–133.

18. R. Srikumar, N.J. Parthasarathy, E.M. Shankar, S. Manikandan, R. Vijayakumar, R. Thangaraj, K. Vijayananth, R. Sheeladevi, and U.A. Rao, "Evaluation of the growth inhibitory activities of Triphala against common bacterial isolates from HIV infected patients," *Phytother Res.*, May 2007, 21(5):476–480.

19. K. Anand, B. Singh, A.K. Saxena, B.K. Chandan, V.N. Gupta, and V.N. Bhardwaj, "3,4,5-THydroxy benzoic acid (gallic acid), the hepatoprotective principle in the fruits of Terminalia belerica: Bioassay guided activity," *Pharmacological Research*, 1997, 36(4):315.

20. K. K Anand, B. Singh, A.K. Saxena, B.K. Chandan, and V.N. Gupta, "Hepatoprotective studies of a fraction from the fruits of Terminalia belerica Roxb. on experimental liver injury in rodents," *Phytotherapy Research*, 1994, 8(5):287.

21. S. Satyanaryanana, M. Savitir, and D. Visweswaram, "Anti-gastric ulcer activity of brucine and Triphala," *Indian Journal of Pharmaceutical Science*, 1994, 56(4):165.

22. K. Elango, B. Suresh, E.P. Kumar, et al., "Pharmacological validation of certain Siddha drugs for their antiulcer and anti-inflammatory activity," International Seminar on Recent Trends in Pharmaceutical Science," Ootacamund, February 1995.

23. K. Kumar and M.Junius, "A spectacular case history of Pyoderma gangrenosum at the Ayurvedic Health Care Centre of South Australia," in P.H. Kulkarn (Ed.) *Biorhythm* (City: Ayurved Acad. Pune, 1995).

24. Nariya M, Shukla V, Jain S, Ravishankar B. Comparison of enteroprotective efficacy of triphala formulations (Indian Herbal Drug) on methotrexate-induced small intestinal damage in rats. Phytother Res. 2009 Aug;23(8):1092-8.

25. P. Paranjpe Patki and B. Patwardhan, "Ayurvedic treatment of obesity: A randomized double-blind, placebo-controlled clinical trial," *Journal of Ethnopharmacology*, 1990, 29(1):1.

26. P. H. Kulkarni and P. Paranjpe, "Clinical assessment of Ayurvedic anti-obesity drugs: A double blind placebo controlled trial," *Journal of Natural and Integrated Medicine*, 1990, 32(1):7.

27. P.H. Kulkarni, "Clinical study of effect of Sukshma (subtle) Triphala Guggulu (TC.3x) in obesity," *Med. Aromat. Plant Abs.*, 1996, 18(5):512.

28. P. Sripathi and R. Tarpanam, "Boon to Drusti Lopa (refractive errors)," Proc. Seminar on Research in Ayurveda and Siddha, New Delhi, CCRAS, March 1995.

29. U.V Sudrik, "Management of Anjananamika in amavastha with Swedana and Sookshma Triphala," *Med. Aromat. Plant Abs.*, 1995, 18(5):514.

30. S.K. Padam, I.S. Grover, and M. Singh, "Antimutagenic effects of polyphenols isolated from Terminalia belerica (Myrobalan) in Salmonella typhimurium," *Indian Journal of Experimental Biology*, 1996, 43(2):98.

31. D. Ghosh, R. Uma, P. Thejomoorthy, and G. Veluchamy, "Hypoglycemic and toxicity studies of Triphala— a Siddha drug," *Journal of Research in Ayurveda and Siddha*, 1990, 11(l–4):78.

32. M.C, Sabu and R. Kuttan, "Antidiabetic and anti-oxidant activity of Terminalia belerica Roxb." *Indian J Exp Biol.*, April 2009, 47(4):270–275.

33. V.K. Pandey and A.K. Sharma, "Evaluation of Vatahari Guggulu and Nadivaspa-Sweda in the management of rheumatic diseases," *Rheumatism*,h22; pg 1-6, 1986.

34. D. Ghosh, P. Thejomoorthy, and G. Veluchamy, "Anti-inflammatory, anti-arthritic and analgesic activities of Triphala," *Journal of Research in Ayurveda and Siddha*, 1989, 10(3–4):168.

35. Srikumar R, Jeya Parthasarathy N, Sheela Devi R.,"Immunomodulatory activity of triphala on neutrophil functions," *Biol Pharm Bull.*, Aug. 2005, 28(8):1398–1403.

36. N. Pratibha, V.S. Saxena, A. Amit, P. D'Souza, M. Bagchi, and D. Bagchi, "Anti-inflammatory activities of Aller-7, a novel polyherbal formulation for allergic rhinitis," *Int J Tissue React.* 2004, 26(1–2):43–51.

37. S. Gopumadhavan, M. Rafiq, M.V. Venkataranganna, and S.K. Mitra, "Antihistaminic and antianaphylactic activity of HK-07, a herbal formulation," *Indian J Pharmacol*, 2005, 37:300–303.

38. **A.H. Gilani, A.U. Khan, T. Ali, and S. Ajmal,** "Mechanisms underlying the antispasmodic and bronchodilatory properties of Terminalia bellerica fruit," *J Ethnopharmacol.*, March 18, 2008, 116(3):528–538. Epub Jan. 16, 2008.

39. G. Deep, M. Dhiman, A.R. Rao, and R.K. Kale, "Chemopreventive potential of Triphala (a composite Indian drug) on benzo(a)pyrene induced forestomach tumorigenesis in murine tumor model system," *J Exp Clin Cancer Res.*, Dec. 2005, 24(4):555–563.

40. International Institute of Rural Reconstruction, *Ethnoveterinary Medicine in Asia: An Information Kit on Traditional Animal Health Care Practices* (Silang, Philippines: IIRR, 1994).

41. H.L Dhar, B.D. Miglani, and D. Dhawan, "Studies on purgative action of an oil obtained from Terminalia belerica," *Indian Journal of Medical Research*, 1969, 57(1):103.

41

Terminalia Chebula

Introduction

Terminalia chebula, known commonly by its Sanskrit name Haritaki, is a plant of great importance in Ayurvedic medicine. It is an ingredient of the popular formulation Triphala, or "three fruits," a rasayana that also contains Terminalia bellerica (Bibhitaki) and Phyllanthus emblica (Amalaki). Haritaki was first mentioned in Chinese medicine in 1061 and also is used in Tibetan medicine, where it is referred to as the "king of medicines." According to legend, it is thought to promote fearlessness.

Haritaki bark has been used in Indian medicine for at least 5,000 years as a remedy for heart ailments and as a digestive aid. The extract obtained from Haritaki fruit has anti-bacterial and anti-fungal properties. This substance inhibits the growth of bacteria and fungi including Escherichia coli. Haritaki also is believed to have a powerful effect on parasites including Amoeba Giardia and many others.

The aerial parts of Haritaki—its fruit, leaves, and stem—are used medicinally in Ayurveda. Haritaki is an aperient, astringent, cardiotonic, carminative, fungicide, laxative, tonic, demulcent, purgative, alterative, febrifuge, anti-asthmatic and anti-dysenteric. It is believed to strengthen the brain and enrich the blood. It also is used to treat bronchitis, burns, conjunctivitis, cough, dysuria, inflammation, leucorrhoea, measles, metritis, prolapse, ulcer, and splenomegaly.

Terminalia has been evaluated to a limited extent for its cardiovascular properties, as well as for its role in cancer therapy. Hepatoprotective, cholesterol-reducing, and anti-oxidant effects also have been described.

Synonymous Names

English: Myrobalan, inknut
Hindi: Hara, harda
Sanskrit: Haritaki

Habitat

Haritaki occurs natively in the sub-Himalayan tract of India. It also is found in Myanmmar, Sri Lanka, and other Asian countries, growing up to elevations of 1500 meters.

Botanical Characteristics

Haritaki is a large deciduous tree that reaches 30 meters in height. Its trunk is as wide as 2.5 meters. The bark is dark brown, often longitudinally cracked, exfoliating in woody scales. The leaves are glabrous, opposite, ovate, or elliptic and up to 20 centimeters long with an acute apex. The flowers are yellowish-white, in terminal spikes, with an unpleasant odor. The fruit is an ovoid hanging drupe, up to 5 centimeters long, yellow to orange-brown in color, sometimes tinged with red or black, and hard when ripe. The seeds are hard and pale yellow.

Chemical Composition

Triterpenoid glycosides: Chebulosides I and II, arjunin, arjunglucoside, 2-Alpha-hydroxyursolic acid and 2-Alpha-hydroxymicromiric acid have been reported.[1,2]

Tannins and polyphenols: Chebulinic acid, chebulin, punicalagin, punicalin, terflavins A, B, C and D, maslinic acid, gallic acid, synergic acid, terchebulin I, 1,2,3,4,6-penta-O-galloyl-beta-D-glucopyranose and others have been isolated.[3]

Pharmacological Activity

Cardiotonic activity:

Mitochondria play a central role in molecular events leading to tissue damage in ischemia. A study was undertaken to examine the role of the alcoholic extract of Haritaki pre-treatment to attenuate the isoproterenol-induced alterations on heart mitochondrial ultrastructure and function in rats. Isoproterenol (ISO)-induced cardiotoxicity was evidenced by a significant rise in the level of lactate and a decrease in enzyme activities of the tricarboxylic acid cycle, mitochondrial respiration, levels of adenosine triphosphate, and oxidative phosphorylation. Intervention with the herbal preparation significantly attenuated these alterations by ISO and retained near normal function of the mitochondria. Electron microscopic studies of the mitochondria further support the isoproterenol-induced deleterious changes and credit the protective effect of Haritaki on mitochondrial structure and energy metabolism.[4] Tests carried out on frog hearts in normal as well as hypodynamic conditions showed extracts from the fruit rind of Terminalia chebula increased the force of contraction and cardiac output without changing the heart rate.[5, 4]

Anti-cholesteremic activity:

Hypercholesterolemia is a major factor in coronary artery disease. A study was conducted to determine the efficacy of the Ayurvedic herbal formulation Triphala on total cholesterol, low density lipoprotein (LDL), very low density lipoprotein (VLDL), high density lipoprotein (HDL) and free fatty acid in experimentally induced hypercholesterolemic rats. Four groups of animals were used for the study: (1) control, (2) Triphala-treated, (3) hypercholesterolemia rats, and (4) Triphala pre-treated hypercholesterolemic rats. The study results showed that total cholesterol, LDL, VLDL, and free fatty acid were reduced significantly in the Triphala-treated hypercholesterolemic rats. These data demonstrated that Triphala formulation was associated with hypolipidemic effects on the experimentally induced hypercholesterolemic rats.[6]

Anti-anaphylactic activity:

A water-soluble fraction of Haritaki was found to be effective with systemic and local anaphylaxis. Systemic and passive cutaneous anaphylaxis was inhibited and serum histamine levels were reduced in a dose-dependent manner. The fraction also significantly inhibited histamine release from rat peritoneal mast cells, indicating that it may possess anti-anaphylactic action.[7] The effects of a water-soluble fraction of Terminalia chebula on systemic and local anaphylaxis extract administered 1 hour before a compound 48/80 injection inhibited compound 48/80-induced anaphylactic shock 100% at doses of 0.01–1.0 g/kg. When the extract was administered 5 or 10 minutes after the compound 48/80 injection, the mortality also decreased in a dose-dependent manner. Passive cutaneous anaphylaxis was inhibited by 63.5+/-7.8% by oral administration of the Haritaki extract. When the extract was used as a pretreatment at concentrations ranging from 0.005 to 1.0 g/kg, the serum histamine levels were reduced in a dose-dependent manner. The Haritaki extract also significantly inhibited histamine release from rat peritoneal mast cells by compound 48/80. The extract, however, had a significant increasing effect on anti-dinitrophenyl IgE-induced tumor necrosis factor-alpha production from the mast cells. These results indicate that Haritaki may possess a strong anti-anaphylactic action.

Anti-mutagenic activity:

The anti-mutagenicity of an aqueous extract of the dry fruit of Terminalia chebula was determined for two direct-acting mutagens—sodium azide and 4-nitro-o-phenylenediamine (NPD). Several strains of Salmonella typhimurium and the S9-dependent mutagen 2-aminofluorene (2-AF) were used. The extract reduced NPD as well as 2-AF induced histidine revertants, but did not have any perceptible effect against sodium azide in the TA100 and TA153S bacterial strains. Pre-incubation studies did show an enhanced inhibitory effect.[8] A study was undertaken to assess the anti-mutagenic properties of the herbal preparation Triphala.[9] The drug was sequentially extracted with water, acetone, and chloroform at room temperature. The study showed that the water extract of Triphala was ineffective in reducing the revertants induced by the mutagens; however, the results with chloroform and acetone extracts showed inhibition of mutagenicity induced by both direct and S9-dependent mutagens. A significant inhibition of 98.7% was observed with the acetone extract against the revertants induced by S9-dependent mutagen, 2AF, in co-incubation mode of treatment.

Anti-bacterial activity:

Gallic acid and its ethyl ester exhibited strong antimicrobial activity against methicillin-resistant strains of Staphylococcus aureus.[10] In another study, an extract of Terminalia chebula showed a potent wide-spectrum anti-bacterial activity against human pathogenic Gram-positive and Gram-negative bacteria.[11] A study was undertaken to evaluate the effect of an aqueous extract of Terminalia chebula on salivary samples and its potential for use as an anticaries agent in the form of mouthwash.[12] A concentrated aqueous extract was prepared from the fruit of Haritaki. A mouth rinse of 10% concentration was prepared by diluting the extract in sterile distilled water. The effectiveness of the mouth rinse was assessed by testing on 50 salivary samples. Salivary samples were collected from subjects assessed to be at high risk for caries. Salivary pH, buffering capacity, and microbial activity were assessed before rinsing, immediately after, and 10 min, 30 min, and 1 hour after rinsing. There was an increase in the pH and buffering capacity and decrease in microbial count. An aqueous extract of Terminalia chebula used as a mouth rinse seems to be an effective anticaries agent. The growth inhibitory activity of materials derived from the fruit of Terminalia chebula was evaluated against six intestinal bacteria by means of an impregnated paper disk agar diffusion method.[13] The butanol fraction of Terminalia chebula extract had profound growth-inhibitory activity at a concentration of 5 mg per disk. The biologically active component isolated from the fruits was identified with a variety of spectroscopic analyses as ethanedioic (oxalic) acid. The growth responses varied in accordance with the bacterial strain, chemical, and dosage tested. In the test with concentrations of 2 and 1 mg per disk, ethanedioic acid showed strong and moderate inhibitory activity against Clostridium perfringens and Escherichia coli, respectively, with no associated adverse effects on the growth of the four tested lactic acid-producing bacteria. Ellagic acid derived from Terminalia chebula fruits exerted a potent inhibitory effect against C. perfringens and E. coli, but little or no inhibition was observed with treatments of behenic acid, P-caryophyllene, eugenol, isoquercitrin, oleic acid, a-phellandrene, 3-sitosterol, stearic acid, a-terpinene, terpinen-4-ol and terpinolene. These results may be an indication of at least one of the pharmacological properties of Terminalia chebula fruits.

The effects of ether, alcoholic, and water extracts of Terminalia chebula on Helicobactor pylori were examined using an agar Helicobacter method on Columbia Agar. Water extracts of the herb showed significant anti-bacterial activity and had a minimum inhibitory concentration and minimum bactericidal concentration of 125 and 150 mg/l, respectively. The extract was active after autoclaving for 30 minutes at 121 degrees C. Plant powder (incorporated in agar) yielded higher values. Water extracts of Haritaki at a concentration of 1-2.5 mg/ml inhibited urease activity of H. pylori. The results show that Haritaki extracts contain one or more heat stable agents with possible therapeutic potential. Other bacterial species also were inhibited by the herbal water extracts.[14] In another study, 54 plant extracts (methanol and aqueous) were assayed for their activity against multi-drug resistant Salmonella typhi. Strong anti-bacterial activity was shown by the methanol extracts of Aegle marmelos, Salmalia malabarica, Punica granatum, Myristica fragrans, Holarrhena antidysenterica, Terminalia arjuna, and Triphala.[15] An examination of the ethyl alcohol extract of the fruiting bodies of Terminalia chebula led to the isolation of two potent antimicrobial substances with effectiveness against even methicillin-resistant strains of Staphylococcus aureus. On the basis of spectroscopic evidence, the two isolates have been identified as gallic acid and its ethyl ester.[16]

Anti-viral activity

Haritaki fruit extract, when orally administered in combination with acyclovir, exhibited a strong anti-HSV-I activity by reducing the virus concentration in the brain and skin more strongly than acyclovir alone.[17] The extract also showed a significant inhibitory activity on HIV-1 reverse transcriptase.

Many medicinal herbs, including Terminalia chebula, have shown action against the herpes simplex virus, and they inhibit replication of the human cytomegalovirus (CMV) and murine cytomegalovirus (MCMV) in-vitro. These anti-CMV activities were examined in an MCMV infection model using immunosuppressed mice. Terminalia chebula significantly suppressed MCMV yields in the lungs of the treated mice compared to the water treatment. Terminalia chebula may be beneficial for the prophylaxis of CMV diseases in immunocompromised patients.[18] Gallic acid and chebulagic acid, isolated from the extract of the fruit of Terminalia chebula, were shown to be the active principles blocking the cytotoxic T lymphocyte (CTL)-mediated cytotoxicity. Gallic acid and chebulagic acid inhibited the killing activity of the CD8+ CTL clone at IC50 values of 30 microM and 50 microM, respectively. Granule exocytosis in response to anti-CD3 stimulation also was blocked by gallic acid and chebulagic acid at the equivalent concentrations.[19]

Ten herbal extracts, including Terminalia chebula, were tested for their effectiveness against anti-herpes simplex virus type 1. Terminalia extract showed a stronger anti-HSV-1 activity in combination with acyclovir than did the other herbal extracts in-vitro. When acyclovir and/or a herbal extract were administered orally at doses corresponding to human use, each of the four combinations significantly limited the development of skin lesions and/or prolonged the mean survival times of the infected mice compared to both the acyclovir and the herbal extract alone. These combinations were not toxic to mice. They reduced virus yields in the brain and skin more strongly than acyclovir alone and exhibited stronger anti-HSV-1 activity in the brain than in the skin, in contrast to the acyclovir treatment by itself. Combinations of acyclovir with historically used herbal medicines showed strong combined therapeutic anti-HSV-1 activity in mice, especially a reduction of the virus yield in the brain.[20] Extracts from 41 plants used in traditional medicines were screened for their inhibitory effects on human immunodeficiency virus-1 reverse transcriptase. Extracts of the fruits of Terminalia, along with five other herbs, showed significant inhibitory activity.[21] Terminalia chebula (Methyl alcohol and water extracts) and Terminalia horrida (Methyl alcohol extract) showed significant inhibitory activity with IC50 of 2-49 mcg/ml.[22] The bioassay-directed isolation of Terminalia chebula fruits yielded four human immunodeficiency virus type 1 (HIV-1) integrase inhibitors: gallic acid and three galloyl glucoses.[23]

Immunomodulatory activity:

The crude extract of a formula containing Terminalia chebula, Tinospora cordifolia, Berberis aristata, and Zingiber officinale showed significant enhancement in humoral immunity. This was measured by hemagglutination titer and cell-mediated immune response, exhibited by inhibition of leucocyte migration.[24] Allergic rhinitis is an immunological disorder and an inflammatory response of nasal mucosal membranes. Allergic rhinitis, a state of hypersensitivity, occurs when the body overreacts to a substance such as pollens or dust. A novel, safe polyherbal formulation (Aller-7) has been developed for treating allergic rhinitis using a unique combination of extracts from seven medicinal plants: Phyllanthus emblica, Terminalia chebula, Terminalia bellerica, Albizia lebbeck, Piper nigrum, Zingiber officinale, and Piper longum.

Because inflammation is an integral mechanistic component of allergy, a study was aimed at determining the anti-inflammatory activity of Aller-7 in various in-vivo models.[25] The efficacy of Aller-7 was investigated in compound 48/80-induced paw edema in Balb/c mice and in Swiss albino mice, carrageenan-induced paw edema in Wistar albino rats, and Freund's adjuvant-induced arthritis in Wistar albino rats. The trypsin inhibitory activity of Aller-7 also was determined and compared with ovo-mucoid. At a dose of 250 mg/kg, Aller-7 demonstrated 62.55% inhibition against compound 48/80-induced paw edema in the Balb/c mice. Under the same conditions, prednisolone at an oral dose of 14 mg/kg exhibited 44.7% inhibition. Aller-7 significantly inhibited compound 48/80-induced paw edema at all three doses of 175, 225, or 275 mg/kg in the Swiss albino mice; the most potent effect was observed at 225 mg/kg. Aller-7 (120 mg/kg, p.o.) demonstrated 31.3% inhibition against carrageenan-induced acute inflammation in the Wistar albino rats, while ibuprofen (50 mg/kg, p.o.) exerted 68.1% inhibition. Aller-7 also exhibited a dose-dependent (150–350 mg/kg) anti-inflammatory effect against Freund's adjuvant-induced arthritis in the Wistar albino rats, and an approximately 63% inhibitory effect was observed at a dose of 350 mg/kg. The trypsin inhibitory activity of Aller-7 was determined using ovomucoid as a positive control. Ovo-mucoid and Aller-7 demonstrated IC50 concentrations at 1.5 and 9.0 microg/ml, respectively. The results demonstrate that this novel polyherbal formulation is a potent anti-inflammatory agent that can ameliorate the symptoms of allergic rhinitis.

Anti-amoebic activity:

The anti-amoebic effects of an ethanolic extract of a formulation including Terminalia chebula, Tinospora cordifolia, Berberis aristata, and Zingiber officinale were studied against experimental cecal amoebiasis in rats (Entamoeba histolytica). The results showed an effective cure rate compared to the controls.[26]

Anti-oxidant activity:

An ethanolic extract of Terminalia leaves significantly inhibited lipid peroxidation in the mouse liver, lung homogenate, and mitochondria, by effectively scavenging oxygen-free radicals and inhibiting red cell hemolysis. Haritaki also produced a significant inhibition in the chemiluminescence of human leucocytes induced by the tissue plasminogen activator. The extract also prevented DNA breaks in human leucocytes induced by TPA and cigarette smoke condensates.[27] The aqueous extract of Terminalia chebula was tested for potential anti-oxidant activity by examining its ability to inhibit gamma-radiation-induced lipid peroxidation in rat liver microsomes and damage to superoxide dismutase enzyme in rat liver mitochondria.[28] The antimutagenic activity of the extract was being examined by following the inhibition of gamma-radiation-induced strand breaks formation in plasmid pBR322 DNA. To understand the phytochemicals responsible for this, HPLC analysis of the extract was carried out, which showed the presence of compounds such as ascorbate, gallic acid and ellagic acid. This was also confirmed by cyclic voltammetry. The plant extract inhibits xanthine/xanthine oxidase activity, and is also an excellent scavenger of DPPH (2,2-diphenyl-1-picrylhydrazyl) radicals. The rate at which the extract and its constituents scavenge the DPPH radical was studied by using a stopped-flow kinetic spectrometer. Based on all these results, it was concluded that the aqueous extract of Terminalia chebula acts as a potent anti-oxidant, and because it is able to protect cellular organelles from the radiation-induced damage, it may be considered as a probable radioprotector. Ethanol extract from the fruit of Terminalia chebula has exhibited significant inhibitory activity on oxidative stress and age-dependent shortening of the telomeric DNA length. In a peroxidation model using tert-Butyl hydroperoxide, the herbal extract showed a notable cytoprotective effect on the HEK-N/F cells with 60.5 +/- 3.8% at a concentration of 50 microg/ml. Terminalia chebula extract exhibited a significant cytoprotective effect against UVB-induced oxidative damage. The lifespan of the HEK-N/F cells was elongated by 40% as a result of continuous administration of 3 microg/ml of the extract, compared to that of the control. These observations were attributed to the inhibitory effect of the Terminalia extract on the age-dependent shortening of the telomere length as shown by Southern blots of the terminal restriction fragments (TRFs) of DNA extracted from the subculture passages.[29]

Anti-diabetic activity:

The aqueous extract of the fruit of Terminalia chebula was evaluated for its anti-diabetic activity in streptozotocin-induced mild diabetic rats, and compared to a known drug, tolbutamide. The oral effective dose of the extract was observed to be 200 mg/kg body weight, which produced a fall of 55.6% in the oral glucose tolerance test.[30] Oral administration of the aqueous extract of Terminalia daily once for 2 months reduced the elevated blood glucose and significantly reduced the increase in glycosylated hemoglobin. The same dose showed marked improvement in controlling the elevated blood lipids, as well as decreased serum insulin level, in contrast to the untreated diabetic animals. The hepatic and skeletal muscle glycogen content decreased by 75% and 62.9%, respectively, in the diabetic controls. These alterations were partly prevented in the treated group when compared to the healthy controls.

The in-vitro studies with pancreatic islets showed that the insulin release was nearly two times more than that in the untreated diabetic animals. The treatment did not have any unfavorable effect on other blood parameters of liver and kidney function tests. LD 50 was found to be above 3 g/kg bw after 15 doses of the extract, because there were no deaths of animals even at this dose, which indicates a high margin of safety. These findings highlight the need for further investigation of possible use of aqueous extract of the fruits of Terminalia chebula to treat diabetes.[31]

A chloroform extract of Terminalia seed powder was investigated for its anti-diabetic activity in streptozotocin-induced diabetic rats using short-term and long-term study protocols. Efficacy of the extract also was evaluated for the protection of renal functions in diabetic rats.[32] The blood glucose-lowering activity of the chloroform extract was determined in streptozotocin-induced diabetic rats, after oral administration at doses of 100, 200, and 300 mg/kg in the short-term study. Blood samples were collected from the eye retro-orbital plexus of rats before and also at 0.5, 1, 2, 4, 6, 8, and 12-hour intervals after drug administration. The samples were analyzed for blood glucose by using glucose-oxidase/peroxidase method using a visible spectrophotometer.

In a long-term study the extract was administered to streptozotocin-induced diabetic rats, daily for 8 weeks. Blood glucose was measured at weekly intervals for 4 weeks. Urine samples were collected before the induction of diabetes and at the end of 8 weeks of treatments and were analyzed for urinary protein, albumin, and creatinine levels. The data was compared statistically using one-way ANOVA with post-hoc Dunnet's t-test. It also produced significant reduction in blood glucose in the long-term study. Significant renal protective activity was observed in the treated rats. The results indicate a prolonged action in reduction of blood glucose by Terminalia chebula, probably mediated through enhanced secretion of insulin from the beta-cells of Langerhans or through extra pancreatic mechanism.

These studies clearly indicate significant anti-diabetic and renal protective effects with the chloroform extract of Terminalia chebula and lend support for its traditional usage.

Studies have shown that chebulagic acid from Terminalia chebula is a potent alpha-glucosidase inhibitor.[34]

Chemo-preventive activity:

Triphala significantly reduced the benzo(a)pyrene induced forestomach papillomagenesis in mice.[35] In the short-term treatment groups, the tumor incidence was lowered to 77.77% by 2.5% and 5% doses of the Triphala mixed diet. In the long-term treatment, the tumor incidence was reduced to 66.66% and 62.50%, respectively, by the 2.5% and 5% Triphala-containing diet. The tumor burden was 7.27 +/- 1.16 in the control group, whereas it was reduced to 3.00 +/- 0.82 by a 2.5% dose and 2.33 +/- 1.03 by a 5% dose of Triphala.

In long-term studies, the tumor burden was reduced to 2.17 +/- 0.75 and 2.00 +/- 0.71 by a 2.5% and 5% diet of Triphala, respectively. Notably, Triphala was more effective in reducing the incidence of tumors than its individual components alone. Triphala also significantly increased the anti-oxidant status of animals, which might have contributed to the chemoprevention. The concomitant use of multiple agents seemed to have a high degree of chemoprevention potential as well.[36]

Nickel, a major environmental pollutant, is a known potent nephrotoxic agent. Terminalia chebula was studied for its chemopreventive effect on nickel chloride-induced renal oxidative stress, toxicity, and cell proliferation response in male Wistar rats.[37] Administration of the nickel chloride to the male Wistar rats resulted in an increase in the reduced renal glutathione content, glutathione-S-transferase, glutathione reductase, lipid peroxidation, H_2O_2 generation, blood urea nitrogen, and serum creatinine, with a concomitant decrease in the activity of glutathione peroxidase. The nickel chloride treatment also induced tumor promotion markers. Prophylactic treatment of rats with Terminalia chebula daily for one week resulted in the diminution of nickel chloride-mediated damage, as evidenced from downregulation of all the parameters studied, with concomitant restoration of glutathione peroxidase activity. This investigation suggests that Terminalia chebula extract could be used as a therapeutic agent for cancer prevention as evidenced from this study, in which it blocked or suppressed the events associated with chemical carcinogenesis.

Gallic acid, 1,2,3,4,6-penta-O-galloyl-p-D-glucopyranose, chebulagic acid, and chebulinic acid, isolated from the methanol fraction of Terminalia chebula fruits, exhibited moderate cytotoxicity against cultured human tumor cell lines.[38]

In an effort to identify a new chemopreventive agent, a study was conducted to investigate the role of Terminalia chebula in preventing ferric nitrilotriacetic acid-induced oxidative stress and renal tumorigenesis in Wistar rats.[39] A single application of Fe-NTA significantly induced oxidative stress and elevated the marker parameters of tumor promotion. However, the pre-treatment of animals with different doses of Terminalia extract (25 and 50 mg/kg body weight) restored the levels of reduced glutathione (GSH) and cellular protective enzymes. Malondialdehyde formation and hydrogen peroxide content also were reduced significantly at both doses. The promotion parameters tested also were significantly suppressed. Terminalia also inhibited N-diethyl nitrosamine initiated renal carcinogenesis by showing a reduction in the number of animals with renal cell tumors and the percentage of incidences of tumors compared to the tumor-induced rats. The study was further confirmed histologically. These results suggest a potential role of Terminalia chebula in protection from Fe-NTA-induced renal carcinogenesis and oxidative damage.

Hepatoprotective activity:

A hepatoprotective compound was isolated from the ethanolic extract of the fruits of Terminalia chebula by consecutive solvent partitioning, followed by silica gel and Sephadex LH-20 column chromatographies.[40] The purified compound was identified as a mixture of chebulic acid and its minor isomer, neochebulic acid, with a ratio of 2:1 by spectroscopic analysis including 1D and 2D NMR and MS spectroscopy. This is the first report on the protection of rat hepatocytes against oxidative toxicity by chebulic acid obtained from Terminalia chebula. The compound exhibited in-vitro a free radical-scavenging activity and ferric-reducing anti-oxidant activity. The isolated rat hepatocyte experiment demonstrated that treating hepatocytes with chebulic acid significantly reduced the tert-butyl hydroperoxide-induced cell cytotoxicity, intracellular reactive oxygen species level, and the ratio of GSSH, oxidized form of glutathione to the over total GSH (GSH + GSSG) (4.42%) compared to that with t-BHP alone.

In another study, 95% ethanolic extract of Terminalia chebula fruit, which was chemically characterized on the basis of chebuloside II as a marker, was investigated for its hepatoprotective activity against anti-tuberculosis drug-induced toxicity. The extract was found to prevent the hepatotoxicity caused by administration of rifampicin, isoniazid, and pyrazinamide in combination in a sub-chronic mode (12 weeks). The hepatoprotective effect of the extract could be attributed to its prominent anti-oxidative and membrane stabilizing activities. Changes in the biochemical observations were supported by the histological profile.[41] A study was conducted to evaluate the protective effects of an aqueous extract of fruit of Terminalia chebula on tert-butyl hydroperoxide-induced oxidative injury observed in cultured rat primary hepatocytes and the rat liver.[42] Treatment and pre-treatment of the hepatocytes with the Terminalia extract both significantly reversed the t-BHP-induced cell cytotoxicity and lactate dehydrogenase leakage. In addition, the Terminalia extract exhibited in-vitro ferric-reducing anti-oxidant activity and 2,2-diphenyl-1-picryhydrazyl free radical-scavenging activities. The in-vivo study showed that pre-treatment with the extract for 5 days before a single dose of t-BHP significantly lowered the serum levels of the hepatic enzyme markers aspartate aminotransferase and alanine aminotransferase, and reduced the indicators of oxidative stress in the liver, in a dose-dependent manner. Histopathologic examination of the rat livers showed that the Terminalia extract reduced the incidence of liver lesions, including hepatocyte swelling and neutrophilic infiltration, and repaired necrosis induced by t-BHP. Based on these results, Terminalia is speculated to have a potential role in preventing hepatic oxidative damage in living systems.

Radioprotective activity:

The aqueous extract of the fruit of Terminalia chebula was evaluated for its anti-oxidant and radioprotective abilities. The Terminalia extract was able to neutralize 1,1-diphenyl-2-picrylhydrazyl, a stable free radical, by 92.9%. The free-radical neutralizing ability of Terminalia was comparable to that of ascorbate 93.5% and gallic acid 91.5% and was higher than that of the diethyldithiocarbamate 55.4%, suggesting the free radical activity of Terminalia. The extract prevented the plasmid DNA pBR322 from undergoing the radiation induced strand breaks.[43] Radiation damage converts the supercoiled form of plasmid to an open circular form. The presence of Terminalia chebula extract during radiation exposure protected the plasmid from undergoing these damages. Administration of the extract prior to whole-body irradiation of the mice resulted in a reduction of peroxidation of membrane lipids in the mice liver, as well as a decrease in radiation induced damage to DNA, as assayed by single-cell gel electrophoresis. The extract also protected the human lymphocytes from undergoing gamma radiation-induced damage to the DNA exposed in-vitro to 2 Gy gamma-radiation. These results suggest the radioprotective ability of Terminalia chebula.

Ethnoveterinary Usage

The fruits are used to treat bloating and as an appetite stimulant, and the seeds are used to treat wounds in ruminants.[44]

Dr. Sodhi's Experience

Before beginning treatment with Haritaki, the practitioner should consider the following:

- Is there constipation?
- Is there a viral infection?
- Is the liver congested?
- Is excess pitta present in the digestive system?

Haritaki almost always is used in Ayurveda for digestive disturbances when excess pitta is present. It has effects very similar to those of Emblica officinalis (amla) and is used for many of same conditions. It can be used for constipation, flatulence, bloating, and as an anti-parasitic. It is an important supplement for people who travel, especially as part of the digestive formula Triphala, which consists of equal parts Emblica officinalis (amalaki), Terminalia bellerica (bibhitaki), and haritaki. It may be used alone when constipation is predominant; otherwise, Triphala is more effective.

Haritaki also is good to use for weight loss in people with pitta dominance. Haritaki helps to stimulate bile production to purge the liver and is used for most liver conditions, usually as part of Triphala. Wherever there is liver congestion, alcoholism, or drug use, Triphala should be used. Triphala rasayana, composed of Triphala plus Tinospora cordifolia (guduchi)—equal parts of all four herbs—is considered to be more powerful than Triphala alone. This extremely powerful combination of anti-oxidants and adaptogenic herbs delays aging, increases longevity, and protects against most diseases.

Haritaki also is a powerful anti-viral. It can be used to treat bladder infections because it helps to eliminate pathogenic microflora such as E. coli.

Herbal Protocol

For viral hepatitis (B, C, or herpes):
> Haritaki, 250 mg extract three times a day

> Liver support herbs should be used, such as: Tinospora cardifolia (guduchi), Picrorrhiza kurnoa (kutki), and Boerhaavia diffusa (purnarnava) extracts, 50 mg of each herb in a proprietory blend of Phyllanthus amarus (bhumyamalaki), Swertia chirayita (kiraata), Calotropis gigantis (ark), Raphanus sativa (malaka), Berberis aristata (daaruCurcuma), Terminalia arjuna (arjun), Terminalia bellerica (bibhitaki), Terminalia chebula (haritaki), Emblica officinalis (amalaki), Solanum nigrum (kakmachi), and Andrographis paniculata (bhuunimb), one or two tablets three times a day

Safety Profile

No adverse effects of Terminalia chebula have been reported in the literature. The maximum tolerated doses of the 50% ethanolic extract of the stem bark and fruit were found to be 25 mg/kg body weight and 100 mg/kg body weight respectively, in adult albino rats.[44]

Dosage

Powder: 1–6 g (higher doses are laxative)
Decoction: 56–112 ml
Extract: 5:1 250 mg once or twice per day

Ayurvedic Properties

Rasa: Madhur, Amal, katu, tikta and kshaya, all rasas (except lavana)
Guna: Laghu (light), ruksha (dry)
Veerya: Ushna (hot)
Vipaka: Madhur (sweet)
Dosha: Pacifies tridosha

Notes

1. C. Singh, "2alpha-hydroxymicromeric acid, a pentacyclic triterpene from Terminalia chebula," *Phytochemistry*, 1990, 29(7):2348. 23–48?

2. A.P. Kundu and S.B Mahato, "Triterpenoidsand their glycosides from Terminalia thebula," *Phytochemistry*, 1993, 32(4):999.

3. See Note 2.

4. S. Suchalatha, P. Srinivasan, and C.S. Devi, "Effect of T. chebula on mitochondrial alterations in experimental myocardial injury," *Chem Biol Interact.*, Sept 20, 2007, 169(3):145-53. Epub June 20, 2007.

5. V.R.C. Reddy, S.V. Ramrnana Kumari, B.M. Reddy, M.A. Anzeem, M.C. Prabhakar, and A.V.N. Appa Rao, "Cardiotonic activity of the fruits of Terminalia chebula," *Fitoterapia*, 1990, 61(6):517.

6. Saravanan S, Srikumar R, Manikandan S, Jeya Parthasarathy N, Sheela Devi R. Hypolipidemic effect of triphala in experimentally induced hypercholesteremic rats. Yakugaku Zasshi. 2007 Feb;127(2):385-8.

7. T.Y Shin. H.J. Jeong, D.K. Kirn, et al., "Inhibitory action of water soluble fraction at Terminalia chebula on systemic and local anaphylaxis," *Journal of Ethnopharmacology*, 2001, 4(2):133.

8. I. S. Grover and B. Saroj, "Antimutagenie activity of T. chebula (myrobalan) in Salmonella typhimurium," *Indian Journal of Experimental Biology*, 1992, 30(4):399.

9. S. Kaur, S. Arora, K. Kaur, and S. Kumar, "The in vitro antimutagenic activity of Triphala—an Indian herbal drug," *Food Chem Toxicol.*, April 2002, 40(4):527–534.

10. S.A. Phadke and S.D. Kulkarni, "Screening of w vitro anti-bacterial activity of Terminalia chebula, Eclipta alba and Odmum sanctum," *Indian Journal of Medical Sciences*, 1989, 43(S):113.

11. See Note 10.

12. U. Carounanidy, R. Satyanarayanan, and A. Velmurugan, "Use of an aqueous extract of Terminalia chebula as an anticaries agent: A clinical study," *Indian J Dent Res.*, Oct–Dec, 2007, 18(4):152–156.

13. H.G, Kim, J.H. Cho, E.Y. Jeong, J.H. Lim, S.H. Lee, and H.S. Lee, "Growth-inhibiting activity of active component isolated from Terminalia chebula fruits against intestinal bacteria," *J Food Prot.*, Sept. 2006, 69(9):2205–2209.

14. F. Malekzadeh, H. Ehsanifar, M. Shahamat, M. Levin, and R.R. Colwell, "Anti-bacterial activity of black myrobalan (Terminalia chebula Retz) against Helicobacter pylori," *Int J Antimicrob Agents*, July 2001, 18(1):85–88.

15. P. Rani and N. Khullar, "Antimicrobial evaluation of some medicinal plants for their anti-enteric potential against multi-drug resistant Salmonella typhi," *Phytother Res.*, Aug. 2004, 18(8):670–673.

16. Y. Sato, H. Oketani, K. Singyouchi, et al., "Extraction and purification of effective antimicrobial constituents of Terminalia thebula Ret2, against nu'thidllin-resistant Siaphyloa Kcus aurcus," *Biological and Pharmaceutical Bulletin*, 1997, 20(4):401.

17. M. Kurokawa, K. Nagasaka, T. Hirabayashi, et al., "Efficacy of traditional herbal medicines in combination with acyclovir against herpes simplex virus type I infection in vitro and in vivo," *Anti-viral Research*, 1995, 27(1-2):19.

18. K. Shiraki, T. Yukawa, M. Kurokawa, and S. Kageyama, "Cytomegalovirus infection and its possible treatment with herbal medicines," *Nippon Rinsho*, Jan. 1998, 56(1):156-60.

19. S. Hamada, T. Kataoka, J.T. Woo, A.Yamada, T. Yoshida, T. Nishimura, N. Otake, and K. Nagai, "Immunosuppressive effects of gallic acid and chebulagic acid on CTL-mediated cytotoxicity," *Biol Pharm Bull.*, Sept. 1997, 20(9):1017–1019.

20. See Note 17.

21. See Note 8.

22. S. El-Mekkawy, M.R. Meselhy, I.T. Kusumoto, S. Kadota, M. Hattori, and T. Namba, "Inhibitory effects of Egyptian folk medicines on human immunodeficiency virus (HFV) reverse transcriptase," *Chemical and Pharmaceutical Bulletin*, 1995, 43(4):641.

23. M. J. Ahn, C.Y. Kim, J.S. Lee, T.G. Kim, S.H. Kim, C.K. Lee, B. B. Lee, C.G. Shin, H. Huh, and J. Kim, "Inhibition of HIV-1 integrase by galloyl glucoses from Terminalia chebula and flavonol glycoside gallates from Euphorbia pekinensis," *Planta Med.*, May 2002, 68(5):457–459.

24. Y.R. Sohni and R.M. Bhatt, "Activity of a crude extract formulation in experimental hepatic amoebiasis and in immunomodulation studies," *Journal of Ethnopharmacology*, 1996, 54(2–3):119.

25. N. Pratibha, V.S. Saxena, A. Amit, P. D'Souza, M. Bagchi, and D. Bagchi, "Anti-inflammatory activities of Aller-7, a novel polyherbal formulation for allergic rhinitis," *Int J Tissue React.*, 2004, 26(1–2):43–51.

26. Y.R. Sohni and R.M. Bhatt, "The antiamoebic effects of crude drug formulation of herbal extracts against Entamoeba histolytica in vitro and in vivo," *Journal of Ethnopharmacology*, 1995, 45(1):43.

27. N. Fu, L. Quan, L. Huang, R. Zhang, and Y. Chen, "Anti-oxidant action of extract of Terminalia chebula and its preventive effect on DNA breaks in human white cells induced by TPA," *Chinese Traditional Herbal Drugs*, 1992, 23(1):26.

28. G. H. Naik, K.I. Priyadarsini, D.B. Naik, R. Gangabhagirathi, H. Mohan, "Studies on the aqueous extract of Terminalia chebula as a potent anti-oxidant and a probable radioprotector," *Phytomedicine*, Sept. 2004, 11(6):530–538.

29. M. Na, K. Bae, S.S. Kang, B.S. Min, J.K. Yoo, Y. Kamiryo, Y. Senoo, S. Yokoo, and N. Miwa, "Cytoprotective effect on oxidative stress and inhibitory effect on cellular aging of Terminalia chebula fruit," *Phytother Res.*, Sept. 2004, 18(9):737–741.

30. Y.K. Murali, P. Anand, V. Tandon, R. Singh, R. Chandra, and P.S. Murthy, "Long-term effects of Terminalia chebula Retz. on hyperglycemia and associated hyperlipidemia, tissue glycogen content and in vitro release of insulin in streptozotocin induced diabetic rats," *Exp Clin Endocrinol Diabetes*, Nov. 2007, 115(10):641–646.

31. See Note 30. **Check all of these "See Notes"**

32. Rao NK, Nammi S. Antidiabetic and renoprotective effects of the chloroform extract of Terminalia chebula Retz. seeds in streptozotocin-induced diabetic rats. BMC Complement Altern Med. 2006 May 7;6:17.

33. See Note 32.

34. H. Gao, Y.N. Huang, G. Gao, and J. Kawabata, "Chebulagic acid is a potent alpha-glucosidase inhibitor," *Biosci Biotechnol Biochem.*, Feb. 2008, 72(2):601–603. Epub Feb. 7, 2008.

35. N.M. Gandhi and C.K. Nair, "Radiation protection by Terminalia chebula: Some mechanistic aspects," *Mol Cell Biochem.*, Sept. 2005, 277(1–2):43–48.

36. G. Deep, M. Dhiman, A.R. Rao, and R.K. Kale, "Chemopreventive potential of Triphala (a composite Indian drug) on benzo(a)pyrene induced forestomach tumorigenesis in murine tumor model system," *J Exp Clin Cancer Res.*, Dec. 2005, 24(4):555–563.

37. L. Prasad, T. Husain Khan, T. Jahangir, and S. Sultana, "Chemomodulatory effects of Terminalia chebula against nickel chloride induced oxidative stress and tumor promotion response in male Wistar rats," *J Trace Elem Med Biol.*, 2006, 20(4):233–239. Epub Oct 2, 2006.

38. S.H. Lee, S.Y. Ryu, S.U. Choi, et al., "Hydrolysable tannins and related compound having cytotoxic activity from the fruits of Terminalia chebula," *Archives of Pharmacological Research*, 1995, 18(2):118.

39. L. Prasad, T.H. Khan, T. Jahangir, and S. Sultana, "Abrogation of DEN/Fe-NTA induced carcinogenic response, oxidative damage and subsequent cell proliferation response by erminalia chebula in kidney of Wistar rats," *Pharmazie*, Oct. 2007, 62(10):790–797.

40. H.S. Lee, S.H. Jung, B.S. Yun, and K.W. Lee, "Isolation of chebulic acid from Terminalia chebula Retz. and its anti-oxidant effect in isolated rat hepatocytes," *Arch Toxicol.*, March 2007, 81(3):211–218. Epub Aug. 24, 2006.

41. S.A. Tasduq, K. Singh, N.K. Satti, D.K. Gupta, K.A. Suri, and R.K. Johri, "Terminalia chebula (fruit) prevents liver toxicity caused by sub-chronic administration of rifampicin, isoniazid and pyrazinamide in combination," *Hum Exp Toxicol.*, March 25, 2006, 25(3):111–118.

42. H. S Lee, N.H. Won, K.H. Kim, H. Lee, W. Jun, and K.W. Lee, "Anti-oxidant effects of aqueous extract of Terminalia chebula in vivo and in vitro," *Biol Pharm Bull.*, Sept. 2005, 28(9):1639–1644.

43. See Note 35.

44. International Institute of Rural Reconstruction, *Ethnoveterinary Medicine in Asia. An Information Kit on Traditional Animal Health Care Practices. Part I, General Information* (Silang, Philippines: IIRR, 1994).

42

Tribulus terrestris

Introduction

Tribulus terrestris is a low-growing herb that has been used in the traditional medicines of China and India for centuries. Known in Ayurveda as Goksura, Tribulus terrestris became well-known in the Western world in the 1990s after Eastern European Olympic athletes reported that taking the herb enhanced their athletic performance.

Having a long history of use for a variety of conditions, Tribulus is believed to have been used in ancient Greece and India as a physical rejuvenation tonic. In China, it has been used for more than 400 years to treat psoriasis, eczema, premature ejaculation, liver disease, and kidney conditions. Other ancient Eastern cultures used Tribulus for its diuretic properties and to treat infections. It also has been used in Eastern European folk medicine for increased muscle strength and sexual potency. Ancient Ayurvedic texts describe Tribulus as soothing to the kidneys and urinary tract.

Tribulus terrestris allegedly was introduced to the United States in the early 1900s with livestock imported from the Europe. Even today it is found growing alongside railroad tracks.

Currently, Tribulus is a component of herbal preparations used to treat conditions affecting the liver, kidney, cardiovascular, and immune systems.

In Ayurvedic tradition, Tribulus is known as a rasayana because of its rejuvenating effects. It is believed to enhance cardiovascular, immune, and sexual health. Because of its effectiveness against bacterial growth, Tribulus terrestris is often used to treat infections. It has been shown to be effective against gram-negative bacteria such as E-coli.

Synonymous Names

English: Puncture vine, Land caltrops, small caltrops
Hindi: Gokharu
Sanskrit: Gokshura, shuuadamshtra, swadukantaka, trikantaka
Bengali: Gokuri

Habitat

Tribulus terrestris is native to southern Asia, southern Europe, Africa, and northern Australia. It grows in warm, tropical regions as well as dry, desert areas in soil in which most plants don't thrive. It also grows widely in the southwestern United States. Tribulus prefers light-textured soils but will grow in a wide range of soil types. In Australia, it is considered to be a weed that hinders cultivated crops and is found in overgrazed pastures, stockyards, roadsides, lawns, and neglected areas.

Botanical Characteristics

Tribulus terrestris is a prostrate herb, with stems up to 2 meters in length. Its leaves are opposite, each consisting of four to eight pairs of spear-shaped leaflets. Long hairs are present on the leaf margins and the lower surfaces. The stems are round and hairy. The flowers have five yellow petals that produce a fruit about a week after they bloom. The fruit is a woody, star-shaped structure 5 to 7 millimeters long and 5 to 6 millimeters wide, which contains seeds with two or three pointed spines. These horn-shaped spines are sharp enough to puncture skin. The long, thin roots have a light scent and are light-brown in color. The taste is described as similar to that of turnips and asparagus.

Chemical Constituents

Tribulus terrestris' active components are believed to be its saponins, which include glucopyranosyl galactopyrans, ruscogenin, protodioscin, hecogenin, and diosgenin. Other components are sterols, steroidal glycosides, flavonoids, fatty acids and tannins.[1,2,3]

Pharmacological Activity

Sexual health activity

For centuries in Ayurvedic tradition, Tribulus terrestris has been used as an aphrodisiac, for erectile dysfunction, and to improve overall sexual health. Independent studies have revealed that Tribulus terrestris extract elevates hormonal levels. Comparative studies have found that tonic properties of Tribulus terrestris are similar to those of ginseng, although the mechanism of action of the two herbs appears to be distinct.

Tribulus elevates testosterone levels by increasing gonadotropin-releasing hormone, which, in turn, stimulates the production of LH and follicle-stimulating hormone. Besides its role in body building, fertility, and libido, testosterone has a positive effect on the immune system and on bone marrow activity, promoting the production of healthy red blood cells.

The hormonal effects of Tribulus terrestris were evaluated in primates, rabbits, and rats to assess the herb's potential in managing erectile dysfunction. Tribulus extract was administered intravenously to primates at a variety of dosages. Rabbits and normal rats were treated orally with 2.5, 5, and 10 mg/kg of Tribulus extract for 8 weeks in the chronic study. In addition, castrated rats were treated orally with either testosterone cypionate or Tribulus biweekly for 8 weeks. Blood samples were analyzed for testosterone, dihydrotestosterone, and dehydroepiandrosterone sulfate (DHEA) levels using radioimmunoassay.[4] Statistically significant increases were observed for all three of the analyzed substances. In rabbits, both testosterone and dihydrotestosterone levels were increased compared to the controls; however, only the increases in dehydroepiandrosterone were statistically significant. In the castrated rats, increases in testosterone levels by 51% and 25% were observed with Tribulus extract that were statistically significant. Tribulus terrestris was shown to increase the levels of some sex hormones, possibly due to the presence of protodioscin in the extract.

These results indicate that Tribulus may be useful in mild to moderate cases of erectile dysfunction.[5] The rodent study described above found Tribulus to be useful as a sex booster.[6,4] Sexual behavior and intracavernous pressure were studied in both normal and castrated mice to further evaluate the role of Tribulus as an aphrodisiac. The adult rats were divided into three groups, including both normal and castrated rats. Group one was treated with distilled water; group two was treated with testosterone; and group three was treated with Tribulus. Compared to the castrated controls, treatment of the castrated rats with either testosterone or Tribulus extract resulted in an increase in prostate weight and intracavernous pressure. There was also mild to moderate improvement in sexual behavior as evidenced by an increase in mounting frequency.

A study was conducted to evaluate the effect of Tribulus on nicotinamide adenine dinucleotide phosphate-diaphorase activity and androgen receptor immuno-reactivity in rat brains.[7] Twenty-four adult male rats were distributed into two groups of 12 each. Group one was treated with distilled water, and Group two was treated with Tribulus terrestris at a dose of 5mg/kg body weight orally, once daily for 8 weeks. At the end of the treatment period, transcardiac perfusion was done with Ringer lactate, 4% paraformaldehyde, and 30% sucrose. Brain tissue was removed, and sections of the paraventricular area of the hypothalamus were taken for immunostaining. There was an increase in both NADPH-d (67%) and androgen receptor (AR) immunoreactivity (58%) in the Tribulus terrestris-treated group. The results were statistically significant compared to the control. Chronic treatment of Tribulus terrestris in rats increases the NADPH-d positive neurons and androgen receptor (AR) immunoreactivity in the paraventricular region. Androgens are known to increase both androgen receptor and NADPH-d positive neurons, either directly or by their conversion to estrogen. The mechanism for the observed increases in androgen receptor and NADPH-d positive neurons observed in this study is probably a result of the androgen-enhancing properties of Tribulus terrestris. These findings add further support to the aphrodisiac claims of the Tribulus. A few other studies failed to show any effect on androgen production.[8, 9, 10, 11]

Other hormone activity

A study was undertaken to observe the effect of Tribulus terrestris extract on melanocyte stimulating hormone (MSH) expression in C57BL/6J mouse hair follicles, and to investigate the role of Tribulus terrestris extract in activation, proliferation, and epidermal migration of dormant hair follicle melanocytes. The aqueous extract of Tribulus terrestris was administered orally in specific pathogen-free C57BL/6J mice at the daily dose equivalent of 1 g/1 kg in adult humans, and the expression and distribution of melanocyte stimulating hormone in the mouse hair follicles were observed with immunohistochemistry.[12] The positivity rate of melanocyte stimulating hormone expression in the hair follicle melanocytes was 75% in the mice treated with the extract—significantly higher than the rate of only 18.75% in the control group (P<0.01). The aqueous extract of Tribulus terrestris can significantly increase melanocyte stimulating hormone expression in the hair follicle melanocytes by activating tyrosinase activity and promoting melanocyte proliferation, melanine synthesis, and epidermal migration of dormant melanocytes. Melanocyte stimulating hormone acts as an anti-inflammatory, regulatory hormone made in the hypothalamus. It controls the production of hormones, modulates the immune system, and controls nerve function. It is made when leptin is able to activate its receptor in the proopio-melanocortin (POMC) pathway. If the receptor is damaged by peripheral immune effects, such as the release of too many pro-inflammatory cytokines, the receptor doesn't work properly and MSH isn't made.

Leptin controls storage of fatty acids as fat, so MSH and leptin may be dependent on each other. Damage to leptin receptors can be similar to insulin resistance. MSH controls hypothalamic production of melatonin and endorphins. MSH deficiency causes chronic fatigue and chronic pain. MSH also controls many protective effects in the skin, gut and mucous membranes of the nose and lung. It also controls the peripheral release of cytokines; when there isn't enough MSH, the peripheral inflammatory effects are multiplied. MSH also controls pituitary function, with 60% of MSH-deficient patients not having enough antidiuretic hormone. These patients are thirsty all the time, urinate frequently, and often have unusual sensitivity to static electrical shocks. Of MSH-deficient patients, 40% won't regulate male hormone production, and another 40% won't regulate control of ACTH and cortisol.

Any illness that begins with excessive production of pro-inflammatory cytokines usually will cause an MSH deficiency. This is the basic mechanism that underlies damage caused by exposure to biologically produced toxins, neurotoxins (biotoxins) made by invertebrate organisms, including fungi (molds), dinoflagellates (ciguatera and Pfiesteria), spirochetes (Lyme disease), blue-green algae (Cylindrospermopsis in Florida and Microcystis throughout the world) and bacteria such as anthrax. Nearly 100% of patients with chronic fatigue syndrome (CFS) have an MSH deficiency.

Anti-bacterial and anti-fungal activity

The anti-microbial activity of organic and aqueous extracts from the fruits, leaves, and roots of Tribulus terrestris was examined against 11 species of pathogenic and non-pathogenic microorganisms—Staphylococcus aureus, Bacillus subtilis, Bacillus cereus, Corynebacterium diphtheriae, Escherichia coli, Proteus vulgaris, Serratia marcescens, Salmonella typhimurium, Klebsiella pneumoniae, Pseudomonas aeruginosa, and Candida albicans—using microdilution method in 96 multiwell microtiter plates.[13] All the extracts from different parts of the plant showed anti-microbial activity against the tested microorganisms. The most active extract against both Gram-negative and Gram-positive bacteria was ethanol extract from the fruits, with a minimal inhibitory concentration (MIC) value of 0.15 mg/ml against B. subtilis, B. cereus, P. vulgaris, and C. diphtheriae. In addition, the same extract from the same plant part demonstrated the strongest antifungal activity against C. albicans with an MIC value of 0.15 mg/ml.

Cardiac activity

The effects of methanolic and aqueous extracts of Tribulus terrestris on rat blood pressure and the perfused mesenteric vascular bed were investigated. The extracts were found to reduce blood pressure in spontaneously hypertensive rats in a dose-dependent manner. The aqueous fraction was shown to be more potent than the methanolic fraction at all doses tested.[14] The methanolic, but not the aqueous, Tribulus extract produced a dose-dependent increase in perfusion pressure of the mesenteric vascular bed. When the perfusion pressure was raised with phenylephrine, the aqueous extract produced a dose-dependent reduction in perfusion pressure at all doses. A low dose of the methanolic extract produced a vasoconstrictor effect, and the higher doses produced dose-dependent reductions in perfusion pressure, A L-NAME (a nonselective inhibitor of nitric oxide synthase used experimentally to induce hypertension) significantly reduced, but did not abolish, vasodilation induced by the extracts. Vasodilator responses to aqueous and methanolic fractions were reduced significantly in preparations in which perfusion pressure was raised with KCl. A combination of KCl and L-NAME abolished the vasodilator responses induced by the extracts. It was concluded that methanolic and aqueous extracts of Tribulus terrestris possess significant antihypertensive activity in spontaneously hypertensive rats. The antihypertensive effects appeared to result from a direct arterial smooth-muscle relaxation, possibly involving nitric oxide release and membrane hyperpolarization. Another study evaluating Tribulus showed that the anti-hypertensive affect of Tribulus might be a result of decreased ACE activity. ACE activity was inversely proportional to Tribulus intake. Interestingly this activity was more pronounced in the kidneys.[15] Isolated rat hearts were subjected to 30 minutes of ischemia followed by 120 minutes of reperfusion using Langendorff's technique. The hearts were assigned to seven groups:

control, ischemia/reperfusion (I/R), treatment with gross saponins from Tribulus terrestris (GSTT) 100 mg/L, treatment with tribulosin (100, 10, and 1 nmol/L), and treatment with a PKC inhibitor (chelerythrine) (1 micromol/L). Infarct size was assessed by triphenyltetrazolium chloride staining. Malondialdehyde (MDA), aspartate aminotransferase (AST), and lactate dehydrogenase (LDH) contents, as well as superoxide dismutase (SOD) and creatine kinase (CK) activities, were determined after the treatment. Histopathological changes in the myocardium were observed using hematoxylin-eosin (H&E) staining. Bcl-2, Bax, caspase-3 and PKC epsilon protein expression were examined using the Western blot test. Apoptosis was observed using terminal deoxynucleotidyl transferase nick-ending labeling(TUNEL) assay.

In another study, Tribulosin treatment significantly reduced MDA, AST, CK, and LDH contents and increased the activity of SOD.[16] The infarct size of I/R group was 40.21% of the total area. Gross saponins from Tribulus terrestris (GSTT) and various concentrations of tribulosin treatment decreased the infarct size to 24.33%, 20.24%, 23.19%, and 30.32% (P<0.01). Tribulosin treatment reduced the myocardial apoptosis rate in a concentration dependent manner. Bcl-2 and PKC epsilon protein expression was increased after tribulosin preconditioning, whereas Bax and caspase-3 expression was decreased. In the chelerythrine group, Bcl-2 and PKCepsilon expression was decreased, whereas Bax and caspase-3 expression was increased. Tribulosin protects myocardium against ischemia/reperfusion injury through PKC epsilon activation.

Pleotropic effects of extract of Tribulus terrestris was investigated, on the lipid profile and vascular endothelium of the abdominal aorta in New Zealand rabbits fed a cholesterol-rich diet.[17] Eighteen rabbits were randomly divided into three groups (n=6 for each). One experimental group (EG-I) was given a cholesterol rich diet, a second experimental group (EG-II) was treated with Tribulus following a cholesterol-rich diet, and a control group was fed a standard diet. Blood samples were collected on day 0 and then at weeks 4 and 12 to determine total serum cholesterol , high density lipid-cholesterol (HDL-C), low density lipid-cholesterol (LDL-C) and triglyceride (TG) levels. Tissues were collected from the abdominal aorta for immunohistochemistry and transmission and scanning electron microscopy. In EG-II, the serum lipid profile was significantly lower than that of EG-I at week 12 with a reduction of TC: 65%; LDL-C: 66%; HDL-C: 64%; and TG: 55%. The ultrastructural analysis revealed that endothelial damage was more prominent in EG-I compared to EG-II. The ruptured endothelial linings and damaged cellular surfaces increased in EG-I compared to EG-II. Dietary intake of Tribulus can significantly lower serum lipid profiles, decrease endothelial cellular surface damage and rupture and may partially repair the endothelial dysfunction resulting from hyperlipidemia. An experiment was designed to determine whether Tribulus saponins relieve left ventricular remodeling after myocardial infarction in a murine hyperlipidemia model.[18] Myocardial infarction and hyperlipidemia models were induced, and high and low doses of Tribulus and simvastatin were administered to the rats. Four weeks later, an echocardiographic observation was performed and the left and right ventricular weight index (LVWI, RVWI) was calculated. The echocardiographic results showed that both the high dose of Tribulus and the simvastatin had a beneficial effect on increasing fractional shortening and ejection fraction (EF), reducing left ventricular end diastolic volume (LVEDV), systolic volume (LVESV), left ventricular dimension end diastole (LVDd) and systole (LVDs), and decreasing LVWI, as compared to those in the hyperlipidemia MI model group (p < 0.05, 0.01). Both medicines had little impact on thickness of the anterior and posterior walls. No significant difference was observed between each treatment group (p > 0.05). Tribulus not only lowered serum lipidemia but also relieved left ventricular remodeling and improved cardiac function in the early stage after MI. In another study, 60 male Wistar rats weighing 280–320 grams were randomly divided into five groups: normal, sham operation model, Tribulus treatment (XNST-T), and Western medicine treatment (WM-T).[19] An acute multi-infarct model in rats was induced by injecting the embolus of blood powder through the right external carotid artery into the internal carotid artery. At 72 hours after ischemia, morphologic change and the expression of tumor necrosis factor-alpha (TNF-alpha) and interleukin-1beta (IL-1beta) in hippocampus section and cortex were observed, and biochemical criteria including the activity of Na+ -K+ -ATPase, lactate dehydrogenase (LDH), superoxide dismutase (SOD), and the content of malondialdehyde (MDA) in the hippocampus were examined. Morphologic changes in the hippocampus and cortex of both the XNST-T and the WM-T groups were milder than in model group. The activity of Na+ -K+ -ATPase, LDH, and SOD in the hippocampus were all decreased significantly in the model group (P <0. 01), and elevated in the XNST group (P <0. 01) as well as in the WM-T group (P <0. 01). The content of MDA in the hippocampus was increased significantly in the model group (P <0. 05), and was reduced in the XNST group (P <0. 05), as well as in the WM-T group (P <0. 01). These results suggest that Tribulus has a protective effect against cerebral ischemic injury.

Renal and urinary health activity

In the Ayurvedic system, Tribulus is believed to be one of the best herbal remedies for the kidneys. It is known to nourish and to strengthen the kidneys and reproductive organs and has been widely used to treat many urinary disorders including urolithiasis, cystitis, renal calculi (kidney stones), incontinence, gout, and impotence. Tribulus has a diuretic effect, and the fruit of Tribulus is believed to promote the flow of urine and to cool and soothe membranes of the urinary tract.

Ethanol extract of Tribulus fruit was tested for its action against artificially induced urolithiasis in albino rats.[20] Results of the study supported claims that Tribulus has a beneficial effect on urinary health. The product UNEX containing the extracts of Boerhaavia diffusa and Tribulus terrestris was studied at two dose levels of 600 and 800 mg/kg body weight (p.o.). Standard drug used was furosemide (20 mg/kg body weight) in a 0.9% sodium chloride solution. Urine volume was recorded for all the groups for 5 hours. The product UNEX exhibited significant diuretic activity at doses of 600 and 800 mg/kg body weight as evidenced by increased total urine volume and the urine concentration of Na + , K + , and Cl–.[19] Another study was conducted to investigate the effects of saponins from Tribulus terrestris on renal carcinoma cells in-vitro and the associated inhibitory mechanisms. The effects of Tribulus extract on the cytotoxicity, morphological changes of apoptosis, cell cycle, and expression of Bcl-2 protein were tested, as well as flow cytometry.[21] This study revealed: (1) a significant cytotoxic effect, observed by the MTT assay; (2) apoptosis, as viewed by Wright's and acridine orange stain assays; (3) an increased distribution of 786-0 on the S phase, and (4) a decrease in the expression of Bcl-2 protein and cyclin D1. These results indicate that saponins from tribulus terrestris can significantly inhibit the growth of 786-0 in vitro, partially by apoptosis.

Analgesic activity

For a long time Tribulus terrestris has been used in traditional medicine for relieving rheumatic pain and as an analgesic plant. In an investigation, the analgesic effect of methanolic extract of this plant on male albino mice was evaluated by formalin and tail-flick test. The results showed that a dose of 100 mg/kg of percolated extract had the highest significant analgesic effect compared to the control group ($P < 0.01$) in formalin and tail flick test.[22] There was no significant difference in the analgesic effect of soxhlet and percolated extract. The analgesic effect of the extract was lower than morphine, 2.5 mg/kg in both tests, and higher than aspirin 300 mg/kg in chronic phase of pain in the formalin test ($P < 0.05$). Pretreatment of animal with naloxone did not change the analgesia induced by the plant extract in both tests; therefore, involvement of the opioid receptor in the analgesic effect of this plant was excluded. Results of the ulcerogenic studies indicate that the gastric ulcerogenecity of the plant extract is lower than the indomethacin in the rat's stomach.

Hepatoprotective activity against mercury

The efficacy of the methanolic fraction of Tribulus terrestris fruit extract on mercury intoxicated mice, Mus musculus, has been studied. At a median-lethal dose of mercuric chloride (12.9 mg/ kg body wt.) administration enhanced the levels of glutamate oxaloacete transaminase (GOT) and glutamate pyruvate transminase (GPT); simultaneously, decreased levels of acid phosphatase (ACP) and alkaline phosphatase (ALT) activities were noted in the liver. As a result of the mercury toxicity, liver cells were damaged, altering their enzymes. The results suggested that oral administration of methanolic fraction of Tribulus terrestris fruit extract (6 mg/kg body wt.) provided protection against the mercuric chloride induced hepatic damage in the mice, M. musculus.[23] In Arabic folk medicine, Tribulus terrestris is used to treat various diseases. An article reported on the protective effects of Tribulus terrestris diabetes mellitus .[24] Diabetes is known to increase the level of reactive oxygen species , which subsequently contributes to the pathogenesis of diabetes. The rats were divided into six groups and treated with saline, or glibenclamide , or Tribulus for 30 days. The rats in group 1 were given saline after the onset of streptozotocin (STZ)-induced diabetes The second diabetic group was administered Glibencalmide (10 mg/kg body weight). The third diabetic group was treated with the Tribulus extract (2 g/kg body weight).

At the end of the experiment, serum and liver samples were collected for biochemical and morphological analyses. The levels of serum alanine aminotransferase (ALT) and creatinine were estimated. In addition, levels of malondialdehyde (MDA) and reduced glutathione (GSH) in the liver were assayed. The Tribulus extract significantly decreased the levels of ALT and creatinine in the serum ($P < 0.05$) in the diabetic groups and lowered the MDA level in the liver ($P < 0.05$) in the diabetic and ($P < 0.01$) non-diabetic groups. On the other hand, the levels of reduced GSH in the liver were significantly increased ($P < 0.01$) in diabetic rats treated with Tribulus. The histopathological examination revealed significant recovery of the liver in the herb-treated rats.

Dr. Sodhi's Experience

Before beginning treatment with Tribulus terrestris, the following should be considered: consider the following:

- Is there kidney dysfunction or failure?
- Are BUN or creatinine levels high?
- Is nephritic syndrome present?
- Is there edema?
- Is there a need for a loop-sparing diuretic?
- Is there any sexual dysfunction in a male? Impotence? Low libido? Infertility?
- Is testosterone low?

- Are there digestive symptoms?

Tribulus terrestris is an effective diuretic, with properties similar to the prescription drug furosemide. Tribulus terrestris can be used whenever a diuretic is needed, for edema, for ascites, and for improving kidney function. It also is mucilaginous, protecting the mucosal lining of the intestines. In ancient times in India, people who drank alcohol on a regular basis used Tribulus to protect the liver and kidneys from alcohol damage. It is used to treat kidney stones, bladder stones, kidney infections, and nephrotic syndrome. In some cases, Tribulus has been known to reverse kidney failure, bringing creatinine and BUN levels back within a normal range.

Tribulus terrestis often is combined with other kidney minerals and herbs such as black asphaltum (shilajit), Crataevus religious (varuna), Arctostaphylos uva ursi, and Didymocarpus pedicellata (shilapushpa). In Ayurveda, it is considered to be a cooling herb. Tribulus acts like testosterone in some respects and promotes male sexual health. It helps to cleanse spermatic fluids and enhances spermatogenesis. Finally, it is used as a body-building agent.

Case Histories

Kidney failure:

A 50-year-old general contractor from California came to our clinic with kidney failure and nephrotic syndrome, hoping to find a way to preserve the kidney function he still had. He wanted to avoid dialysis if at all possible. We put him on the following herbal protocol:

For kidney support:

Didymocarpus pedicellata (shilapushpa) and Saxifraga ligulata (pashanabhedi) extracts, 200 mg each, with 50 mg each of Rubia cordifolia (manjistha), Ocimum santum (tulsi), Achyranthes aspera (aparamarga), black asphaltum (Shilajit), Cyperus rotundus (motha), Arctostaphylus uva ursi extracts, 50 mg each, and Crataeva religiosa (varuna) extract, 100 mg, plus 200 mg magnesium aspartate and 50 mg of vitamin B6, in a proprietary blend of cranberry extract, Tribulus terrestris (gokhru), Mimosa pudica, Dolichos B, and Equisetum arvense: to be taken three times a day.

For inflammation: Curcumin longum extract, 500 mg: three times a day.

For elevated eosinophils: Withania somnifera 500 (1000) mg: three times a day.

For elevated cholesterol (characteristic of nephritic syndrome): Guggulids 250 mg one capsule three times a day.

We also prescribed probiotics to improve gastrointestinal function and help clear phosphates and chlorides more efficiently in the digestive tract. As a further supplement for high cholesterol, we prescribed fish oil, 1000 mg, to be taken three times a day. We also had him do Panchakarma (detoxification treatment) for 3 weeks. When this patient first came to our clinic, his creatinine was 9.4 and his BUN level was 75. After 3 weeks of the herbal protocol and the panchakarma, his creatinine had dropped to 3.2 and his BUN was back to normal. He was happy with the results, and he continued to progress well at home.

In another case, a senator from Seattle who had a less severe case of kidney failure visited our clinic. His creatinine level, which was 3.6 when we first saw him, dropped back to normal within a month after beginning the above protocol.

Staghorn kidney disease:

A 76-year-old man came to see one of my colleagues in our clinic in India with a blood pressure of 190/120 mm Hg and creatinine at 11.0. Kidney imaging showed that he had staghorn kidneys. Immediately he was put on the kidney protocol described above, along with 100 mg each of Convolvulus pluricaulis (shankhapushpi) and Tribulus terrestris (gokhru), with 50 mg of Rauwolfia serpentina (sarpagandha) and 25 mg Rosa vinca (sadafuli), for blood pressure. To help dissolve his kidney stones, we had him put lemon or lime juice in his drinking water.

We observed the patient closely, and after 2 weeks his creatinine had dropped 3.5. After another 1½ months, his creatinine was 1.2, and a second diagnostic imaging revealed that he had phosphate stones. These stones are very soft, so they did not cause pain when his kidneys released them.

Delayed male development:

A 16-year-old boy, 5 feet 9 inches tall, weighing 170 pounds, came to see me because he had large breasts and small genitals. His testicles were the size usually found on boys around 7 or 8 years of age, and his penis was still quite short. He had no secondary sexual characteristics, no chest, underarm, or pubic hair. We ordered hormone panels and found that his testosterone was 70, as compared to the lowest normal value of 240. He wanted to take testosterone, and it was difficult to convince him that this was not the best choice, as it can lead to testicular shrinkage if used on a long-term. We convinced him to try an Ayurvedic protocol for 2 months and put him on the following treatment plan:

For low testosterone:
Withania somnifera (ashwagandha) 175 mg extract, Tribulus terrestris (gokhru) 50 mg extract, Shilajit (black asphaltum) 25 mg, Saw palmetto, 25 mg extract, Muira puma 20 mg extract, in a proprietary blend of Crocus sativus (Kumkuma), Emblica officinalis (amalaki), Piper longum (Pippli), Glycyrrhiza glabra (yastimadhu), Bacopa monniera (indriya brahmi), Sida cordifolia (bala), Mucuna pruriens (kapikachu), and Spilanthes acmella (akarkara): to be taken three times a day, along with 25 mg DHEA per day.

For genitourinary health:
Didymocarpus pedicellata (shilapushpa) and Saxifraga ligulata (pashanabhedi) extracts, 100 mg each, with 25 mg each of Rubia cordifolia (manjistha), Ocimum sanctum (tulsi), Achyranthes aspera (aparmarga), Black asphaltum (Shilajit), Cyperus rotundus (motha), Arctostaphylus uva ursi extracts, 25 mg each, and Crataeva religiosa (varuna) extract, 50 mg, plus 100 mg magnesium aspartate and 25 mg of vitamin B6, in a proprietary blend of cranberry extract, Tribulus terrestris (gokshura), Mimosa pudica, Dolichos B, and Equisetum arvense: to be taken taken three times a day.

For mood and mental health:
Withania somnifera 500 mg, three times a day, Mucuna pruriens (kapikachu) extract 250 mg in a proprietary blend of Centella asiatica (brahmi) and Valeriana Wallichii (tagara).to be taken three times a day.

We also advised the patient to exercise daily, and to lift weights to improve his testosterone level. We recommended a kapha-building diet, increasing his intake of nuts, seeds, fish, chicken and oils.

Two months later, his testosterone level had jumped to 354, well within the normal range, but he still had breasts because he had not followed his exercise program. We explained that exercise, in addition to building muscle, increases testosterone. Once he began to exercise, his breasts shrank.

Low libido with infertility:

A 34-year-old Indian man came to our clinic complaining that he had no sexual desire and was extremely fatigued. He and his wife were trying to conceive a child and had been unable to do so. He had many symptoms of digestive dysfunction, including diarrhea, constipation, and flatulence. He had been given several prescription medications to treat microbial infections, but nothing had helped. We tested him for anti-gliadin antibodies and tissue transglutaminase and found that he had gluten intolerance. We also checked his free testosterone and found that it was extremely low at 129.

We gave him the protocol described above for male health, and added the following supplements for his enteropathy:

> Digestive enzymes: Curcuma longum (Haridra), 500 mg, to be taken three times a day with coconut milk; Triphala, equal parts Emblica officinalis (amalaki), Terminalia bellerica (bibhitaki), and Terminalia chebula (haritaki), 500 mg three times a day; a multivitamin; and probiotics, 100 billion organisms per day for the first week, then 30 billion. In addition, we had him remove all gluten from his diet.

In 3 months, the patient's testosterone level had risen to 436. He reported having renewed sexual desire and was enjoying sexual interactions more. His energy also had improved. When we last spoke, he and his wife still had not conceived, but they had adopted a child from India. Prior to bringing her to the United States, they had stayed in India with her for 3 months so she could become accustomed to them in her own environment. They are still hoping to have a biological child someday.

Herbal Protocols

For dialysis support:

> Didymocarpus pedicellata (shilapushpa) and Saxifraga ligulata (pashanabhedi) extracts, 200 mg each, with 50 mg each of Rubia cordifolia (manjistha), Ocimum sanctum (tulsi), Achyranthes aspera (aparamarga), Black asphaltum (Shilajit), Cyperus rotundus (motha), Arctostaphylus uva ursi extracts, 50 mg each, and Crataeva religiosa (varuna) extract, 100 mg, plus 200 mg magnesium aspartate and 50 mg of vitamin B6, in a proprietary blend of cranberry extract, Tribulus terrestris (gokshura), Mimosa pudica, Dolichos B, and Equisetum arvense: to be taken three times a day.

In addition to the above, liver support herbs should be used, such as: Tinospora cordifolia (guduchi), Picrorrhiza kurroa (kutki), and Boerhaavia diffusa (Punarnava) extracts, 50 mg of each herb in a proprietary blend of Phyllanthus amarus (bhumyamalaki), Swertia chirayita (kiraata), Calotropis gigantic (ark), Raphanus sativa (malaka), Berberis aristata (daaruharidra), Terminalia arjuna (arjun), Terminalia bellerica (bibhitaki), Terminalia chebula (haritaki), Emblica officinalis (amalaki), Solanum nigrum (kakmachi), and Andrographis paniculata (bhuunimb).

Be careful not to load the kidneys too much. Magnesium, phosphates and salicylates are of particular concern and should be monitored carefully.

Safety Profile

Tribulus terrestris seems to be generally safe, with the following exceptions:

It may have a diuretic effect. Caution is advised when the herb is used with other diuretics. Tribulus also may lower blood glucose levels. Thus, caution is advised for patients taking glucose-lowering medications. Patients taking drugs for diabetes by mouth or insulin should be monitored closely when using Tribulus, as adjustments in medications may be necessary.

Tribulus also has been found to have blood pressure-lowering effects and may affect patients taking drugs that alter blood pressure. Tribulus may increase levels of steroid hormones. Pregnant and nursing women, along with those having hormone dependent conditions such as breast or prostate cancer, may not use Tribulus.

Dosage

Tribulus terrestris is often taken at a dose between 85 to 250 mg three times daily, with meals.

Ayurvedic Properties

Guna: Guru, snigdha
Rasa: Madhura
Veerya: Sheeta
Vipaka: Madhura
Dosha: Vat and Pit shamak, kaph nisarak

Notes

1. E. Bedir, I.A. Khan, and L.A. Walker, "Biologically active steroidal glycosides from Tribulus terrestris," *Pharmazie*, 2002, 57(7):491–493.
2. J. Conrad, D. Dinchev, I. Klaiber, et al., "A novel furostanol saponin from Tribulus terrestris of Bulgarian origin," *Fitoterapia*, 2004, 75(2):117–122.
3. E. De Combarieu, N. Fuzzati, M. Lovati, et al., "Furostanol saponins from Tribulus terrestris," *Fitoterapia*, 2003,74(6):583–591.
4. K. Gauthaman, et al., "Sexual effects of puncturevine (Tribulus terrestris) extract (protodioscin): an evaluation using a rat model," *Journal of Alternative and Complementary Medicine*, 2003, 9(2): 237–265.
5. K. Gauthaman and A.P. Ganesan, "The hormonal effects of Tribulus terrestris and its role in the management of male erectile dysfunction—an evaluation using primates, rabbit and rat," *Phytomedicine.*, Jan. 2008, 15(1–2):44–54.
6. K. Gauthaman, et al. "Aphrodisiac properties of Tribulus terrestris extract (Protodioscin) in normal and castrated rats," *Life Sciences*, 2002, 71(12):1385–1396.
7. Gauthaman K, Adaikan PG. "Effect of Tribulus terrestris on nicotinamide adenine dinucleotide phosphate-diaphorase activity and androgen receptors in rat brain," *J. Ethnopharmacol.*, Jan. 4, 2005, 96(1–2):127–132.
8. V.K Neychev and V.I. Mitev, "The aphrodisiac herb Tribulus terrestris does not influence the androgen production in young men, *Journal of Ethnopharmacology*, 2005, 101(1–3), 319–323.
9. G.A Brown, M.D. Vukovich, E.R. Martini, et al., "Effects of androstenedione-herbal supplementation on serum sex hormone concentrations in 30- to 59-year-old men," *Int J Vitam.Nutr.Res*, 2001,71(5):293–301.
10. Martino-Andrade AJ, Morais RN, Spercoski KM, Rossi SC, Vechi MF, Golin M, Lombardi NF, Greca CS, Dalsenter PR."Effects of Tribulus terrestris on endocrine sensitive organs in male and female Wistar rats," *J Ethnopharmacol.*, Sept. 23, 2009.

11. M. L Kohut, J.R. Thompson, J. Campbell, et al., "Ingestion of a dietary supplement containing dehydroepiandrosterone (DHEA) and androstenedione has minimal effect on immune function in middle-aged men," *J Am Coll Nutr.*, 2003, 22(5):363–371.

12. L.Yang, J.W. Lu, J. An, and X. Jiang, "Effect of Tribulus terrestris extract on melanocyte-stimulating hormone expression in mouse hair follicles," *Nan Fang Yi Ke Da Xue Xue Bao*, Dec. 2006, 26(12):1777–1779.

13. F.A Al-Bayati and H..F. Al-Mola, "Anti-bacterial and antifungal activities of different parts of Tribulus terrestris L. growing in Iraq," *J Zhejiang Univ Sci B.*, Feb. 2008, 9(2):154–159.

14. O.A. Phillips, K.T. Mathew, and M.A. Oriowo, "Antihypertensive and vasodilator effects of methanolic and aqueous extracts of Tribulus terrestris in rats," *J Ethnopharmacol.*, April 2006, 104(3):351–355. Epub Nov. 9, 2005.

15. A. M. Sharifi, R. Darabi, and N. Akbarloo, "Study of antihypertensive mechanism of Tribulus terrestris in 2K1C hypertensive rats: role of tissue ACE activity," *Life Sci.*, Oct. 24, 2003, 73(23):2963–2971.

16. S. Zhang, H. Li, and S.J. Yang. "Tribulosin protects rat hearts from ischemia/reperfusion injury," *Acta Pharmacol Sin.*, June 2010, 31(6):671–678.

17. M.A. Tuncer, B. Yaymaci, L. Sati, S. Cayli, G. Acar, T. Altug, and R. Demir, "Influence of Tribulus terrestris extract on lipid profile and endothelial structure in developing atherosclerotic lesions in the aorta of rabbits on a high-cholesterol diet," *Acta Histochem.*, 2009, 111(6):488–500.

18. Y. Guo, D. Z, H.J. Shi Yin, and K.J. Chen, "Effects of Tribuli saponins on ventricular remodeling after myocardial infarction in hyperlipidemic rats," *Am J Chin Med.*, 2007, 35(2):309–316.

19. J, Zhang Y.L. Zhang, J.L. Lou, H. Zheng X.M. Liu, R. Hao, and Q.F. Huang, "Protective effects of Xinnao shutong capsule on acute cerebral ischemic injury of multiple infarcts in rats," *Zhongguo Zhong Yao Za Zhi*, Dec. 2006, 31(23):1979–1982. I think this is okay

20. M. Li, W. Qu, Y. Wang, H. Wan, et al., "Hypoglycemic effect of saponin from Tribulus terrestris," *Zhong.Yao Cai.*, 2002, 25(6):420–422.

21. Yang HJ, Qu WJ, Sun B. "Experimental study of saponins from Tribulus terrestris on renal carcinoma cell line," *Zhongguo Zhong Yao Za Zhi*, Aug. 2005, 30(16):1271–1274.

22. M.R. Heidari, M. Mehrabani, A. Pardakhty, P. Khazaeli, M. J, Zahedi, M. Yakhchali, and M. Vahedian, "The analgesic effect of Tribulus terrestris extract and comparison of gastric ulcerogenicity of the extract with indomethacine in animal experiments," *Ann N Y Acad Sci.*, Jan. 2007, 1095:418–427.

23. G. Jagadeesan and A.V. Kavitha, "Recovery of phosphatase and transaminase activity of mercury intoxicated Mus musculus (Linn.) liver tissue by Tribulus terrestris (Linn.) extract," *Trop Biomed.*, June 2006, 23(1):45–51.

24. A. Amin, M. Lotfy, M. Shafiullah, and E. Adeghate, "The protective effect of Tribulus terrestris in diabetes," *Ann N Y Acad Sci.*, Nov. 2006, 1084:391–401.

Trigonella foenum-graecum

Introduction

Trigonella foenum-graecum, or Fenugreek, is a plant indigenous to the Mediterranean region, Ukraine, India, and China. Fenugreek seeds have long been prized for their medicinal properties. The ripe, dry seeds have been used for thousands of years in Arabian, Greek, Indian, and Chinese medicine. Crushed or powdered, Fenugreek seeds can be used externally and applied as poultices for boils, hives, ulcers, and eczema. Internally, Fenugreek seeds have been used to reduce blood sugar, to increase lactation, and to treat pellagra, appetite loss, indigestion, dyspepsia, bronchitis, fever, hernia, impotence, vomiting, and stomach ulcers.

Fenugreek is much used in herbal medicine in many areas of the world. The seeds are highly nourishing and are given to convalescents. Research has shown that the seeds can inhibit cancer of the liver, lower cholesterol levels, and have an anti-diabetic effect. Fenugreek seed and leaves also have anti-inflammatory, anti-tumor, carminative, demulcent, deobstruent, emollient, expectorant, febrifuge, laxative, parasiticidal, and restorative properties. Fenugreek seeds yield a strong mucilage and, therefore, are useful in treating stomach ulcers. For external use, Fenugreek seeds are ground into a powder and used as a poultice for abscesses, boils, ulcers, and burns.

In recent years, Fenugreek seed has received attention in medical research for its anti-diabetic activity. Research scientists at India's National Institute of Nutrition discovered that ground Fenugreek seeds reduced fasting blood sugar levels in patients with type 1 diabetes. These patients also showed improvement in their blood cholesterol levels.[1] Israeli scientists have confirmed this with normal and sugar-control patients, and several animal studies have documented the same. Other studies have established anti-inflammatory effects of the seeds and strong activity against abnormal growths.

Synonymous Names

Latin: Trigonella foenum-graecum
English: Fenugreek, Bird's foot, Greek hay-seed
Hindi: Methi
Sanskrit: Methika, Jyoti, Chandrika, Mantha
Other Names: Venthium, Kairavi, Vallari, Uluva, Methun

Habitat

Fenugreek is native to North Africa and the countries on the eastern shores of the Mediterranean. The herb is cultivated in India, Africa, Egypt, Morocco, and occasionally in England. It is cultivated in open areas, and its seeds are collected in autumn.

Botanical Characteristics

Fenugreek is an erect, strongly aromatic, annual herb, which grows to heights of 24 to 32 inches. The flowers are yellowish and pea-like, and the leaves are trifoliate. The seeds are brownish, about 1/8 inch long, oblong, rhomboidal, with a deep furrow dividing them into two unequal lobes. The seeds occur in 10 to 20 long, narrow, sickle-like pods.

Chemical Composition

The chemical composition of Fenugreek seed is:

- Carbohydrates, 45% to 60%: mainly mucilaginous fiber (galactomannans);
- Proteins, 20%–30% proteins high in lysine and tryptophan;
- Fixed oils (lipids): 5%–10%
- Alkaloids: Pryridine-type alkaloids mostly trigonelline, choline, gentianine, and carpaine.
- Flavonoids: Apigenin, luteolin, orientin, quercetin, vitexin, and isovitexin.
- Free amino acids: 4-hydroxyisoleucine, arginine, histidine, and lysine.
- Other constituents: Calcium, iron, saponins, glycosides yielding steroidal sapogenins on hydrolysis (diosgenin, yamogenin, tigogenin, neotigogenin); cholesterol and sitosterol, vitamins A, B1, C, and nicotinic acid; and volatile oils (n-alkanes and sesquiterpenes).

Pharmacological Activity

Anti-inflammatory and analgesic activity

The analgesic and anti-inflammatory effects of Fenugreek were examined in a partially purified fraction of the seed extract. The analgesic effects of graded doses of the fraction were evaluated in mice against acetic acid-induced writhing (chemically induced pain) and the hot-plate method (thermally induced pain). The analgesia produced by Fenugreek seed extract was compared with the standard analgesics pentazocine and diclofenac sodium. The acute anti-inflammatory activity of fraction also was evaluated in carrageenan-induced rat paw edema model and compared with diclofenac sodium. The Fenugreek extract showed highly significant, dose dependent analgesic activity against thermally as well as chemically induced pain compared to the control group. A seed extract at a dose of 40 mg/kg showed significant analgesic activity compared to diclofenac sodium and pentazocine. Fenugreek also produced marked acute anti-inflammatory activity in the rats. These results suggest that the water-soluble fraction of Fenugreek has significant analgesic and anti-inflammatory potential, as reflected by the parameters investigated.[2]

Anti-diabetic activity

The anti-diabetic activity of Fenugreek has been attributed to the presence of an unusual amino acid, 4-hydroxyisoleucine, which has been demonstrated to have insulinotropic and anti-diabetic properties in animal models. The effect of 4-hydroxyisoleucine on liver function and blood glucose was examined in two rat models of insulin resistance. One study group was fructose-fed, and the second group had streptozotocin-induced type 2 diabetes. In the fructose-fed group, levels of glucose and liver damage marker aspartate transaminase were significantly elevated compared to the controls. Alanine transaminase was elevated slightly, and all markers were restored to near control values after treatment with 4-hydroxyisoleucine at 50 mg/kg per day for 8 weeks. This prolonged exposure to 4-hydroxyisoleucine was well tolerated in the control animals and did not alter levels of glucose or liver damage markers significantly. In the diabetic rats, treatment with 4-hydroxyisoleucine did not affect glucose or liver damage markers, but did improve HDL-cholesterol. These findings indicate the usefulness of 4-hydroxyisoleucine as a well-tolerated treatment for insulin resistance, both directly as a hypoglycemic and also as a protective agent for the liver.[3] A study was conducted to determine the effects of galactomannan (GAL), a soluble dietary fiber extracted from Fenugreek seeds, on blood lipid and glucose responses in sucrose-fed rats.[4] The rats were randomly assigned to one of three high sucrose diets: 10% cellulose (control), 7.5% cellulose + 2.5% GAL, and 5% cellulose + 5% GAL. This diet was continued for 4 weeks. After 3 weeks, an oral glucose tolerance test was performed on each rat. A week later, blood samples were collected to determine the effect on blood lipids. A significant reduction in glycemic response was observed in the 5% GAL group, compared with that of the control and the 2.5% GAL groups. The plasma level of insulin also was significantly reduced in the 5% GAL-fed rats. These animals also showed a reduction in body weight gain that corresponded to the reduced food intake. All of the GAL-fed rats had significantly reduced plasma levels of triglycerides and total cholesterol in association with a reduction in epididymal adipose weight. Overall, this study demonstrated that feeding galactomannan isolated from Fenugreek seeds has the potential to alter glycemic and lipidemic status and reduce abdominal fat in normal rats. Previous studies have reported that a preparation of a dialysed aqueous extract of Fenugreek seeds stimulates the insulin signaling pathway.[5] A subsequent study was conducted to investigate the long-term effects of this preparation on blood glucose level and body weight, and the short-term effect on serum insulin and hepatic enzymes, under experimentally-induced diabetic conditions. The multiple dose effects of the extract on the glucose level and body weight was studied in alloxan-diabetic mice.[6] Intraperitoneal administration of Fenugreek seed extract for 5 consecutive days reduced hyperglycemia in the diabetic mice on Day 5 of treatment. This effect was sustained for 10 days. The extract-induced hypoglycemic effect showed no accompanying reduction in overall body weight, compared to the diabetic mice, in which body weight was reduced significantly. The single- dose effects of the extract on hepatic glucokinase and hexokinase enzymes was studied in streptozotocin-induced diabetic mice. Intraperitoneal administration of Fenugreek decreased blood glucose levels significantly in the diabetic mice, with an effect comparable to that achieved by insulin injection. This effect was associated with a significant enhancement in the liver enzyme activities on par with that of insulin. In the normal mice, Fenugreek seed extract improved the intraperitoneal glucose tolerance accompanied by a reduction in serum insulin concentration. These results are indicative of an extra-pancreatic mode of action of the extract. Fenugreek seed extract corrects metabolic alterations associated with diabetes by exhibiting insulin-like properties, and has a potential for clinical applications.

In a clinical trial, 69 patients with type 2 diabetes mellitus whose blood glucose levels were not well controlled by oral sulfonylureas hypoglycemic drug were randomly assigned to the treated group (46 cases) and the control group (23 cases), and were given Trigonella foenum-graecum or a placebo three times per day, 6 pills each time, for 12 weeks, respectively.[7] Meanwhile, the patients continued taking their original hypoglycemic drugs. The following indexes—including effects on traditional Chinese medicine (TCM) symptoms, fasting blood glucose, 2-h post-prandial blood glucose (2h PBG), glycosylated hemoglobin (HbA1c), clinical symptomatic quantitative scores , body mass index (BMI), as well as hepatic and renal functions—were observed and compared before and after treatment. The efficacy on TCM symptoms was obviously better in the treated group than that in the control group

(P<0.01), and there were statistically remarkable decreases in aspects of fasting blood glucose, 2h post-prandial blood glucose, HbA1c, and clinical symptomatic quantitative scores in the treated group compared to those in the control group (P<0.05 or P<0.01). No significant difference was found in BMI, hepatic, and renal functions between the two groups (P>0.05). Combined therapy of Trigonella foenum-graecum with sulfonylureas hypoglycemic drug could lower the blood glucose level and ameliorate clinical symptoms in the treatment of type 2 diabetes mellitus and the therapy was relatively safe. HOMA model was used in mild to moderate type 2 diabetes mellitus in a double-blind placebo-controlled study.[8] Twenty five newly diagnosed patients with type 2 diabetes (fasting glucose < 200 mg/dl) were randomly divided into two groups. Group I (n=12) received 1 gram/day hydroalcoholic extract of fenugreek seeds, and Group 2 (n=13) received the usual care (dietary control, exercise) and placebo capsules for 2 months. At baseline, both groups were similar in anthropometric and clinical variables. The oral glucose tolerance test, lipid levels, fasting C-peptide, glycosylated hemoglobin, and HOMA-model insulin resistance also were similar at baseline. In Group 1, as compared to Group 2 at the end of 2 months, fasting blood glucose (148.3 +/- 44.1 to 119.9 +/- 25 versus 137.5 +/- 41.1 to 113.0 +/- 36.0) and 2-hour post-glucose blood glucose (210.6 +/- 79.0 to 181.1 +/- 69 versus 219.9 +/- 41.0 to 241.6 +/- 43) were not different. But the area under curve of blood glucose (2375 +/- 574 versus 27597 +/- 274) and insulin (2492 +/- 2536 versus 5631 +/- 2428) was significantly lower (p < 0.001). The HOMA model derived insulin resistance showed a decrease in percent beta-cell secretion in Group 1 compared to Group 2 (86.3 +/- 32 vs. 70.1 +/- 52) and an increase in percent insulin sensitivity (112.9 +/- 67 vs 92.2 +/- 57) (p < 0.05). Serum triglycerides decreased, and HDL cholesterol increased significantly in group 1 as compared to group 2 (p < 0.05). Adjunct use of Fenugreek seeds improved glycemic control and decreases insulin resistance in mild type-2 diabetic patients. There is also a favorable effect on hypertriglyceridemia.

Anti-obesity activity

One study investigated the effects of repeated administration of a Fenugreek seed extract on the eating behavior of overweight subjects.[9] Thirty-nine healthy overweight male volunteers completed a 6-week double-blind randomized placebo-controlled parallel trial of a fixed dose of a Fenugreek seed extract. The main endpoints were energy intake (dietary records and meal test), weight, fasting and post-absorptive glucose and insulin, appetite/satiety scores, and oxidative parameters. Daily fat consumption, expressed as the ratio of fat reported energy intake/total energy expenditure (fat-REI/TEE), was significantly decreased in the overweight subjects who were administered the Fenugreek seed extract compared to those receiving the placebo (fat-REI/TEE 0.26 +/- 0.02 vs. 0.30 +/- 0.01, respectively; P = 0.032). There was a significant decrease in the insulin-to-glucose ratio in the subjects treated with Fenugreek seed extract relative to the placebo group (0.89 +/- 0.09 versus. 1.06 +/- 0.10 mUI mmol(-1), respectively; P = 0.044). No significant effect was observed on weight, appetite/satiety scores, or oxidative parameters. The repeated administration of a Fenugreek seed extract slightly but significantly decreased dietary fat consumption in healthy overweight subjects in this short-term study.

Cholesterol and other lipid metabolism

Fenugreek seed was evaluated for this potential on the experimental induction of cholesterol gall stones in laboratory mice.[10] Cholesterol gall stones were induced by maintaining the mice on a high cholesterol diet (0.5% cholesterol) for 10 weeks. Fenugreek seed powder was included at 5%, 10%, and 15% in this diet. The dietary Fenugreek significantly lowered the incidence of cholesterol gall stones in these mice; the incidence was 63%, 40%, and 10% in the 5%, 10%, and 15% Fenugreek groups, respectively, compared to 100% control group. The anti-lithogenic influence of fenugreek is attributable to its hypocholesterolemic effect. Serum cholesterol level was decreased by 26%–31% by the dietary Fenugreek, and hepatic cholesterol was lowered by 47%–64% in these high cholesterol-fed animals. As a result of dietary Fenugreek, biliary cholesterol was 8.73–11.2 mmol/L compared to 33.6 mmol/L in the high-cholesterol feeding without Fenugreek. The cholesterol saturation index in the bile was reduced to 0.77–0.99 in the Fenugreek treatments compared to 2.57 in the high-cholesterol group.

Anti-cancer activity

In recent years, various dietary components that can potentially be used for the prevention and treatment of cancer have been identified. Researchers tried to demonstrate that extract from the seeds of the plant Trigonella foenum graecum are cytotoxic in-vitro to a panel of cancer cells but not normal cells.[11] Treatment with 10–15 ug/mL of Trigonella foenum-graecum for 72 hours was growth inhibitory to breast, pancreatic, and prostate cancer cell lines (PCa). When tested at higher doses (15–20 ug/mL), continued to be growth inhibitory to PCa cell lines but not to either primary prostate or hTert-immortalized prostate cells. At least part of the growth inhibition is a result of induction of cell death, as seen by incorporation of Ethidium Bromide III into the cancer cells exposed to Trigonella foenum-graecum. Molecular changes induced in PCa cells are: in DU-145 cells, downregulation of mutant p53, and in PC-3 cells, upregulation of p21 and inhibition of TGF beta induced phosphorylation of Akt. The surprising finding of the studies is that death of cancer cells occurs despite growth stimulatory pathways being simultaneously upregulated (phosphorylated) by Trigonella foenum-graecum.

Safety Profile

Fenugreek traditionally has been considered safe and well-tolerated. There are rare reports of dizziness, diarrhea, gas, facial swelling, numbness, difficulty breathing (after inhalation from occupational exposure), fainting, increased risk of bleeding, reduction of blood sugars, reduction of serum potassium levels, and alteration of thyroid hormone levels.

Dr. Sodhi's Experience

I have used Fenugreek seeds with success in hypertension, obesity, perimenopausal, menopausal, and Type 1 and type 2 diabetes. Patients are asked to soak one tablespoon of Fenugreek seeds at night so they can chew the seeds in the morning. The seeds are slightly bitter, and some people have not developed a taste for this. But the seeds also may be placed in smoothies for better palatability. Fenugreek is a precursor for all the hormones. Traditionally, it has been used as a uterine cleanser after delivery of babies. Fenugreek seeds also have galactogogue action. Females who use Fenugreek seeds for 40 days after delivery reduce their pregnancy fat, reduce their waist line, and promote milk production at the same time. In Type 1 and type 2 diabetes, Fenugreek can be added with each meal for better blood sugar control.

Dosage

   Fluid extract: 1:1 (g/ml): 6 ml.
   Tincture: 1:5 (g/ml): 30 ml.
   Native extract: 3-4:1 (w/w): 1.5-2 g.

Ayurvedic Properties

Guna: Laghu and snighdha
Rasa: Madhura, katu
Virya: Ushna
Vipaka: Katu

Notes

1. J. Carper, *Food—Your Miracle Medicine: How Food Can Prevent and Cure Over 100 Symptoms and Problems* (New York:? HarperCollins, 1994), p. 423. See this http://books.google.com/books/about/Food_your_miracle_medicine.html?id=QVQtAQAAMAAJ

2. S. Vyas, R.P., R.P. Agrawal, P. Solanki, and P. Trivedi, "Analgesic and anti-inflammatory activities of Trigonella foenum-graecum (seed)," *Acta Pol Pharm.*, July-Aug. 2008, 65(4):473–6.

3. M.R. Haeri, M. Izaddoost, M.R. Ardekani M.R. Nobar, and K.N. White, "The effect of fenugreeek 4-hydroxyisoleucine on liver function biomarkers and glucose in diabetic and fructose-fed rats," Phytother Res., Aug. 4, 2008.

4. A. Srichamroen, C.J. Field, A.B. Thomson, and T.K. Basu, "The modifying effects of galactomannan from Canadian-grown fenugreek (Trigonella foenum-graecum L.) on the glycemic and lipidemic status in rats," *J Clin Biochem Nutr.*, Nov. 2008, 43(3):167–174. Epub Oct. 31, 2008.

5. M.V.Vijayakumar and M.K. Bhat, "Hypoglycemic effect of a novel dialysed feungreek seeds extract is sustainable and is mediated, in part, by the activation of hepatic enzymes," *Phytother Res.*, April 2008, 22(4):500–505.

6. See Note 5.

7. F.R. Lu, Y. Qin, L. Gao, H. Li, and Y. Dai, "Clinical observation on Trigonella foenum-graecum L. total saponins in combination with sulfonylureas in the treatment of type 2 diabetes mellitus," *Chinese Journal of Integrative Medicine*, March 14, 2008, 14(1):56–60.

8. A. Gupta, R. Gupta, and B. Lal, "Effects of Trigonella foenum-graecum seeds on glycemic control and insulin resistance in type 2 DM; a double blind placebo controlled study," *Journal of the Association of Physicians of India*, Nov. 2001, 49:1057–1061.

9. H. Chevassus, J.B. Gaillard, A. Farret, F. Costa, I. Gabillaud, E. Mas, A.M. Dupuy, F. Michel, C. Cantié, E. Renard, F. Galtier, and P. Petit, "A fenugreek seed extract selectively reduces spontaneous fat intake in overweight subjects," *Eur J Clin Pharmacol.*, May 2010, 66(5):449–455.

10. R.L Reddy and K. Srinivasan, "Fenugreek seeds reduce atherogenic diet-induced cholesterol gallstone formation in experimental mice," *Can J Physiol Pharmacol.*, Nov. 2009, 87(11):933–943.

11. S. Shabbeer, M. Sobolewski, R.K. Anchoori, S. Kachhap, M. Hidalgo, A. Jimeno, N. Davidson, M.A. Carducci, and S.R. Khan, "Fenugreek: A naturally occurring edible spice as an anticancer agent," *Cancer Biol Ther.*, Feb. 2009, 8(3):272–278.

Withania Somnifera

Introduction

Withania somnifera, or Ashwagandha, is a shrubby plant cultivated in India, parts of East Asia, and Africa that offers tremendous potential as an energizing medicinal herb. Ayurvedic practitioners have used the roots of this plant for centuries with success as a tonic to increase vitality and longevity, as well as to treat health conditions as diverse as tumors and arthritis. Laboratory studies have begun to confirm what Ayurvedic practitioners have known for years—that Withania somnifera deserves attention as an herbal therapy to ease or even eliminate many of today's common health problems.

Sometimes referred to as "Indian ginseng" because of its stimulating effects, Ashwagandha is used to calm the mind, relieve weakness and nervous exhaustion, build sexual energy, and promote healthy sleep. In Ayurvedic practice, the herb is considered to be a rasayana, which means that it acts as a tonic for vitality and longevity. It also is classified as an adaptogen,[1] meaning that it assists the body's immune and other defense mechanisms in coping with stress factors.

Traditionally, Ashwagandha has been used as an aphrodisiac, a liver tonic, an anti-inflammatory agent, an astringent, and to treat bronchitis, asthma, ulcers, emaciation, insomnia, and senile dementia. Clinical trials and animal research support the use of Ashwagandha for anxiety, cognitive and neurological disorders, inflammation, and Parkinson's disease.

Less well-established but potentially exciting properties of Withania somnifera are its anti-inflammatory and anti-carcinogenic effects, and its ability to stabilize mood and brain function. The chemopreventive properties of Ashwagandha make it a potentially useful adjunct for patients undergoing radiation and chemotherapy. Ashwagandha also is used therapeutically for patients with nervous exhaustion, insomnia, and debility as a result of stress, and as an immune stimulant in patients with low white blood cell counts.

Encouraging research indicates that Ashwagandha may provide significant anti-inflammatory effects that could ease the symptoms of many rheumatic diseases such as osteoarthritis. As Western medical practitioners become more receptive to the possible contributions of non-Western medical traditions, Ashwagandha may begin to be used as part of multi-layered medical therapies to replace or lower the dosage of modern drugs that have problematic side-effects.

Synonymous Names

In addition to its Indian name Ashwagandha, Withania somnifera is also known as winter cherry, Indian ginseng, Ajagandha, Kanaje

Hindi: Asgandh
Sanskrit: Ashwagandha

It belongs to the Solanaceae, or nightshade, family.

Habitat

Withania somnifera grows natively in India and parts of Asia, Africa, and North America. It is grown fairly easily in sunny locations with well-drained soil. Although by nature it is a perennial, Ashwagandha may be grown as an annual and will blossom and bear fruit in its first year when grown from seed.

Botanical Characteristics

Withania somnifera is an erect shrub that grows to a height of about 2 feet. Its stem and branches are covered with tiny star-shaped hairs. The root, the part that is most valuable for medicinal uses, is fairly long and tuberous, with two or three lateral roots slightly smaller in size. The roots are grayish yellow with longitudinal wrinkles and a soft center mass with scattered pores. They are characterized by a strong odor—hence the Indian name for the plant, which translates as "horse's smell."

The plant flowers throughout the year. Its leaves are simple and ovate in shape, measuring about 10 centimeters long. The leaves are alternate in arrangement. The plant's flowers resemble others of the nightshade family. They are small, greenish-yellow blooms borne in short axillary clusters. The fruit is a smooth, red enclosed berry, about 6 millimeters in diameter. Ashwagandha's shoots and seeds are used in India as a thickener for food and milk.

Chemical Composition

Laboratory analysis has revealed more than 35 chemical constituents contained in the roots of Withania somnifera.[2] The biologically active chemical constituents are alkaloids (isopellertierine, anferine), steroidal lactones (withanolides, withaferins), saponins containing an additional acyl group (sitoindoside VII and VIII), and withanoloides with a glucose at carbon 27 (sitonidoside XI and X). Withania somnifera is also rich in iron.

The roots of Withania somnifera consist primarily of compounds known as withanolides, which are believed to account for its extraordinary medicinal properties. Withanolides are steroidal and bear a resemblance, both in action and appearance, to the active constituents of Asian ginseng (Panax ginseng) known as ginsenosides.[3] Ashwagandha's withanolides have been researched in a variety of animal studies examining their effect on numerous conditions, including immune function and even cancer.

Chemical analysis of Ashwagandha shows its main constituents to be alkaloids and steroidal lactones. Among the various alkaloids, withanine is the main constituent. The other alkaloids are somniferine, somnine, somniferinine, withananine, pseudo-withanine, tropine, pseudo-tropine, 3-a-gloyloxytropane, choline, cuscohygrine, isopellertierine, anaferine, and anahydrine. Two acyl steryl glucosides— sitoindoside VII and sitoindoside VIII—have been isolated from the root. The leaves contain steroidal lactones, commonly called withanolides. The withanolides have a C28 steroidal nucleus with a C9 side chain with a six-membered lactone ring.[4]

An overview presented in the journal *Molecules* gives an overview of the chemical structures of triterpenoid components and their biological activity, focusing on two novel activities: (1) tumor inhibition and antiangiogenic properties of withaferin A, and (2) the effects of withanolide A on Alzheimer's disease.[5]

Further chemical analysis has shown the presence of the following: anaferine (alkaloid), anahygrine (alkaloid), beta-sisterol, chlorogenic acid (in leaf only), cysteine (in fruit), cuscohygrine (alkaloid), iron, pseudotropine (alkaloid), scopoletin, somniferinine (alkaloid), somniferiene (alkaloid), tropanol (alkaloid), withanine (alkaloid), withananine (alkaloid) and withanolides A-Y (steroidal lactones).[6,7]

Pharmacological Activity

Centuries of Ayurvedic medical experience using Withania somnifera have revealed it to have pharmacological value as an adaptogen, antibiotic, abortifacient, aphrodisiac, astringent, anti-inflammatory, deobstruent, diuretic, narcotic, sedative, and tonic. Ashwagandha has been found to:

- provide potent anti-oxidant protection[8]
- stimulate the activation of immune system cells, such as lymphocytes and phagocytes[9,10]
- counteract the effects of stress and generally promote wellness.[11]

Anti-stress activity

A study conducted by the Institute of Basic Medical Sciences at Calcutta University examined the effects of Ashwagandha on chronic stress in rodents. For a period of 21 days, the animals received a mild electric shock to their feet. The resulting stress on the animals produced hyperglycemia, glucose intolerance, an increase in plasma corticosterone levels, gastric ulcerations, male sexual dysfunction, cognitive deficits, immunosuppression, and mental depression.[12]

Researchers using Withania somnifera discovered that the animals given the herb an hour before the footshock experienced a significantly reduced level of stress. This research confirms the theory that Ashwagandha has a significant anti-stress adaptogenic effect.[13]

Research conducted at the Department of Pharmacology, University of Texas Health Science Center indicated that extracts of Ashwagandha produce GABA-like activity, which may account for the herb's anti-anxiety effects.[14] GABA (Gamma Amino-Butyric Acid) is an inhibitory neurotransmitter in the brain. Its function is to decrease neuron activity and inhibit nerve cells from over-firing. This action produces a calming effect. Excessive neuronal activity can lead to restlessness and insomnia, but GABA inhibits the number of nerve cells that fire in the brain and helps to induce sleep, uplift mood, and reduce anxiety.

Ashwagandha traditionally has been used to stabilize mood in patients with behavioral disturbances. Research has revealed that the herb produces an anti-depressant and anti-anxiety effect in rodents that is comparable to the anti-depressant drug imipramine and the anti-anxiety drug Lorazepam (Ativan).[15] In fact, Ashwagandha is one of the most widespread tranquillizers used in India, where it holds a position of importance similar to ginseng in China. Ashwagandha acts mainly on the reproductive and nervous systems, having a rejuvenative effect on the body, and is used to improve vitality and aid recovery after chronic illness.[16]

In one study, employees with moderate to severe anxiety of longer than 6 weeks' duration were randomized based on age and gender to receive naturopathic care (n = 41) or standardized psychotherapy intervention (n = 40) over a period of 12 weeks.[17] Blinding of investigators and participants during randomization and allocation was maintained. Participants in the naturopathic care group received dietary counseling, deep breathing relaxation techniques, a standard multi-vitamin, and the herbal medicine Ashwagandha (Withania somnifera) (300 mg b.i.d. standardized to 1.5% with anolides, prepared from root). The other group received psychotherapy along with matched deep-breathing relaxation techniques and a placebo. The primary outcome measure was the Beck Anxiety Inventory (BAI). Secondary outcome measures included the Short Form 36 (SF-36), Fatigue Symptom Inventory (FSI), and Measure Yourself Medical Outcomes Profile (MY-MOP) to measure anxiety, mental health, and quality of life, respectively. The participants were blinded to the placebo-controlled intervention, and the 75 participants (93%) were followed for 8 or more weeks in the trial. The BAI scores decreased by 56.5% (p<0.0001) in the naturopathic care group and 30.5% (p<0.0001) in the psychotherapy group. Naturopathic care and Ashwgandha group significantly improved mental health, concentration, fatigue, social functioning, vitality, and overall quality of life and serious adverse reactions were observed in either group.

In a rat model of chronic stress syndrome, Withania somnifera and Panax ginseng extracts were compared and contrasted for their abilities to relieve some of the adverse effects of chronic stress. The research results showed that both Ashwagandha and Panax ginseng decreased the frequency and severity of stress-induced ulcers, reversed stress-induced inhibition of male sexual behavior, and inhibited the effects of chronic stress on retention of learned tasks. Both botanicals also reversed stress-induced immunosuppression, but only the Withania extract increased peritoneal macrophage activity. Withania somnifera, however, has an advantage over Panax ginseng in that the former does not appear to result in "ginseng-abuse syndrome," a condition characterized by high blood pressure, water retention, muscle tension, and insomnia.[18]

Anti-oxidant activity

Researchers from Banaras Hindu University in Varanasi, India, have discovered that some of the chemicals found in Withania somnifera are powerful anti-oxidants. Studies conducted on rats' brains showed the herb produced an increase in the levels of three natural anti-oxidants — superoxide dismutase, catalase, and glutathione peroxidase. These findings are consistent with the therapeutic use of Withania somnifera as an Ayurvedic rasayana. The anti-oxidant effect of active principles of Withania somnifera root may explain the reported anti-stress, cognition facilitating, anti-inflammatory and anti-aging effects produced by them in experimental animals, and in clinical situations. Propoxur (2-isopropoxyphenyl N-methylcarbamate) is widely used as an acaricide in agriculture and public health programs. Sub-chronic exposure to propoxur can cause oxidative stress, immuno-suppression, and exhibit inhibitory effect on cholinesterase activity. Oral administration of propoxur (10 mg/kg b.wt.) in rats resulted in a significant reduction of brain and blood acetylcholinesterase activity. Oral treatment of Withania somnifera exerts a protective effect and attenuates acetylcholinesterase inhibition and cognitive impairment caused by sub-chronic exposure to propoxur.[19]

Anti-carcinogenic activity

Ashwagandha is reported to have anti-carcinogenic effects. Research on animal cell cultures has shown that the herb decreases the levels of the nuclear factor kappaB, suppresses the intercellular tumor necrosis factor, and potentiates apoptotic signaling in cancerous cell lines.[20]

One of the most exciting of the possible uses of Ashwagandha is its capacity to fight cancers by reducing the size of tumors.[21,22] Ashwagandha was evaluated for its anti-tumor effect in urethane induced lung tumors in adult male mice.[23] Of the mice that were fed urethane, 100% developed cancer. Of the mice that were fed Ashwagandha along with the carcinogen, only 25% developed cancer. The mice that were fed Ashwagandha and didn't develop cancer had normal, healthy-looking lungs. Withania somnifera showed protective effects on gentamicin-induced nephrotoxicity in male Wistar rats. Gentamycin-induced nephrotoxicity was ameliorated by Withania somnifera, as evidenced by biochemical parameters. Urea, creatinine, uric acid, non-protein nitrogen, urinary protein, N-acetyl-beta-D-glucosaminidase, thiobarbituric acid reactive substance, and hydroperoxides were decreased markedly, with an increase in glutathione peroxidase, superoxide dismutase, catalase, and reduced glutathione in liver and kidney tissues. Histopathologically, liver and kidney cellular integrity was protected by Withania somnifera.

Notch signaling pathways play a crucial role in the development of colon cancer. Withaferin-A, a bioactive compound derived from Withania somnifera, inhibits Notch-1 signaling and down regulates pro-survival pathways, such as Akt/NF-kappaB/Bcl-2, in thHCT-116, SW-480, and SW-620, in colon cancer cell lines. Withaferin-A downregulated the expression of mammalian target of the rapamycin-signaling components, pS6K and p4E-BP1, and activated c-Jun-NH(2)-kinase-mediated apoptosis in colon cancer cells. Withferin A showed promising targeted chemotherapy as well as chemoprevention in colon cancer.[24]

In another study, withaferin A inhibited growth of human breast cancer cells in culture and in-vivo in association with apoptosis induction and largely inhibited cell migration and invasion of breast cancer cells even after IL-6-induced activation of STAT3, which is a therapeutic advantage of withaferin A.[25] Withaferin A treatment caused G2 and mitotic arrest in human breast cancer cells, both in estrogen-independent MDA-MB-231 and estrogen responsive MCF-7 cell lines. This may be one of the antiproliferative mechanisms of withferin-A against human breast cancer cells.[26]

Heat-shock proteins are increased in many solid tumors and hematological malignancies. Intracellular heat shock proteins are highly expressed in cancerous cells and are essential to the survival of these cell types. Heat shock protein 90 (Hsp90) is especially responsible for the transformation of cells to cancerous forms.[27] Targeting Hsp90 with inhibitors would degrade these oncogenic proteins and serve as useful anticancer agents. Withaferin A exhibited potent antiproliferative activity against pancreatic cancer cell lines Panc-1, MiaPaCa2 and BxPc3 by inhibiting Hsp90 by 30-58% through ATP-independent mechanism[28]

Glioma is a type of tumor that starts in the brain or spine arising from glial cells. Glial cells serve four main functions: (1) to surround neurons and hold them in place, (2) to supply nutrients and oxygen to neurons, (3) to insulate one neuron from another, and (4) to destroy pathogens and remove dead neurons.

Alcoholic extract of Ashwagandha leaves containing Withaferin A, Withanone, and Withanolide A inhibited the proliferation of glioma cell lines in a dose-dependent manner and changed their morphology toward the astrocytic type, which has a role in the repair and scarring process of the brain and spinal cord.[29]

Expression of hsp70 family protein (mortalin), glial cell differentiation marker (glial fibrillary acidic protein), and neural cell adhesion molecule showed changes subsequent to the treatment with water extract of Ashwagandha leaves extract. This supports its anti-proliferative, differentiation-inducing and anti-metastasis for glioma.[30]

Withaferin-A (WA), also has shown radiosensitizing properties. C57BL mice bearing B16F1 tumors were treated with fractionated radiotherapy (RT, 2 Gy x 5 days/week, 4 weeks), withaferin-A (15 mg/kg, i.p., 5 days/week, 3 weeks), local hyperthermia (HT, 43ºC once a week, 3 weeks) and their combinations. Another group was given acute radiotherapy (40 Gy), withaferin A (40 mg/kg), hyperthermia treatment (43º C, 30 min), and their combinations. Acute radiotherapy and hyperthermia treatment produced 50% partial response, which increased to 62.5% with a combination of withaferin-A. In the fractionated regimen, a combination of radiotherapy, hyperthermia, and withaferin-A resulted in 100% partial response.[31]

A combination of paclitaxel with Withania somnifera effectively treated benzo(a)pyrene-induced lung cancer in mice by offering protection from reactive oxygen species damage, suppressing cell proliferation and enhancing the action of chemotherapy.[32]

Azoxymethane-induced colon cancer was normalized by Withania somnifera in experimental mice.[33] Standardized Withania somnifera induced apoptosis by activating both intrinsic and extrinsic signaling pathways by activation of caspase-9, caspase 8, caspase-3, and PARP cleavage. Poly (ADP-ribose) polymerase (PARP) is a family of proteins involved in a number of cellular processes involving mainly DNA repair and programmed cell death. Withania inhibited the expression of pStat-3 with selective stimulation of Th1 immunity, as evidenced by enhanced secretion of IFN-gamma and IL-2. It also enhanced the proliferation of CD4(+)/CD8(+), NK cells along with an increased expression of CD40/CD40L/CD80 and T cell activation.[34] Withaferin A showed similar results in human leukemia U937 cells.[35]

Withaferin A has shown strong growth-inhibitory effect on several human leukemic cell lines and on primary cells from patients with lymphoblastic and myeloid leukemia in a dose-dependent manner, showing no toxicity on normal human lymphocytes and primitive hematopoietic progenitor cells. Withferin-A induced apoptosis was mediated by an increase in phosphorylated p38MAPK expression, which further activated downstream signaling by phosphorylating ATF-2 and HSP27 in leukemic cells. The RNA interference of p38MAPK protected normal cells from Withferin-A induced apoptosis.[36] P38 mitogen-activated protein kinases (p38MAPK) constitute a class of mitogen-activated protein kinases that are responsive to stress stimuli, such as cytokines, ultraviolet irradiation, heat shock, and osmotic shock, and are involved in cell differentiation and apoptosis.

Similarly, in prostate cancer cells Withania somnifera treatment significantly downregulated the gene and protein expression of pro-inflammatory cytokines IL-6, IL-1beta, chemokine IL-8, Hsp70 and STAT-2, and a reciprocal upregulation was observed in gene and protein expression of p38 MAPK, PI3K, caspase 6, Cyclin D, and c-myc. Also, the treatment significantly modulated the JAK-STAT pathway that regulates both the apoptosis process and MAP kinase signaling. These studies outline several functionally important classes of genes, which are associated with immune response, signal transduction, cell signaling, transcriptional regulation, apoptosis, and cell cycle regulation, providing an effective chemopreventive agent in prostate cancer progression.[37]

Withania somnifera reduces tumor cell proliferation while increasing overall animal survival time. Further, it has been shown to enhance the effectiveness of radiation therapy while potentially mitigating undesirable side-effects. Withania somnifera also reduces the side-effects of chemotherapeutic agents cyclophosphamide and paclitaxel without interfering with the tumor-reducing actions of the drugs. These effects have been demonstrated in-vitro on human cancer cell lines, and in-vivo on animal subjects. Given its broad spectrum of cytotoxic and tumor-sensitizing actions, Withania somnifera presents itself as a novel complementary therapy for integrative oncology care.[38]

Anti-inflammatory activity

Research has explored the capacity of Ashwagandha to ease the symptoms of arthritis and other inflammatory conditions These studies have proven that the herb acts as an effective anti-inflammatory agent. Its naturally occurring steroidal content has shown more potent anti-inflammatory action than hydrocortisone.[39] Rats given powdered root of Withania somnifera orally one hour before being given injections of an inflammatory agent over a 3-day period showed that Withania produced anti-inflammatory responses comparable to that of hydrocortisone sodium succinate.[40]

Chronic inflammatory diseases results from dysregulation of pro-inflammatory cytokines (tumor necrosis factor and interleukin-1beta) and pro-inflammatory enzymes that mediate the production of prostaglandins (cyclooxygenase-2) and leukotrienes (e.g. lipooxygenase), together with the expression of adhesion molecules and matrix metalloproteinases, and hyperproliferation of synovial fibroblasts. Nuclear factor-kappaB is a regulator of all these factors. Withanoloids have been shown to suppress activation of NF-kappaB.[41,42]

Pure root powder of Withania somnifera showed potent inhibition of inflammation in a Pristane induced model of lupus. It showed a potent inhibitory effect on proteinuria, nephritis, and other inflammatory markers.[43]

In an inflammatory bowel disease rat model, gel of Withania somnifera extract applied rectally normalized the intestinal mucosa back to healthy normal tissue.[44]

The effectiveness of Ashwagandha in a variety of rheumatologic conditions may result in part from its anti-inflammatory properties.

Anti-aging activity

Ashwagandha was tested for its anti-aging properties in a double-blind clinical trial. A group of 101 healthy males, 50–59 years old, was given the herb at a dosage of 3 grams daily for one year. The subjects experienced significant improvement in hemoglobin, red blood cell count, hair melanin, and seated stature. Their serum cholesterol decreased, and nail calcium was preserved. Of the research subjects, 70% reported improvement in sexual performance and seated posture.[45]

Withanone, a component of Withania somnifera, has both anti-cancer and anti-aging activities and points to the molecular link between aging and cancer.[46]

In a double-blind, randomized, placebo-controlled trial, the effects of Withania somnifera root and leaf extract were evaluated for treating stress related health conditions. The participants were randomly assigned to Withania somnifera root and leaf extract (125 mg QD, 125 mg BID, or 250 mg BID) or placebo groups. Stress levels were assessed at Days 0, 30, and 60, using a modified Hamilton anxiety (mHAM-A) scale. Biochemical and clinical variables were measured at days 0 and 60. Of the 130 subjects enrolled, 98 completed the study. Between days 0 and 60, the Withania somnifera extract 125 mg QD group decreased significantly more than the placebo for the mean Hamilton anxiety score, serum cortisol, serum C-reactive protein, pulse rate, and blood pressure, and increased significantly for mean serum DHEAS and hemoglobin. Other Withania somnifera extract treatment groups had greater dose-dependent responses in these parameters and had significantly greater responses compared to the placebo in mean fasting blood glucose, serum lipid profiles, and cardiac risk ratios.[47]

Cardioprotective activity

Ashwagandha has been evaluated in clinical studies with human subjects for its diuretic, hypoglycemic, and hypocholesterolemic effects.[48] Six type 2 diabetes mellitus subjects and six mildly hypercholesterolemic subjects were treated with a powder extract of the herb for 30 days. A decrease in blood glucose comparable to that which would be caused by administration of a hypoglycemic drug was observed. Significant increases in urine sodium, urine volume, and decreases in serum cholesterol, triglycerides, and low-density lipoproteins also were seen.

Pre-treatment of rats with Withania reduced myocardial damage, as evidenced by histopathologic evaluation. The anti-oxidant and anti-apoptotic properties may be a contributing factor in cardioprotection.[49]

A combination of niacin-bound chromium (0.45%), standardized extract of Withania somnifera extracts (10.71%), caffeine (22.76%), D-ribose (10.71%), and selected amino acids such as phenylalanine, taurine, and glutamine (55.37%) have been shown to have cardioprotective properties. The hearts of male and female rat were subjected to 30 minutes of global ischemia followed by 2 hours of reperfusion at 30 and 90 days of treatment. Cardiovascular functions, including heart rate, coronary flow, aortic flow, left ventricular developed pressure, and infarct size, were monitored. The levels of myocardial adenosine triphosphate (ATP), creatine phosphate (CP), and phospho-adenosine monophosphate kinase (p-AMPK) were analyzed at the end of 30 and 90 days of treatment. Significant improvement was observed in all parameters in the treatment groups compared to the controls.[50]

Thyroid-stimulating activity

Animal studies have shown that Ashwagandha may have an effect on thyroid activity. An aqueous extract of dried Withania root was given to mice daily for 20 days. Significant increases in serum T4 were observed, indicating that the plant has a stimulating effect at the glandular level. Withania somnifera also may stimulate thyroid activity indirectly via its effect on cellular anti-oxidant systems. Ashwagandha may be a useful botanical in treating hypothyroidism.[51,52]

Metformin is a frequently used medication for type 2 diabetes, but it causes hypothyroidism, and steroids make diabetes worse. However, oral administration with either Withania somnifera (1.4 g/kg) or Bauhinia purpurea (2.5 mg/kg) extract along with dexamethasone and metformin elevated the concentrations of circulating T3 and T4 back to normal in diabetic model animals. The plant extracts also corrected the ratio and concentration of lipids.[53]

Anti-diabetic activity

The effect of an aqueous extract of Withania somnifera on insulin sensitivity in non-insulin-dependent diabetes mellitus (NIDDM) rats was studied. NIDDM was induced by a single intraperitoneal injection of streptozotocin (100 mg/kg) to 2-day-old rat pups. Extract of Withania somnifera (200 and 400 mg/kg) was administered orally once a day for 5 weeks after the animals were confirmed as diabetic 75 days after a streptozotocin injection. Significant increases in blood glucose, glycosylated haemoglobin (HbA(1)c), and serum insulin levels were observed in the NIDDM control rats. Treatment with Withania reduced the elevated levels of blood glucose, HbA(1)c, and insulin in the NIDDM rats. The glucose tolerance test showed improvement in the rats treated with Withania. The treatment significantly improved the insulin sensitivity index.[54]

Immunomodulatory activity

A series of animal studies demonstrated Ashwagandha to have profound effects on the healthy production of white blood cells. It is an effective immunoregulator and chemoprotective agent.[55,56] Ashwagandha also inhibited delayed-type hypersensitivity reactions and enhanced phagocytic activity of macrophages compared to a control group.

Nitric oxide has been determined to have a significant effect on macrophage cytotoxicity against microorganisms and tumor cells. Iuvone et al. demonstrated that Withania somnifera increased nitric oxide production in mouse macrophages in a concentration-dependent manner. This effect was attributed to increased production of inducible nitric oxide synthase, an enzyme generated in response to inflammatory mediators and known to inhibit the growth of many pathogens.[57,58,59]

Tea prepared from Withania somnifera, Glycyrrhiza glabra, Zingiber officinale, Ocimum sanctum, and Elettaria cardamomum was studied for immunoenhancing natural killer (NK) cell activity after consumption of fortified tea compared with regular tea in two independent double-blind intervention studies. Both studies were conducted in India with healthy volunteers (age > or = 55 years) selected for a relatively low baseline NK cell activity and a history of recurrent coughs and colds. Natural tea significantly improved the NK cell activity of the volunteers compared to a population consuming regular tea. These results were validated in an independent crossover study with 110 volunteers.[60]

A study was done to investigate the immunologic effects of Ashwagandha (Withania somnifera) on four types of immune cells in a human sample to determine the immunologic mechanism. Five participants consumed 6 mL of an Ashwagandha root extract twice daily for 96 hours. Ashwagandha was administered with anupana (whole milk). Peripheral blood samples were collected at 0, 24, and 96 hours and compared for differences in cell surface expression of CD4, CD8, CD19, CD56, and CD69 receptors by flow cytometry. Significant increases were observed in the expression of CD4 on CD3+ T cells after 96 hours. CD56+ NK cells also were activated after 96 hours, as evidenced by expression of the CD69 receptor. At 96 hours of use, mean values of receptor expression for all measured receptor types were increased over the baseline, indicating that a major change in immune cell activation occurred across the sample.[61]

Research also has shown Ashwagandha to have stimulatory effects, both in-vitro and in-vivo, on the generation of cytotoxic T lymphocytes, and a demonstrated potential to reduce tumor growth.[62] The chemopreventive effect was demonstrated in a study of Ashwagandha root extract on induced skin cancer in Swiss albino mice given Ashwagandha before and during exposure to the skin cancer-causing agent (7,12-dimethylbenz[a]anthracene).[63] A significant decrease in incidence and average number of skin lesions was demonstrated compared to the control group. In addition, levels of reduced glutathione, superoxide dismutase, catalase, and glutathione peroxidase in the exposed tissue returned to near normal values following administration of the extract. The chemopreventive activity is thought to be due in part to the anti-oxidant and free radical scavenging activity of the extract.

Withanolide A improved chronic stress-induced alterations on a T lymphocyte subset distribution in experimental Swiss albino mice.[64] Stress disturbs the homeostatic state and brings about behavioral, endocrine, and immunological changes. The chronic suppression induced by stress depresses immune functioning and increases susceptibility to diseases. Oral administration of Withanolide caused significant recovery of the stress-induced depleted T cell population, causing an increase in the expression of IL-2 and IFN-gamma, a signature cytokine of Th1 helper cells, and a decrease in the concentration of cortisol in the stressed experimental animals. It also reversed the restraint stress-induced increase in plasma alanine aminotransferase (ALT), aspartate aminotransferase (AST), and hepatic lipid peroxidation levels, and improved the restraint stress-induced decrease in hepatic glutathione (GSH) and glycogen levels, showing significant anti-stress action.

The leaf extract of Withania demonstrated its usefulness in Th 1 immunity weakness for chronic infectious diseases.[65]

Withania somnifera root powder was investigated for its in-vivo and in-vitro immunomodulatory properties. It showed potent inhibitory activity toward the complement system, mitogen-induced lymphocyte proliferation, and delayed-type hypersensitivity reaction, and did not have a significant effect on humoral immune response in rats. Withania could be a candidate for development as an immunosuppressive medicine for the inflammatory diseases.[66]

Cystic fibrosis is one of the most common autosomal genetic disorders in humans. This disease is caused by mutations within a single gene, coding for the cystic fibrosis transmembrane conductance regulator (CFTR) protein. Cystic fibrosis patients usually have chronic lung infection and associated inflammation from opportunistic microbes such as Pseudomonas aeruginosa, Haemophilus influenzae, and Staphylococcus aureus. This eventually leads to deterioration of lung function and death in most cystic fibrosis patients. Control of inflammation and infection in cystic fibrosis patients is critical in managing the disease. Anti-inflammatory agents and antibiotics are frequently prescribed to control inflammation and infections. However, most of the anti-inflammatory agents in cystic fibrosis have severe limitations because of adverse side-effects and resistance to antibiotics. Because Withferin-A blocks PAF-induced activation of NfkappaB, it may provide a new direction in treatment of cystic fibrosis because of its anti-inflammatory and immune modulatory properties.[67]

Nephroprotective effect

Administration of aqueous root extract of Withania somnifera has shown to protect kidneys from dehydration induced nephrotoxicity.[68] Gentamycin induced nephrotoxicity has been reversed by root extract of Withania somnifera.[69]

Neuroprotective activity

Alzheimer's disease is an irreversible neurodegenerative disorder with symptoms of confusion, memory loss, and mood swings. The beta-amyloid plaque plays a significant role in the development of Alzheimer's disease. The cell death caused by beta-amyloid has been negated by withanamide treatment. Withanamide is present in the fruit of Withania. Molecular modeling studies showed that withanamides A and C uniquely bind to the active motif of beta-amyloid and have the ability to prevent the fibril formation.[70]

Parkinson's disease is a degenerative disorder of the central nervous system. The motor symptoms of Parkinson's disease result from the death of dopamine-generating cells in the substantia nigra, a region of the midbrain. The cause of this cell death is unknown. In Parkinson's disease model mice, in which the mice were treated with 1-methyl-4-phenyl-1,2,3,6-tetrahydropyridine (MPTP) for 4 days to show biochemical and physiological abnormalities similar to patients with Parkinson's disease, the addition of Withania reversed the damages done by MPTP by increasing levels of dopamine, 3,4-dihydrophenyacetic acid, homovanillic acid, glutathione, and glutathione peroxidase, and lowering the lipid perosidation (TBARS) markers.[71]

Huntington's disease is another genetically inherited neurodegenerative disorder that results from the destruction of neurons in the basal ganglia, and oxidative stress has been implicated in its pathogenesis. Administration of Withania somnifera root extract (100 and 200 mg/kg) dose-dependently restored biochemical alterations induced by chronic 3-Nitropropionic treatment ($P < .05$), suggesting a neuroprotective.[72]

The treatment options for improving the balance in degenerative cerebellar ataxias are few. Ayurvedic texts have described diverse treatment regimens for this disease. A study was done to determine the change in balance indices, if any, by dynamic posturography (Biodex Balance System, USA) in progressive cerebellar ataxia following Ayurvedic treatment. The researchers performed a preliminary open labeled study on 10 patients diagnosed with progressive cerebellar ataxia. The patients were treated over a one-month period. The treatment consisted of Shirobasti (therapeutic retention of medicament over the scalp) in male patients and Shirodhara (pouring a steady stream of medicament on the forehead) in female patients with Dhanvantaram tailam (medicated oil) for 45 minutes daily, followed by Abhyanga (methodical massage) with Dhanvantaram tailam and a steam bath for 14 days. Along with these treatments, the patients were prescribed Maharasnadi kashayam 15 ml three times daily, a herbal combination Dhanvantaram capsule 101, and Ashwagandha one 500 mg tablet three times daily, for one month. The patients improved as assessed on the Biodex balance system before and after the treatment.[73]

Spinal cord injuries are difficult to treat. Studies have demonstrated that the active constituents, withanolide A, withanoside IV, and withanoside VI, restored pre-synapses and post-synapses, in addition to both axons and dendrites in cortical neurons after Abeta (25–35)-induced injury. In-vivo, oral withanolide A, withanoside IV, and withanoside VI (10 micromol/kg/day for 12 days) improved Abeta (25–35)-induced memory impairment, neurite atrophy, and synaptic loss in the cerebral cortex and hippocampus in mice. Oral treatment with withanoside IV improved locomotor functions in mice having spinal cord injury. In the mice treated with withanoside IV (10 micromol/kg/day for 21 days), the axonal density and peripheral nervous system myelin level increased.[74]

Sominone, an aglycone of withanoside IV, after a single i.p. injection of sominone into normal mice, could memorize scenery information better than the control mice. Sixty minutes after the sominone injection, RET (glial cell receptor) phosphorylation was increased, particularly in the hippocampus of the mice. After the memory tests, the densities of axons and dendrites were increased in the hippocampus by administration of sominone. Sominone could reinforce the morphological plasticity of neurons by activation of the RET pathway and thus enhance memory.[75]

Management of addictions and side effects

Opiate withdrawal is associated with morphological changes of dopamine neurons. A study investigated morphine withdrawal in rats that were chronically treated with Withania somnifera extract along with morphine or saline. Withania somnifera extract treatment reduced the severity of the withdrawal syndrome when given during chronic morphine but not during withdrawal. Pre-treatment with Withania somnifera extract protects against the structural changes induced by morphine withdrawal.[76]

Withania somnifera can play a critical role in addiction to morphine, alcohol, and benzodiazepines. Withdrawal symptoms are scary, and the individuals usually end up going back to the addiction. Ethanol withdrawal anxiety was markedly antagonized by administration of Withania somnifera.[77]

Catalepsy induced by administration of haloperidol was reversed significantly by a combination of Withania somnifera, Ocimum sanctum, Camellia sinensis, Triphala, and Shilajit by increasing superoxide dismutase levels.[78]

Other therapeutic benefits

Ashwagandha have shown to be effective in the treatment of osteoarthritis,[79] inflammation,[80] stroke,[81] infertility from chronic stress,[82] and tardive dyskinesia.[83] Ashwagandha has been shown to be a potential antimicrobial agent with anti-fungal activity and moderate anti-bacterial activity against Staphylococcus aureus and Pseudomonas aeruginosa bacteria strains.[84]

Platelets and fibrin play an important role in allergies and allergic asthma. Listeria monocytogenes infected mice were used as asthma models; the asthmatic mice were treated with the anti-inflammatory plant Withania somnifera, separately and in combination with selenium. Hydrocortisone was used as positive control. The results indica' that the control mice possessed major thick fibers, minor thin fibers, and tight, round activated platelets with typical pseudopodia formation.[86] Minor fibers of the asthmatic mice have a net-like appearance covering the major fibers, whereas the platelets form loosely connected, granular aggregates. Hydrocortisone makes the fibrin more fragile, and platelet morphology changes from a tight activated platelet to a more granular activated platelet, not closely fused to each other. In the study, Withania somnifera in combination with selenium did not affect the fragility of the fibrin and reversed the formation of the dense minor net-like layer over the major fibers, and the platelets formed a dense aggregate. The asthmatic mice treated with selenium showed a dense minor fibrin layer; however, the platelets formed a dense aggregate. These findings suggest a positive role of Withania and selenium in allergies and allergic asthma.

Aqueous extracts of Withania somnifera root powder showed a chondroprotective effect on damaged human osteoarthritic cartilage matrix in 50% of the patients. Withania showed inhibition of the gelatinase activity of the collagenase type 2 enzyme.[87]

Withania somnifera extract protected mice from a lethal dose of Listeria monocytogenes when administered prophylactically at 100, 250, and 500 mg/kg for 10 days, with survival rates up to 30%. It also prevented the myelosuppression and the splenomegaly caused by infection.[88]

A combination of Withania somnifera, Camellia sinensis, Ocimum sanctum, Shilajit, and Triphala protected against aspirin and pyloric ligation induced ulceration. The results were comparable to omeprazole in preventing ulcer formation.[89]

A combination of Withania somnifera, Tribulus terrestris, Mucuna pruriens, and Argyreia speciosa has been used for several years for its bio-stimulating, revitalizing, and fertility enhancing effects. Acute oral toxicity reveals that the product is safe up to a dose of 5000 mg/kg.[90]

Dr. Sodhi's Experience

Over many years of observation, I have concluded that the full potential of Ashwagandha as a medicinal herb has yet to be realized. Especially in its use as an anti-inflammatory to relieve the symptoms of rheumatic disorders, much more remains to be discovered.

During my second year of medical school, a 70-year-old male neighbor in considerable pain from osteoarthritis in his knees requested urgent help. After 3 weeks of drinking one tablespoon of Ashwagandha boiled in milk on a nightly basis, he reported no pain, increased energy, and renewed ability to walk long distances.

The possibilities for treatment success with patients suffering from rheumatic disorders is especially encouraging, as Withania somnifera potentially could replace steroids and other drugs that involve serious side-effects.

I also have observed impressive results using Ashwagandha to treat anxiety, depression, and stress. This feature could make it useful for overstressed young workers who find themselves experiencing panic attacks and tachycardia.

Also, I have had phenomenal success using Ashwagandha to treat patients with multiple myeloma. I used the herb to treat a 70-year-old with neck and back pain. Touching her back was like touching concrete. It appeared that she had osteoporotic fractures. An x-ray showed punched holes along the spine, which is typical of multiple myeloma. The patient's husband had died with multiple myeloma after being treated with thalidomide and chemotherapy. The female subject refused to see a doctor because of what had happened to her husband, but I convinced her to try Ashwagandha because of the natural steroids it contains. After 9 months of treatment, the patient's x-rays were normal and she had resumed walking with no pain.

I believe that Ashwagandha has great potential as a replacement therapy not only to replace steroids but also to replace commonly used drugs such as prednisone and dexamethasone. I have treated hundreds of patients who were able to stop taking such medications after beginning treatment with Ashwagandha. In addition, I have had excellent success using Ashwagandha in treating rheumatoid arthritis, psoriatic arthritis, polymyalgia rheumatica, and asthma.

As a final example, a 29-year-old patient came to the clinic with a history of idiopathic thrombocytopenia purpura. She had been treated repeatedly with loading doses of prednisolone, which put her into remission for some time, and then she would return for treatment. She was experiencing serious side-effects from the steroids and now did not want to be on steroids. She was given a hypoallergenic and pitta pacifying diet. I put her on a standardized extract of Ashwagandha 1000 mg three times per day, standardized extract of Triphala 500 mg three times per day, along with 500 mg three times per day of licorice extract.

- For insomnia, Ashwagandha can be mixed with valerian root and oyster shell. As a general nerve tonic, especially for hypoglycemia or low blood pressure, Ashwagandha is combined with goksura.
- For chronic fatigue, Ashwagandha may be combined with another great Ayurvedic tonic herb—Shatavari (Asparagus racemosa), licorice, amla (Emblica myrobalan) or minerals, especially calcium and magnesium.
- In treating impotence, Ashwagandha can be used alone or combined with fried mucuna seeds. For weak lungs, Ashwagandha may be combined with Sida cordifolia (Bala).
- To stimulate milk production in nursing mothers, Ashwagandha may be combined with Asparagus racemosus along with licorice, taken three times daily.
- As a nerve tonic, Ashwagandha may be combined with Bacopa monnieri, Centella asiatica, and Mucuna pruriens in equal parts. This is also especially good for hypoglycemia and low blood pressure.

Safety Profile

Ashwagandha is a safe and gentle herb when used in recommended doses; however, certain safety precautions should be noted. Ashwagandha has a mildly depressant effect on the central nervous system, so patients should avoid alcohol, barbiturates, or any other sedatives while being treated.[91]

Large doses of Ashwagandha may possess abortifacient properties; therefore, it should not be taken by pregnant women. The herb should not be used during severe and acute inflammatory conditions because these may be the result of acute infections.

Side-effects

Ashwagandha is generally safe when taken in the prescribed dosage range; however, large doses have been shown to cause gastrointestinal upset, diarrhea, and vomiting. Sedation may be a side-effect with some Withania somnifera products, depending on the dosage and extract potency. When side-effects become a problem during treatment with Withania somnifera, it may be beneficial for patients to take breaks from using it. For example, the herb could be used three or four times a week rather than daily. Those experiencing drowsiness after taking the herb may try using it before bedtime rather than during the day.

Drug/herb interaction

Ashwagandha should not be taken with sedatives or anti-anxiety drugs without supervision by a medical practitioner. Caution should be exercised in these cases, and there may be a need to adjust the dosages of each of the therapies periodically.

In treating gastric and duodenal ulcers, Withania somnifera should not be taken on an empty stomach. For stress ulcers, it may be taken with other ulcer-healing herbs.

Dosage

A typical maintenance dose of Ashwagandha is 3 to 6 grams daily of the dried root powder, 300–500 mg of an extract standardized to contain 1.5 percent withanolides, or 6–12 ml of a 1:2 fluid extract per day.

The root is taken in a 30-gram dosage for general debility, consumption, malnourishment in children, senile debility, rheumatic and arthritic conditions, nervous exhaustion, fatigue, brain-gag, memory weakness, senile dementia, muscular weakness, spermatorrhea, and leucorrhea. Normally this can be taken as a powder 10 grams three times daily mixed with warm milk or water, or as a 1-to-5 alcoholic extract, one or two tablespoons three times daily.

Ayurvedic Properties

The roots of Withania somnifera are used extensively in Ayurveda. In the Ayurvedic tradition, Withania somnifera is categorized as a rasayana, which means that it is useful to promote physical and mental health, to provide a defense against diseases and adverse environmental factors, and to slow the aging process.

Guna: Laghu (light) and snigdha (unctuous)
Rasa: tikta, kashaya and madhur
Vipaka: Madhur
Virya: ushna
Karma: Vatapittahara, Kaphashamak, balyam, vajikarana tonic, adaptogen, relaxing nervine, post-partum tonic, immunomodulant, astringent, galactogogue, diuretic, thermogenic

Notes

1. Author?, "Withania somnifera," *Alternative Medicine Review,* Oct. 13, 2008. It is a compilation so no authors were listed.
2. R.P. Rastogi and B.N. Mehrotra, *Compendium of Indian Medicinal Plants*: Vol. 6. (New Delhi, India: Central Drug Research Institute, 1998).
3. A. Grandhi, "Comparative pharmacological investigation of ashwagandha and ginseng," *Journal of Ethnopharmacology* (Ireland), 1994, 3:131–135.
4. A. Padmawar, *Withania Somnifera*, monograph for Anruta Herbals, Ltd., This is fine. This how it was referenced in previous articles
5. M.H. Mirjalili, E. Moyano, M. Bonfill, R.M. Cusido, and J. Palazón, "Steroidal lactones from Withania somnifera, an ancient plant for novel medicine," *Molecules*, July 3, 2009, 14(7):2373–2393.
6. X. Tong, H. Zhang, and B.N.Timmermann, "Chlorinated withanolides from Withania somnifera," *Phytochem Lett.*, Dec. 2011, 4(4):411–414.
7. M. Elsakka, E. Grigorescu, and U. Stanescu, et al., "New data referring to chemistry of Withania somnifera species," *Rev Med Chir Soc Med Nat Iasi*, 1990, 94:385–387. Please see http://www.ncbi.nlm.nih.gov/pubmed/2100857
8. A.M. Abou-Douh, "New withanolides and other constituents from the fruit of Withania somnifera," *Arch Pharm*, 2002, 335:267–276.
9. H. Wagner, H. Norr, and H. Winterhoff, "Plant adaptogens," *Phytomed*, 1994:1:63–76.
10. B. Singh, A.K. Saxena, B.K.Chandan, et al., "Adaptogenic activity of a novel, withanolide-free aqueous fraction from the root of Withania somnifera (Part 1)," *Phytother Res*, 2001,15:311–318.
11. B. Singh, B.K. Chandan, and D.K. Gupta, "Adaptogenic activity of a novel withanolide-free aqueous fraction from the roots of Withania somnifera Dun. (Part II)," *Phytother Res.*, May 2003, 17(5):531–536.
12. S.K. Bhattacharya and A.V. Muruganandam, "Adaptogenic activity of Withania somnifera: An experimental study using a rat model of chronic stress," *Pharmacol Biochem Behav.*, June 2003, 75(3):547–555.
13. A. Bhattacharya, S. Ghosal, and S.K. Bhattacharya, "Anti-oxidant effect of Withania somnifera glycowithanolides in chronic footshock stress-induced perturbations of oxidative free radical scavenging enzymes and lipid peroxidation in rat frontal cortex and striatum," *J Ethnopharmacol* 2001,74:1–6.
14. A.K. Mehta, P. Binkley, S.S. Gandhi, and M.K. Ticku, "Pharmacological effects of Withania somnifera root extract on GABA receptor complex," *Indian J Med Res.*, Aug. 1991, 94:312–315.
15. R. Archana and A. Namasivayam, "Antistressor effect of Withania somnifera," *J Ethnopharmacol*, 1999, 64:91–93.
16. S. Bhattacharya, R. Goel, R. Kaur, and S. Ghosal, "Anti-stress activity of Sitoindosides, VII and VIII: New acylsterylglucosides from Withania somnifera," *Phytotherapy Res*, 1987, 1:32–39.
17. K. Cooley, O. Szczurko, D. Perri, E.J. Mills, B. Bernhardt, Q, Zhou, and D. Seely, "Naturopathic care for anxiety: A randomized controlled trial," *PLoS One*, Aug. 31, 2009, 4(8):e6628 This is how the authors wanted the article to be cited S.K. Bhattacharya, A. Bhattacharya, K. Sairam, and S. Ghosal, "Anxiolytic-anti-depressant activity of Withania somnifera glycowithanolides: An experimental study," *Phytomedicine*, 2000, 7:463–469.
18. C.S. Yadav, V. Kumar, S.G. Suke, R.S. Ahmed, P.K. Mediratta, and B.D. Banerjee, "Propoxur-induced acetylcholine esterase inhibition and impairment of cognitive function: Attenuation by Withania somnifera," *Indian J Biochem Biophys.*, April 2010, 47(2):117–120.
19. H. Ichikawa, Y. Takada, S. Shishodia, B. Jayaprakasam, M.G. Nair, and B.B. Aggarwal, "Withanolides potentiate apoptosis, inhibit invasion, and abolish osteoclastogenesis through suppression of nuclear factor-kappaB (NF-kappaB) activation and NF-kappaB-regulated gene expression," *Molecular Cancer Therapeutics*, June 2006, 5(6):1434–1445.
20. J. Prakash, S.K. Gupta, and A.K. Dinda, "Withania somnifera root extract prevents DMBA-induced squamous cell carcinoma of skin in Swiss albino mice," *Nutr Cancer* 2002, 42:91–97.
21. B. Jayaprakasam, Y. Zhang, N. Seeram, and M. Nair, "Growth inhibition of tumor cell lines by withanolides from Withania somnifera leaves," *Life Sci*, 2003,74:125–132.

22. T. Jeyanthi and P. Subramanian, "Protective effect of Withania somnifera root powder on lipid peroxidation and anti-oxidant status in gentamicin-induced nephrotoxic rats," *J Basic Clin Physiol Pharmacol*, 2010, 21(1):61–78.

23. S. Koduru, R. Kumar, S. Srinivasan, M.B. Evers, and C. Damodaran, "Notch-1 inhibition by Withaferin-A: A therapeutic target against colon carcinogenesis," *Mol Cancer Ther.*, Jan. 2010, 9(1):202–210.

24. J. Lee, E.R. Hahm, and S.V. Singh, "Withaferin A inhibits activation of signal transducer and activator of transcription 3 in human breast cancer cells," *Carcinogenesis*, Aug 19, 2010.

25. S.D, Stan, Y. Zeng, and S.V. Singh, "Ayurvedic medicine constituent withaferin A causes G2 and M phase cell cycle arrest in human breast cancer cells," *Nutr Cancer.*, 2008, 60 (Suppl 1):51–60.

26. C. Didelot, D. Lanneau, M. Brunet, et al. (2007), "Anti-cancer therapeutic approaches based on intracellular and extracellular heat shock proteins," *Curr. Med. Chem.*, 14(27): 2839–2847.

27. Y. Yu, A. Hamza, T. Zhang, M. Gu, P. Zou, B. Newman, Y. Li, A.A. Gunatilaka, C.G. Zhan, and D. Sun, "Withaferin A targets heat shock protein 90 in pancreatic cancer cells," *Biochem Pharmacol.*, Feb. 15, 2010, 79(4):542–551.

28. N. Shah, H. Kataria, S.C. Kaul, T. Ishii, G. Kaur, and R. Wadhwa, "Effect of the alcoholic extract of Ashwagandha leaves and its components on proliferation, migration, and differentiation of glioblastoma cells: Combinational approach for enhanced differentiation," *Cancer Sci.*, Sept. 2009, 100(9):1740–1747.

29. Hardeep Kataria, Navjot Shah, Sunil C. Kaul, Renu Wadhwa, and Gurcharan Kaur, "Water Extract of Ashwagandha Leaves Limits Proliferation and Migration, and Induces Differentiation in Glioma Cells," *Evidence-Based Complementary and Alternative Medicine*, vol. 2011, Article ID 267614, 12 pages, 2011. G. Kalthur and U.D. Pathirissery, "Enhancement of the response of B16F1 melanoma to fractionated radiotherapy and prolongation of survival by Withaferin A and/or hyperthermia," *Integr Cancer Ther.*, Aug. 16, 2010.

30. P. Senthilnathan, R. Padmavathi, V. Magesh, and D. Sakthisekaran, "Chemotherapeutic efficacy of paclitaxel in combination with Withania somnifera on benzo(a)pyrene-induced experimental lung cancer," *Cancer Sci.*, July 2006, 97(7):658–664.

31. G. Muralikrishnan, S. Amanullah, M.I. Basha, A.K. Dinda, and F. Shakeel, "Modulating effect of Withania somnifera on TCA cycle enzymes and electron transport chain in azoxymethane-induced colon cancer in mice," *Immunopharmacol Immunotoxicol.*, Sept. 2010, 32(3):523–527.

32. F. Malik, A. Kumar, S. Bhushan, D.M. Mondhe, H.C. Pal, R. Sharma, A. Khajuria, S. Singh, G. Singh, A.K. Saxenam, K.A. Suri, G.N. Qazi, and J. Singh, "Immune modulation and apoptosis induction: Two sides of antitumoural activity of a standardised herbal formulation of Withania somnifera," *Eur J Cancer*, May 2009, 45(8):1494–1509.

33. J.H. Oh, T.J.Lee, S.H. Kim, Y.H. Choi, S.H. Lee, J.M. Lee, Y.H.Kim, J.W. Park, and T.K. Kwon, "Induction of apoptosis by withaferin A in human leukemia U937 cells through down-regulation of Akt phosphorylation," *Apoptosis*, Dec. 2008, 13(12):1494–1504.

34. C. Mandal, A. Dutta, A. Mallick, S. Chandra, L. Misra, R.S. Sangwan, and C. Mandal, "Withaferin A induces apoptosis by activating p38 mitogen-activated protein kinase signaling cascade in leukemic cells of lymphoid and myeloid origin through mitochondrial death cascade," *Apoptosis.*, Dec. 2008, 13(12):1450–1464.

35. R. Aalinkeel, Z. Hu, B.B. Nair, D.E. Sykes, J.L. Reynolds, S.D. Mahajan, and S.A. Schwartz, "Genomic analysis highlights the role of the JAK-STAT signaling in the anti-proliferative effects of dietary flavonoid 'Ashwagandha' in prostate cancer cells," *Evid Based Complement Alternat Med.*, Jan 10, 2008.

36. M. Winters, "Ancient medicine, modern use: Withania somnifera and its potential role in integrative oncology," *Altern Med Rev.*, Dec. 2006, 11(4):269–277.

37. K. Anbalangan and J. Sadique, "Influence of an Indian medicine (Ashwagandha) on acute-phase reactants in inflammation," *Indian Journal of Experimental Biology*, 1981, 19:245–249.

38. V.H. Begum and J. Sadique, "Long-term effect of herbal drug Withania somnifera on adjuvant-induced arthritis in rats," *Indian J Exp Biol*, 1988, 26: 877–882.

39. D. Khanna, G. Sethi, K.S. Ahn, M.K. Pandey, A.B. Kunnumakkara, B. Sung, A. Aggarwal, and B.B. Aggarwal, "Natural products as a gold mine for arthritis treatment," *Curr Opin Pharmacol.*, June 2007, 7(3):344–351. e-pub May 1, 2007.

40. H. Ichikawa, Y. Takada, S. Shishodia, B. Jayaprakasa, M.G.Nair, and B.B. Aggarwal, "Withanolides potentiate apoptosis, inhibit invasion, and abolish osteoclastogenesis through suppression of nuclear factor-kappaB (NF-kappaB) activation and NF-kappaB-regulated gene expression," *Mol Cancer Ther.*, June 2006, 5(6):1434–1445.

41. U. Minhas, R. Minz, P. Das, and A. Bhatnagar, "Therapeutic effect of Withania somnifera on pristane-induced model of SLE," *Inflammopharmacology*, Dec. 13, 2011.

42. P. Pawar, S. Gilda, S. Sharma, S. Jagtap, A Paradkar, K. Mahadik, P. Ranjekar, and A. Harsulkar, "Rectal gel application of Withania somnifera root extract expounds anti-inflammatory and muco-restorative activity in TNBS-induced inflammatory bowel disease," *BMC Complement Altern Med.*, April 18, 2011, 11:34.

43. K. Bone, *Clinical Applications of Ayurvedic and Chinese Herbs* (Queensland, Australia: Phytotherapy Press, 1996), pp. 137–141.

44. N. Widodo, N. Shah, D. Priyandoko, T. Ishii, S.C. Kaul, and R. Wadhwa, "Deceleration of senescence in normal human fibroblasts by withanone extracted from ashwagandha leaves," *J Gerontol A Biol Sci Med Sci.*, Oct. 2009, 64(10):1031–1038. This is fine see this http://www.ncbi.nlm.nih.gov/pubmed/19587106

45. A. Biswajit, H. Jayaram, M. Hazra, A. Mitra, B. Abedon, and S. Ghosal, "A standardized Withania somnifera extract significantly reduces stress-related parameters in chronically stressed humans: A double-blind, randomized, placebo-controlled study, *JANA*, Dec. 2008, 11(1): 50–56.

46. B. Andallu and B. Radhika, "Hypoglycemic, diuretic and hypocholesterolemic effect of winter cherry (Withania somnifera) root," *Indian Journal of Experimental Biology* 2000, 38:607–609.

47. I.R. Mohanty, D.S. Arya, and S.K.Gupta, "Withania somnifera provides cardioprotection and attenuates ischemia-reperfusion induced apoptosis," *Clin Nutr.*, Aug. 2008, 7(4):635–642.

48. M. Thirunavukkarasu, S. Penumathsa, B. Juhas, L. Zhan, M. Bagchi, T. Yasmin, M.A. Shara, H.S. Thatte, D. Bagchi, and N. Maulik, "Enhanced cardiovascular function and energy level by a novel chromium (III)-supplement," *Biofactors*, 2006, 27(1–4):53–67.

49. S. Panda ahd A. Kar, "Withania somnifera and Bauhinia pupurea in the regulation of circulating thyroid hormone concentrations in female mice," *J Ethnopharmacol*, 1999, 67:233–239.

50. S. Panda and A. Kar, "Changes in thyroid hormone concentrations after administration of ashwaganda root extract to adult male mice," *J Pharm Pharmacol*, 1998, 50:1065–1068.

51. R. Jatwa and A. Kar, "Amelioration of metformin-induced hypothyroidism by Withania somnifera and Bauhinia purpurea extracts in type 2 diabetic mice," *Phytother Res.*, Aug. 2009, 23(8):1140–1145.

52. T. Anwer, M. Sharma, K.K. Pillai, and M. Iqbal, "Effect of Withania somnifera on insulin sensitivity in non-insulin-dependent diabetes mellitus rats," *Basic Clin Pharmacol Toxicol.*, June 2008, 102(6):498–503.

53. G. Kuttan, "Use of Withania somnifera Dunal as an adjuvant during radiation therapy," *Indian J Exp Biol*, 1996, 34:854–856.

54. M. Ziauddin, N. Phansalkar, P. Patki, et al., "Studies on the immunomodulatory effects of Ashwagandha," *J Ethnopharmacol*, 1996, 50:69–76.

55. L. Davis and G. Kuttan G., "Immunomodulatory activity of Withania somnifera," *J Ethnopharmacol*, 2000, 71:193–200.

56. T. Iuvone, G. Esposito, F. Capasso, and A. Izzo, "Induction of nitric oxide synthase expression by Withania somnifera in macrophages," *Life Sci*, 2003, 72:1617–1625.

57. C. Bogdan, "Nitric oxide and the immune response," *Nature Immunol*, 2001, 2:907–916.

58. J. Bhat, A. Damle, P.P. Vaishnav, R. Albers, M. Joshi, and G. Banerjee, "In vivo enhancement of natural killer cell activity through tea fortified with Ayurvedic herbs," *Phytother Res.*, Jan. 2010, 24(1):129–135.

59. J. Mikolai, A. Erlandsen, A. Murison, K.A. Brown, W.L. Gregory, P. Raman-Caplan, and H.L. Zwickey, "In vivo effects of Ashwagandha (Withania somnifera) extract on the activation of lymphocytes," *J Altern Complement Med.*, April 2009, 15(4):423–430.

60. L. Davis and G. Kuttan, "Effect of Withania somnifera on CTL activity," *J Exp Clin Cancer Res*, 2002, 21:115–118.

61. J. Prakash, S.K. Gupta, and A.K. Dinda, "Withania somnifera root extract prevents DMBA-induced squamous cell carcinoma of skin in Swiss albino mice," *Nutr Cancer*, 2002, 42:91–97.

62. K. Kour, A. Pandey, K.A. Suri, N.K. Satti, K.K. Gupta, and S. Bani, "Restoration of stress-induced altered T cell function and corresponding cytokines patterns by Withanolide A.," *Int Immunopharmacol.*, Sept. 2009, 9(10):1137–1144.

63. S. Khan, F. Malik, K.A. Suri, and J. Singh, "Molecular insight into the immune up-regulatory properties of the leaf extract of Ashwagandha and identification of Th1 immunostimulatory chemical entity," *Vaccine*, Oct 9, 2009, 27(43):6080–6087.

64. M. Rasool and P. Varalakshmi, "Immunomodulatory role of Withania somnifera root powder on experimental induced inflammation: An in vivo and in vitro study," *Vascul Pharmacol.*, June 2006, 44(6):406–410.

65. R. Maitra, M.A. Porter, S. Huang, and B.P. Gilmour, "Inhibition of NFkappaB by the natural product Withaferin A in cellular models of cystic fibrosis inflammation," *J Inflamm (Lond)*, May 13, 2009, 13, 6:15.

66. K. Das, T.T. Samanta, P. Samanta, and D.K. Nandi, "Effect of extract of Withania somnifera on dehydration-induced oxidative stress-related uremia in male rats," *Saudi J Kidney Dis Transpl.* Jan 2010, 21(1):75–80.

67. See Note 23.

68. B. Jayaprakasam, K. Padmanabhan, and M.G. Nair, "Withanamides in Withania somnifera fruit protect PC-12 cells from beta-amyloid responsible for Alzheimer's disease," *Phytother Res.*, June 2010, 24(6):859–863.

69. S. RajaSankar, T. Manivasagam, V. Sankar, S. Prakash, R. Muthusamy, A. Krishnamurti, and S. Surendran, "Withania somnifera root extract improves catecholamines and physiological abnormalities seen in a Parkinson's disease model mouse," *J Ethnopharmacol..* Sept. 25, 2009, 125(3):369–373. E-pub Aug 8, 2009

70. P. Kumar and A. Kumar, "Possible neuroprotective effect of Withania somnifera root extract against 3-nitropropionic acid-induced behavioral, biochemical, and mitochondrial dysfunction in an animal model of Huntington's disease," *J Med Food.*, June 2009, 12(3):591–600.

71. S.J. Sriranjini, P.K. Pal, K.V. Devidas, and S. Ganpathy, "Improvement of balance in progressive degenerative cerebellar ataxias after Ayurvedic therapy: A preliminary report," *Neurol India.*, Mar–Apr 2009, 57(2):166–171.

72. C. Tohda, "Overcoming several neurodegenerative diseases by traditional medicines: The development of therapeutic medicines and unraveling pathophysiological mechanisms," *Yakugaku Zasshi*, Aug. 2008, 128(8):1159–1167.

73. C. Tohda and E. Joyashiki, "Sominone enhances neurite outgrowth and spatial memory mediated by the neurotrophic factor receptor, RET," *Br J Pharmacol.*, Aug. 2009, 157(8):1427–1440.

74. S. Kasture, S. Vinci, F. Ibba, A. Puddu, M. Marongiu, B. Murali, A. Pisanu, D. Lecca, G. Zernig, and E. Acquas, "Withania somnifera prevents morphine withdrawal-induced decrease in spine density in nucleus accumbens shell of rats: A confocal laser scanning microscopy study," *Neurotox Res.*, Nov. 2009, 16(4):343–355.

75. G.L. Gupta and A.C. Rana, "Effect of Withania somnifera Dunal in ethanol-induced anxiolysis and withdrawal anxiety in rats," *Indian J Exp Biol.*, June 2008, 46(6):470–475.

76. V. Nair, A. Arjuman, P. Dorababu, H.N. Gopalakrishna, R.U. Chakradhar, and L. Mohan, "Effect of NR-ANX-C (a polyherbal formulation) on haloperidol induced catalepsy in albino mice," *Indian J Med Res.*, Nov. 2007, 126(5):480–484.

77. R.R. Kulkarni, P.S. Patki, and V.P. Jog, et al., "Treatment of osteoarthritis with a herbomineral formulation: A double-blind, placebo-controlled, cross-over study," *J Ethnopharmacol*, 1991, 33:91–95.

78. K. Anbalangan and J. Sadique, "Influence of an Indian medicine (Ashwagandha) on acute-phase reactants in inflammation," *Indian Journal of Experimental Biology*, 1981, 19:245–249.

79. G. Chaudhary, U. Sharma, N. Jagannathan, and Y. Gupta, "Evaluation of Withania somnifera in a middle cerebral artery occlusion model of stroke in rats," *Clin Exp Pharmacol Physiol*, 2003, 30:399–404.

80. A.A. Mahdi, K.K. Shukla, M.K. Ahmad, S. Rajnder, S.N. Shankhwar, V.Singh, and D. Delela, "Withania somnifera improves semen quality in stress related male fertility," *Evidence Based Complementary Alternative Medicine*, Sept. 29, 2009.

81. S.K. Bhattacharya, D. Bhattacharya, and K. Sairam, "Ghosal S. effect of Withania somnifera glycowithanolides on a rat model of tardive dyskinesia," *Phytomedicine*, 2002, 9:167–170.

82. G. Kuttan, "Use of Withania somnifera Dunal as an adjuvant during radiation therapy," *Indian J Exp Biol*, 1996, 34:854–856.

83. N.A. Ali, W.D. Julicch, C. Kusnick, and U. Lindequist, "Screening of Yemeni medicinal plants for anti-bacterial and cytotoxic activities," *J Ethnopharmacol*, 2001, 74:173–179.

84. E. Pretorius, H.M. Oberholzer, W.A. Vieira, and E. Smit, "Ultrastructure of platelets and fibrin networks of asthmatic mice exposed to selenium and Withania somniferamm," *Anat Sci Int.*, Sept. 2009, 84(3):210–217.

85. V.N. Sumantran, A. Kulkarni, S. Boddul, T. Chinchwade, S.J. Koppikar, A. Harsulkar, B. Patwardhan, A. Chopra, and U.V. Wagh, "Chondroprotective potential of root extracts of Withania somnifera in osteoarthritis," *J Biosci.*, March 2007, 32(2):299–307.

86. S.T. Teixeira, M.C. Valadares, S.A. Gonçalves, A. de Melo, and M.L. Queiroz, "Prophylactic administration of Withania somnifera extract increases host resistance in Listeria monocytogenes infected mice," *Int Immunopharmacol.*, Oct. 2006, 6(10):1535–42.

87. V. Nair, A. Arjuman, H.N. Gopalakrishna, P. Dorababu, P.V. Mirshad, D. Bhargavan, and D. Chatterji, "Evaluation of the anti-ulcer activity of NR-ANX-C (a polyherbal formulation) in aspirin & pyloric ligature induced gastric ulcers in albino rats," *Indian J Med Res.*, Aug. 2010, 132:218–223.

88. A. Riaz, R.A. Khan, S. Ahmed, and S. Afroz S., "Assessment of acute toxicity and reproductive capability of a herbal combination," *Pak J Pharm Sci.*, July 2010, 23(3):291–294.

89. A.A. Aphale, A.D. Chhibba, N.R. Kumbhaakarna, et al., "Subacute toxicity study of the combination of ginseng (Panex ginseng) and ashwagandha (Withania somnifera) in rats: A safety assessment," *Indian J Physiol Pharmacol*, 1998, 42:299–302.

ABOUT THE AUTHOR

The first Ayurvedic and Board certified licensed Naturopathic Physician in the United States, Dr. Sodhi has seen thousands of patients in his 34 years of clinical practice from all over the world. His keen intuition and exceptional training in multiple modalities has set him apart in the treatment and management of general family medicine and chronic disease alike. With his unique training and perspective, he has become a distinguished educator of patients as well as physicians, contributes to a growing body of evidence in support of integrative practices in medicine as a writer, speaker, educator and advocate and grounds this knowledge firmly in the ancient and science-proven art that is Ayurvedic medicine.

He and his brothers have founded and grown an Ayurvedic supplement company that serves countless individuals worldwide through its time tested, clinically relevant, physician respected line of products that support patients and consumers in the pursuit and maintenance of optimal health. Ayush Herbs, Inc. is an Internationally recognized company having won numerous awards for its innovation and contribution as a company well-grounded in Ayurvedic concepts coupled with the latest research and technology and is considered one of the premier Ayurvedic companies in the United States and elsewhere.

INDEX

abortion, spontaneous, case history, 365
abortifacient / uterotonic activity
    Adhatoda vasica, 3–4
    Ashwagandha, 437, 449
    bitter melon, 261
Acanthaceae family, 25
acne
    cystic, case history, 157
    Solanum nigrum treatment, 383
ACTH (adrenocorticotrophic hormone), 32
adaptogenic properties / adaptogens
    Amla, 320–321
    Ashwagandha, 437, 438
    Gotu kola 122
    Picrorhiza kurroa, 328
    Piper longum, 340
    Shankhapushpi, 163
    Shilajit, 370, 372–373
    Triphala, 400
    Tulsi, 289
Adhatoda vasica, 1
    abortifacient, 3–4
    allergy treatment, 3
    for asthma, 3, 5
    chemicals in, 2
    for parasites / insects, 3, 5
    for respiratory conditions, 1, 3, 5
    for tuberculosis, 1, 2, 5
    for ulcers, 4
    wound healing, 4
Aegle marmelos. *See also* Bael
    aegeline study, 18
    anti-bacterial, anti-viral, anti-parasitic, and anti-fungal, 11–12
    anti-fertility activity, 19–20
    cardioprotective activity, 16–17
    chemoprotective activity, 15–16
    diabetes treatment, 9, 12–14
    diarrhea / IBS uses, 10–11
    ophthalmic activity, 18
    respiratory tract activity, 19–20
    Shigella treatment, 11
    ulcer treatment with luvagetin, 17
    uses of fruit, leaves, bark, and roots, 9
aging, anti- / longevity
    Amla, 312
    Ashwagandha, 437, 443
    Gotu effect, 122
    Ocimum extract, 297
    Shilajit, 372
    Triphala, 395
AIDS (acquired immunodeficiency syndrome), Aegle marmelos treatment, 12
air potato, 205
alcoholism, Triphala for, 414
Aller-7 for allergic rhinitis, 388–389, 409
Alzheimer's studies and treatments. *See also* dementia / Alzheimer's
    Curcuma longa / curcumin, 184
    Shilajit, 370
    Withania somnifera, 438, 446–447
amoebic dysentery, Bael to treat, 20
alkaloids
    in Adhatoda vasica, 2
    in Bael leaves, 10
    in bitter melon, 258
    in Brahmi, 74
    in Piper longum, 338
    in Piper nigrum, 346
    in Varuna, 170
allergies, treating
    Adhatoda vasica, 3
    Centella asiatica, 130
    Inula racemosa, 253–254
    licorice, 236–237
    Picrorhiza kurroa, 330
    Pippli protocol for food allergies, 342
    Shilajit, 369
Ambroxol, 3
Amla, 311. *See also* Phyllanthus emblica
    aging-related disorders, 312
    anti-aging 311, 317–319 (also see anti-oxidant and connective tissue activity)
    anti-bacterial, 311, 313–314
    anti-carcinogenic, 314–315
    anti-diabetic, 315–316
    anti-viral / HIV, 312–313
    astringent, 311
    case histories
        corneal ulcers, 321–322
        pancreatitis, 322
        peptic ulcers, 321, 323
        prostatitis, 322–323
    cholesterol lowering, and protocol, 314, 323
    digestive system disorders, 312
    hepatoprotective, 316
    hypocholesterolemic, 314
    metabolic disorders, 312
    Phyllemblin, anti-oxidant 317–318
    polyphenols, 312
    neurasthenia, 312

pancreatitis, 317
protocols
    eye care / cataracts, 323
    hair growth, 323
    leucorrhea and bacterial vaginosis, 323
    metal toxicity, 323
    ulcers, 323
respiratory conditions, 311, 312
toxicity protection, 316
Vitamin C in, 311, 321
wound healing, 318–319
analgesic activity of Tribulus terrestris, 423–424
anaphylaxis, Haritaki study, 406–407
Andrographis paniculata
    and andrographolides, 26
    anti-carcinogenic activity, 26–28
    anti-diarrhea treatment, 31
    anti-fertility activity, 33
    anti-inflammatory activity, 32–33
    anti-ulcerogenic activity, 30
    anti-viral /HIV activity, 28
    cardioprotective activity, 31–32
    as common cold treatment, 28–29
    fever-reducing activity, 29–30
    for immune support, 25
    liver / hepatoprotective / hepatitis activity, 33–34, 35
    as malaria treatment, 30–31
    respiratory activity, 34
    sedative effect of, 34
anemia, Shilajit treatment, 373
angioplasty, Andrographis, 31–32
anorexia remedy, Picrorhiza kurroa, 327
anti-amoebic activity of berberine, 88–89
anti-atherosclerotic acitivity of Neem, 57
anti-bacterial activity. *See also* anti-microbial
    Adhatoda vasica, 4–5
    Amla, 311, 313–314
    Cyperus rotundus, 195
    Inula racemosa, 253
    Neem, 56
    Piper longum, 339
    Shatavari, 45–46
anti-carcinogenic activity. *See* cancer
anti-depressants
    Aegle marmelos, 18–19
    Ashwagandha, 448
    berberine, 90–92
    Boswellia gum resin, 110
    Centella asiatica, 126
    Shankhapushpi, 164
anti-fungal activity
    Ashwagandha, 447

Asparagus racemosus, 46
Aspergillus flavus, 55
Azadirachta indica, 55
berberine, 89
Cedrus deodara, 139
Cyperus rotundus, 195
Inula racemosa, 253
antihepatotoxic
    Eclipta alba, 212
    Shatavari root, 45
anti-inflammatory activity. *See also* inflammation
    Aegle marmelos, 17–18
    Andrographis paniculata, 32–33
    Ashwagandha, 437, 442–443, 448
    Azadirachta indica, 48
    berberine, 89
    Berberis aristata, 87
    Boswellia serrata, 103, 105–106
    Cedrus deodara, 138–139
    Cissus quadrangularis, 146
    Curcuma, 175, 176–179
    Eclipta alba, 214
    Fenugreek, 430
    Glycyrrhizin, 233–234
    Guggul, 152, 156
    licorice, 233
    Manjistha, 362
    mustak, 196
    Nigella, 278
    Phyllanthus amarus, 305–306
    Picrorhiza kurroa, 327, 328
    Pippli / piperine, 339, 348, 349
    Pterocarpus marsupium, 357–358
    Shilajit, 371
    Sida cordifolia, 377, 378
    Swertia chirayita, 392
    Tulsi, 291–292
    Varuna, 169, 171
    Vijaysar, 357
anti-microbial activity
    Ashwagandha, 447
    asiaticoside, 129
    Bael, 11, 20
    Brahmi, 79
    Curcuma, 179–180
    Didymocarpus, 202
    Dioscorea, 208
    Embelin, 222
    Inula racemosa, 253
    licorice, 232
    Neem, 56
    Ocimum oils, 290–291

    Piper nigrum, 348
    Pterocarpus marsupium, 358
    Swertia chirayita, 392
    Terminalia bellerica, 396-397
    Tribulus terresris, 420
anti-mutagenic activity
    Curcuma, 180
    Glycyrrhiza glabra, 232
    Triphala, 397
anti-oxidant activity
    Aegle marmelos, 12-14
    Amla, 311, 317
    Ashwagandha, 437, 440
    Bacopa monnieri, 73
    Brahmi, 75, 78
    Cedrus deodara, 138
    Curcuma, 178, 180
    Didymocarpus pedicellata, 201-202
    Embelia ribes, 221, 222-223
    licorice, 230-231
    Madder, 363
    Mucuna pruriens, 271-272
    mustak, 196-197
    Picrorhiza kurroa, 330-331
    Piper nigrum, 349
    Shilajit, 373
    Terminalia leaves, 410
    Triphala, 396
    Tulsi, 289, 291
    Varuna, 172
anti-seizure activity, Centella asiatica, 128
anti-spasmolytic activity, Cedrus deodara, 138
anti-tumor activity
    Embelia ribes, 220-221
    Neem, 59
anxiety treatments
    Ashwagandha, 448
    Bacopa monnieri, 73, 77
    Boswellia, 110
    Gotu kola, 126
aphrodisiacs
    Amla, 311
    Ashwagandha, 437, 438
    licorice, 227
    Mucuna, 267
    Sida cordifolia, 377
    Tribulus terrestris, 418
apoptosis, 197, 358. *See also* cancer
appetite, Swertia to stimulate, 389
aromatherapy, Cedrus deodara, 137
arthritis treatment. *See also* osteoarthritis; rheumatism
    Ashwagandha, 437, 449

    Boswellia, 103, 104-105
        case histories, 111-112
    Centella asiatica, 124
    Curcuma, 175
    Guggul, 157-158 (case studies)
    Nigella, 278
    Shankhapushpi, 163
    Shilajit, 369
Ashwagandha, 437. *See also* Withania somnifera
    anti-oxidant, 440
    anti-carcinogenic, 440-442
    anti-inflammatory, 442-443, 448
    anti-stress / anti-anxiety, 439-440, 448
    immunomodulatory, 444-446
    longevity and anti-aging, 437, 444
    mutltiple myeloma case history, 448
    sexual energy, 437
    side-effects, 449
    thyroid-stimulating, 444
    tonic for vitality and longevity, 437
asiaticoside study, 123
Asparagus / Asparagaceae, 42
Asparagus racemosus, 41. *See also* Shatavari
    case history: osteoporosis with low estrogen, 47-49
Aspergillus flavus fungus, 55, 139
Asteraceae family, 251
asthma / bronchial asthma treatments
    Adhatoda vasica, 3, 5
    Aegle marmelos (Bael), 9
    Andrographis paniculata, 32
    Ashwagandha, 437, 447-448, 449
    bitter melon, 257
    Boswellia, 108, 115-116
    Cissus quadrangularis, 143
    Curcuma, 180
    glycyrrhizin, 237
    Guggul, case history, 159
    Inula extract, 253
    Nigella, 278-280
    Ocimum, 292
    Pippli, 340
    Picrorhiza kurroa, 330
    Piper longum, 338-339, 341
    Swertia chirayita, 389
    Terrminalia bellerica. 399
astringents
    Amla, 311
    Ashwagandha, 437, 438
    Bala, 377
    Brahmi, 73
    Neem bark and fruit, 53

Pterocarpus bark, 353
Terminalia bellerica, 395
atherosclerosis
    Amla treatment, 314
    Guggal treatment, 156
    Picrorhiza kurroa, 330
atorvastatin, 17
auto-immune disease, studies and treatment
    Brahmi, 81
    Curcuma, 185-186
    Gotu kola plant, 130
    Guggul action, 156
Azadirachta indica, 53. *See also* Neem
    case histories
        chicken pox, 67
        eczema treatment, 65-66, 67
        Lyme disease, 66
        MRSA, 66-67
    chemical composition, 54
    protocols, 67
Azadirachta indica leaf extract (AAILE), 59

Bacopa monnieri. *See also* Brahmi
    amnesia treatment, 76-77
    anti-anxiety, 77
    brain tonic, 73, 81, 164
    for diarrhea, 10
    and morphine withdrawal, 80, 82
bacterial vaginitis, Neem treatment protocol, 68
Bael. *See also* Aegle marmelos
    anti-microbial uses, 11, 20
    bark, 9, 21
    calming effect, 20
    as diabetes treatment, 12-14
    fruit, 9, 10, 15, 20, 21, 17, 18, 21
    for jaundice, 9
    leaves, 9, 10, 11, 13, 15, 19, 21
    radioprotective effects, 14-15
    roots /root bark, 9, 16, 17, 21
    veterinary usage, 20
Bala, 377, 380. *See also* Sida cordifolia
    aphrodisiac, 377
    cardiac / heart stimulant, 377, 379
bdellium, 151
benzodiazepines, 76
Berberis aristata, 87. *See also* berberine; Daruhaldi; Rasaunt
    case histories
        gall stones, 93
        liver support, 93
    chemical constituents, 88
    protocols, 93-94

berberine, 88
    anti-amoebic, 88-89
    anti-bacterial activity, 90
    anti-depressant study, 90-92
    anti-diarrheal, 88
    anti-fungal, 89
    anti-platelet activity, 90
    Leishmania treatment, 89-90
Bhringaraj, 211. *See also* Eclipta alba
Bibhitaki, 395. *See also* Terminalia bellerica; Triphala
bile. *See also* liver
    Adhatoda experiment in animals, 4
    Andrographis paniculata activity, 33
    Daruhaldi to increase, 92
    Haritaki to stimulate, 413-414
bioavailability enhancement of Trikatu, 339, 345, 348, 350
bioflavonoids
    as renal protective, 178-179
    Vijaysar source, 354
bitter melon uses, 257. *See also* Momordia charantia
    anti-cancer, 259-261
    anti-fertility, 261
    anti-viral, 261-262
    asthma, 257
    chemical composition, 258
    cholesterol reduction, 259
    diabetes / hepatoprotective, 257, 258
    gastrointestinal problems, 257
    hypertension, 257
    infections, 257
    parasites / worms, 257
    wound healing, 257
black cumin seeds. *See also* Nigella sativa
    digestion promotion, 277
    parasitic infections, 278
    respiratory and inflammatory diseases, 278-279
black nightshade, 383, 384
bleeding control
    Adhatoda vasica, 1
    Amla, 312
    Curcuma, 184
    Glycyrrhiza glabra, 235
blood pressure effect, Gotu kola, 125. *See also* cardiotonic effect; high blood pressure
blood sugar / blood glucose. *See* diabetes
Boerhaavia diffusa, 97-98. *See also* Punarnava
    anti-cancer activity, 99
    diuretic activity, 98
bone
    healer, Cissus quadrangularis, 143, 144-145, 147
    resorption, Punarnava to inhibit, 98

Boswellia serrata / boswellic acids (BA), 103
    anti-asthmatic activity, 108
    anti-carcinogen studies, 108–110
    anti-inflammatory activity, 105–106, 111
    arthritis activity, 104–106
    case histories and protocols
        allergic dermatitis, 116
        bronchial asthma, 115–116
        Crohn's disease, 113–114, 115
        encephalitis, 115
        fibrosis, 111
        glioblastoma, 114–115
        juvenile rheumatoid arthritis, 112
        polymyalgia rheumatica, 112–113
        psoriatic arthritis, 113
        rheumatoid and psoriatic arthritis, 111-112, 115
        shoulder pain, 111
        ulcerative colitis, 114
        and boswellic acids (BA), 103, 105–106, 108
    and Crohn's disease treatment, 106–107
    dermatological activity, 110. *See also* skin
    gastrointestinal activity, 106–108
    gum resin, 104, 105–106, 108, 110
    neuronal activity, 110
Brahmi. *See also* Bacopa monnieri
    as anti-oxidant, 78
    bronchodilatory activity, 78
    cardioprotective activity, 79
    chemicals in, 74
    cognitive support for children, 75
    drug interactions, 82
    gastrointestinal activity, 78–79
    memory and cognitive function, 73, 74–76, 165
    protocols
        inflammation and immune modulation, 81
        liver support, 81
        lupus, 81
        scleroderma, 81
brain tonics / function, 73, 81, 122, 127, 164, 437. *See also* cognitive activity
bronchodilatory effect
    Adhatoda vasica, 2
    Brahmi, 78
    Punarnava, 100
burns, Curcuma protocol, 188

cancer / chemoprotection / carcinogenic activity
    Aegle marmelos, 15
    Amla, 314–315
    Andrographis paniculata, 26–28
    Ashwagandha, 437, 440–442
    bitter melon, 259–261
    Boerhaavia, 99
    Boswellia, 108–110
    Brahmi, 81
    case history, 299
    Cedrus deodara, 138
    Centella asiatica, 129
    Commiphora mukul, 151
    Curcuma, 176, 181–185
    Dioscorea bulbifera, 206
    Embellia ribes, 223
    Fenugreek, 429, 433
    Guggulsterone, 154–155
    Inula racemosa, 254
    licorice, 231–232
    Lupeol, 169
    Manjistha, 363
    Mucuna pruriens, 267
    Neem, 59-63
    Ocimum, 292
    Phyllanthus amarus, 306–307
    Piper longum, 338
    Piper nigrum, 346–348
    prostate, studies and protocol, with Curcuma, 183, 188
    Pterocarpus marsupium, 358
    Shatavari, 45, 46
    Sida cordifolia, 380
    Solanum nigrum, 384–385
    Swertia chirayita, 392–393
    Trigonella foenum, 433
    Triphala, 400, 411, 413
    Varuna (for pancreatic cancer), 171–172
Candida / candidiasis treatments
    Amla, 313–314
    Asparagus racemosus, 46
    Azadirachta indica, 55
    Pippoli case history and protocol, 340–341
    Tribulus terresris, 420
carcinogenesis. *See* cancer
cardioprotective activity
    Aegle marmelos, 16–17
    Andrographis paniculata, 31–32
    Ashwagandha, 437, 443–444
    Curcuma longa, 186
    Embelia ribes, 221–222
    Guggul, 153
    Inula racemosa, 251, 252–253
    Neem, 63
    Nigella sativa, 283–284
    Ocimum sanctum, 293
    Phyllanthus amarus, 305
    Shatavari root, 45

Tribulus terresris, 420–422
cardiotonic effect
    Gotu kola, 124–126
    Haritaki, 406
    Ptercarpus marsupium, 357
    Tulsi, 289
cardiovascular conditions. *See also* cardioprotective
    Terminalia bellerica, 396
    Tribulus terrestris, 417
cataract treatment. *See* eye
catarrh in infants, Eclipta alba, 211
Cedrus deodara, 137. *See also* deodara
    anti-cancer activity, 138
    anti-fungal activity, 139
    anti-inflammatory activity, 138–139
    anti-oxidant activity, 138
    anti-spasmolytic activity, 138
Centella asiatica, 121. *See also* Gotu kola
    allergy treatment, 130
    anti-cancer, 129
    anti-depressant, 126
    anti-fertility, 129
    anti-seizure, 128
    arthritis treatment, 124, 125
    brain tonic, 127, 164
    cognitive and neuroprotective properties, 127
    colitis treatment, 126–127
    dermatological activity, 129-130
    physical performance, increased, 128–129
    wound-healing studies, 122–123, 130
central nervous system (CNS) activity and studies
    Andrographis paniculata, 34
    Azadirachta indica, 57
    Centella asiatica, 127
    Eclipta alba, to ease aggression, 213
    Sida cordifolia, 379–380
    Swertia chirayita, 391
Charaka Samhita, 289
chirayita. *See* Swertia chirayita
chlamydia, Rausasnt treatment, 89
cholagogue activity of Adhatoda vasica, 4
cholera
    berberine inhibiting, 89
    Piper nigrum treatment 345
    Pterocarpus marsupium, 353
    Terminalia bellerica, 397
cholesterol lowering properties
    Amla, and case history 314, 323
    bitter melon, 259
    Boswellia, 110
    curcuma, 186
    Dioscorea bulbifera, 206

    Fenugreek, 429, 432–433
    Guggul, and case history, 153, 156, 156, 159
    Gymnema, 246
    Ocimum sanctum, 294
    piperine, 339
    Pterocarpus marsupium, 357
    Rubia cordifolia, 364
    Shilajit, 373
chorioepithelioma, 34–35
chronic inflammatory diseases, case history, 157–158
Cissus quadrangularis, 143
    anti-inflammatory and analgesic activity, 146
    anti-ulcer properties, 147
    bone-healing activity and case history, 144–145, 147–148
    chemical composition, 144
    obesity and weight loss, 146–147
    osteoporosis and case history, 145–146, 147
    periodontal regeneration, 145
cognitive activity. *See also* central nervous system
    Brahmi, 74–76, 80–81
    Gotu kola, 127, 130
    Ocimum, 297
    piperine, 349
    Shilajit, 370–371
colds, 345. *See also* common cold
colic treatments, 257, 312, 383
colitis
    Bael treatment, 20
    Centella asiatica treatment, 126–127
    Curcuma protocol, 188
    Guggul treatment and case history, 152, 158–159
collagen support, 130, 319. *See also* auto-immune; skin
Commiphora mukul, 151. *See also* Guggul
    case histories
        chronic inflammatory diseases, 157–158
        cystic acne, 157
        hyperlipidemia, 156
        stroke, 157
common cold remedies
    Andrographis paniculata, 28–29
    curcuma, 175
    Nigella, 277
    Tulsi, 289
constipation relief
    Amla, 312
    Curcuma protocol, 188
    Embelia ribes, 219
    Haritaki, 413
    Piper nigrum, 345
contraceptive
    Embelia ribes, 219, 220, 224

Neem, 65
Convolvulus pluricaulis, 163. *See also* Shankhapushpi
COPD, Pippli protocol, 341
coronary artery disease, Triphala study, 406
cortisol, 32, 163, 251
Crataeva nurvala, 169. *See also* Varuna
Crohn's disease
    Bael to treat, 20
    Boswellia serrata treatment, 105, 106–107
        case study and protocol, 113–114, 115
    Curcuma study, 177
    Guggul, and case history, 152, 158–159
Curcuma longa / curcumin, 175
    Alzheimer's study, 184
    anti-asthmatic activity, 180
    anti-cancer studies, 181–183
    anti-inflammatory activity, 176–179
    anti-microbial activity, 179–180
    anti-mutagenic activity, 180
    anti-oxidant activity, 180
    anti-ulcer activity, 184
    cardiac activity, 186
    chemical composition, 176
    cholesterol reduction, 186
    female reproduction, 186–187
    hepatoprotective activity, 180–181
    hypoglycemic activity, 184
    immune modulation and immunostimulant studies, 184–186
    neurological studies, 183–184
    protocols, 187–188
    rheumatoid arthritis study, 176
Cyperus rotundus, 195, 197–198. *See also* mustak
cystic fibrosis
    Amla treatment, 320
    Pippli treatment, 340
    Withania study, 446

Daruhaldi, 87–88. *See also* Berberis aristata; berberine; Rasaunt
    gall bladder cleansing, 92–93
    hepatoprotective, 89
    ophthalmic tincture, 90
    protocols, 93–94
        conjunctivitis, 93
        skin ulcers / boils, 94
        weaning, 93
deafness, Bael to treat age-related, 20
dementia / Alzheimer's activity. *See also* Alzheimer's
    Ashwagandha, 437
    Ocimum sanctum, 297
    Shilajit, 370

deodara, 137, 138. *See also* Cedrus deodara
depression. *See* anti-depressants
dermatitis. *See also* skin
    Boswellia protocol, 116
    Centella asiatica studies, 129
    Curcuma protocol, 188
DHEA levels, 109
diabetes, studies and treatment. *See also* type 2 diabetes
    Amla, 311, 315–316
    Bael, 9, 12–14
    Berberis aristata, 92
    bitter melon / Momordica, 257, 258, 262
    curcumin study, 184
    Embelia ribes, 221
    Fenugreek, 429, 430–432, 433
    Guggulsterone, 155
    Gymnema research, 244–246
    Inula extract, 253
    Mucuna pruriens / velvet bean, 267, 270–271
    mustak, 196
    Neem, 67–68
    Ocimum sactum (Tulsi), 294
    Phyllanthus amarus, 306
    Pterocarpus marsupium, 354
    protocol, 263
    Shilajit, 371
    Withania somnifera, 444
diabetic cardiomyopathy (DCM), Aegle marmelos to treat, 17
diabetic nephropathy, Picrorhiza kurroa to treat, 330
dialysis support, protocol, 426
diarrhea relief
    Aegle marmelos, 10–11
    Amla, 311
    Andrographis paniculata, 31
    Bacopa monnieri, 10
    Bael, 10–11, 20
    berberine, 88
    Cyperus rotundus, 195, 198
    Dioscorea bulbifera, 205
    Eclipta alba, 211
    mustak, 198
    Piper nigrum, 345
    Pterocarpus bark, 353
    Terminalia bellerica, 395
Didymocarpus pedicellata, 201–202
digestion, improving
    Amla, 312
    Haritaki, 413
    Nigella, 277, 285
    Piper longum, 340, 350

Piper nigrum, 350
Shankhapushpi, 163
Tulsi, 289
Dioscorea bulbifera, 205
    anti-cancer, 206
    antimicrobial 208
    cholesterol lowering, 206
    chemical composition, 206
    estrogenic, 207–208
    in hormone manufacture, 205
    hypoglycemic, 206–207
    pain relief, 208
    poisonous nature, 205
    syphilis treatment, 205
diphtheria treatment, Eclipta alba, 211
diuretic
    Ashwagandha, 437
    Gotu kola, 122
    Mucuna pruriens, 267
    Punarnava, 98
    Tribulus terrestris, 424, 426
dopamine / L-dopa, 267, 268, 269
DPT (diphtheria, tetanus, pertussis) vaccine, 45
dropsy, Bael for, 9
dysentery treatment
    Bael, 20
    Dioscorea bulbifera, 205
    Mucuna pruriens, 267
    Shankhapushpi, 163
    Solanum nigrum, 383
dyspepsia treatment
    Amla, 321
    Adhatoda vasica, 4
    Dioscorea bulbifera, 205
    Embelia ribes, 219
    Neem flowers, 53
    Pippli protocol, 341
    Shilajit, 369

Eclipta alba, 211, 212
    anti-inflammatory, 214
    case history, 215
    chemical composition, 212
    hair growth, 214–215
    hepatoprotective activity, 212
    high blood pressure, 212–213
    immunomodulation activity, 214
    malaria, anti-, 213
    pain treatment, 211, 214
E.coli bacterial infections, treating
    Amla, 313
    Andrographis paniculata, 31

bitter melon, 261
Embelia ribes, 219
Haritaki, 405, 407, 414
Neem, 56
Shatavari, 45
Tribulus terrestris, 417, 420
eczema, treatment with Neem, 67
Embelia ribes / Embelin, 219
    analgesic, 222
    anti-diabetic, 221
    anti-microbial, 222
    anti-oxidant, 222–223
    anti-tumor, 220–221
    cardioprotective, 221–222
    chemical composition, 220
    chemoprotective, 223
    contraceptive, 220
    insecticidal, 223
    periodontal treatment, 223
    worm control, 219, 221
Emblica officianalis. *See also* Amla; Phyllanthus emblica
    cystic fibrosis treatment, 320\
    in digestive formula, 413
    extract in cancer studies, 315
    liver, fruit extract for, 316–317
encephalitis, and treatment, 115, 232
Entamoeba histolytica, 88, 89, 261, 339
ephedrine / ephedra ban, 377, 378
epilepsy treatment
    Brahmi, 73
    curcumin, 175
    Piper nigrum, 345
    anti-epileptic
    Shankhapushpi, 164
Euphorbiaceae family, 311
eczema, treatment
    Neem, 67
    Solanum nigrum, 383
    Tribulus terrestris, 417
eye disorders / treatments
    Amla case histories, 321, 323
    Bael, 14
    conjunctivitis and protocols, 93, 188, 205
    Curma protocol, 188
    Ocimum sanctum, 298, 356
    Pterocarpus marsupium, 356–357
    Rasaunt treatment, 87
    Triphala, 397
    Tulsi, 289

fatigue / chronic fatigue
    Amla for, 312

Ashwagandha, 449
Shankhapushpi for, 163
female reproductive and menopausal activity,
    contraception; childbirth, lactation, hormone
    imbalance
    Adhatoda vasica for uterine contractions 1
    Ashwagandha, 449
    black cumin, 277
    Curcuma, 186–187
    Dioscorea bulbifera, 207–208
    Fenugreek, 433
    Phyllanthus amarus, 308
    Shatavari, 41, 42, 43, 46
    Varuna, 169
Fenugreek, 429. See also Trigonella foenum-graecum
    anti-cancer, 433
    anti-diabetic, 429, 430–432
    anti-inflammatory and analgesic activity, 430
    anti-obesity, 432
    cancer inhibitor, 429
    cholesterol, 432–433
    Fenugreefemalek, 433
    hypertension, 433
    obesity, 433
fertility / infertility activity
    Aegle marmelos, 19–20
    Andrographis paniculata, 33
    Centella asiatica, 129
    male studies / case history using Mucuna, 272–273, 274
    Neem, 58, 68
    Phyllanthus amarus, 308
    Piper longum, 342
    Shilajit, 369
fever reducers
    Andrographis paniculata , 29–30
    Picrohiza, 328
    Shankhapushpi, 163
    Swertia chirayita, 389
fibromyalgia, case history, 158
flatulence treatment
    Amla, 321
    Embelia ribes, 219
    Haritaki, 413
    Punarnava, 100
flavonoids
    in Adhatoda vasica, 2
    in Bergeris aristata, 88
    in Brahmi, 74
    in licorice, 228, 230
    in Varuna, 170
food allergies, protocol with Pippli, 342
free radical inhibition. See also anti-oxidant

of Bael, 15
of Brahmi, 73, 78
of Shilajit, 373
fungus, See anti-fungal

galactogogue activity of Shatavari, 43, 46
gall bladder
    Andrographolide stimulation, 33–34
    Daruhaldi cleansing, 92–93
gastrointestinal activity
    Boswellia serrate, 106–108
    bitter melon, 257
    Brahmi, 78–79
    Shatavari, 43, 46
gemfibrozil, 17
Gentianaceae family, 390
Giardia
    Bael to treat, 20
    berberine to treat, 88, 89
    Neem to treat, 67
glycoside, Shatavari as, 42
Glycyrrhiza glabra / glycyrrhizin, 227–228, 233–234
    anti-inflammatory activity, 233
    anti-mutagenic, 232
    anti-viral activity, 232. See also licorice
    asthma study, 237
    bleeding management, 235
    hormonal uses, 234–235
    immune modulation, 233
    stroke studies, 235–236
Goksura, 417. See also Tribulus terrestris
gonorrhea, Ocimum sanctum to treat, 296
Gotu kola, 121–122
    anti-ulcerogenic activity, 123–124
    anxiety and insomnia activity, 126
    cardiotonic and venous activity, 124–125
    dermatological activity. 129–130
    immunomodulatory activity, 124
    tuberculosis effectiveness, 124
    wound-healing activity, 121, 122–123, 130
gout. See arthritis
Guggul / Guggulsterone / guggul gum, 151. See also
    Commiphora mukul
    anti-cancer, 154–155
    anti-diabetic, 155
    anti-inflammatory activity, 152
    cancer treatment and studies, 151, 154–155
    cardioprotective, 153
    chemical composition, 152
    for cholesterol lowering, 151, 153
    for obesity, 151, 152
    for osteoarthritis, 151, 154

Gurmar, 243, 247. *See also* Gymnema sylvestre
Gymnema sylvestre, 243
    anti-diabetic, 243, 244–246
    anti-obesity, 246–247
    case histories, 247–248
        blood pressure, 248
        diabetic, 247–248
        chemical composition, 244
        cholesterol reduction, 246
    safety with other drugs, 248

hair enhancement / growth
    Amla, and case history, 312, 323
    Eclipta alba, 211, 214–215
Haritaki, 405–406. *See also* Terminalia chebula; Triphala
    anti-bacterial, 405, 407–408
    anti-fungal, 405
    anti-oxidant, 410
    anti-viral activity, 408, 414 (case study)
    digestive disturbances, 413
    anti-viral, 408
    cardiotonic, 406
heart disease, Shilajit treatment, 369. *See also* cardioprotective
Helicobacter pylori
    Brahmi treatment, 78-79
    protocol, 341–342
    Terminalia chebula study, 408
hemorrhoids, Embelia ribes treatment, 219
hepatitis / hepatoprotective activity. *See also* liver
    Andrographolides, 34, 35
    case history, 262–263
    Curcuma, 180–181
    Darauhaldi, 89
    herbal protocol with Haritaki, 414
    Manjistha, 362
    Momordica, 262
    Neem treatment and protocol, 57–58, 68
    Phyllanthus amarus activity, 304–305
    Picrorhiza kurroa, 328–330, 331
    Punarnava, 98
    Sida cordifolia, 378
    Solanum nigrum, 385-386
    Swertia chirayita, 391
    Terminalia bellerica, 395, 397
    Terminalia chebula, 412–413
    Tribulus terrestris (against mercury), 423
    Tulsi, 289
herpes treatment
    with Gotu kola, 129
    Neem, 65, 67
    Swertia chirayita, 392

Terminalia chebula, 4
high blood pressure, treating
    with Andrographis paniculata, 32
    Eclipta alba, 212–213
    with Gotu kola, 121, 125-126
    case history / protocol, 248
HIV/AIDS
    Amla fruit activity, 312–313
    Andrographis paniculata treatment, 28
    Haritaki frut extract, 408
    licorice treatment, 232
    Momordica treatment, 262
    Phyllanthus amarus activity, 305
    Terminalia bellerica, 395, 396
"Holy Basil," 299
hormones. *See also* cortisol
    ACTH, 32
    Dioscorea, 205
    estrogenic, 207–208
    Fenugreek, 433
    glycyrrhizin, 234–235
    noradrenaline (brain), 32
    stress, adrenaline and cortisol, 163, 251
    Tribulus terrestris, 419–420
H.pylori protocol, 188
Huntington's disease, study, 446–447
hyperlipidemia / hypolipidemia, 17, 246. *See also* cardioprotective; cholesterol
    case history using Guggul, 156–157
hypertension action. *See also* high blood pressure
    bitter melon, 257
    Cyperus rotundus, 195
    Fenugreek, 433
    Piper nigrum, 349
hyperthyroidism
    Ashwagandha to counteract, 444
    Guggal protocol, 159–160
    Shankhapushpi for, 163
hypoglycemic effect / studies. *See also*
    bitter melon, 258–259
    Dioscorea bulbifera, 206–207
    Neem, 54-56
    Orimum sanctum, 294
    Phyllanthus amarus, 308
    Sida cordifolia, 379
    Terminalia bellerica, 397
hypolipidemic activity of Terminalia bellerica, 396

imipramine, 19, 126
immune support / immunomodulatory activity
    Aegle marmelos, 18
    Amla, 317, 321

Andrographis paniculata, 25, 27
Ashwagandha, 437, 444–446
of boswellic acids, 108
Brahmi, 81
Curcuma, 184–186
Eclipta alba, 214
Glycyrrhiza glabra, 233–234
Gotu kola, 124
Neem, 59–63
Ocimum sanctum, 295
Picrorhiza kurroa, 331
Pippli effect, 338
Shankhapushpi, 163
Shatavari, 44–45
Triphala, 398
Tulsi case history, chemotherapy, 299
Terminalia bellerica, 395
Terminalia chebula, 409
Tribulus terrestris, 417
Indian Echinacea, 25
Indian ginseng, 41, 437
Indian gooseberry, 311
"Indian Viagra," 371
infertility and impotence, 369, 447. See also fertility
inflammation. See also anti-inflammatory; allergies
Adhatoda vasica, 3, 5
Ashwagandha, 442
Bacopa, 73, 81
bitter melon, 257
Boswellia to reduce, 103, 105–106, 111
Curcuma, 175, 187–188
Eclipta alba, 214
Inula britannica, 254
Rasaunt (for external), 87
Shilajit, 369
inflammatory bowel disease (IBD), 184
influenza case history with Pippli, 341
insect repellents / insecticides
Adhatoda vasica, 5
Azadirachta indica, 53
Cedrus deodara, 137
Curcuma, 175
Embelia ribes, 223
Neem, 63, 64, 67
Tulsi, 289
insomnia treatments
Ashwagandha, 437, 439–440, 449
Gotu kola, 126
Piper nigrum, 345
insulin regulation. See also diabetes
marmelose, 13
bitter melon, 258-259

licorice, 230
Ocimum plant, 294
Withania somnifera, 444
Inula racemosa, 251
allergy, 253–254
anti-microbial, 253
asthma, 253
diabetes, 253
cancer, 254
cardioprotective, 252–253
inflammatory conditions, 254
skin diseases, 251
tuberculosis, 251
irritable bowel syndrome (IBS)
Bael to treat, 10–11, 20
Brahmi to treat, 78–79

jaundice, Bael for, 9

kidney infection / diseases, treatment. See also renal; urinary
Andrographolide, 34
Didymocarpus pedicellata, 201–202
Picrorhiza kurroa protection, 331–332
Punarnava, 99, 100
Shilajit, 369, 371
Tribulus terrestris, 417, 424–425
Withania somnifera, 446
Klebsiella pneumonia treatment
Neem oil, 56
Tribulus terresris, 420

Laksha Guggulu, 146, 160
Lamiaceae family, 289
laxatives
Amla, 311
Daruhaldi, for children, 87
Embelia ribes, 219
Punarnava, 100
Tulsi, 289
Varuna, 169
L-dopa /dopamine, 267, 268, 269
lectins, to treat infectious diseases, 11
Leishmania
berberine treatment, 89–90
Swertia treatment, 391
leprosy treatment
with bitter melon, 257
with Gotu koa, 121, 122
with Shilajit, 369
leptospirosis, 34
leukemia treatments

Andrographis, 26-28
Terminalia bellerica, 395
licorice, 227. *See also* Glycyrrhiza glabra
    allergy treatment, 236–237-
    anti-oxidant activity, 230–231
    cancer prevention, 231–232
    chemical composition, 228
    cholesterol reduction, 229
    hepatoprotective activity, 230
    obesity control, 230
    safety profile, 237–238
    ulcer treatment, 229
licorice flavonoid oil (LFO), 238
Liliaceae family, 42
lipid metabolism, 364, 395, 432–433. *See also* cholesterol
liver disorders / support
    alcohol-induced, 328
    Amla, 316
    Andrographis treatment, 33–34, 35
    Ashwagandha, 437
    Brahmi protocol, 81
    Curcuma treatment, 175, 180-181
    Daruhaldi, 89
    Eclipta alba, 212, 215
    licorice treatment, 227, 230–231
    Neem activity, 57–58
    Picrorhiza kurroa, 327, 328–330, 332
    Pippli / piperine, 339, 349
    Punarnava, 98, 100
    Rasaunt treatment, 87
    Solanum nigrum, 385–386
    Swertia chirayita, 389, 391
    Tribulus terrestris, 417
L-dopa. *See* dopamine
longevity. *See* aging
long pepper, 337, 342, 345. *See also* Piper longum; Piper nigrum
Lorazepam, 77
lupus
    case history, 158
    protocol, 81–82
lung. *See* respiratory
Lyme disease, Neem for, 65, 66

Madder, 363. *See also* Manjistha
    anti-oxidant, 363
    food color, 366
malaria treatment
    Andrographis, 30–31
    Azadirachta indica, 53, 65, 67
    Curcuma, 175
    Eclipta alba, 213

mustak, 196
Tulsi, 289
Swertia, 389
male
    aphrodisiac, 371–372
    benign prostatic hypertrophy, Shilajit, 369
    delayed development case history, 425
    erectile dysfunction, 130, 419
    impotence and sexual debility
        Ashwagandha, 449
        Cyperus Rotundus treatment, 195
        Mucuna pruriens treatment, 267, 274
        Shatavari treatment, 41, 46
    infertility and low libido, case history, 425–426
    premature ejaculation, Tribulus terrestris, 317
Manjistha. *See also* Rubia cordifolia, 361
    anti-allergic, 361
    anti-oxidant, 363-364
    anti-psoriatic activity, 364
    blood purifier, 361
    case history, spontaneous abortion, 365
    chemical composition, 362
    hepaoprotective, 362
    rheumatism, 361
    urinary health, 361
marmin, 19–20
melancholia, Bael for, 9
memory, 163, 213, 369, 370. *See also* cognitive activity
Meniere's disease, Bael to treat, 20
Merasingi, 243. *See also* Gymnema sylvestre
metabolic disorders. *See* diabetes
Metformin. *See* Type 2 diabetes, 444
Momordica charantia, 257. *See also* bitter melon
    anti-cancer 259
    anti-fertility 261
    anti-genotoxic activity, 261
    anti-helmintic activity, 261
    anti-viral, 262
    diabetes activity and protocol, 258–259, 262, 263
    hepatitis B and HIV, 262
    parasites, 262
morphine toxicity and withdrawal, 80, 82
mosquito repellent, Neem for, 63–64. *See also* insect repellent
MRSA, 66–67, 180
Mucuna pruriens, 267–268. *See also* velvet bean
    anti-oxidant activity, 271–272
    anti-venom activity, 270
    male fertility studies, 272–27
    Parkinson's disease
        case history, 273–274
        treatment with dopamine, 268–269

safety profile, 275
tardive dyskinesia treatment, 269–270
multiple myeloma case, 448
mustak, 195. *See also* Cyperus rotundus
    anti-diabetic, 196
    anti-diarrheal, 198
    anti-inflammatory, 196
    anti-malarial, 196
    anti-oxidant, 196–197
    anti-pyretic, 196
    chemical composition, 196
    Cytoprotective, 197
    obesity control, 196

Neem, 53. *See also* Azadirachta indica
    analgesic activity, 57
    anti-atherosclerotic activity, 57
    anti-bacterial activity, 56
    anti-fertility activity, 58–59
    anti-fungal activity, 55–56
    anti-inflammatory activity, 58
    anti-pyretic activity, 57
    anti-tumor activity, 59–63
    anti-ulcerogenic activity, 57
    anti-viral activity, 56
    anxiolytic activity, 57
    bark as astringent, 53
    cardioprotective activity, 63
    central nervous system activity, 57
    constituents, 54
    flowers for dyspepsia, 53
    hepatprotective activity, 57–58
    immune modulating activity, 59, 61–63
    insecticidal activity, 63–64, 67
    for parasite treatment, 20
    twigs for teeth cleaning, 53
Neem leaf preparation (NLP) for immune modulation, 59–62
Neem leaf glycoprotein (NLGP) for immune activation, 61
Neem oil, for topical, 62–63, 68
"Nepali Neem," 389
nescafé (coffee bean), 267
neurasthenia, Amla for, 312
neurological / neuroprotective activity. *See also* central nervous system activity
    Asparagus racemosus, 46
    Centella asiatica, 127–128
    Cyperus rotundus, 197–198
neurotransmitter dopamine, 267, 268, 269
neutrophils (PMN), studies with Curcuma, 184–185
Nigella sativa, 277
    analgesic activity, 284–285
    anti-asthmatic, 278–280
    anti-cancer, 280–282
    anti-inflammatory / arthritis activity, 278
    cardioprotective activity, 283–284
    chemical composition, 277–278
    common cold, 277
    gastroprotective / Thymoquinone, 282–283
    immune system, 277
    liver and kidney function, 277, 282
    neuroprotective / spinal cord, 282
    opioid addiction, 285
    skin conditions, 277
nightshade family, 438
nootropic, Ocimum extract as, 297
NSAID (non-steroidal anti-inflammatory drugs), 103

obesity / weight loss activity
    Cissus quadrangularis, 146–147
    Fenugreek, 432, 433
    Guggul, 151, 152
    Gymnema, 246–247
    licorice, 229-230
    mustak, 196
    Shilajit, 369
    Sida cordifolia, 378
    Terminalia bellerica and Triphala, 397
Ocimum sanctum, 289–290. *See also* Tulsi
    anti-asthmatic, 292
    anti-carcinogenic, 292–293
    anti-dementia, 297
    anti-genotoxic, 297
    anti-gonorrhea activity, 296
    anti-microbial activity, 290
    anti-psychotic, 297
    cardioprotective, 293–294
    case history, 300
    cataract activity, 298
    cholesterol reduction, 294
    dementia and Alzheimer's activity, 297
    generalized anxiety disorder (GAD) studies, 296
    gonorrhea treatment, 296
    hypoglycemic, 294–295
    hypolipidemic, 294
    immunomodulatory, 295
    radioprotection, 295
    stress reducer, 296
    ulcer activity, 298
    wound-healing, 296–297
oncology support, Didymocarpus, 202. *See also* cancer
ophthalmic activity. *See also* eye disorders
    Bael leaves / Aegle marmelos fruit, 9, 18
    Rasaunt, 90
    Terminalia bellerica, 397

opioid / opiate addiction, withdrawal, 447
    Nigella, 285
    Withania somnifera, 447
osteoarthritis
    Ashwagandha, 438, 447, 448
    Boswellia study, 104–105
    Guggul case history, 158
    Guggul gum, 151
osteoporosis
    Amla, 312
    Cissus quadrangularis studies, 145–146
    Curcuma protocol, 187–188

pain treatment
    Boswellia, 111
    Dioscorea bulbifera, 208
    Eclipta alba, 211, 214
    Mucuna pruriens, 267
    Nigella sativa, 284-285
    Solanum nigrum, 383, 386
    Tulsi, 289
pancreatitis, treatments
    Amla, 317, 322
    curcumin, 178
parasites / parasitic treatments. *See also* worms
    Adhatoda vasica, 3
    Bael, 20
    bitter melon, 257. 262
    black cumin, 277
    Embelia ribes, 219, 223
    Haritaki, 405, 413
    Neem, 20, 53, 67
    Nigella, 278
    Pippli protocol, 341
    Shilajit, 369
Parkinson's disease
    Ashwagandha treatment, 437, 446
    case history, 273–274
    curcumin study, 183
    Levodopa treatment, 267, 269
    Mucuna study, 268–269
    velvet bean treatment, 267, 268–269
periodontal
    Cissus quadrangularis regeneration, 145
    Embellia ribes, prevention, 223
pests. *See* insect repellents
Phyllanthus amarus, 303
    anti-cancer, 306-307
    anti-fertility, 308
    anti-inflammatory, 305–306
    anti-ulcer activity, 308
    cardioprotective, 305
    chemical composition, 304
    chemoprotective studies, 306–307
    diabetes activity, 306
    hepatoprotective, 304–305
    hypoglycemic effect, 308
Phyllanthus emblica, 311. *See also* Amla
phytochemicals
    Andrographis paniculata as source, 26
phytotherapy for managing diabetes, 13
Picrorhiza kurroa, 327
    anti-cancer, 331
    anti-oxidant activity, 330–331
    asthma prevention, 330
    digestive tone, 327
    kidney protection, 331–332
    liver / hepatoprotective agent / hepatitis, 327–330
    skin treatments, 327
    urinary tract tone, 327
Piper longum / Pippli / piperine, 337, 342. *See also* long pepper
    anti-asthmatic, 338–339
    antibacterial, 339
    anti-cancer, 338
    anti-inflammatory, 339
    bioavailability, 339
    case histories and protocols
        candidiasis, 340–341
        childhood asthma, 341
        decreased white blood cell count, 341
        dyspepsia and gastric inflammation, 341
        food allergies and hypochlorhydria, 342
        gastrointestinal disturbances, 341
        heliobacter phlori, 341–342
        influenza, 341
        lung weakness and COPD, 341
        parasitic infections, 341
        upper respiratory infections, 341
    chemical composition, 338
    cholesterol inhibition, 339
    hepatoprotective, 339
    immunomodulatory activity, 338
    Salmonella activity, 339–340
    stimulant effects, 338
Piper nigrum / piperine / peppercorn, 345
    anti-cancer, 346–348
    anti-convulsant, 348
    antihypertensive, 349
    anti-inflammatory, 349
    anti-oxidant, 349
    anti-spasmodic, 349
    bioavailability enhancement, 348

chemical constituents, 346
cognitive function, 349
hepatoprotective, 349
spices, 345, 350
thermogenic agent, 348
vitamin and mineral source, 346
pituitary gland and ACTH, 32. *See also* brain
platelet activating factor (PAF), Manjistha, 362
polio virus, Neem treatment, 55, 56
prednisolone, 103, 449
pregnancy termination
    Punarnava for, 100
    Neem, 58
prostatitis case history, 322–323
psoriasis. *See also* skin conditions
    Rubia cordifolia treatment, 364
    Solanum nigrum, 383
    Tribulus terrestris, 417
psychosis / schizophrenia, Ocimum study, 297
Pterocarpus marsupium / pterostilbene, 353. *See also* Vijaysar
    anti-cancer, 358
    anti-diabetic, 354–357
    anti-inflammatory, 357–358
    antimicrobial, 358
    chemical constituents, 354
Punarnava / punarvavoside / punarvavasava, 97, 100, 101. *See also* Boerhaavia diffusa
    cardiotonic, 357
    chemical constituents, 97–98
    congestive heart failure treatment, 100
    liver and kidney treatment, 100
    radioprotective effect, 99
Pushkaramoola, 251. *See also* Inula Racemosa
pyelonephritis, 34

quercetin as renal protective, 178
quinones, in Manjistha, 362

radioprotective effects /radiotherapy, 99
    Bael, 14–15
    Centella, 129
    Curcumin, 178
    Ocimum sanctum, 295
    Punarnava, 99
    Terminalia chebula, 413
rasayana
    Amla, 311
    Ashwagandha, 437, 450
    Eclipta alba, 211
    licorice, 227
    Pippli, 340

    Shilajit, 369, 372
    Shankhapushpi as, 165
    Triphala, 395, 398, 400, 405, 414
    Tribulus, 417
Rasaunt, 87, 89. *See also* Berberis; berberine
renal function. *See also* kidney; urinary system
    curcumin study, 178–179.
    Didymocarpus pedicellata activity, 202
    Picrorhiza kurroa, 331
    Tribulus terresris, 422
respiratory conditions, treatment
    Adhatoda vasica, 1, 3, 5
    Aegle marmelos, 19–20
    Ashwagandha, 437
    Amla, 311, 312
    Andrographis paniculata, 34
    Asparagus racemosus, 4
    curcumin, 175
    marmin, 19–20
    Pippli, 338
    Punarvava, 100
    Tulsi, 289
Reye's syndrome, Neem and, 68
Rifampin therapy, 34
rheumatism / rheumatoid arthritis treatments
    Adhatoda vasica, 3, 5
    Ashwagandha, 448, 449
    Bacopa monnieri, 80, 81
    Boswellia, 103, 111-112
    Curcuma, 176
    Daruhaldi, 87
    Guggul case history, 158
    Mucuna pruriens, 267
    Neem, 53
    Picrorhiza kurroa, case history, 332
    Sida cordifolia, 377
Rubia cordifolia, 361. *See also* Madder; Manjistha
    red dye, 361
    urolithiasis, protective against, 364
rutaceae family, 10

Salmonella treatment
    bitter melon, 261
    Piper longum, 339–340
    Shatavari, 45
    Terminalia bellerica, 396–397
saponins, 74
scabies treatment with Neem, 55–56
sciatica, Sida cordifolia for, 377
scleroderma protocol, 81
Scopolamine, 76
Scrophulariaccae family, 73

sexual health / energy
    Ashwagandha, 437
    Tribulus terrestris, 418–419
Shankhapushpi, 163. *See also* Convolvulus pluricaulis
    anti-ulcer, 165
    brain tonic / anti-depressant, 164
    chemical composition, 163–164
    immunomodulatory, 165
    mental disturbances, 165
Shatavari / Shatavarins, 41, 42. *See also* Asparagus racemosus
    anti-bacterial activity, 45–46
    anti-cancer activity, 45, 46
    antihepatotoxic activity, 45
    cardioprotective activity, 45
    cooling effect for fevers and inflammation, 49
    galactogogue activity, 43, 46
    gastrointestinal activity, 43–44
    immunomodulatory activity, 44–45
    uterotonic activity, 42
Shigella
    Bael to treat, 11–12
    Shatavi to treat, 45–46
Shilajit, 369
    adaptogenic activity, 372–373
    anti-anemia, 373
    anti-diabetic, 371
    anti-inflammatory, 371
    chemical composition, 370
    cognitive activity, 370–371
    high-altitude problems, alleviating, 373
    male sexual debility, 371–372
    pharmacological activity, 370
    ulcer activity, 371
    urinary / kidney function, 371
Shilpushpa, 201–202
Sida cordifolia, 377. *See also* Bala
    anti-cancer, 380
    anti-inflammatory and analgesic, 378
    cardiac activity, 379
    central nervous system activity, 379
    chemical composition, 378
    hepatoprotective activity, 378
    obesity activity, 378
skin conditions / disorders / bites
    Amla, 318–320
    Berberis aristata protocol, 93
    boswellic acid treatment, 110
    Cedrus deodara treatment, 137
    curcumin, 175
    Cyperus rotundas treatment, 195
    cystic acne, case history, 157
    Eclipta alba for, 211

    Gotu kola for, 121, 129–130
    Inula for, 251
    Manjistha, 365
    Neem for, 53, 65, 67
    Nigella oil, 277
    Brahmi for, 81
    Piper nigrum, 345
    Pterocarpus leaves, 353
    Rasaunt for, 87
    Rubia cordifolia for psoriasis, 364
    Solanum nigrum, 383
sleep. *See* insomnia
Solanaceae family, 438
Solanum nigrum, 383
    anti-cancer, 384–385
    anti-ulcer, 385
    chemical composition, 384
    digestive disorders, 383
    hepatoprotective, 385–386
    skin conditions, 383
spinal cord injury, Nigella treatment, 282
stress aids
    Ashwagandha, 437, 439–440, 447, 448
    Tulsi, 289
    hormones adrenaline and cortisol, 163, 251
    Ocimum sanctum, 296, 299
    Punarnava activity, 98–99
stroke treatments
    Ashwagandha, 447
    Commiphora mukul case history, 157
    Glycyrrhiza glabra activity, 235–236
stomach disorders. *See* digestion
Sucralfate, 165
Surasa. *See* Ocimum sanctum; Tulsi
Swertia chirayita, 389
    anti-inflammatory, 392
    anti-viral /Herpes simplex, 392
    cancer, 392–393
    central nervous system depressant, 391
    chemical composition, 390–391
    liver disorders, 389, 391
    skin problems, 389
    ulcers, 391
syphilis treatment, Sioscorea, 205

tannic acid / tannins
    Amla fruit 311
    Bael fruit, 10
    Bibhitaki, 400
    Haritaki, 405, 406
    Tribulus terrestris, 418
    Varuna, 170

tardive dyskinesia (TD), Mucuna to treat, 269
Terminalia bellerica, 395, 405. *See also* Triphala
    anti-allergic, 398-399
    anti-asthmatic, 399–400
    anti-microbial activity, 396–397
    anti-mutagenic, 397
    anti-ulcer, 397
    anti-viral / HIV, 395, 396
    cardiovascular activity, 396
    chemical composition, 396
    hepatoprotective activity, 397
    hypolipidemic activity, 396
    for longevity, 395
    rejuvenator, 395
Terminalia chebula, 405. *See also* Haritaki; Triphala
    anti-amoebic, 409–410
    anti-anaphylactic, 406-407
    anti-bacterial activity, 407
    anti-mutagenic, 407
    anti-oxidant, 405, 310
    anti-viral / herpes and HIV, 408–409
    cancer therapy, 405
    Cardiotonic, 406
    cardiovascular properties, 405
    cholesterol, reducing, 405
    hepatoprotective, 405, 412–413
    immunomodulatory activity, 409
    radioprotective, 413
thyroid stimulant
    Ashwagandha, 444
    Guggul as, 156
tonsillitis, Andrographis paniculata to treat, 34
toothache treatment
    Eclipta alba, 211
    Piper nigrum, 345
    Pterocarpus bark, 353
toxicity: treatment / detoxification, 323, 350
    Amla, 316
    Bala, 379
    Brahmi, 80
tranquilizers
    Cyperus rotundus, 195
    Shankhapushpi 163
Tribulus terrestris, 417–418
    analgesic activity, 422–423
    anti-bacterial and anti-fungal activity, 420
    cardiac activity, 420–422
    chemical components, 418
    diuretic properties, 417
    hepatoprotective activity against mercury, 423
    hormone activity, 419–420
    kidney failure / disease, case histories, 424–425

    liver disease treatment, 429
    mercury, activity against, 423
    sexual health, 418–419
    urinary / renal health, 422
Trichomonas vaginalis, 88, 89
Trikatu, bioavailability enhancement, 339, 345, 348, 350
Trigonella foenum-graecum, 429, 433. *See also* Fenugreek
Triphala, 311, 323, 400, 405. *See also* Terminalia chebula
    for alcoholism, 414
    anti-cancer, 400, 411
    anti-inflammatory, 398
    anti-mutagenic, 407
    anti-oxidant, 396
    anti-ulcer, 397
    in digestive formula, 413
    hypoglycemic, 397–398
    for liver disorders and gastrointestinal problems, 395, 414
    obesity control, 397
    opthalmic, 397
    with Terminalia bellerica, 395
triterpenes, 74, 169, 170, 171, 172, 228
tuberculosis treatments
    Adhatoda vasica, 1, 2, 5
    Andrographis paniculata, 34
    Gotu kola, 124
    Mucuna pruriens, 267
    Shilajit, 369
Tulsi, 289–290. *See also* Ocimum sanctum
    Cardioprotective, 293-294
    case history, chemotherapy, 299
    essential oil, 290, 299
        analgesic, 295
        anti-bacterial, 299
        anti-inflammatory, 291–292
        anti-oxidant activity, 291
turmeric, 175
type 2 diabetes, treatment. *See also* diabetes
    Aegle marmelos, 12-14
    Ashwagandha, 443–444
    Azadirachta indica, 54–55
    Guggul, 155
    Metformin medication, 444
    Pterocarpus marsupium, 356

ulcer treatments
    Adhatoda vasica, 4
    Aegle marmelos, 17
    Amla, 321, 323
    Andrographis paniculata, 30
    Asparagus racemosus, 43–44
    Azadirachta indica, 57

Cissus quadrangularis, 147
Curcuma, 184, 188
Cyperus rotundas, 195, 197
Eclipta alba, 211
Fenugreek, 429
Gotu kola, 123–124
licorice, 227
Ocimum sanctum, 298
Phyllanthus amarus, 308
Shankhapushpi, 163
Shilajit, 371
Sida cordifolia, 379
Solanum nigrum, 385
Swertia chirayita, 391
Terminalia bellerica and Triphala, 397
upper respiratory tract infection (URTI)
    Andrographis paniculata treatment, 28–29
urinary system and disorders. *See also* kidney
    Punarnava treatment, 100
    Shilajit treatment, 369, 371
    urolithiasis, Rubia cordifolia treatment, 364
    Varuna treatment, 169
    Tribulus terresris 417
vaginal infection protocols, 68, 93
Varahi, 205
Varuna, 169. *See also* Crataeva nurvala
    anti-inflammatory activity, 171
    anti-lithic studies, 170–171
    anti-oxidant activity, 172
    chemical composition, 170
    pancreatic cancer activity, 171–172
vascular studies / venous insufficiency, using Gotu kola, 124–125, 131
vasicine / vasicinone treatment of Adhatoda vasica, 2, 3, 4
velvet bean, 267. *See also* Mucuna pruriens
    chemical composition, 268
    for nervous system disorders, 267
    Parkinson's disease treatment, 268–269
    safety profile, 275
veterinary uses
    Adhatoda vasica, 5
    Amla, 320
    Bael, 20
    berberine, 92
    Brahmi, 81
    Cedrus deodara, 139
    Cissus quadrangularis, 147
    Curcuma, 187
    Daruhaldi, 92
    Embelia ribes, 223
    Glycyrrhiza glabra, 237
    Gotu kola, 130

Guggul, 155
Manjistha, 364
mustak, 196, 198
Neem, 64
Ocimum sanctum, 298–299
Piper longum, 340
Piper nigrum, 349–350
Terminalia bellerica, 400
Terminalia chebula, 413
Varuna, 172
vidanga, 219, 223. *See also* Embelia ribes
Vijaysar, 353, 358–359. *See also* Pterocarpus
    anti-diabetic, 353, 354–355, 359
    case history, 359
water hyssop, 73. *See also* Bacopa; Brahmi
weight loss. *See also* obesity
    Haritaki for, 413–414
    Vijaysar for, 359
    using Guggulsterone, 151
Withania somnifera / withanolides / withanamide, 437. *See also* Ashwagandha
    addiction management / morphine withdrawal, 447
    anti-aging, 443
    anti-inflammatory, 443
    asthma and allergy management, 447–448
    botanical characteristics, 438
    chemical composition, 438–439
    nephroprotective effect, 446
    neuroprotective activity, 446–447
    pharmacological activity, 439
    side-effects, 449
    for Type 2 diabetes, 444
worm treatment: ringworm / tapeworm / roundworm / pinworm / asarides. *See also* parasites
    bitter melon, 257
    case history / protocol, 224
    Embelia ribes, 219, 221
    Mucuna pruriens, 267
    Nigella, 278
    Picrorhiza kurroa, 327
wound-healing
    Amla, 318–319
    Adhatoda vasica, 4
    Bacopa monniera, 79, 81
    bitter melon, 257
    Gotu kola / Centella, 121, 122–123, 130
    licorice, 227
    Ocimum sanctum, 296–297